MEDICINAL CHEMISTRY

MEDICINAL CHEMISTRY

NORMA DUNLAP
DONNA M. HURYN

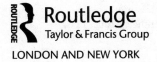

Routledge
Taylor & Francis Group

LONDON AND NEW YORK

Garland Science
Vice President: Denise Schanck
Senior Editor: Summers Scholl
Assistant Editor: Claudia Acevedo-Quiñones
Senior Production Editor: Georgina Lucas
Senior Digital Production Editor: Natasha Wolfe
Illustrator and Cover Design: Matthew McClements, Blink Studio, Ltd.
Copyeditor: Heather Whirlow Cammarn
Typesetter: NovaTech
Proofreader: Susan Wood
Indexer: Nancy Newman

About the Authors

Norma Dunlap is Professor of Chemistry at Middle Tennessee State University, where she specializes in synthetic organic chemistry and medicinal chemistry. Her research, done primarily with undergraduates, is focused on design and synthesis of bioactive peptidomimetics. She holds a Ph.D. in organic chemistry from the University of Wyoming and was an NIH postdoctoral fellow at the University of Pennsylvania. She began her career as a Senior Research Scientist at Hoffmann-La Roche, in drug discovery. After moving to academia, she was a Lecturer at Vanderbilt University before moving to Middle Tennessee State University.

Donna M. Huryn is Research Professor in the School of Pharmacy at the University of Pittsburgh where her research focuses on medicinal chemistry projects on novel drugs to treat cancer and neurodegenerative diseases. She holds a Ph.D. from the University of Pennsylvania where she is also Adjunct Professor of Chemistry. She started her career in industry at Hoffmann-LaRoche and then Wyeth Research before joining academia. She is a Fellow of the American Chemical Society.

First published 2018 by Garland Science

2 Park Square, Milton Park, Abingdon, Oxfordshire OX14 4RN
52 Vanderbilt Avenue, New York, NY 10017

Routledge is an imprint of the Taylor & Francis Group, an informa business

First issued in paperback 2019

ISBN 978-0-8153-4556-5 (pbk)

Library of Congress Cataloging-in-Publication Data
Names: Dunlap, Norma K., author. | Huryn, Donna M., author.
Title: Medicinal chemistry / Norma K. Dunlap, Donna M. Huryn.
Description: New York, NY : Garland Science, Taylor & Francis Group, LLC, [2018]
Identifiers: LCCN 2017039687 | ISBN 9780815345565
Subjects: LCSH: Pharmaceutical chemistry. | Chemotherapy.
Classification: LCC RS403 .D86 2018 | DDC 615.1/9--dc23
LC record available at https://lccn.loc.gov/2017039687

PREFACE

This textbook is an overview of the subject of medicinal chemistry within the context of drug design and discovery. Both of us were trained as synthetic organic chemists and had our "first" careers in medicinal chemistry departments at major pharmaceutical companies. Upon moving into academia, we both took on teaching a one-semester class in medicinal chemistry. Anyone who has taught this type of course quickly realizes the difficulty in bringing together the many aspects that comprise this subject, such as organic chemistry, pharmacology, and biochemistry, as well as introducing therapeutic areas in medicinal chemistry in just one semester. After teaching this course for many years using various review articles as text, as well as material written ourselves, we decided to write this textbook. We have tried to write a text that includes the historical background of drug discovery but emphasizes modern practices in design, discovery, and development. We focus on drug targets and how current knowledge of these targets drives medicinal chemistry and drug discovery. While it is not possible to cover all therapeutic areas in a one-semester text, selected areas and classes of drugs are also included. Overall, we intend for this text to meet the need for a modern, one-semester textbook that ties together the many different aspects of medicinal chemistry as it is currently practiced.

The target audience is primarily upper-level undergraduate students and beginning graduate students in organic chemistry and medicinal chemistry. Other students who might find the text useful include pharmacy students and anyone planning to pursue a career in the drug discovery field. In addition to science majors, we have had students from fields as diverse as finance, engineering, and biomedical ethics take our courses, all with a common interest in learning about drug discovery. The book should also be useful for professional scientists, such as chemists, biologists, and patent professionals, who are just entering the drug discovery field and may not have had direct experience with medicinal chemistry. It is expected that those using this textbook have a basic knowledge of organic chemistry as well as basic biology.

To present this broad subject in a way that is logical and covers essential topics in a one-semester format, our approach is to divide the text into three sections. PART I, Drug Discovery and Development: the first five chapters cover historical background in drug discovery, as well as the modern drug discovery and development process, with an emphasis on medicinal chemistry strategies used in various phases. These chapters give the essential background of hit and lead discovery, modifications driven by knowledge of both target and pharmacophore structure, common medicinal chemistry strategies, and the central importance of pharmacokinetics. They provide the background that subsequent chapters build upon. PART II, Classes of Drug Targets: Chapters 6–9 focus on the major drug targets, namely, their structure and function and how medicinal chemists approach each. Examples of specific drugs developed for each type of target are included. Targets include receptors and ion channels, enzymes, protein–protein and lipid interactions, and nucleic acids. Each of those is broken down into more specific classes of important drug targets. These chapters can be covered in any order but reference topics in Chapters 1–5. PART III, Selected Therapeutic Areas: the final chapters, 10–13, are devoted to selected important therapeutic areas. While there are many more chapters that could have been written on additional areas of interest, these topics were selected as examples that tie together components introduced in the earlier chapters and represent both historically important agents and future opportunities. Those topics included are anti-cancer, antibacterial, and antiviral drugs and drugs acting on the central nervous system. A subset of Chapter 13 is devoted to drugs of abuse, informed by student interest on this topic. Any of these last chapters on specific therapeutic areas can be considered optional or used independently, but they also rely on the material covered in Chapters 1–9.

In writing this book, we have tried to emphasize modern practices, while also retaining some historical background as a way to show progress in the field and to help explain complex concepts. Full color figures are used throughout to identify key structural features and highlight specific points of significance. Key terms are highlighted in boldface type and are further explained in an expanded glossary. Each chapter ends with problems divided into review questions and application questions. Review questions are based on understanding material presented in the chapter, whereas application problems require critical thinking skills to apply previously covered concepts to new problems. Some application problems ask the student to research a topic, intending to provide relevant experience to students. Answers to review questions are printed in the back of the book. Each chapter also includes two case studies on individual drugs that highlight relevant subjects in those chapters. While some are historical examples, most case studies focus on compounds and recently developed drugs.

ACKNOWLEDGMENTS

We gratefully acknowledge the contributions of the following scientists and instructors for their advice and critique in the development of this book:

Galia Blum (The Hebrew University), Justin M. Chalker (Flinders University), Amber F. Charlebois (SUNY Geneseo), Emily Dykhuizen (Purdue University), Steven M. Firestine (Wayne State University), Lekh Nath Sharma Gautam (St. Jude Children's Research Hospital), George Greco (Goucher College), Wayne C. Guida (University of Southern Florida), Geneive Henry (Susquehanna University), David Hunt (The College of New Jersey), William Maio (New Mexico State University), Paul L. Ornstein (Roosevelt University), Timothy S. Snowden (The University of Alabama), Erika A. Taylor (Wesleyan University), Nanette Wachter (Hofstra University), Simon Ward (University of Sussex).

Special thanks go to Jay Kostman for reviewing the text, particularly for providing expert feedback on antiviral and antibacterial chapters; to Stephen Kostman and Emily Rizzo for text preparation; and to Chelsea Harmon and Melissa Grenier for review of the text and preparation of answer keys. We are grateful for the input of many students over the past years. Finally, our thanks also go to the people at Garland Science, especially to senior editor Summers Scholl and assistant editor Claudia Acevedo-Quiñones for their enthusiasm, support, and guidance for this project. Senior Production Editors Natasha Wolfe and Georgina Lucas have been very helpful in guiding completion of the project, and we thank Matt McClements for his excellent artwork.

Norma Dunlap
Donna M. Huryn
July 2017

RESOURCES FOR INSTRUCTORS AND STUDENTS

The teaching and learning resources for instructors and students are available online. The instructor resources on the Garland Science website are password-protected and available only to adopting instructors. The student resources on the Garland Science Website are available to everyone. We hope these resources will enhance student learning and make it easier for instructors to prepare dynamic lectures and activities for the classroom.

Instructor Resources

Instructor Resources are available on the Garland Science Instructor Resource area, located at www.garlandscience.com. The website provides access not only to the teaching resources for this book but also to all other Garland Science textbooks. Adopting instructors can obtain access to the site from their sales representative or by emailing science@garland.com.

Art of Medicinal Chemistry

The images from the book are available in two convenient formats: PowerPoint® and JPEG. They have been optimized for display on a computer. Figures are searchable by figure number, by figure name, or by keywords used in the figure legend from the book.

Answer Keys to Application Questions

Answers to application questions are available to qualified instructors.

Student Resources

The resources for students are available on the Medicinal Chemistry Student Website, located at www.garlandscience.com.

Journal Club

The Journal Club recommends journal articles that complement topics in the textbook to improve students' critical analysis of research and to promote a better understanding of the research process. These are examples taken from the recent literature and include early-stage experimental compounds as well as compounds that are at the clinical trial stage. Each Journal Club document provides background information on the chosen paper as well as questions and discussion points to stimulate in-class discussion. We have found that primary literature is very helpful in exposing upper-level students to research articles, giving students practice in comprehension of real-life research questions, and in teaching them how all aspects of medicinal chemistry come together in drug development. Answers will be provided to instructors only.

CONTENTS

PART I

DRUG DISCOVERY AND DEVELOPMENT

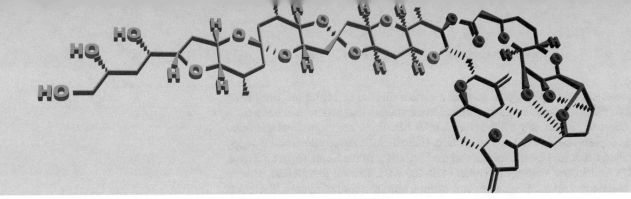

Historical perspective and overview of drug discovery

1

LEARNING OBJECTIVES

- Understand how medicinal chemistry is defined.
- Become familiar with the historical progression of therapeutics from plant preparations to single, pure substances.
- Learn how organic chemistry contributed to the identification and synthesis of drugs.
- Describe how scientists' understanding of drug action in the body has evolved over time.

Even before we are born, we are under assault by foreign organisms and by defects in our bodies that ultimately may lead to an overwhelming variety of diseases and conditions. We fight back by means of our immune system and various repair mechanisms, and when these prove insufficient, we rely on external substances: medicines. **Medicinal chemistry** is the branch of chemistry that focuses on the design, synthesis, and development of new medicines or drugs. Hidden in this simple definition are several areas of science, including organic chemistry, biochemistry, and pharmacology. The vast majority of drugs are small organic molecules, as opposed to inorganic molecules or macromolecules such as proteins. Hence, in order to study these drugs, an understanding of the structure and nature of functional groups present in organic compounds is required. To understand how drugs exert their action in a living system, it is also necessary to have a basic understanding of **pharmacology**, the study of drug action. The process of how new drugs are designed involves examining drug–macromolecule interactions at a molecular level, which includes some aspects of biochemistry. Overall, the process of drug discovery and development in medicinal chemistry includes the iterative process of understanding drug–target interactions, designing improved analogs, synthesizing new molecules, and evaluating compounds.

HISTORICAL PERSPECTIVE OF THE PRACTICE OF MEDICINAL CHEMISTRY

Medicinal chemistry has been practiced, in some form or another, for thousands of years, progressing from the use of certain plants or plant parts through preparation of semi-pure plant extracts to isolation of pure active molecules and finally to the invention of molecules specifically designed to treat a certain disease or condition. Until fairly recently, our source of medicines was limited to substances that occurred in nature.

Between approximately 3000 BC and 1000 AD, there are numerous recorded instances of plants being used to treat disease. These include descriptions of the poppy plant (called Gil or Joy) by ancient Sumerians (3000 BC), in the Ebers Papyrus (Egypt, 1550 BC), and in the writings of Galen (129–199 AD). During this period, special priests, shamans, and medicine men and women administered medicine. There was an aura of mystery and religion involved in their knowledge of the magical plants that could heal, prolong life, and treat pain and other symptoms of disease. Many of these substances are still used today, either in their crude plant form or as the pure active component of the plant.

During the early part of the second millennium, scientists began to realize that a specific ingredient in the plant was responsible for its beneficial activity; therefore, there was a focus on obtaining semi-pure and standardized plant preparations to be used as medicines. In this time period, publications of **herbals** and **pharmacopeias** appeared, which are written collections of descriptions of plants useful for medicinal purposes. These publications listed plants that had been used for thousands of years and described treatments using those plants for specific conditions. Some important examples include an herbal published in Switzerland in 1470 by Bartholomeus Anglicus; the *Nuovo Receptario Composito*, published in Venice in 1498; the *First London Pharmacopoeia*, published in 1618; and *The Divine Husbandman's Materia Medica Classic*, published in 1596 in China. These various publications provided specific information on the use and preparation of various plants that have been used for thousands of years, a number of which are still used today. During this time period, the Swiss physician Paracelsus (1493–1541), in particular, attempted to find the healing element in both organic and inorganic pharmaceutical preparations. Some specific examples of medicinal plants and their uses are summarized in **Table 1.1**.

As can be seen by the examples in Table 1.1, there is a long history of the use of medicinal plants, going back to the earliest recorded history. While most were used to treat specific medical conditions, others, such as *Erythroxylum coca*, were used as stimulants or euphorics. Some others originated from the arrow poisons (known as woorara) used as a paralytic to hunt animals for centuries in South America. In the 1800s, animal studies using woorara, carried out by Sir Benjamin Brodie and others, showed that the heart kept beating while the animal became paralyzed, eventually leading to use of the active ingredient, tubocurarine, in anesthesia.

The science of chemistry moved into a more modern understanding of the composition of materials between the 1700s and the 1900s. With this expansion of the field of chemistry, there was a focus on the isolation of pure compounds and attributing biological activity to specific substances even though the structure was often unknown. By the late 1800s, the knowledge of organic compounds had advanced to a basic understanding of functional group arrangements, along with the correct assignment of many structures. This period also marked the introduction of the first semisynthetic drugs: those prepared by chemical derivatization of natural products.

1.1   Many medicines were originally isolated from plants

Many early medicines fall into the category of nitrogen-containing plant products called **alkaloids**. The first alkaloid obtained in pure form was morphine, isolated by Serturner from a type of poppy plant (*Papaver somniferum*) in 1805 and named for Morpheus, the Greek god of dreams. It became widely used both to treat pain and as a cough suppressant. Many other medicinally active plant ingredients were isolated during this period. For example, Pierre Pelletier and Jean Caventou isolated colchicine from the autumn crocus in 1820, Friedrich Gaedcke isolated cocaine in 1855, and Nagayoshi Nagai isolated ephedrine from ma huang in 1887. Another example is the isolation of salicylic acid from willow bark. Salicin, originally isolated from the bark in 1826 by Johann Buchner, is an aryl glycoside. Crude isolation in this case involved preparation of a simple tea or aqueous extract of willow bark and leaves, followed by further extraction and crystallization.

Table 1.1   Examples of medicinal plants, historical documentation of their use and active ingredient

Plant (common name)	Historical mention	Use	Active agent	
Papaver somniferum (opium poppy)	3000–300 BC (Sumeria, Egypt, Greece, China) 1500s (Paracelsus in Switzerland): laudanum (~12% morphine)	analgesic	morphine	
Dichroa febrifuga (Chang shan or Chinese quinine)	2735 BC (China); one of the "50 fundamental herbs" in traditional Chinese medicine	malaria, fever	febrifugine	
Ephedra sinica (ma huang)	2735 BC (China)	cough, asthma	ephedrine	
Cinchona (fever tree)	1600s (South America); brought to Europe by Jesuit missionaries	malaria, fever	quinine	
Colchicum autumnale (autumn crocus)	AD 300 (Egypt) AD 560 (Arabia); source of hermodactyls (medicinal roots) early 1900s (England)	joint pain, gout, rheumatism	colchicine	
Erythroxylum coca "the divine plant of the Incas"	AD 600 (South America); used by the Moche and Inca civilization, possibly as early as 3000 BC 1596 (Spanish explorers mention its effects)	stimulant and euphoric	cocaine	
Chondrodendron tomentosum (ourari/woorara = "killer of birds")	1516 (South America); brought to England by Walter Raleigh, after visiting Guyana	paralytic in anesthesia (originally used for hunting)	tubocurarine	
Salix alba (willow)	500 BC (Greece: Hippocrates; Sumeria, Assyria) 1700s (Native Americans) 1763 (England)	pain, fever	salicylic acid	
Digitalis purpurea (foxglove)	1250 (Wales) 1785 (England)	cardiac stimulant	digoxigenin	

Poppy photo by Réginald Hulhoven/Wikimedia Commons, CC BY-SA 1.0. Quinine photo by Wouter Hagens/Wikimedia Commons, CC BY-SA 3.0. Ephedra photo by Lazare Gagnidze/Wikimedia Commons, CC BY-SA 4.0. Coca photo by Geoff Gallice/Wikimedia Commons, CC BY 2.0. Chondrodendron photo by Alex Popovkin/Flickr, CC BY 2.0. Salix alba photo by Ladislav Luppa/Wikimedia Commons, CC BY-SA 3.0. Digitalis purpurea drawing by Elisabete Ferreira/Wikimedia Commons, CC BY-SA 3.0.

Many active plant products contain either a basic amine or a carboxylic acid, and isolation procedures rely on liquid–liquid extractions with sequential basic and acidic aqueous solutions. The isolation of ephedrine outlined below is a typical procedure for isolating an amine:

Step 1: The *Ephedra sinica* (ma huang) plant material is harvested, dried, and powdered, and the powder is partitioned between a two-phase mixture of benzene and cold aqueous sodium carbonate. In basic solution, the amine of ephedrine is not protonated and the compound resides in the organic (benzene) layer. The basic aqueous layer contains various water-soluble compounds, debris, and any organic acids, which are deprotonated at high pH and therefore water-soluble.

Step 2: The two layers are separated, and the benzene solution is extracted with dilute HCl. This treatment protonates the amine, making ephedrine charged, and it is partitioned into the aqueous layer. Any unwanted non-basic organic compounds remain in the benzene layer.

Step 3: The aqueous layer from the previous step is combined with chloroform, and then potassium carbonate is added to "free base" the amine. This converts ephedrine back to its amine form, rendering it organic-soluble once again. The organic layer is collected, and the chloroform is evaporated to provide solid ephedrine with minimal impurities.

Step 4: The purest forms of solids are usually crystalline materials, and many amines crystallize easily as salts. The ephedrine in this case was treated with oxalic acid and crystallized as its oxalate salt. Nagai obtained a 2% yield (based on plant material) of the pure ephedrine salt following this procedure (**Figure 1.1**).

Although historically plants were the earliest sources for medicines, in the 1900s bacteria and molds became important sources as well. The type of isolation procedure outlined in Figure 1.1 works well for many compounds containing basic amines, as long as they are stable to extraction conditions with strong base and strong acid. In contrast to ephedrine, some sensitive compounds such as penicillin cannot be isolated in this manner. In fact, the development of penicillin was temporarily abandoned in 1932 because of difficulty in isolation of the pure compound.

Until the 1940s, nearly all drugs were isolated directly from plants as the natural products or were simple derivatives, such as esters, of natural products, with most having some origin in herbal and medicinal plant lore. In the late 1900s, natural product isolation as a source of drugs became a less frequent approach; however, there was still interest in finding new drugs or leads from plant and animal sources, often through government initiatives. One example was the International Cooperative Biodiversity Groups project (ICBG) launched by the National Institutes of Health (NIH), the National Science Foundation (NSF), and the U.S. Agency for International Development in 1993. This program supported partnerships between academic institutions, private enterprises, and local populations in countries where medicinal plants are found. The goal of this initiative was to identify new drugs to treat a variety of diseases by both random and targeted collection of plants and plant extracts, based on ethnobotanical information from local healers.

1.2 Semisynthetic drugs are prepared from natural products

A **semisynthetic compound** is one that is derived from a natural product but undergoes additional chemical modification, usually requiring only a few synthetic steps. The earliest reported semisynthetic drug is acetylsalicylic acid (aspirin), derived from salicylic acid by acetylation with acetic anhydride. In 1829, Henri Leroux isolated approximately 25 g of salicin from 1 kg of willow bark. Nine years later, Raffaelle Piria converted salicin to β-D-glucopyranose and the oxidation product, salicylic acid. Salicylic acid is generated upon ingestion of salicin and is the active ingredient in willow bark. Salicylic acid, however, was too irritating to the stomach to be useful, and the acetate was first prepared by Charles Gerhardt in 1853 as a less irritating form of the drug. Although Gerhardt did not pursue marketing the drug, in 1897 Felix Hoffmann, a chemist working for Bayer Pharmaceuticals in Germany, prepared some of the acetate for his father, who

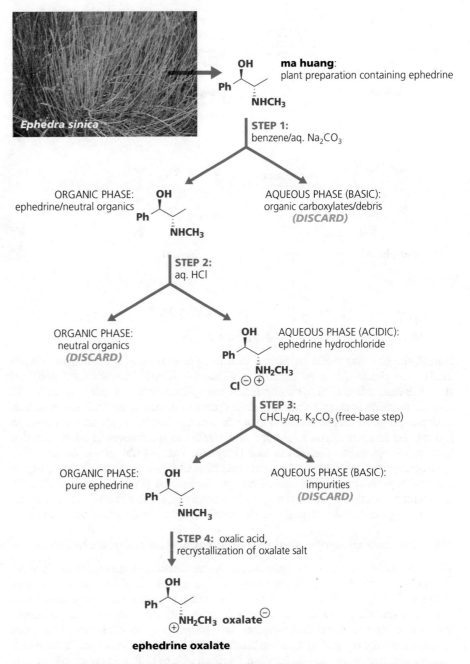

Figure 1.1 Procedure for isolation of ephedrine from ma huang. Step 1: The crude plant preparation is partitioned between benzene and aqueous base (ephedrine is shown in red). Step 2: The organic phase is extracted with aqueous acid. Step 3: Base is added to the aqueous phase to free-base ephedrine; the next step is extraction of the free base into organic solvent and evaporation to solid ephedrine. Step 4: Recrystallization as the oxalate salt. Photo by Lazare Gagnidze/Wikimedia Commons, CC BY-SA 4.0.

was suffering from arthritis. Acetylsalicylic acid was marketed by Bayer Pharmaceuticals in 1900 as aspirin (**Figure 1.2**). Aspirin is still widely used to alleviate pain and fever, as well as for the prevention of cardiovascular disease and stroke.

Another early example of a semisynthetic drug is heroin, which is the bis(acetate) of morphine. The drug was first synthesized in England in 1874 by C. R. Alder Wright by the reaction of morphine with acetic anhydride. It was later prepared by Hoffmann (the inventor of aspirin) and dubbed heroin after the German word for heroic. Heroin was mistakenly believed to be a less addictive form of morphine and was marketed by Bayer as a cure for morphine addiction until 1910, when it became clear that it was rapidly converted to morphine and was, in fact, even more addictive.

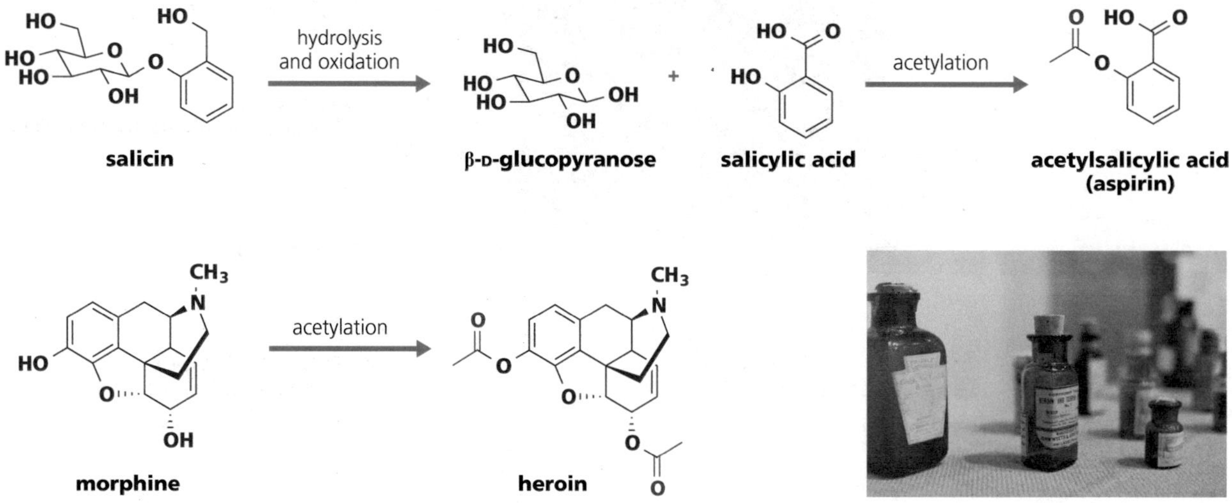

salicin   →(hydrolysis and oxidation)→   β-D-glucopyranose   +   salicylic acid   →(acetylation)→   acetylsalicylic acid (aspirin)

morphine   →(acetylation)→   heroin

OVERVIEW OF THE PRACTICE OF MEDICINAL CHEMISTRY IN THE MODERN ERA

During the last 100 years, medicinal chemistry has become a branch of science in its own right. The most significant advances were in the identification and structure elucidation of active compounds, the appreciation that drugs interact with specific proteins such as enzymes and receptors to elicit a beneficial effect, and in understanding the molecular interactions between a drug molecule and its target. In just the last 50 years alone, there have been tremendous advances in our knowledge of drug targets such as enzymes and receptors. With combinations of improved spectroscopic technology and computer graphics, as well as advances in imaging, we can now "see" a drug as it interacts with a specific enzyme or protein. This technology allows for the design of new drugs based on observable interactions, whereas in the past, the approach to developing new drugs was based on empirical observations.

Figure 1.2 Semisyntheses of aspirin and heroin. The hydroxy group of salicylic acid (generated from hydrolysis and oxidation of salicin) and both hydroxyl groups of morphine react with acetic anhydride to form the acetate esters (shown in red). (Photo by Karen Neoh/Flickr, CC BY 2.0.)

1.3   Identification of complex structures began in the early 1900s

The early 1900s witnessed an explosion in the elucidation of structures of bioactive molecules. Earlier, substances were described by the methods by which they were isolated, their appearance, and simple characterization such as melting point, rather than their specific chemical structures. Without the benefit of modern spectroscopic methods, these complex structures were solved primarily by use of elemental analyses, degradation studies, and simple functional group manipulations to deduce which functional groups were present. For example, from 1902 to 1907, early work in Germany by four separate laboratories identified the empirical formula of morphine as well as some features of the structure. Natural products isolated from the poppy plant included morphine ($C_{17}H_{19}NO_3$), codeine ($C_{18}H_{21}NO_3$), and thebaine ($C_{19}H_{21}NO_3$). Simple analysis of acid–base properties showed that while morphine possessed a phenolic (acidic) alcohol, codeine and thebaine did not (**Figure 1.3A**). The presence of a methylated basic nitrogen in each was also indicated. Methylation of the phenol group of morphine provided codeine, and oxidation of the alcohol of codeine to a ketone, followed by formation of the methyl enol ether, afforded thebaine. Other important common structural features identified were the presence of an alkene and the fact that degradation of each afforded a phenanthrene structure (based on three fused benzene rings). On the basis of knowledge that the three core structures were related and further studies of the properties and reactions of these compounds, a pentacyclic structure for morphine was proposed in 1902 (shown in **Figure 1.3B**). Soon after, in 1907, a bridged rather than a fused ring system was suggested. This structure was accepted as correct for nearly 20 years until, in 1923, Sir Robert Robinson published the structure in which the bridge junction is at C13 rather than C5 and the alkene is between C7 and C8 rather

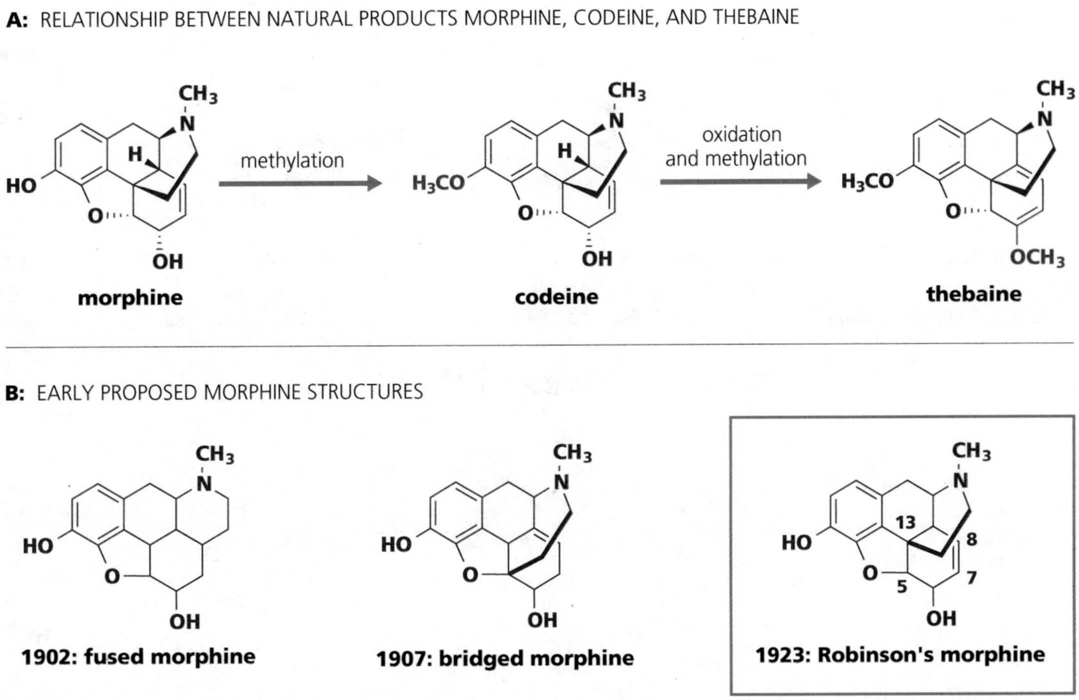

A: RELATIONSHIP BETWEEN NATURAL PRODUCTS MORPHINE, CODEINE, AND THEBAINE

B: EARLY PROPOSED MORPHINE STRUCTURES

1902: fused morphine

1907: bridged morphine

1923: Robinson's morphine

Figure 1.3 Elucidation of morphine structure. A: Relationship between the natural products morphine, codeine, and thebaine; structural differences in each step are shown in red. B: Initially proposed morphine structure containing fused ring system; structure modified to bridged structure; and correct structure, [which modifies the ring fusion and double-bond positions compared to 1907 structure].

than C8 and C9. Ultimate confirmation that Robinson's structure was correct came in the 1950s with Marshall Gates's independent synthesis of morphine.

Overall, elucidation of the structure of morphine took approximately 30 years and the work of many scientists from independent laboratories. **Figure 1.4** illustrates additional medically active compounds (many listed in **Table 1.1**) that were isolated and whose structures were elucidated during this period.

Since the early 1900s, purification procedures have been greatly improved with the advent of modern chromatographic methods. Sources of natural products have also expanded beyond plant materials to include products from bacteria, fungi, and marine sources. In addition, the development of infrared spectroscopy (IR), nuclear magnetic resonance spectroscopy (NMR), and mass spectrometry (MS) allows use of very small quantities of material to rapidly determine the presence of functional groups, molecular connectivity, and accurate masses, respectively. With these spectroscopic methods, as well as advances in X-ray crystallography, complex structures are now identified much more quickly and with greater confidence. For example, the complex structures of taxol, isolated from yew trees in 1967, and of calicheamicin, isolated in 1987 from soil microbes, were solved within just a few years of their isolation and the characterization of their potent anti-proliferative activity. Mansukh Wani and Monroe Wall at Research Triangle Institute reported the structure of taxol (**Figure 1.5**) in 1971 using NMR, IR, and MS, along with X-ray crystallography of a simple derivative. Scientists at Lederle Laboratories used classical degradation studies as well as spectroscopy and X-ray crystallography to solve the structure of the highly complex ene-diyne known as calicheamicin γ1 (see Figure 1.5) in 1992. Taxol (paclitaxel) is currently approved for the treatment of certain cancers. Calicheamicin γ1 is too toxic to be used as a stand-alone agent, but a derivative was conjugated to an antibody, and that compound (gemtuzumab ozogamicin) is now approved to treat certain types of acute myeloid leukemia.

1.4 Advances in total synthesis allow access to natural products and analogs

Once methods to reliably elucidate the structures of biologically active natural products were readily available, the synthesis of those structures and their analogs became feasible. Development of a **total synthesis**, the complete synthesis from

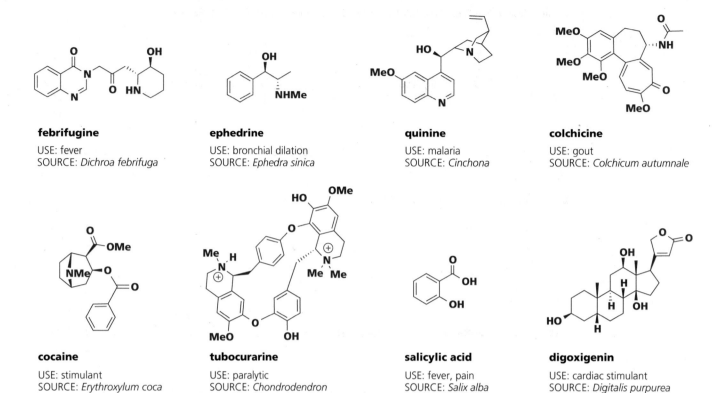

febrifugine

USE: fever
SOURCE: *Dichroa febrifuga*

ephedrine

USE: bronchial dilation
SOURCE: *Ephedra sinica*

quinine

USE: malaria
SOURCE: *Cinchona*

colchicine

USE: gout
SOURCE: *Colchicum autumnale*

cocaine

USE: stimulant
SOURCE: *Erythroxylum coca*

tubocurarine

USE: paralytic
SOURCE: *Chondrodendron tomentosum*

salicylic acid

USE: fever, pain
SOURCE: *Salix alba*

digoxigenin

USE: cardiac stimulant
SOURCE: *Digitalis purpurea*

simple starting materials, of a natural product is desirable and important for a number of reasons:

- Isolations can be time-consuming and expensive and may give variable results.

- Very large amounts of materials (kilograms) may be required to produce milligrams of the isolated product.

- Access to materials may be restricted due to either climatic or political conditions.

- Independent synthesis of the natural product serves to confirm the structure.

- Synthesis provides reliable access to new and unnatural analogs.

- Synthesis can be a source of large quantities of material.

There is, of course, no difference between a natural compound and a synthetic one. They are chemically identical in all respects, including stereochemistry. Often, analogs of natural products, which have variations in the functional groups and sometimes in the core skeleton, maintain biological activity and in some cases provide an improvement over the original structure. Developing a synthesis of the natural product allows for a much larger and more diverse array of analogs than might be available directly from the natural product itself. For example, semisynthetic compounds such as aspirin and heroin are available by simple esterification of the alcohol functional groups present in the natural products. Since the number and reactivity of the functional groups in a given natural product can limit the number

Figure 1.4 Examples of isolated active components. These structures were elucidated in the early 1900s, and their uses and plant sources are listed.

Figure 1.5 Structures of taxol and calicheamicin γ1. Taxol and calicheamicin γ1 are two recent examples of structurally complex bioactive natural products. Taxol binds and stabilizes microtubules and inhibits cell proliferation. The ene-diyne portion (shown in red) of calicheamicin γ1 is responsible for its ability to cause cleavage of DNA.

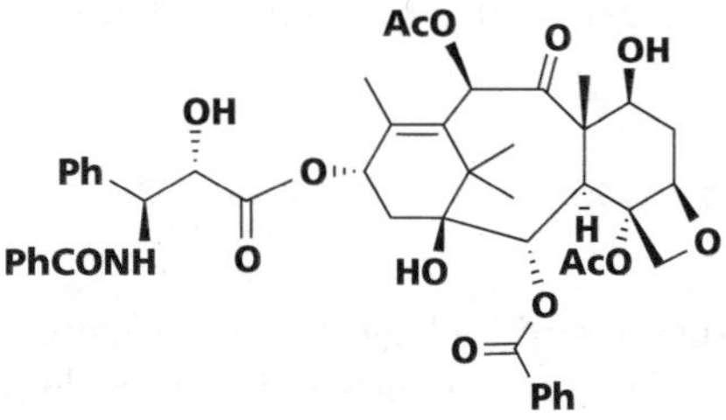

taxol

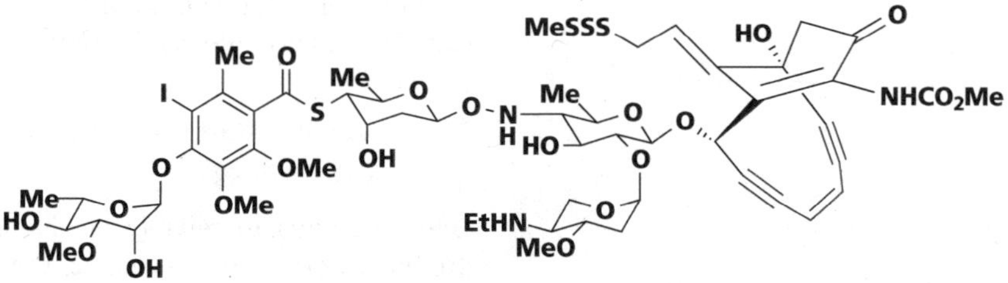

calicheamicin γ1

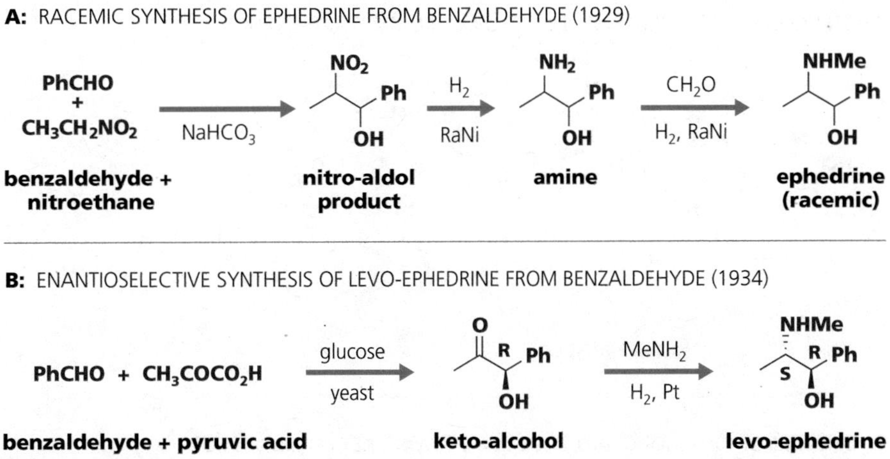

Figure 1.6 Syntheses of ephedrine. A: Racemic synthesis from benzaldehyde. A nitro-aldol (Henry) reaction between nitroethane and benzaldehyde is followed by reduction of the nitro group to an amine; reductive amination with formaldehyde generates racemic ephedrine. B: Enantioselective synthesis from benzaldehyde and pyruvate. Enzymes in fermenting glucose catalyze condensation of the starting materials to give a keto-alcohol with the *R*-configuration; reductive amination with methylamine affords levo-ephedrine selectively.

A: RACEMIC SYNTHESIS OF EPHEDRINE FROM BENZALDEHYDE (1929)

B: ENANTIOSELECTIVE SYNTHESIS OF LEVO-EPHEDRINE FROM BENZALDEHYDE (1934)

and diversity of analogs that may be prepared by semisynthesis, modification of intermediates used in a total synthesis can be used to even further expand the analogs prepared. It can also provide optical isomers that are inaccessible from the natural product. For example, two syntheses of ephedrine, one providing the racemic form and one providing the natural (levo) stereoisomer, are shown in **Figure 1.6**.

Although the synthesis of ephedrine requires only a few steps, some total syntheses can be quite lengthy. For example, the first synthesis of morphine (by Gates) required 28 steps and afforded racemic material in only 0.0014% yield (see **Figure 1.7** for synopsis). A more efficient biomimetic synthesis was reported by Kenner Rice in 1980; it led to morphine in 18 steps with 11% yield. The first enantioselective total synthesis, one that did not rely on a step to resolve stereoisomers, was not accomplished until 1993. That synthesis, reported by Larry Overman, began with an enantioselective ketone reduction and proceeded in 24 steps with 5% yield.

A more recent example can be seen surrounding the efforts toward total synthesis of halichondrin B, an anti-tumor product isolated from the marine sponge *Halichondria okadai* in 1986. Very limited quantities of the natural product were available from natural sources; therefore, a number of chemistry labs have investigated and published on their efforts to synthesize this highly complex molecule. The first total synthesis of halichondrin B was reported by Yoshito Kishi in 1992, with the longest linear sequence requiring 47 steps (see **Figure 1.8** for a synopsis; synthesis of intermediates not shown). Intermediates prepared during a total synthesis are routinely tested to determine which segments of the structure are essential for biological activity. These efforts indicated that fragments of the right side of halichondrin B exhibited significant anti-proliferative activity. This fragment

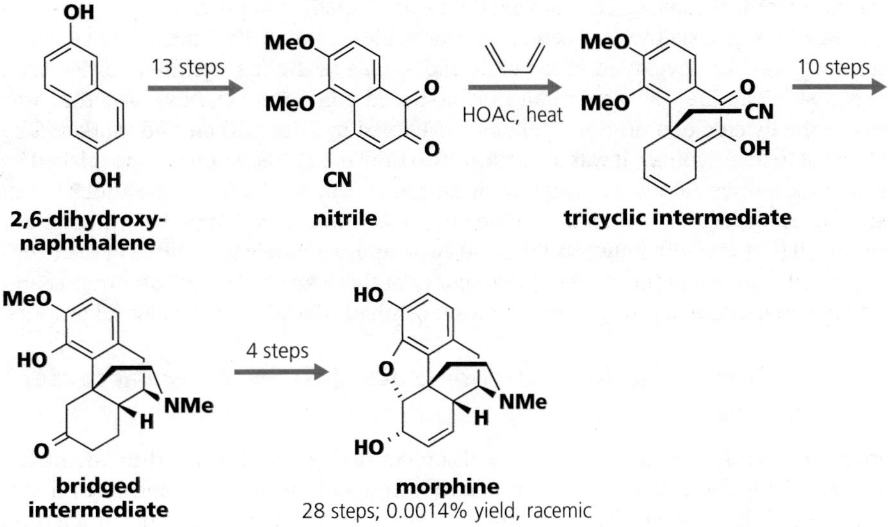

Figure 1.7 Outline of Gates's synthesis of morphine. Starting with 2,6-dihydroxynaphthalene, 13 steps adjust the oxidation level and add the two-carbon nitrile that will become the nitrogen-containing ring. A Diels–Alder reaction affords a tricyclic intermediate. Ten more steps are required to form the bridged intermediate, and then four final steps are required to provide morphine.

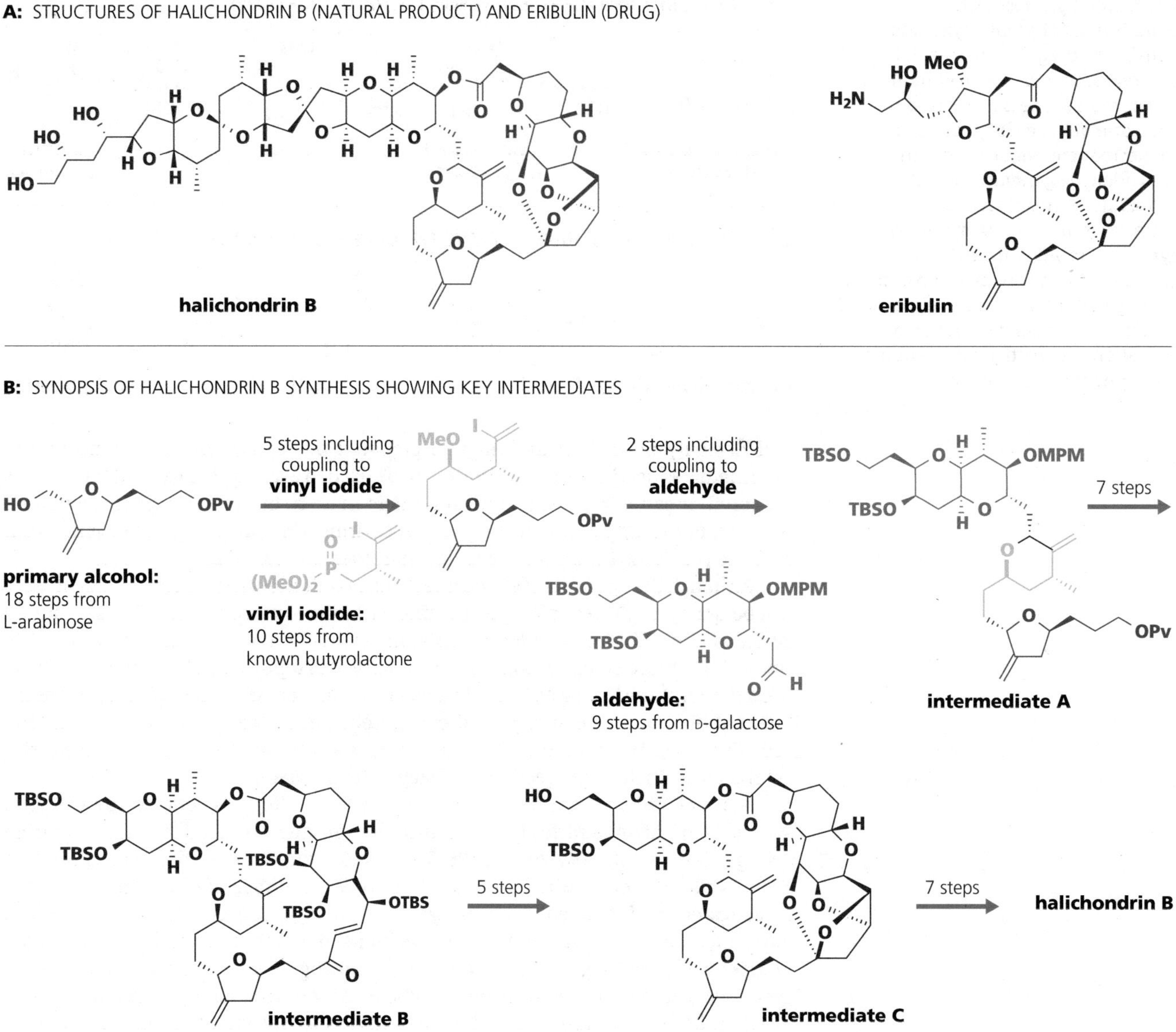

A: STRUCTURES OF HALICHONDRIN B (NATURAL PRODUCT) AND ERIBULIN (DRUG)

halichondrin B

eribulin

B: SYNOPSIS OF HALICHONDRIN B SYNTHESIS SHOWING KEY INTERMEDIATES

primary alcohol:
18 steps from
L-arabinose

vinyl iodide:
10 steps from
known butyrolactone

aldehyde:
9 steps from D-galactose

intermediate A

intermediate B

intermediate C

halichondrin B

was further modified and resulted in the anti-cancer agent eribulin. Development of a synthesis of this complex natural product led to the generation of a related but unnatural anti-cancer agent, showing the value of such an approach.

In addition to synthesis of natural products, the synthesis of medicines not derived from nature also developed in the early 1900s. One of the first synthetic drugs used was arsphenamine (Salvarsan), an arsenic-based compound (whose structure was not correctly elucidated until much later) developed by Paul Ehrlich and marketed by Hoechst to treat syphilis. It was used from 1910 until the 1940s, when it was replaced by much safer drugs. Another early synthetic drug, developed in 1935, was the antibacterial sulfanilamide, which is generated in the body after administration of the synthetic dye prontosil (**Figure 1.9**). Between 1981 and 2014, approximately two-thirds of the drugs approved were small molecules. The majority of these are synthetic compounds and about a quarter are natural products or semi-synthetic derivatives of a natural product.

1.5   Medicinal chemistry currently is based on the molecular causes of disease

In the not-so-distant past, diseases or disorders were often attributed to witchcraft, possession by the devil, or immoral behavior. It is only in more recent times that it was proved that certain diseases were caused by an infectious agent or an aberrant

Figure 1.8 Total synthesis of halichondrin B and identification of eribulin. A: Structures of halichondrin B and eribulin, a drug derived from an intermediate prepared during a total synthesis of the natural product. The moiety (right side) of halichondrin B from which eribulin was derived is shown in red. B: Synopsis of halichondrin B synthesis. Three fragments, the primary alcohol (violet), vinyl iodide (green), and aldehyde (pink), are combined to give intermediate A. Seven steps convert A to intermediate B; five steps are required to form the spiroacetal intermediate C; and seven final steps prepare halichondrin B.

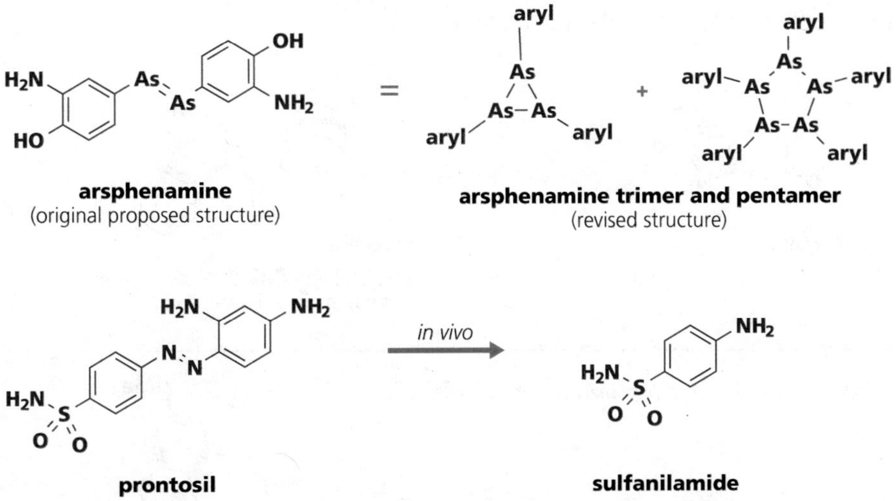

Figure 1.9 Examples of early synthetic drugs. Arsphenamine was used to treat syphilis: the proposed As=As structure (left) was revised in 2005 and shown to consist of a mix of trimer and pentamer structures. The antibacterial sulfanilamide is produced *in vivo* by cleavage of the azo bond (N=N) of the synthetic dye prontosil.

arsphenamine
(original proposed structure)

arsphenamine trimer and pentamer
(revised structure)

prontosil

sulfanilamide

physiological process. For instance, the germ theory of disease, although suggested in some cultures for many hundreds of years, was not widely accepted until the 1800s. Studies of human physiology in the twentieth century led to the basis of our current understanding of many conditions. Most recently, developments in DNA technology and sequencing of the human genome allowed the identification of genomic changes, and therefore the corresponding changes at the protein level, that are associated with disease.

Almost all drugs interact with a specific **macromolecular target**. The three major classes of targets are enzymes, receptors, and the nucleic acids DNA and RNA (these, and others, will be discussed in detail in Chapters 6–9). Ehrlich introduced one of the most important concepts in modern medicinal chemistry in 1897 when he proposed the side-chain theory to explain how bacterial toxins might interact with antitoxins through a specific chemical character of the cells. In 1900, he replaced the side-chain term with **receptor** and defined it as a specific chemical entity that could interact with drugs. He also introduced the concept of a **magic bullet** to target specific bacteria. This idea, that a drug could kill bacteria by specific interactions, without damaging the patient's cells, led to his development of Salvarsan, described above. The receptor concept was further advanced by John Langley, a British physiologist who studied the autonomic nervous system. He observed that a solution of jaborandi (an extract from a South American shrub), which contains the alkaloid pilocarpine, decreased the heartbeat of frogs when injected, but the heartbeat could then be increased by dosing with atropine, another natural product isolated from a plant called deadly nightshade (**Figure 1.10A**). Eventually, it was recognized that pilocarpine was a muscarinic receptor agonist (activator) and atropine was a muscarinic receptor antagonist (blocker): both compounds affected the same receptor but with opposite results.

Later in his career, in 1905, he observed a similar antagonistic action between nicotine and curare (**Figure 1.10B**). Injection of nicotine into a chicken led to a contraction of denervated leg muscle; injection of the plant extract curare, which contains tubocurarine, abolished the contraction. This work led to the concept that drugs interact with a specific receptive substance on the muscle cells.

Receptor theory was not fully accepted until the 1930s, and with the late 1940s came the recognition that multiple subtypes of the same receptor could exist. This appreciation explained how similar compounds could exhibit different types of activities and portended a focus on selectivity for one receptor subtype over another, with the hope of developing drugs with fewer side effects. The first receptors were not actually isolated until the 1970s, and in just the last 40 years, there have been tremendous advances in our knowledge of drug targets such as enzymes and receptors.

The history of enzymes parallels that of receptors, with Wilhelm Kühne's proposal of the term enzyme in 1878 to describe the component involved in fermentation of sugar to alcohol, and in 1907, Eduard Buchner named that specific enzyme zymase. Emil Fischer proposed the **lock and key hypothesis** to explain how a substrate interacts with an enzyme by fitting into a specific geometric shape as a key (substrate)

A: STRUCTURES OF PILOCARPINE AND ATROPINE

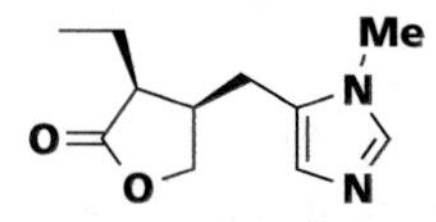

pilocarpine

EFFECT: decreases heart rate

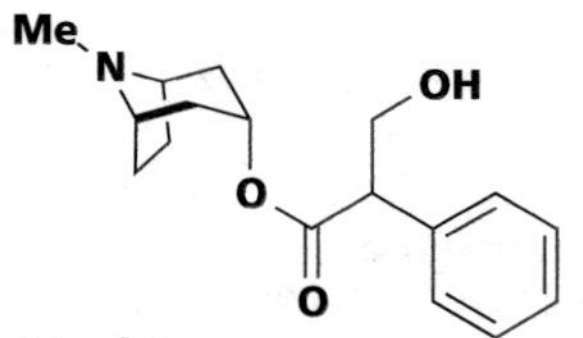

atropine

EFFECT: blocks effect of pilocarpine; result is increased heart rate

B: STRUCTURES OF NICOTINE AND TUBOCURARINE

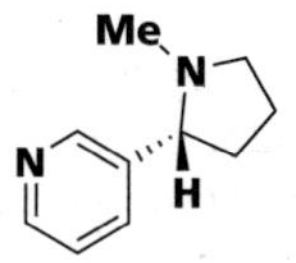

nicotine

EFFECT: muscle contraction

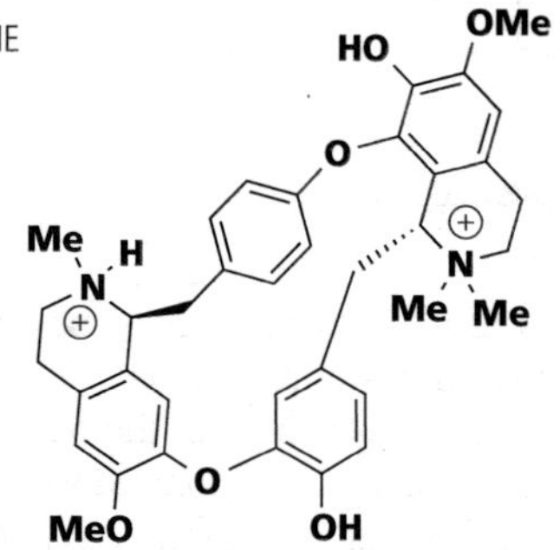

tubocurarine

EFFECT: blocks effect of nicotine; result is muscle relaxation

Figure 1.10 Antagonistic compounds. A: Structures of pilocarpine and atropine, which led to Langley's proposal of receptor theory based on their effect on heart rate: pilocarpine decreases heart rate, while atropine blocks the effect of pilocarpine. B: Structures of nicotine and tubocurarine, the active species in curare: curare blocks the effect of nicotine.

does in a lock (enzyme). Identification and isolation of a number of enzymes followed throughout the 1900s, culminating with the report by David Phillips and colleagues of the first X-ray crystal structure of lysozyme in 1965 and followed a few years later (1969) by the first synthesis of an enzyme (ribonuclease) in a laboratory.

With combinations of technologies like X-ray crystallography, NMR spectroscopy, or cryo-electron microscopy together with computer graphics, we can now "see" a drug as it interacts with a specific enzyme or protein. In many cases, an X-ray crystal structure can allow for the design of new drugs based on observable interactions. Although there are far fewer X-ray structures of receptors than of enzymes, molecular modeling of receptors has also streamlined the process of drug discovery.

SUMMARY

While the remainder of this text will focus on current drug discovery practices, it is also important to review how the practice of medicinal chemistry began. Until the nineteenth century, medicines were, for the most part, either crude or semi-pure plant preparations. Even now, there is continuing interest in **ethnopharmacology**, or the use of plants to treat diseases in native populations. In the mid-to-late 1900s, natural products continued to make important contributions as starting points for new drugs, particularly in both cancer and antibacterial drug discovery. With the rise of the scientific method, and the development of modern chemistry, came isolation and structural identification of the active components. This coincided with the development of synthetic compounds as medicines. New technologies, including synthetic biology and engineered biosynthesis, provide access to novel products with a natural origin. Continued research into the active agents and mechanism of action of traditional plant-based medicines, such as cannabis, will also provide new avenues for medicinal chemistry research.

In the twentieth century, numerous advances were made in the understanding of mechanism and the molecular basis of disease. All of this has led to the modern process of drug discovery, which is based on the idea of developing drugs to act with a specific biochemical mechanism to treat diseases. Most recently, advances in understanding diseases and diagnosis have provided access to precision medicine. For example, genetic testing of tumors allows specific treatment protocols to be designed that will be most effective for a particular patient.

CASE STUDY 1   DISCOVERY OF ARTEMISININ

The discovery of the antimalarial drug artemisinin began in 1967 in China as a response to outbreaks of quinine-resistant malaria among the North Vietnamese during the Vietnam War. A research project (Project 523) was initiated at a number of institutes throughout the country to find new effective medicines, both by synthetic approaches and by screening traditional Chinese medicines. At the Institute of Chinese Materia Medica, Youyou Tu screened over 2000 extracts and identified 640 that were active. About 380 extracts were screened in a mouse model of malaria infection. Extracts from *Artemisia annua* L., a species of wormwood known in China as qinghao, inhibited growth of the disease-causing organism, *Plasmodium falciparum*, by 68%; however, the results were not reproducible in later experiments.

By consulting the ancient literature (*A Handbook of Prescriptions for Emergencies* by Ge Hong, 284–346 AD), she found that the recommended extraction procedure was to "immerse a handful of qinghao with two liters of water, wring out the juice and drink it all". This information led to the idea that heating in the traditional extraction procedure was destroying the active component and might be responsible for the modest and irreproducible activity. Separation of the extract by typical acid extraction afforded acidic and neutral portions. Removal of the acidic portion of the extract left the neutral organic extract, which was nontoxic in assays and showed 100% inhibition of growth of the organism. Pure crystals were obtained and the structure was confirmed by X-ray crystallography in 1979 as an unusual sesquiterpene lactone containing an endoperoxide (**Figure 1.11**).

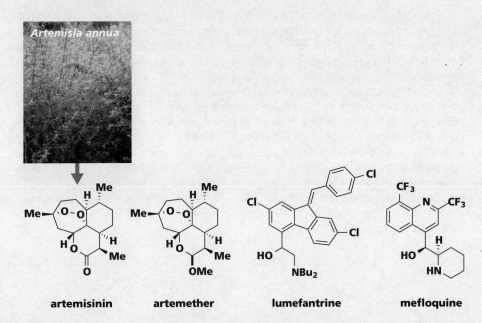

Figure 1.11 Structures of artemisinin and other antimalarial drugs. (Photo by Mark Tuschman, Novartis AG.)

Artemisinin acts rapidly but has a short half-life, and it is now used in combination with the synthetic drug mefloquine to treat malaria. The reduced derivative, artemether, is also commonly used in combination with the synthetic antimalarial drug lumefantrine.

This case study represents a relatively modern example of the discovery of a natural product as a new drug from an ancient remedy. Youyou Tu was recognized for this work with the 2015 Nobel Prize in Physiology or Medicine.

CASE STUDY 2   DISCOVERY OF INGENOL MEBUTATE

Ingenol is a diterpene that was recently approved as a treatment for actinic keratosis, a pre-cancerous skin condition. This natural product was first isolated during studies of *Croton tiglium*, the seed extracts of which are known as croton oil. This plant is a member of the Euphorbiaceae family. Interest in croton oil came from its known toxicity, mainly skin irritation. The methanol-soluble fraction of croton oil is called croton resin and contains 11 compounds responsible for the toxic and irritant properties. In the 1940s, croton oil and croton resin was used by Isaac Berenblum in mouse skin irritant studies and led to the two-stage model of skin carcinogenesis. In this widely used model, a tumor initiator is needed for carcinogenesis, and addition of a tumor promoter leads to progression to cancer. Phorbol esters, a series of diesters of fatty acids, were the naturally occurring compounds identified as the tumor promoters, or co-carcinogens found in croton oil and croton resin. The tumor promoter phorbol triacetate is a widely used research compound in the study of cancers (**Figure 1.12**).

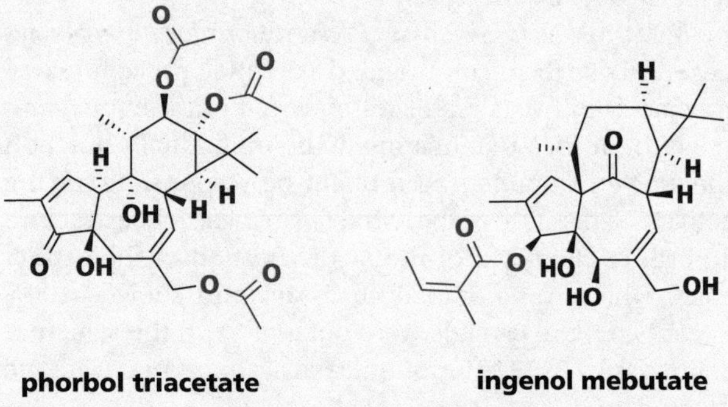

phorbol triacetate   **ingenol mebutate**

Figure 1.12 Structures of phorbol triacetate and ingenol mebutate. Esters are shown in red.

Studies of other members of the Euphorbiaceae family led to isolation of seed oils that were less irritating than croton oil. Ingenol was originally reported in 1968, with the structure confirmed by X-ray crystallography in 1970. It has since been isolated from a number of other plants in the genus *Euphorbia*. The esters of ingenol are less active than the structurally related phorbol esters.

The related plant *Euphorbia peplus* contains ingenol mebutate, the C-3 angelate ester of ingenol. This plant, known commonly as petty spurge, radium weed, or milkweed, has been used since the 1800s as a home remedy for skin conditions. Reports of use to treat basal cell carcinoma in the 1980s, as well as home use to treat actinic keratosis, led to pursuit of its development. A gel formulation was approved as an alternative to both imiquimod (Zyclara) and 5-fluorouracil gels, both of which have some undesirable side effects, including severe skin irritation, and are not completely effective. Ingenol mebutate was introduced in 2012, based on data from clinical trials of a 0.05% gel preparation that showed clearance rates of 75%, with mild skin irritation as the most common side effect.

REVIEW QUESTIONS

1. Describe two advances that were made in the field of medicinal chemistry during the period from 1700 to 1900.

2. Give two examples of semisynthetic drugs and the corresponding natural products.

3. What major advances were proposed by Ehrlich and Langley?

4. What are some reasons for the development of a total synthesis of a bioactive natural product?

5. Describe how recent advances in small-molecule NMR and MS have impacted the field of natural product drug discovery.

6. Describe the impact of X-ray crystallography on modern medicinal chemistry.

7. Review Figure 1.1.

   (a) If the product of interest contained an acid functional group rather than a secondary amine, how would the flowchart change?

   (b) Draw a modified flowchart in Figure 1.1 to show how one could isolate salicylic acid in general terms.

APPLICATION QUESTIONS

1. The isolation of taxol was reported in 1971(Wani MC, Taylor HC, Wall ME et al. [1971] Plant antitumor agents. VI. Isolation and structure of taxol, a novel antileukemic and antitumor agent from *Taxus brevifolia*. *J Am Chem Soc* 93:2325–2327). Summarize the isolation procedure and important features of the structural identification.

2. Cocaine was first isolated in 1860 by Niemann, who also made note that it "numbed the tongue." About 20 years later, von Anrep recognized its use as a local anesthetic after trials on both animals and himself. By the late 1800s, cocaine was in use both as an anesthetic and as a stimulant, with Freud promoting its use as an antidote to morphine addiction. Freud, and many others, became addicted to cocaine, and a search for a better local anesthetic led to the synthetic caine anesthetics. The first of these was amylocaine in 1903, and the second was novocaine in 1905.

   (a) Identify two structural features that are common to cocaine, amylocaine, and novocaine.

   (b) On the basis of your knowledge of organic chemistry, propose a synthesis of novocaine, beginning with toluene and using *N,N*-diethylethanolamine.

3. Explain some of the challenges of using medications directly from plant sources (such as roots and leaves).

4. Research and identify two approved drugs that are natural products and that are commercially produced directly from isolation of the natural product.

5. Research and identify two approved drugs that are natural product derivatives and that are commercially produced through semisynthesis.

6. Research and identify two approved drugs that are natural products or close derivatives and that are commercially produced through total synthesis.

7. Research and identify two approved drugs that are natural products and that are commercially produced through fermentation.

8. The Nobel Prize in Physiology or Medicine has been awarded to several scientists specifically for their contributions to medicinal chemistry. Identify these scientists and describe their contributions.

FURTHER READING

A general source for active components of many herbal preparations:

Varro T & Foster S (1999) The Honest Herbal: A Sensible Guide to the Use of Herbs and Related Remedies, 4th ed. The Haworth Herbal Press.

Aspirin

Mahdi JG (2010) Medicinal potential of willow: A chemical perspective of aspirin discovery. *J Saudi Chem Soc* 14:317–322.

Bentley R (1873) A Manual of Botany: Including the Structure, Classification, Properties, Uses and Functions of Plants. J & A Churchill.

Brodie BC (1811) Experiments and observations on the different modes in which death is produced by certain vegetable poisons. *Philos Trans R Soc London* 101:178–208.

Morphine

Pschorr R & Einbeck H (1907) Zur konstitution des morphins. Uber die konstitution des oxymethylmorphimethins. *Ber Dtsch Chem Ges* 40:1980–1983.

Knorr L & Horlein H (1907) Uber die haftstellen des stickstoffhaltigen nebenringes im kodein und uber die konstitution der morphiumalkaloide. XII. Mittellung: zur kenntnis des morphins von Ludwig Knorr. *Ber Dtsch Chem Ges* 40:3341–3355.

Robinson R & Gulland JM (1923) The morphine group. Part I. A discussion of the constitutional problem. *J Chem Soc C* 123:980–998.

Gates M & Tschudi G (1952) The synthesis of morphine. *J Am Chem Soc* 74:1109–1110.

Halichondrin

Aicher TD, Baszek KR, Fang FG et al. (1992) Total synthesis of halichondrin B and norhalichondrin B. *J Am Chem Soc* 112:3162–3164.

Dong C-G, Henderson JA, Kaburagi Y et al. (2009) New syntheses of E7389 C14–C35 and halichondrin C14–C38 building blocks: reductive cyclization and oxy-Michael cyclization approaches. *J Am Chem Soc* 131:15642–15646.

Damle NK & Frost P (2003) Antibody-targeted chemotherapy with immunoconjugates of chalicheamicin. *Curr Opin Pharmacol* 3:386–390.

Maehle A-H, Prull C-R & Halliwell RF (2002) The emergence of the drug receptor theory. *Nat Rev Drug Discovery* 1:638–641.

Top Pharmaceuticals: From Aspirin to Viagra and More. (2005) *Chem Eng News* 83:1–162.

Case studies

Miller LH & Xinzhuan S (2011) Artemisinin: discovery from the Chinese herbal garden. *Cell* 146:855–858.

Tu Y (2011) The discovery of artemisinin (qinghaosu) and gifts from Chinese medicine. *Nat Med* 17:1217–1220.

Keating GM (2012) Ingenol mebutate gel 0.015% and 0.05% in actinic keratosis. *Drugs* 72:2397–2405.

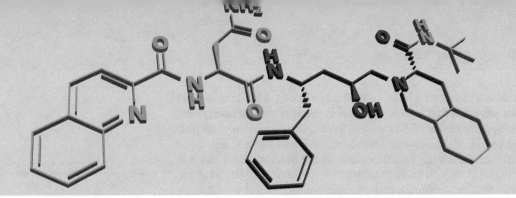

Drug discovery: hit and lead identification

2

LEARNING OBJECTIVES

- Understand the concept of hits and leads in the context of drug discovery.
- Become familiar with the types of assays used for hit characterization.
- Describe various sources of hits and leads.
- Explain how modern small-molecule libraries are constructed.
- Understand the different high-throughput screening processes.
- Learn common tools and strategies used to recognize high-quality hits.

How do we go about finding a cure for cancer, or treatments for AIDS or heart disease, or remedies for any other conditions that affect us? As described in Chapter 1, until the early 1900s, most drugs were products of nature and were based on historical and cultural use of plant or animal materials. Today a number of different strategies are used to discover new drugs. Some new drugs are closely related to older drugs or historical plant products, while others arise from serendipitous observations of effects in humans. The most common strategy in the modern era, however, is to start at a much earlier stage with compounds that exhibit some effect in a biological assay and then, through a process of optimization, eventually develop a compound that exhibits all the appropriate properties of a drug candidate. This chapter will highlight the multiple different pathways to a drug candidate, with a focus on the strategies used to identify the earliest starting points.

OVERVIEW OF DRUG DISCOVERY PROCESS

Today, the most common method of drug discovery is a process that starts by identifying a small-molecule starting point (a hit) and then optimizes its biological, physical, and pharmaceutical properties to generate a lead, and eventually a drug candidate, through an iterative process of design, synthesis, and testing. For the sake of consistency and clarity, a **hit** is defined as a small molecule of confirmed structure and purity that exhibits biological activity at some defined threshold (typically <20 µM) in a particular biological test. Since not all hits are useful starting points for medicinal chemistry, the term **validated hit**, which connotes stricter criteria, is sometimes used to describe a molecule that has reproducible, dose-dependent biological activity after its resynthesis and works through a desirable mechanism of action.

For example, in development of a drug to treat hepatitis C, a hit may be any substance of a known structure that is 90% pure and is capable of decreasing viral load in infected cells by a defined level (such as 50%) at a concentration of 20 µM. A validated hit would be one of the hits that was identified above but had also been resynthesized and retested. Its activity would be **dose-dependent**, meaning there is a change in potency with a change in concentration: a concentration of 50 µM of the compound would show greater inhibition, and a concentration of 5 µM would show less inhibition. In some cases, additional characterization of the molecule's mechanism of action may also have been performed to verify that the activity was due to a virus-specific mechanism and not due to non-specific effects.

Hit triage, the process of evaluating hits, eliminating some and validating others, is the first step toward identification of those compounds that are most likely to be optimized into drug candidates. Validated hits are often the starting points for medicinal chemistry activities, and they evolve through a **hit-to-lead process**, during which the goal is to characterize their attributes and liabilities and to identify and prioritize those that are most likely to be improved further during the optimization process. The product of this process, a **lead** (or **lead series** if a set of structural analogs is identified), is typically defined as a compound that exhibits the following qualities:

- potency (often <1 µM)
- some degree of selectivity toward designated or related biological targets or pathways
- a lack of promiscuity against unrelated targets
- evidence of emerging structure–activity relationships (SAR)
- appropriate pharmaceutical and physical properties such as solubility, permeability, and stability
- accessibility by either isolation, semisynthesis, or synthesis

Continuing with the theoretical drug to treat hepatitis C, the hit-to-lead process surrounding the validated hit that inhibited the enzyme at 20 µM would have been approached on multiple levels. Structural modification of one of the validated hits through preliminary medicinal chemistry activities may have led to a new compound with inhibition at 1 µM, which would have illustrated evidence of a correlation between structural modifications and activity and at the same time proved that analogs were synthetically accessible. This lead would have been evaluated in a number of assays to evaluate its physical properties (stability, aqueous solubility, permeability), and those properties would be deemed acceptable. In addition, biological testing to further characterize its mode of action, as well as selectivity, would have been performed and proven that its mechanism was virus-specific and the lead had an acceptable selectivity index. When a drug is developed from a lead, chemists, biologists, and other scientists work together in the process of **lead optimization**, wherein modifications of the structure are made in an effort to improve activity and selectivity, reduce toxicity, and optimize physical and pharmaceutical properties. The process of lead optimization ultimately results in a **clinical candidate**, which is a compound with activity and safety levels sufficient for testing in humans and that is appropriate for development into a drug. The process of **drug development** focuses on characterization of the clinical candidate in a series of animal tests, as well as development of the drug substance through optimization of its synthesis and development of an appropriate formulation. **Clinical trials** prove the efficacy and safety of a candidate in human subjects and are required for regulatory approval by a government agency such as the U.S. Food and Drug Administration (FDA). If successful, these studies ultimately result in approval of the molecule as a **drug** (Figure 2.1).

It should be noted that a molecule might enter into this process at any stage. For example, natural products such as paclitaxel may enter into the process at the stage of lead or clinical candidate. Drugs that have found an unexpected use at the time of clinical trials may enter the pipeline as a clinical candidate and be **repurposed**, that is, used for a different disease than was originally intended. However, most molecules require the entire progression of activities. Lead optimization to generate a clinical

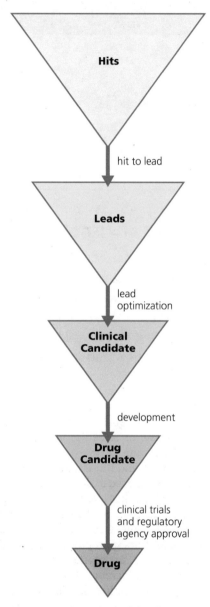

Figure 2.1 Overview of the drug discovery process, showing progression from a large number of hits to identification of a drug. The hit-to-lead process generates leads. The lead optimization process improves potency, safety, and properties of the lead compounds in order to generate clinical candidates. Clinical candidates undergo extensive testing in animals; formulations and syntheses are developed to provide a drug candidate, which is tested in clinical trials. Successful clinical trials and regulatory approval are required before a compound becomes a drug.

candidate, as well as medicinal chemistry strategies, the development process, clinical trials, and the approval process, are described in Chapters 3–5. The earliest aspect of the drug discovery process is initial identification of hits and leads from a variety of sources, which is the subject of this chapter.

IDENTIFICATION OF HITS AND LEADS

The entire process of hit and lead discovery relies on identification of bioactivity, regardless of the sources of hits and leads and where they enter the drug discovery pipeline. Prior to the mid-1900s, discovery of medicines was predominantly based on determination of bioactivity in either animals or humans (*in vivo*) or, in the case of antibacterial drugs, on inhibition of bacterial growth. With the knowledge that specific macromolecular targets such as enzymes and receptors are involved in diseases, discovery shifted to testing for activity in enzyme or receptor assays (*in vitro*). **Drug targets** are the macromolecules, most often proteins or nucleic acids, that the drug affects in the body.

2.1   Various types of assays are used in screening for hit and lead identification

In the modern era, an essential component of hit and lead identification is the availability of a biological assay that detects and measures the effects or activity of a small molecule in a biological system. These assays range in complexity and relevance from those that measure an effect, such as death of a cancer cell at one extreme, to those that work at the molecular level and measure the interactions between two proteins that may initiate a cascade of further events. In the latter case, the outcome measures a phenomenon that is quite remote from the final desired event; in the former case, the death of a cancer cell is the exact desired final outcome of a potential drug. Drug discovery efforts typically start by using one or several assays to identify and characterize small molecules with specific effects. While a variety of different technologies have been applied to these assays, most fall within four categories:

1. **Enzymatic or biochemical assays** typically monitor formation of the product of an enzymatic reaction. In many cases the enzyme itself is isolated and purified, and the assay measures its inhibition (or activation) by detecting, directly or indirectly, the amount of product formed. The nature of enzymes allows a thorough characterization of the kinetics of the reaction and of any inhibitors or activators identified.

2. **Binding assays** detect interaction between two molecules. Under physiological conditions, this binding event often initiates a cascade of biological responses, and therefore measuring binding can identify molecules that either mimic the same response or perhaps inhibit the downstream events. The binding event can occur between a small molecule and a macromolecule, like a protein, enzyme, or nucleic acids, or between two macromolecules, such as two partner proteins or DNA and a transcription factor. It is not necessary for the macromolecule binding partner(s) to be isolated and purified for the binding event to be measured.

3. **Functional assays** generally measure downstream effects of a binding event. Examples include those that measure changes in levels of certain ions or endogenous molecules such as cyclic adenosine monophosphate (cAMP), transcription events, and protein levels.

4. **Phenotypic assays** measure changes in phenotype or an effect in a complex system, regardless of the specific molecular target. They can be performed in cells and even in higher organisms such as yeast, zebrafish, and flies. Examples include assays that monitor whether a molecule can cause the death of a cancer cell through a specific mechanism such as apoptosis, can protect cells against infection by virus or bacteria, or can repair a defect in genetically altered zebrafish. In the broadest sense, most animal models can be considered phenotypic screens. For example, the historical examples of atropine and nicotine described

in Chapter 1 measured changes in heart rate or contraction of a muscle after application of certain compound. These assays reflected a specific phenomenon that was the result of a complex mechanism.

The specific strategies and assays used to identify hits and leads will depend on a variety of factors. These may include the specific disease, the level of understanding of the disease and its causes, and (when available) the nature of the drug target, as well as the available knowledge surrounding that target and any of its ligands.

SOURCES OF HITS AND LEADS IN DRUG DISCOVERY: COMPOUNDS WITH KNOWN BIOACTIVITY

Traditional sources for hits and leads include plant metabolites and microbial products, as well as the natural ligands for enzymes and receptors found in our bodies. Others include bioactive compounds reported in the scientific literature, in addition to clinical observations that identify unexpected activity in known bioactive compounds. While drug discovery based on natural products still occurs today, it is less common than in the past. Examples include the first statins for lowering cholesterol, such as lovastatin; cancer drugs such as paclitaxel (Taxol®); and immunosuppressants such as sirolimus. An analysis of small-molecule drug approvals in the recent past shows that natural products or natural product derivatives account for 33% of the new drug approvals. Of the remaining 66% that are synthetic drugs, about half can trace their origin or inspiration to a natural product. Examples include atorvastatin, which evolved from knowledge of the important structural features of lovastatin and compactin, and ixabepilone, a semisynthetic cancer drug that is an analog of the natural product epothilone.

2.2   Plant-based sources are the starting points for many drugs

Plants were the earliest source of medicines, and today many of those same active compounds are still used. In some cases the active component of the plant material is an approved drug, but more often that compound has been the lead for a less toxic or more potent derivative. Ephedrine, described in Chapter 1, is a natural product from the plant *Ephedra sinica* with stimulant properties and was the starting point used to develop the drugs amphetamine, methamphetamine, and methylphenidate. While methamphetamine is no longer an approved drug due to its addictive properties, amphetamine and methylphenidate are used to treat attention-deficit hyperactivity disorder (ADHD) (**Figure 2.2**).

In a similar fashion, meperidine and fentanyl were developed on the basis of the structure of morphine, the analgesic isolated from the opium poppy. A more recent example is paclitaxel (Taxol®) isolated from the Pacific yew tree, whose activity was first detected in a phenotypic screen of an extract. Paclitaxel itself is used as an anti-cancer drug and also provided the starting point for analogs such as docetaxel and cabazitaxel, both drugs approved to treat certain cancers.

Screening of crude plant extracts typically is a slow process involving heating in an organic solvent, followed by fractionation by liquid–liquid extraction into increasingly polar solvents. Purification of each subfraction by multiple chromatographic steps ultimately provides pure compounds. Bioassays, most often phenotypic assays, are done at each level of purification to identify the active fractions. Once pure compounds are obtained, it may take considerable effort to elucidate novel structures.

The modern techniques that are common today to rapidly assay for activity against pure macromolecular targets (biochemical and binding assays) are not readily applicable to crude extracts that often contain 10–100 compounds. Some problems include a lack of knowledge of the concentrations of active components and the need to remove unwanted compounds, such as tannins and chlorophyll, that cause interference with the assay. However, there has been increasing recognition that there are also many advantages to natural products, including high diversity, druglike properties, and evolutionary selection for biochemical specificity. **Figure 2.3** shows some of the diverse

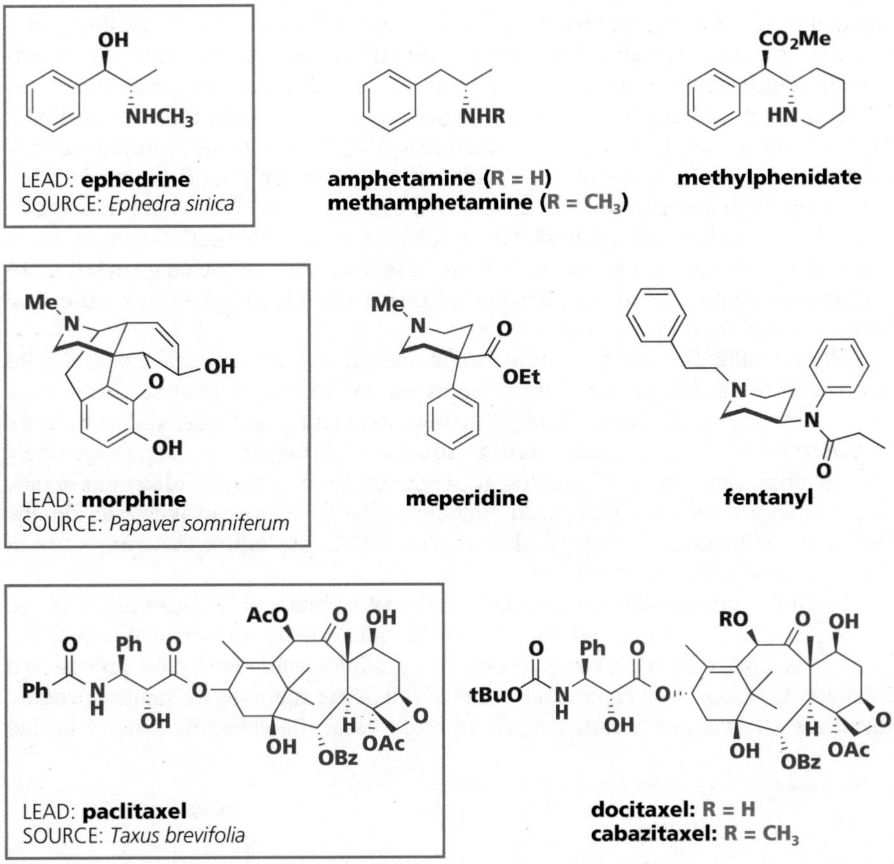

Figure 2.2 Structures of pharmacologically active natural products from plant sources and their synthetic or semisynthetic derivatives. Ephedrine led to amphetamine, methamphetamine, and methylphenidate; morphine led to meperidine and fentanyl; and paclitaxel led to docitaxel and carbazitaxel. Areas highlighted in red indicate common structural features of the original natural product and derived analogs.

LEAD: **ephedrine**
SOURCE: *Ephedra sinica*

amphetamine (R = H)
methamphetamine (R = CH₃)

methylphenidate

LEAD: **morphine**
SOURCE: *Papaver somniferum*

meperidine

fentanyl

LEAD: **paclitaxel**
SOURCE: *Taxus brevifolia*

docitaxel: R = H
cabazitaxel: R = CH₃

structures of compounds, all plant-derived natural products, including paclitaxel, vincristine, and podophyllotoxin, that exhibit anti-tumor activity by binding to the same macromolecular target, microtubules.

Newer techniques to access these natural products include the field of combinatorial biosynthesis, which has developed to generate analogs of natural products by genetic manipulation of the biosynthetic machinery of the organism. In addition, advances have been made in the preparation of prefractionated samples of plant extracts that are adapted to the newer screening methods, allowing for rapid testing of natural products as mixtures of a few compounds.

2.3 Microbes and higher animals may be sources for hits, leads, and drugs

In addition to plants, microbes are an important source of pharmacologically active compounds, with the first compounds having been isolated from fermentation broths in the early 1900s. Penicillin G is the product of a mold, and the cephalosporin β-lactam antibacterial drugs are also microbial products. Cephalosporin C was

Figure 2.3 Structurally diverse anti-tumor natural products. Vincristine, paclitaxel, and podophyllotoxin all bind to the protein tubulin, although at different sites.

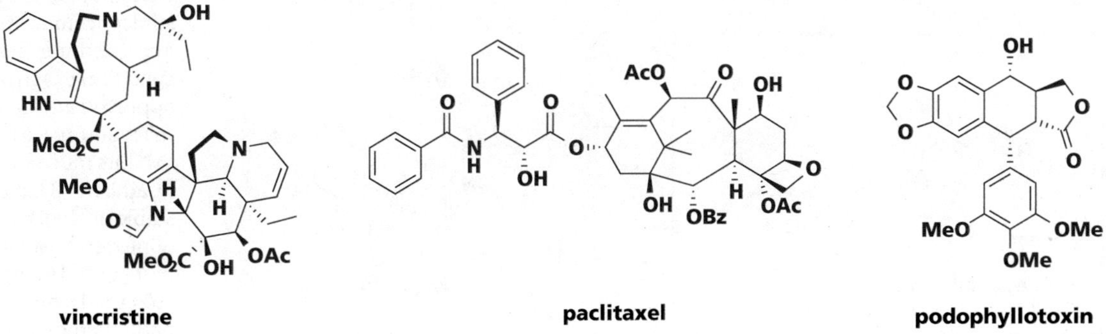

vincristine

paclitaxel

podophyllotoxin

isolated from a fungus, and its structure was modified for improved stability and a broader spectrum of activity to afford compounds such as the third-generation cephalosporin cefotaxime (**Figure 2.4**). Doxorubicin, a metabolite from a soil fungus, has been used for many years as an anti-cancer agent but is cardiotoxic. The synthetic analog mitoxantrone is slightly less potent but has significantly lower cardiotoxicity. A more recent example is that of the epothilones, a class of compounds isolated from a slime bacterium that grows in soil. Several of the natural epothilones have undergone clinical trials, and they have provided the inspiration for semisynthetic analogs such as ixabepilone, an approved cancer treatment. In this case, the only change in structure is from the lactone of epothilone B to the lactam of ixabepilone, which makes the drug less susceptible to degradation.

Higher animals, such as insects, amphibians, and even mammals, can also be sources of drugs. Magainins and cecropins are antimicrobial peptides from frogs and silk moths, respectively. Although there have been no drugs derived from these peptides to date, they have been used as structural starting points for potential new antibacterial compounds. Ziconotide, the ω-conotoxin peptide found in cone snails, is an example of a peptide from an animal source that is in use as an analgesic. Finally, Premarin, a mixture of conjugated estrogens that is prescribed for symptoms of menopause, is isolated from horses.

Natural products will continue to be a source of hits and leads. In many of the historical examples described, the natural product already exhibited many of the properties required of a lead or even a clinical candidate and entered the process at a relatively late stage (see Figure 2.1). Some of the newer methods for natural product discovery allow a much earlier entry. In these cases, liabilities uncovered during

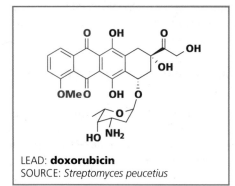

LEAD: **cephalosporin C**
SOURCE: *Cephalosporium acremonium*

cefotaxime

LEAD: **doxorubicin**
SOURCE: *Streptomyces peucetius*

mitoxantrone

LEAD: **epothilone B**
SOURCE: *Sorangium cellulosum*

ixabepilone

Figure 2.4 Examples of pharmacologically active natural products from microbial sources and their synthetic or semisynthetic derivatives. Cephalosporin C was the lead for cefotaxime, which has improved stability and a broader spectrum of activity. Doxorubin, an approved anti-cancer agent, led to mitoxantrone, a compound that exhibits much less cardiotoxicity. Epothilone B led to ixabepilone, a more stable analog, which is the only approved agent in this class. Areas highlighted in red indicate common structural features of the original natural product and derived analogs.

hit-to-lead or lead optimization activities can be addressed with the synthesis of improved analogs that are inspired by natural products. Disadvantages of relying on natural products as a source include the limited number of natural products with the desired biological activity, limited quantities, and the potential challenge of modifying the structure of complex natural products.

2.4 Hits and leads are often based on natural ligands

With a greater understanding of physiology came an additional source of hits and leads for drug discovery and less of a reliance on natural products. Once the physiological effects of macromolecules such as enzymes, receptors, and ion channels and their relationship to disease became understood, so did the concept and importance of **natural ligands**. These are the physiologically relevant molecules, often peptides or small molecules, that bind to or interact with a macromolecule to initiate a biological response. For drug discovery projects that target the biological response mediated by a macromolecule–natural ligand interaction, the natural ligand is an excellent starting point as a hit or lead. This strategy for drug design uses the structural features of the natural ligand as a starting point to develop new compounds that bind at the same site. Once bound, the new molecule may either give a similar effect as the natural ligand or inhibit the effect of the natural ligand. The former is desirable when the disease is caused by a deficiency of the ligand, and the latter is desirable when the disorder is caused by overactivity of the enzyme or receptor.

The anti-ulcer drug cimetidine, which blocks the H_2 subtype of histamine receptors, is one example of a drug that was developed by this strategy. The natural ligand for the H_2 receptor is histamine, and binding between histamine and the H_2 receptor stimulates gastric acid secretion. Cimetidine, a synthetic analog of histamine, binds to the H_2 receptor and prevents histamine from binding, which ultimately leads to a reduction in stomach acid secretion (**Figure 2.5**).

In applying this strategy to develop enzyme inhibitors, the natural substrate is the original inspiration, and it is often modified to afford a novel inhibitor that is recognized by the active site of the enzyme but is not acted upon. For example, when a protease enzyme cleaves the amide bond of a peptide substrate, a **peptidomimetic** is designed that mimics the substrate but does not contain a cleavable bond. Human immunodeficiency virus (HIV) protease is an essential enzyme unique to the virus, and its inhibition results in non-infectious virus. The HIV protease inhibitor saquinavir

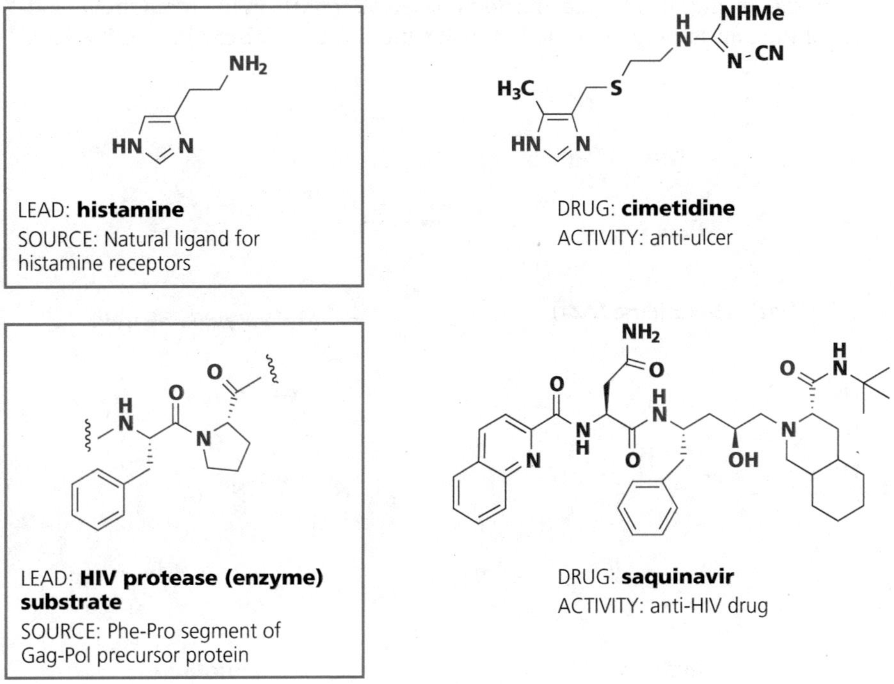

LEAD: **histamine**
SOURCE: Natural ligand for histamine receptors

DRUG: **cimetidine**
ACTIVITY: anti-ulcer

Figure 2.5 Examples of drugs derived from natural ligands such as neurotransmitters or enzyme substrates. The natural ligand of the H_2 receptor, histamine, led to cimetidine, an anti-ulcer agent. The Phe-Pro segment of the Gag-Pol substrate of the enzyme HIV protease led to saquinavir. Areas highlighted in red indicate common structural features of the original natural ligand and derived drug.

LEAD: **HIV protease (enzyme) substrate**
SOURCE: Phe-Pro segment of Gag-Pol precursor protein

DRUG: **saquinavir**
ACTIVITY: anti-HIV drug

was designed, in part, on the basis of the Phe-Pro segment of the substrate (the Gag-Pol precursor protein), which is recognized by the enzyme.

The advantage to using a natural ligand or enzyme substrate as the starting point for hits and leads is that the derived structures are typically already active toward the target. In addition, a significant amount may be known about the ligand and how it binds to the receptor or enzyme, allowing rapid progress in drug design. A disadvantage to this approach is that it will typically generate compounds that are similar in structure to the natural ligand, and the derived analogs may not be selective toward one form of macromolecule versus other forms that utilize the same natural ligand. Obviously, this approach is limited by knowledge of the natural ligand and is not useful when the substrate or ligand is unknown. Today, this approach has expanded beyond enzymes and receptors and is applied to natural ligands that constitute one of the partners in protein–protein interactions that initiate some biological signal.

2.5   Compounds with reported bioactivity are important sources of hits and leads

While natural ligands can be the inspiration for new structures with improved profiles, compounds that have previously been reported in the literature to exhibit activity against a certain target or class of targets are also useful starting points. Similar to the strategy based on natural ligands, this approach relies on previous knowledge of the small molecule's biological activity and often results in compounds that already exhibit activity toward the desired target. In other cases, selectivity for one target can be manipulated into selectivity toward another when starting with a nonselective bioactive compound.

One example of a hit discovered in this fashion is azidothymidine (AZT), which was the first drug approved to treat AIDS (**Figure 2.6**). This nucleoside, lacking the 3-hydroxy group of natural nucleosides, had been synthesized in the 1960s by Jerome Horwitz at the Michigan Cancer Foundation as a potential cancer drug, but it was ineffective in an animal model. Later, a publication in 1974 reported antiviral activity against a mouse retrovirus, attracting only academic interest, since at that time retroviruses were not known to cause any human diseases. In the 1980s, HIV was identified as being a retrovirus, and scientists working with AZT at Burroughs Wellcome had it tested for activity at the National Cancer Institute. Other known 3-deoxynucleosides were also the subject of scientific attention, including eventual drugs such as dideoxyinosine (ddI).

Another example of hit identification based on reports in the literature includes some of the kinase inhibitors used to treat cancer. An early Bcr-Abl tyrosine kinase

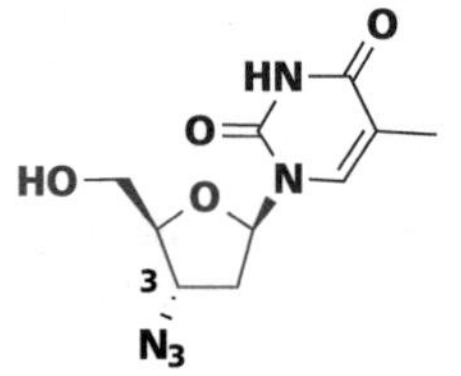

azidothymidine (AZT)

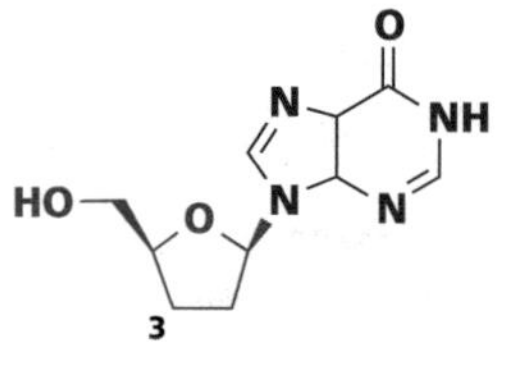

dideoxyinosine (ddI)

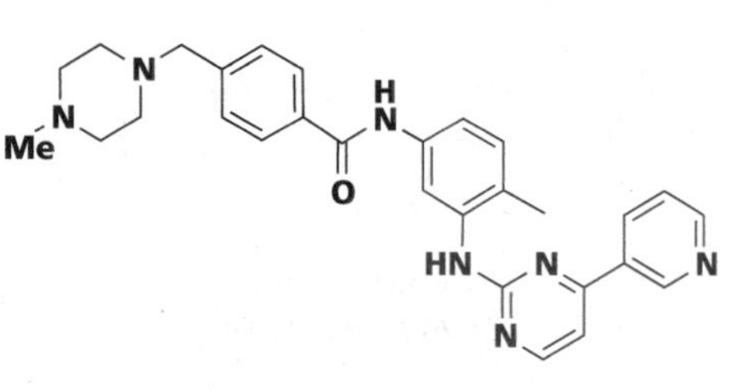

imatinib

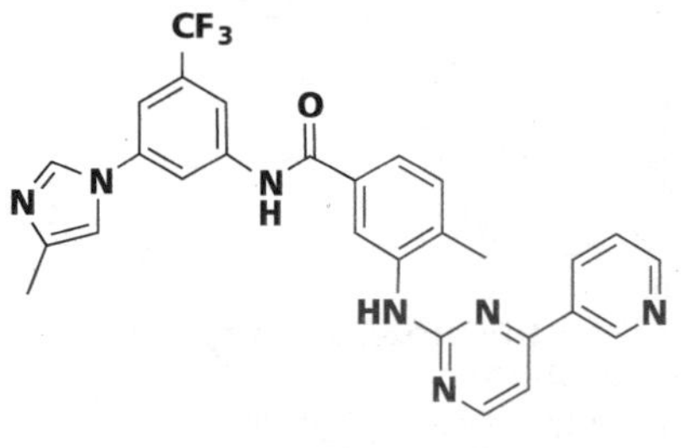

nilotinib

Figure 2.6 Structures of known bioactive compounds that led to new drug approvals. AZT, originally reported as an anti-cancer agent in the 1960s and approved to treat AIDS in 1987. Other previously reported 3-deoxynucleosides such as ddI also became approved AIDS drugs. Imatinib, a kinase inhibitor approved to treat certain cancers, became the lead for nilotinib, another approved anti-cancer agent. Common features are shown in red.

inhibitor drug is imatinib, which was approved in 2001 to treat certain types of cancer. On the basis of an X-ray structure of imatinib in the enzyme target, the structure was modified to give nilotinib, which is more potent than imatinib.

The literature is a rich source of hits and leads for drugs, and this emphasizes the value of published research. In some cases, the compounds may be identified but their value as drugs may not be realized until many years later. AZT and ddI, both originally synthesized in the 1960s as potential anti-cancer agents, are two such representatives. In other cases, new information in an emerging area may allow one hit or lead to be rapidly modified to generate an improved analog.

2.6 Clinical observations may uncover unexpected activities of known bioactive compounds

While most of the examples discussed previously focus on deriving new compounds with similar activity to that of the original source, serendipity has also played a role in developing new drugs. A number of well-known drugs or drug candidates that were being tested for one indication were found to have unexpected, beneficial side effects that eclipsed their original intended use, with some examples shown in **Figure 2.7**. Perhaps one of the more widely known drugs that falls into this category is minoxidil. Minoxidil was patented in 1967 by Upjohn as an anti-hypertensive agent and approved in 1979 to treat high blood pressure. Some patients taking it noticed that they had unusually thick hair growth on their arms and backs. The drug was reformulated as a cream that could be applied to the scalp and remarketed as a hair-growth promoter. A recent, similar instance is bimatoprost. It was originally used as eye drops to treat glaucoma, but had the side effect of promoting eyelash growth, and is now approved for that cosmetic use.

Sildenafil (Viagra®) is probably the most remarkable example of a drug being developed on the basis of side effects observed during clinical trials. Originally developed by Pfizer as a potential treatment for angina, it has revolutionized the treatment of erectile dysfunction, an unexpected use that was noted during its clinical trials for cardiovascular disease. This success of sildenafil led to the development of numerous other drugs (for example, vardenafil and tadalafil) that work through the same mechanism.

Another important, early example is the anti-diabetic drug carbutamide. This sulfonylurea was originally developed as an analog in the class of sulfonamide antibacterial drugs. During clinical trials, it was observed that carbutamide caused hypoglycemia. This observation led to its eventual use to treat diabetes; carbutamide was the first member of the important family of anti-diabetic sulfonylureas.

Drugs that are repurposed on the basis of clinical observations often progress through clinical trials rapidly because they have already passed the numerous safety and regulatory hurdles required for administration to humans. Furthermore, if a beneficial side effect is noticed by patients, it is often robust enough to be significant and a true effect rather than an idiosyncratic response. Thus, the path to approval and market may be much shorter than typical.

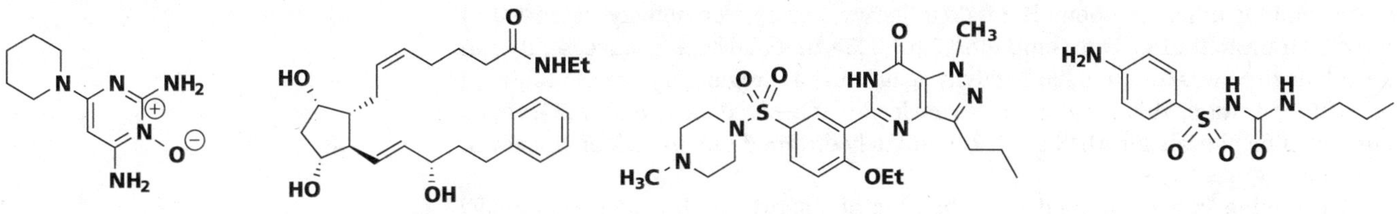

Figure 2.7 Examples of drugs identified by clinical observations. Minoxidil was approved to treat hypertension, and a side effect was hair growth. Bimatoprost was approved to treat glaucoma, and a side effect was eyelash growth. Sildenafil was in clinical trials for treatment of angina, and a side effect was relief of erectile dysfunction. Carbutamide was in clinical trials for antibacterial activity, and a side effect was hypoglycemia.

minoxidil

ORIGINAL USE: hypertension (1979)
CURRENT USE: hypertension and hair growth promoter (1988)

bimatoprost

ORIGINAL USE: glaucoma (2003)
CURRENT USE: glaucoma and eyelash growth (2008)

sildenafil

ORIGINAL INTENDED USE: angina
CURRENT USE: erectile dysfunction (1996)

carbutamide

ORIGINAL INTENDED USE: antibacterial
CURRENT USE: anti-diabetic (1950s)

SOURCES OF HITS AND LEADS IN DRUG DISCOVERY: SYNTHETIC LIBRARIES

When the basis of a drug discovery project was a natural product, a natural ligand, or a known bioactive compound, the starting point already exhibited some level of desirable biological activity, as well as some of the necessary properties of a clinical candidate. With advances in molecular biology, protein science, and physiology came a greater understanding of the molecular basis of disease. This understanding led to a shift in drug discovery strategies from relying on compounds that already had known bioactivity as starting points to searching for new compounds that exhibited specific biological activity. Today, a common practice is **library screening**, which typically involves testing many compounds simultaneously in order to identify starting points for drug discovery. These compounds are often members of synthetic libraries (but can also be natural products as described above) that number between a few hundred to millions of compounds. Unlike the previous approach, the vast majority of compounds tested will be inactive. For the purposes of this discussion, synthetic libraries will be classified into two general categories: legacy libraries and combinatorial libraries.

2.7   Legacy libraries contain compounds from prior discovery campaigns

Legacy libraries consist of compounds that have been synthesized in the past, often as part of a medicinal chemistry optimization effort, and retained for testing in the future. These libraries, from both industry and academia, have historically provided some important hits and/or drugs.

The chances of developing a drug are quite small. On average, for every 10,000 compounds that are synthesized as part of a medicinal chemistry or drug discovery effort, only one becomes a drug. Samples are saved and stored for possible future use and are often included in legacy libraries. These libraries can be particularly useful when molecules for one target are synthesized and retained but then later are tested against a related target. This strategy was applied by some pharmaceutical companies to rapidly identify inhibitors of HIV protease, a member of the family of aspartic proteases. Many companies had previously generated compounds to target another aspartic protease called renin that is involved in blood pressure regulation. Most of these compounds did not advance and became part of a legacy library. When the HIV protease was characterized as an aspartic protease, screening compounds originally synthesized to inhibit the enzyme renin led to potent hits very quickly. Compounds from legacy libraries that target a specific protein class are often used as a focused library set.

While there were reasonable expectations for activity in the renin/HIV protease example, in some cases activity is observed for a compound that would not ordinarily have been expected to have that particular type of activity. One example of this is the benzodiazepine Tat inhibitor Ro 5-3335. Hoffmann-La Roche, like most other firms, instituted an anti-HIV program in the late 1980s. Having a large focused library of benzodiazepines due to their interest in anxiolytic drugs, Roche scientists screened these, among other compounds in their legacy library, for activity against Tat-directed transactivation. One compound, Ro 5-3335, that had been unsuccessful as an anxiolytic drug was found to have activity against the Tat regulatory protein required for HIV replication. This compound was the lead that evolved into Ro 24-7429, which entered clinical trials for AIDS but was ultimately dropped due to lack of efficacy in humans (**Figure 2.8**).

Nevirapine is a compound that chemists at Boehringer Ingelheim originally prepared as a potential blocker of muscarinic receptors and was included in their legacy library. Although it was inactive in that assay, several years later it was found to be active in an HIV reverse transcriptase assay and to have anti-HIV activity. This compound was the first nonnucleoside reverse transcriptase inhibitor approved. A final example is topiramate, which was originally prepared at McNeil Laboratories as a synthetic intermediate. A sample was added to the company library, and it was

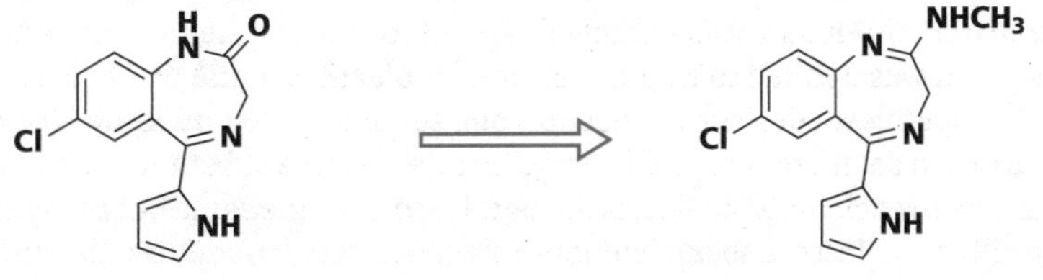

Figure 2.8 Examples of hits obtained from legacy libraries. Ro 5-3335, originally synthesized as an anti-anxiety agent, was later identified as a hit in a screen for inhibiting HIV Tat-mediated transactivation, and led to the clinical candidate Ro 24-7429. Nevirapine is an anti-HIV agent that was originally prepared as a muscarinic antagonist. Topiramate, a synthetic intermediate, became a library sample and was eventually approved to treat epilepsy.

LEAD: **Ro 5-3335**
inactive as anti-anxiety drug (1960s)
anti-HIV activity: 1980s

CLINICAL CANDIDATE: **Ro 24-7429**
anti-HIV activity

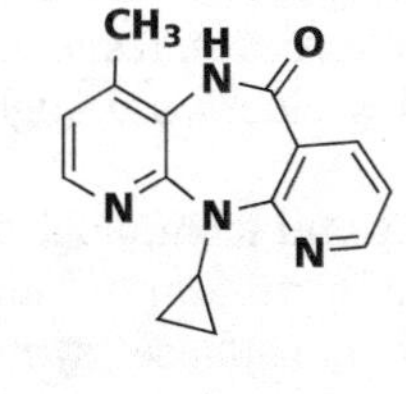

nevirapine
inactive as muscarinic antagonist (1960s)
active: anti-HIV drug (1980s)

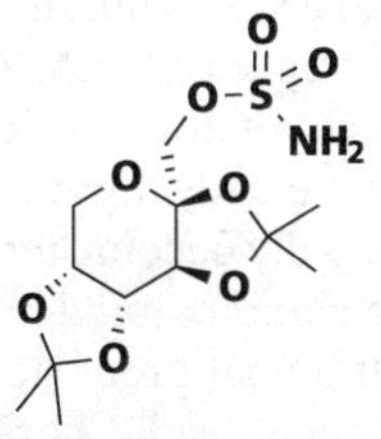

topiramate
synthesized as synthetic intermediate (1979)
active: anti-epileptic drug (1996)

screened for various types of activity. It was selected for screening in a phenotypic assay for seizures, where it exhibited anticonvulsant activity. Topiramate was ultimately marketed as an anti-epileptic drug almost 20 years after its original synthesis.

2.8 Combinatorial libraries are sets of closely related analogs that can be prepared by parallel or split-pool synthesis

In addition to legacy libraries, **combinatorial libraries** are also frequently used as a source of hits and leads. They began to be introduced in the early 1990s and are used as a way to supplement legacy libraries with large numbers of synthetic compounds. They are characterized by their production through rapid synthesis of large numbers of compounds. Note that the term combinatorial library has come to have many meanings. For the purposes of this discussion, it is defined as a relatively large library (>100) of structurally related compounds, regardless of the method of synthesis.

A focal point of these libraries was the appreciation of chemical diversity and the understanding that legacy libraries will be biased toward historical targets rather than future targets. Several recent analyses have indicated the enormity of the chemical universe of small molecules that could be used as starting points for drug discovery efforts. By limiting the number of heavy (that is, non-hydrogen) atoms to C, N, O, and F, the number of potential druglike compounds is over 110 million when stereoisomers are considered. If 30 heavy atoms are used, the number soars to 10^{60}. However, the number of compounds that have been synthesized and are available for testing is far smaller. Therefore, efforts have been, and continue to be, directed toward the synthesis of unique compounds that sample new, previously unexplored chemical diversity space to address new biological targets.

With the advent of new techniques to prepare combinatorial libraries (termed combinatorial synthesis) in the 1990s, numerous libraries were produced by pharmaceutical and biotechnology firms, academic groups, and companies whose main purpose was the synthesis of libraries. These libraries were often based on specific chemistries and were designed such that the resultant molecules were novel and predicted to exhibit druglike properties. A more recent strategy for the synthesis of libraries is based on **diversity-oriented synthesis** (DOS), focusing on diversity of the small molecules generated and efficiency of synthesis.

Combinatorial chemistry was initially designed for the synthesis of peptides in the mid-1980s and was applied to traditional small molecules in the early 1990s. It is the systematic, repetitive, covalent connection of a set of different building blocks of various structures to each other to yield a large array of diverse substituents around a common scaffold. In each individual step, the bond formed is the same but the specific substituents will differ. The number of compounds generated depends on the number of building blocks used and the number of reaction steps. In a tripeptide example, using 20 amino acids in each coupling step would generate $20 \times 20 \times 20 = 20^3$ or 8000 unique tripeptides. This tactic leads to large chemical libraries that have been synthesized on a variety of materials, such as resins or silica chips (solid phases), or in solution. In a way, combinatorial chemistry mimics nature in the use of these building blocks. Peptides, DNA, and oligosaccharides are all prepared in nature from the building blocks of amino acids, nucleotides, and monosaccharides, respectively. Indeed, most of the early libraries used amino acids as building blocks, although the chemistry has rapidly become more sophisticated.

To produce combinatorial libraries, a variety of strategies and technologies can be employed. The final products can be prepared either as a mixture or as isolated individual products; solid-phase, fluorous phase, or solution-phase synthetic methods can be used; and anywhere from tens to thousands of compounds can be prepared at one time. When a solid-phase approach is used, the initial building blocks are linked to a resin. The linked resin is then reacted with sets of building blocks successively until the reaction sequence is completed. Cleavage from the resin affords the final products. The two general approaches to combinatorial synthesis are split-pool synthesis and parallel synthesis. Descriptions of each, making use of solid-phase technology, are given below.

In a **split-pool synthesis**, compounds are typically assembled on beads of a resin by a repetitive sequence of combine, divide, and couple. This process is illustrated in **Figure 2.9**.

Three pots containing resin, represented by spheres, are coupled to building blocks A, B, and C in three separate reactions to give resin–A, resin–B, and resin–C as starting points. These are combined (pooled) to give a mixture of the three monomers (first box in Figure 2.9) The mixture is then divided (split) into three equal portions to give three new pots, theoretically containing equimolar amounts of each monomer. A coupling reaction is then carried out in each pot (a unique reagent for each pot) to add the second set of building blocks, D, E, and F. Each resulting pot contains a mixture of three unique dimers (nine compounds total). These are then combined and divided into three pots, which are coupled to building blocks G, H, and I to give three pots, each containing nine unique trimers, for a total of 27 chemically unique trimers. The process is continued for as long as desired to generate mixtures of final products.

Figure 2.9 Diagram of split-pool combinatorial synthesis on a solid phase. The synthesis begins with three building blocks to prepare 27 compounds. A mixture of the first three building blocks A–C linked to a solid support (resin, represented by spheres) is divided, and then each sample is coupled individually to the second set of building blocks D–F to give three sets of three (nine) dimers. These three mixtures are combined, divided into three, and each mixture coupled to a third set of building blocks G–I to give three sets of nine trimers (27 trimers).

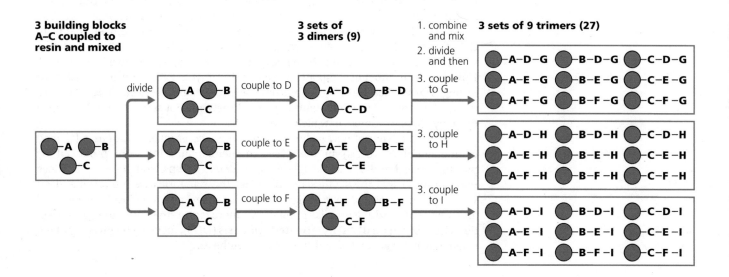

An early example of a series of compounds generated by a split combinatorial synthesis is shown in **Figure 2.10A**. Chemists at Affymax generated a series of proline derivatives in a search for novel angiotensin-converting enzyme (ACE) inhibitors to treat high blood pressure. The library was synthesized on a resin to give substituted proline derivatives that varied four different substituents (R^1, R^2, Z, and Ar) on the five-membered ring and one (R^3) on the nitrogen amide. The four basic steps were as follows:

Step 1: Coupling of protected amino acids (containing the R^1 group) to the resin via an ester linkage

Step 2: Removal of protecting group and condensation of the amine with aromatic aldehydes (containing the Ar group) to form imines

Step 3: 1,3-Dipolar cycloaddition of azomethine ylides (generated from the imines) to various olefins substituted with Z (electron-withdrawing) and R^2 groups to form the five-membered ring

Step 4: Acylation of the amine with various acid chlorides (containing the R^3 group)

Over 400 unique compounds, including stereoisomers, were synthesized from the building blocks shown in Figure 2.10A. The compounds were tested for their ability to inhibit ACE, and one of the library compounds was threefold more potent than captopril, a widely used ACE inhibitor.

A: COMBINATORIAL SYNTHESIS OF ACE INHIBITORS

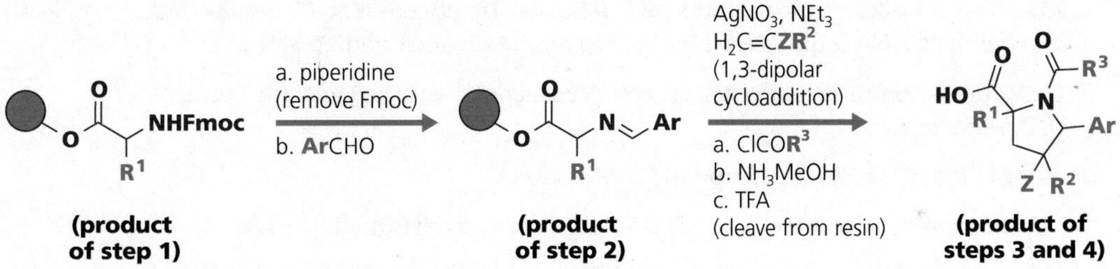

VARIABLES:
R^1 = H, Me, *i*Bu, Bn
Ar = Ph, 2-MePh, 2-OMePh, 2-OTBSPh
Z = CN, CO_2Me, CO_2tBu, COMe
R^2 = H, Me
R^3 = CH_2SAc, CH_2CH_2SAc, $CH(CH_3)CH_2$SAc

B: STRUCTURES OF CAPTOPRIL AND LIBRARY HIT

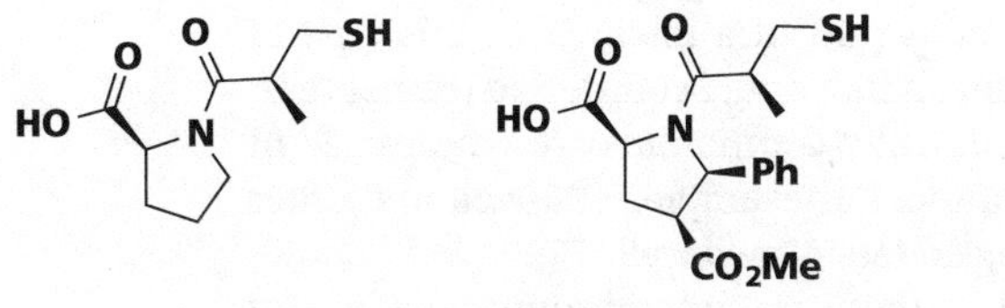

captopril

LIBRARY HIT:
3x more potent inhibition of ACE than captopril

Figure 2.10 Combinatorial synthesis of ACE inhibitors using a split-pool synthesis strategy. A: Step 1 (not shown) gives resin (shown as a sphere) with an ester linkage to Fmoc-protected amino acid. Step 2 consists of (a) removal of the Fmoc protecting group followed by (b) condensation of free amine with aromatic aldehyde (ArCHO) building block to give an imine. Step 3 is a 1,3-dipolar cycloaddition using a terminal olefin. Step 4 consists of (a) acylation of the amine followed by (b) cleavage of the R3 thioester SAc and (c) cleavage from the resin. B: Structures of captopril, an approved ACE inhibitor, and library hit.

In any split-pool synthesis, the final mixtures can be screened for biological activity. If they were prepared on a solid phase, compounds could be assayed either while still attached to a resin or after removal from the solid support. **Deconvolution** of the library, or isolation and identification of the active component, is not trivial, and a number of methods have been developed to facilitate this process. These include co-synthesis of either a DNA sequence or peptide that can be identified by degradation; synthesis and testing of sublibraries where one component is fixed in each sublibrary, allowing identification of the active species by a process of elimination; tagging of pools of libraries; or the separation of individual beads into wells for identification by mass spectrometry and/or NMR.

One powerful technique for library deconvolution is the use of labeling to create **DNA-encoded libraries** (DEL). This technology was first described in 1992 by Sydney Brenner and Richard Lerner, who synthesized a 10^5-member peptide library as a proof of concept. At each synthetic step, a DNA oligomer is co-synthesized and serves as a barcode for the ultimate identification of active hits. During a DNA encoded synthesis, the following steps occur:

- Each building block is attached to a linker that terminates with a short stretch of a specific DNA sequence.

- Each linker–building block is further extended by a specific short DNA sequence that is a tag for that individual building block.

- These are combined to give a mixture of tagged building blocks and split into groups for the next reaction cycle.

- The second building block is reacted, followed by attachment of the second specific short DNA sequence, which is a tag for the second building block.

- This process continues with each reactant or reaction being tagged with a unique DNA sequence.

- At the end of all steps, the compounds are assayed.

- Any hit compounds, as well as their DNA tags, are cleaved from the linker.

- The unique DNA tag sequences are amplified by polymerase chain reaction (PCR) and decoded to reveal the identity of the component of each synthetic step.

A specific example of a DNA-encoded library is shown in **Figure 2.11**. Scientists at GlaxoSmithKline synthesized a focused library of over 4 billion triazines in a search for compounds that inhibit the enzyme aggrecanase, which may be useful to treat osteoarthritis. Four synthetic steps, plus those to attach a DNA oligomer code at each step, were carried out to provide the triazines, which were diversified at four positions. From this extensive library, several hits were identified. One hit example, shown in the figure, was modified to give a lead compound.

In a **parallel synthesis**, deconvolution is not necessary since each individual compound is prepared separately, rather than as part of a mixture. In this type of combinatorial synthesis, each reaction is run on an individual compound (rather than one reaction being run on multiple compounds), and compounds are synthesized in separate vessels, on various phases, or in solution. For example, a 96-well microtiter plate can be used, with different reagents being added to each well. **Figure 2.12** shows a schematic of a spatially addressable parallel synthesis using solid support chemistry on a 4×4 plate. Four different building blocks (A–D) are linked to a resin (red sphere) and each placed in separate columns of wells of a microtiter plate. A second set of four building blocks (E–H) is then added, a separate building block for each row of wells, to give 16 new compounds. Each compound can be identified by its location on the plate.

Parallel synthesis requires more discrete reactions to provide the same number of compounds than a split-pool synthesis, but it can provide larger quantities of each, and compounds are prepared individually rather than as mixtures. Although libraries prepared this way typically produce fewer compounds than those from a split-pool synthesis, a major advantage is the fact that the identity of the active compound is known immediately from its specific location.

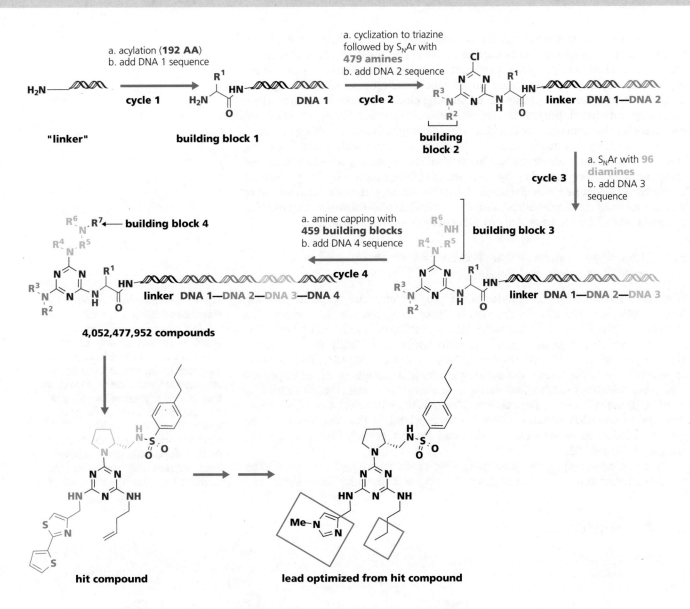

Figure 2.11 DNA-encoded library synthesis of 4 billion triazines. Each synthetic step is one color-coded cycle. Cycle 1: Amide linkage of 192 amino acid building block 1 (red) to linker (black) and attachment of DNA sequence 1 (red). Cycle 2: Cyclization of core triazine (common to all in library), followed by aromatic substitution with 479 amine building block 2 (blue) and attachment of DNA sequence 2 (blue). Cycle 3: Aromatic substitution with 96 diamine building block 3 (green) and attachment of DNA sequence 3 (green). Cycle 4: Amine capping with 459 building block 4 (purple) and attachment of DNA sequence 4 (purple). Cleavage from linker gives hit compound and its corresponding DNA sequence, which is used to determine its structure; a lead compound was generated from the hit by modification of two structural elements (in boxes).

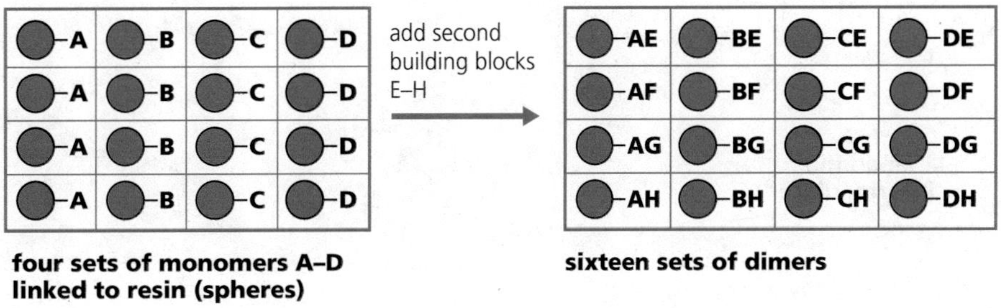

Figure 2.12 Diagram of a parallel combinatorial synthesis. Spheres represent resin linked to four different building blocks, A–D. Each column in a 4 X 4 plate contains one specific building block. Reaction with a second building block (E–H), one to each row, gives 16 compounds, each in a separate location.

In practice, various platforms for parallel synthesis have been applied and developed. For example, in Mario Geysen's multipin technology, the first building blocks are attached to polyethylene pins that fit into the wells of a microtiter plate, where the second coupling steps are carried out. Another technique is Richard Houghten's teabag method, where the initially linked building blocks are sealed in polyethylene mesh bags and labeled. They can be combined into one container for deprotection and then separated out into separate containers for coupling to the next building blocks.

The use of large synthetic combinatorial libraries became widespread beginning in the 1990s. While traditional combinatorial libraries provide a large number of compounds for testing in a relatively short period of time, they are, by design, focused on the synthesis of one molecular scaffold. A newer strategy involves the synthesis of diverse molecules, rather than those aimed at a specific biological target or a particular molecular scaffold, with the goal of providing unique structural templates.

2.9   Diversity-oriented synthesis is another strategy used in designing synthetic libraries

While traditional combinatorial libraries will produce only one particular scaffold, diversity-oriented synthesis (DOS) requires a specific type of reaction strategy that leads to multiple, diverse chemical backbones, depending on reaction conditions. This requires a synthetic sequence that is both high-yielding and, ideally, stereoselective. These sequences can be carried out either in solution or on a solid phase. Two common approaches are to use a variety of building blocks in a cascade or multicomponent reaction or to start with a common intermediate and apply various reaction conditions to afford diverse structures. For example (**Figure 2.13A**), Peter Wipf and co-workers developed a cascade reaction yielding dicyclopropylamines that, depending on the specific reaction conditions, can be converted stereoselectively into four different azaspirocyclic scaffolds.

In a second example, this time using solid-phase techniques (**Figure 2.13B**), Stuart Schrieber and co-workers began with a common enamine intermediate and

Figure 2.13 Examples of diversity-oriented synthesis. A: Wipf's cascade sequence to give four different scaffolds. Substituted alkynes are converted in four steps to a series of dicyclopropylamines as a common intermediate, and a cascade reaction then is used to prepare four diverse scaffolds. B: Schrieber's solid-phase synthesis produces five alkaloid-like scaffolds: under five different sets of reaction conditions, one enamine intermediate can generate five diverse scaffolds after cleavage from the resin.

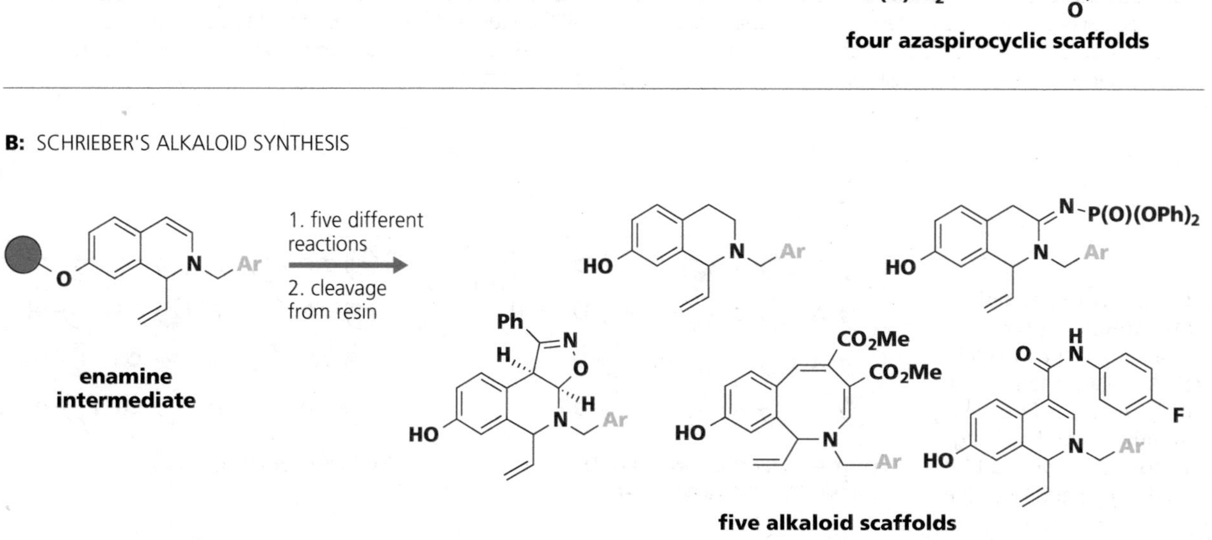

A: WIPF'S SYNTHESIS OF AZASPIROCYCLES

B: SCHRIEBER'S ALKALOID SYNTHESIS

applied various reaction conditions to produce five different alkaloid scaffolds. Diversity-oriented libraries have the potential to generate novel scaffolds and structures that may bind to sites on proteins that are not accessible to more standard chemical structures.

METHODS FOR SCREENING COMPOUND LIBRARIES

The traditional approach for assaying compounds involved evaluating each compound individually, usually in a phenotypic assay, which was a time-consuming process. Advances in protein biochemistry, molecular biology, imaging, miniaturization, and computer science have led to capabilities for rapid screening. Currently, this typically incorporates robotics and extensive computational capabilities. Furthermore, the synthesis and availability of large combinatorial libraries have led to strategies for screening large numbers of compounds, so that many compounds are assayed nearly simultaneously. These capabilities allowed a shift away from strategies that relied on natural products, natural ligands, known bioactive compounds, and serendipity as starting points. **Screening** involves testing or assaying a specific collection (library) of small molecules. The libraries are most often synthetic but may also be natural products, or crude plant or microbial extracts, or even virtual compounds.

Screening is currently the most common method to identify hits and leads. In this strategy, several different tactics can be applied depending on the specific project and target. Often, an unbiased set of small molecules (usually up to millions of compounds) is tested in an assay to identify those that have the desired biological effect. This section describes three main categories: high-throughput screening, fragment-based screening, and virtual screening. In all instances, once tested, the data are analyzed, and those compounds with the desired activity at a certain threshold define a set of small molecules that are considered hits.

2.10 High-throughput screening assays large numbers of compounds by a variety of different techniques

High-throughput screening (HTS) has become a mainstay of drug discovery efforts. It typically relies on a miniaturized *in vitro* assay and is performed robotically in microtiter plates. Capacity ranges from medium-throughput (tens of thousands of compounds) to high-throughput (hundreds of thousands of compounds) to ultra-high-throughput (millions of compounds in a few weeks). In most instances a random assortment of compounds is screened; however, when there is considerable knowledge about a specific biological target, a **focused screening** approach can be taken. In this case, the compounds assayed are not random but in fact are known or predicted to have some activity against the biological target. Often the number of compounds assayed in a focused screen is smaller than in a random screen. HTS assays often screen for inhibitors or activators of some defined macromolecular target protein (enzyme or receptor), but they can also test for modulators of entire pathways or identify molecules that correct defects in cells or organisms. Many times the output of an HTS assay is a biological result at one concentration (for example, percent inhibition at a concentration of 10 µM), but sophisticated protocols can also be employed so that HTS outputs generate complete dose–response curves, providing further efficiencies in the process.

All assays require the detection of a signal that provides information about the results of the assay. For example, in an enzymatic or biochemical assay, the product of the reaction must be detected and quantified in some manner. Similarly, in a phenotypic assay, the phenotype must be observed and quantified. Numerous detection methods and technologies have been developed and applied to HTS assay development that are rapid, robust, efficient, cost-effective, and safe. Two examples of common methods used to detect the product of an enzymatic assay in HTS are described in detail. One example is a fluorescence intensity (FLINT) assay, where enzyme-mediated cleavage of a fluorescent substrate leads to a signal, and inhibition of the enzyme would result in a decreased signal. **Figure 2.14A** illustrates one example

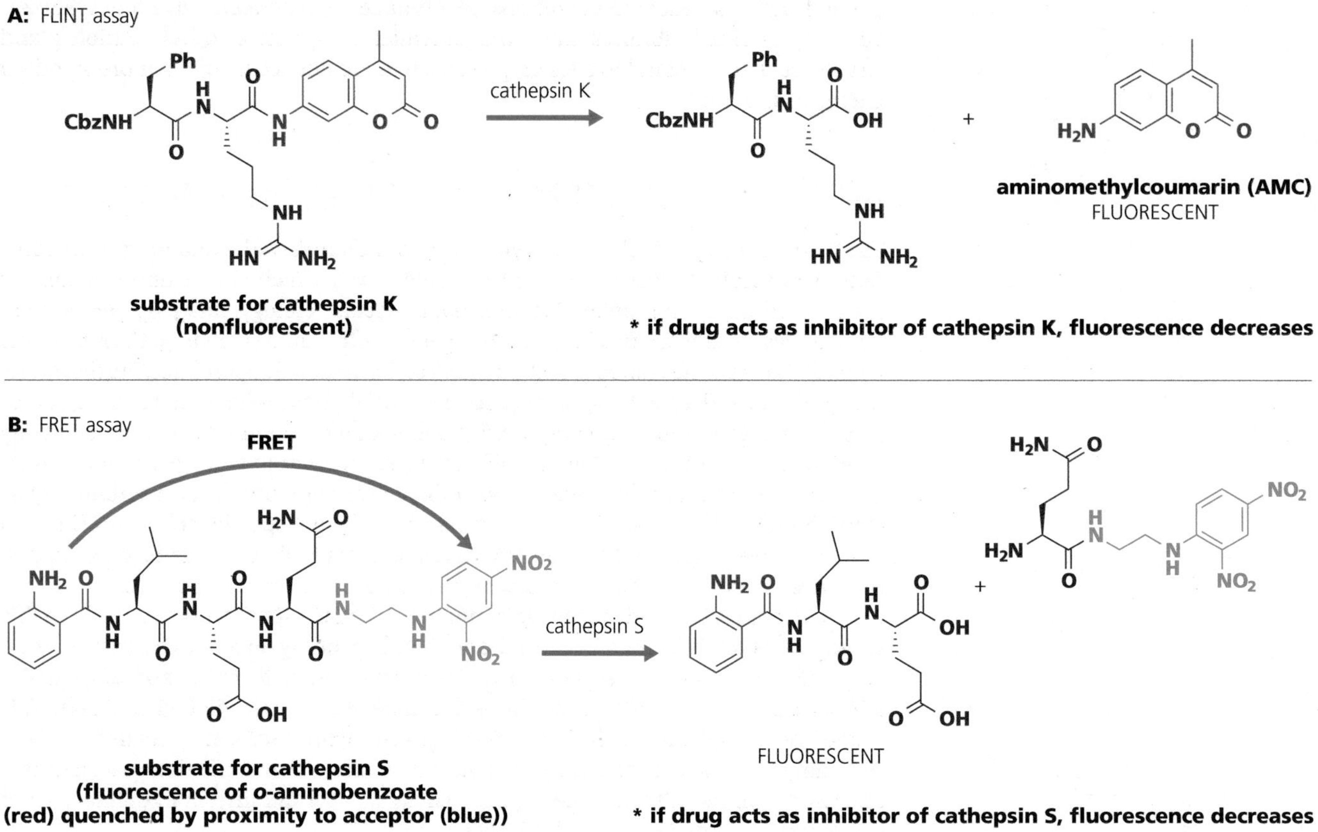

A: FLINT assay

substrate for cathepsin K
(nonfluorescent)

aminomethylcoumarin (AMC)
FLUORESCENT

* if drug acts as inhibitor of cathepsin K, fluorescence decreases

B: FRET assay

substrate for cathepsin S
(fluorescence of *o*-aminobenzoate
(red) quenched by proximity to acceptor (blue))

FLUORESCENT

* if drug acts as inhibitor of cathepsin S, fluorescence decreases

of a substrate developed specifically to detect the activity of the enzyme cathepsin K. The substrate itself is not fluorescent, but the cleavage product, aminomethylcoumarin (AMC), is highly fluorescent. Therefore, when the enzyme is active, the substrate is cleaved, AMC is formed, and high fluorescence can be detected; when the enzyme is inhibited, little or no fluorescence is observed. Importantly, the degree of inhibition is directly related to the amount of AMC formed and therefore can be related to the amount of fluorescence detected, which in turn reflects the potency of the inhibitor.

Similarly, a fluorescence (or Förster) resonance energy transfer (FRET) assay also relies on optical differences between the substrate of the enzymatic reaction and its product. In this type of assay readout, the substrate contains a fluorescent donor and acceptor. In the example shown in **Figure 2.14B**, the *o*-aminobenzoic acid moiety (red) in the substrate is fluorescent, and *N*-(2,4-dinitrophenyl)ethylenediamine (blue) is an acceptor moiety. Within the context of the substrate, the donor–acceptor pair is in close proximity. Upon excitation at a certain wavelength, the acceptor captures the emission energy from the donor, and no signal is observed. When the substrate is cleaved by the action of the enzyme, in this case cathepsin S, the acceptor and donor moieties are no longer in the same molecule. The distance between them increases, the efficiency of the capture decreases, and therefore a strong fluorescence signal is detected.

Other technologies that are often used include assays that detect changes in proximity of two molecules; assays that detect specific molecules such as products of enzymatic reactions, or molecules or ions produced in response to receptor binding; and assays that detect physical changes (for example, molecular weight or optical properties) observed upon binding of a small molecule to a macromolecule.

The overall process for HTS, using an example of a fluorescence assay, is outlined in **Figure 2.15**.

Even though HTS can be used to screen tens of thousands, or even millions, of compounds, most often as individual molecules but sometimes as mixtures, the false-positive rate can be as high as (or even higher than) 50%. This lack of reproducibility is due to many factors including poor quality of compounds in the screening library, lack of assay reproducibility, and assay interference mechanisms, among many others. For

Figure 2.14 Two examples of assays that monitor the production of a fluorescent product. A: In a FLINT assay, the nonfluorescent substrate is cleaved by the enzyme cathepsin K to generate two products, one of which (AMC, shown in red) is highly fluorescent. B: In a FRET assay, the fluorescent donor portion of the substrate (red) is in close proximity to the acceptor portion (blue) and no signal is observed due to FRET. Cleavage by the enzyme generates two products that are no longer in proximity, and therefore the fluorescence of the donor is not quenched and can be detected.

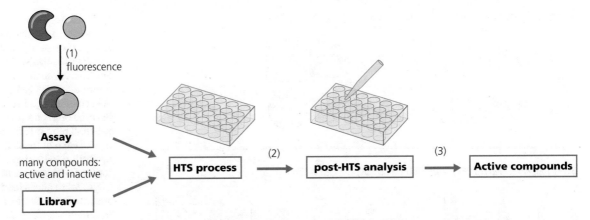

Figure 2.15 Schematic of HTS process based on an assay using fluorescence-based detection. (1) Assay that detects fluorescence is identified for use. (2) Many compounds in a library are assayed in microtiter plates by HTS. (3) Post-HTS analysis identifies hits (active compounds) on the basis of observed fluorescence in individual wells

this reason, HTS campaigns require a significant post-HTS effort aimed at confirming active compounds (discussed later in this chapter). Advantages of the strategy of screening synthetic libraries include the fact that the small molecules identified may be distinct from the natural ligand and synthetically accessible, in contrast to natural products, whose availability may be limited.

2.11 Fragment-based screening detects direct binding to a protein target

High-throughput screening based on fluorescence or related detection methods has the advantage of rapidly screening large numbers of compounds, typically of molecular weight between 300 and 600, and detecting those that are highly active (1 μM–1 nM). However, two significant disadvantages are the large number of false positives identified and the fact that the mechanism of action of the hit, and its mode of binding, may not be known. **Fragment-based screening** (FBS) is based on the concept of identifying smaller fragments (up to about 300 MW) that can bind to a specific protein target even with only modest (millimolar) affinity. By identifying compounds that bind directly to a specific protein target, FBS avoids many of the false positives that are generated in typical HTS approaches. In some instances, the specific binding site on the target protein can even be localized. Once hits are identified, however, they are of low potency. In order to optimize them, when several fragment-sized hits that bind to different sites are identified, they can then be combined; alternatively, single fragments can be grown into hits that occupy multiple binding sites, thereby increasing potency. The general process is outlined in **Figure 2.16**.

One requirement of fragment-based screening is the availability of an isolated enzyme or protein, and often high-resolution structural data (such as NMR or X-ray) of the target macromolecule. The method to detect binding to specific sites on that target usually involves some biophysical change. Fragment-based screening begins with smaller collections of compounds than HTS, but any hits identified are validated by the knowledge that they bind directly to the target of interest. The process of fragment-based screening was pioneered at Abbott Laboratories in the 1990s, using NMR techniques. The idea was based on changes in two-dimensional NMR spectra that are apparent when a compound binds to a macromolecule target. Comparison of spectra in the presence and absence of one or more fragments identifies those that exhibit binding to the target. Other common detection methods include X-ray crystallography, where protein crystals are soaked with various fragments and structures are solved that contain bound fragments, and surface plasmon resonance (SPR), which can detect weak binding to a protein. While fragment-based screening

A: FOUR FRAGMENT LIBRARIES (MW < 300) AS DIVERSE AS POSSIBLE

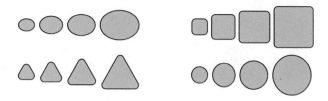

B: THREE FRAGMENTS SHOW ACTIVITY IN DRUG TARGET ASSAY

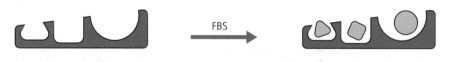

binding pocket of target   **each fragment binds, but weakly**

C: OPTIMIZED FRAGMENTS

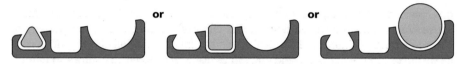

each fragment binds tightly to target

D: EITHER COMBINE OR GROW FRAGMENTS TO FIT BINDING POCKET

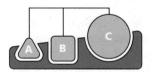   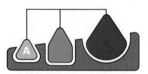

EXAMPLE 1: **combine the three fragments (A, B, and C)**   EXAMPLE 2: **grow one of the fragments (A) to fill other pockets**

Figure 2.16 Schematic of fragment-based screening and optimization. A: Four diverse fragment libraries (depicted as ovals, triangles, rectangles, and circles), each containing multiple members (depicted by size differences) are screened against a protein target. B: Three of the fragments show weak (>1 mM) binding and are considered hits. C: Each of those three fragments is optimized to bind more tightly to the target. D: Fragments may be combined or grown to give a lead compound; shown are the three optimized fragments combined (left) and one optimized fragment (A) grown (right).

has a number of advantages, there are also some limitations having to do with the conversion of low-potency binding fragments into higher-potency drug hits and leads. In order to combine or grow these low-affinity fragments into high-quality leads, a significant amount of synthetic work is often required to identify the optimal linker length, position, and structure in order to generate a molecule that binds as expected.

Since the introduction of FBS in the 1990s, this technique (also called FBDD for fragment-based drug discovery) has been very successful in generating compounds that have advanced to clinical trials. The first drug to reach the market using this strategy was vemurafenib, an anti-tumor drug that targets a mutant form of the protein kinase B-Raf, found in 60% of all melanomas. Vemurafenib, approved in 2011, was developed at Plexxikon in a program that relied on X-ray crystallography FBS. Although the ultimate target was a specific kinase, B-Raf, the project was initiated by a biochemical screen for inhibitors of five diverse kinases using a library of 20,000 fragmentlike (MW = 150–350) compounds. Compounds that inhibited at least three of the five kinases progressed further. From a library of 20,000 compounds, screening at a specific concentration of 200 μM against the three kinases led to 238 compounds with suitable activity (inhibition by >30%). At the time of screening, conditions for crystallizing the target kinase, B-Raf, were not yet optimized, so initial crystal structures were solved with a similar kinase enzyme. Attempts at co-crystallization with one of the kinases, PIM-1, led to solution of over 100 co-structures with bound fragments and showed how one fragment, 7-azaindole, bound to the ATP binding site with modest affinity at ~200 μM. Synthesis of substituted 7-azaindoles led to the 3-aminophenyl analog with improved, albeit still modest, binding affinity (100 μM), and further optimization led to vemurafenib. This is an example where an identified fragment was grown into the final drug (**Figure 2.17A**).

Another example of a molecule developed by FBS is that of the matrix metalloprotease-2 and -9 (MMP-2 and -9) inhibitor ABT-518 (**Figure 2.17B**). Scientists at Abbott identified two fragments using NMR, each with weak binding. One fragment, a biphenyl nitrile (shown in blue), was linked to the other fragment, a hydroxamic acid (shown in red), to provide a compound with improved binding (57 μM) compared to the initial fragments. Further rounds of optimization provided the clinical candidate ABT-518, which entered development as an anti-tumor agent. This is an example where fragments were combined to generate leads that eventually evolved into a drug candidate.

2.12 Virtual libraries can be screened by computational algorithms

Virtual screening (VS), also called *in silico* screening, is defined as assaying by computer and predicting activity, rather than experimentally screening genuine compounds to identify potential hits. The advantage of this approach is that a virtual library of millions of compounds can be screened in a very short period of time at a much lower cost than other methods. However, subsequent testing in the laboratory is always required after the initial virtual screening activities are complete, in order to confirm activity. For comparison, screening a library of a million compounds could take several weeks by HTS, using the most sophisticated equipment, but only a few days with VS. Libraries of compounds are generated computationally and can

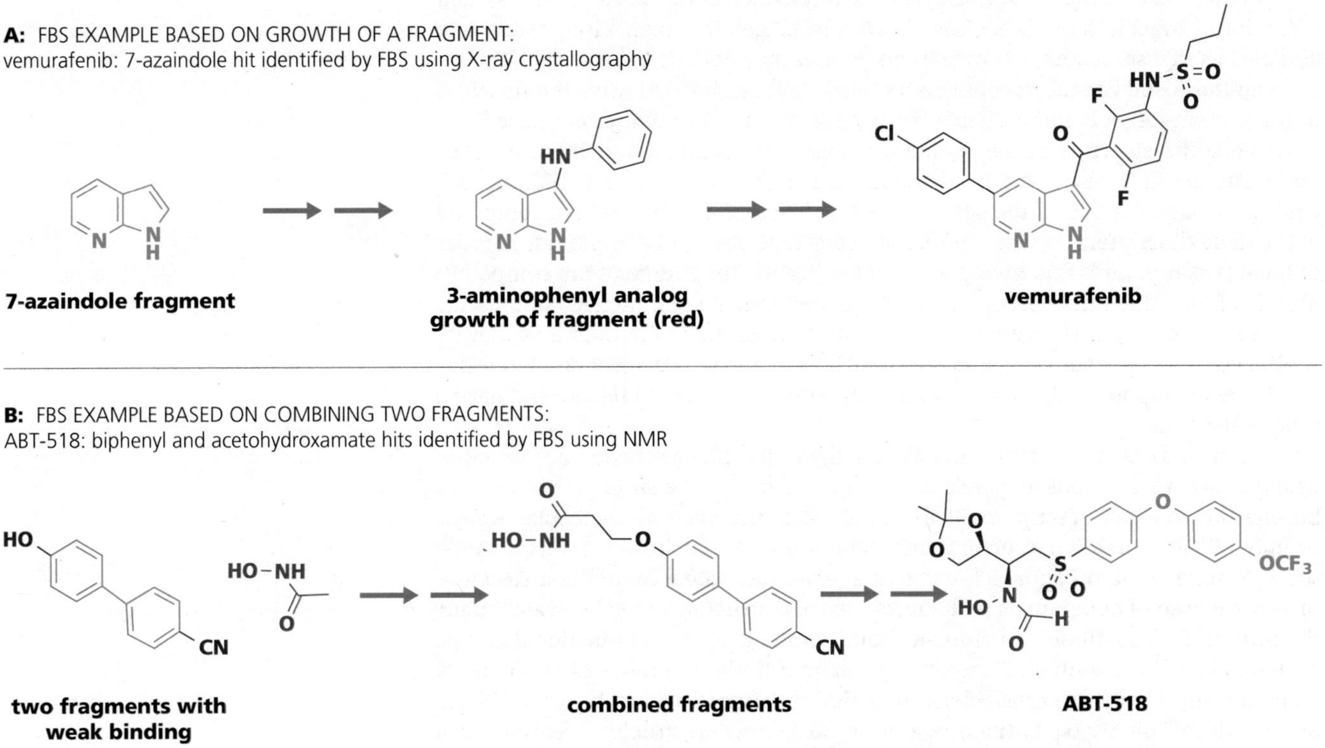

A: FBS EXAMPLE BASED ON GROWTH OF A FRAGMENT:
vemurafenib: 7-azaindole hit identified by FBS using X-ray crystallography

7-azaindole fragment

3-aminophenyl analog growth of fragment (red)

vemurafenib

B: FBS EXAMPLE BASED ON COMBINING TWO FRAGMENTS:
ABT-518: biphenyl and acetohydroxamate hits identified by FBS using NMR

two fragments with weak binding

combined fragments

ABT-518

Figure 2.17 Two examples of drugs or clinical candidates based on hits identified by fragment-based screening. A: 7-Azaindole (blue) was identified by FBS and shown by X-ray crystallography to bind to the ATP site of the kinase PIM-1. The fragment was grown to generate a 3-aminophenyl (shown in red) analog and eventually optimized to generate vemurafenib, a drug approved to treat melanoma. B: Two fragments, a biphenyl nitrile (blue) and a hydroxamic acid (red), were identified by FBS for inhibitors of MMP-2 and -9. They were combined and further optimized to generate ABT-518, which entered clinical trials as an anti-cancer agent.

consist of known compounds or even theoretical compounds. Some examples of electronic files of available small-molecule libraries that can be used for VS include ZINC (University of California San Francisco, UCSF), PubChem (National Center for Biotechnology Information, NCBI), and DrugBank (University of Alberta and The Metabolomics Innovation Centre), all of which may be accessed for free. Other libraries that also contain virtual compounds include the GDB-17 database, which contains over 100 billion molecules with up to 13 atoms containing the heavy atoms C, N, O, S, and Cl. Compounds screened are often computationally filtered for those that fit defined requirements for druglike properties, and then they may be computationally profiled for potential liabilities. These liabilities include the chances of cytochrome P450 interactions (an indication of toxicity) and hERG liabilities (an indication of cardiac toxicity), among many others. Further filtering may incorporate knowledge of the binding site, to eventually generate a selection of virtual hits. Virtual screening can be categorized according to two approaches.

Structure-based virtual screening is an approach that can be applied when a three-dimensional protein structure, co-structures of the protein and a binding partner, or homology models are known. These structures have often been determined by X-ray crystallography, NMR, or other means. The process known as **docking** involves computationally fitting sets of compounds into a model of the binding site of a protein. Compounds are first minimized so that only low-energy conformations are represented, and then they are docked into the active site and scored to compute how well each one fits on the basis of shape, size, and key interactions. Those with the best scores receive higher priority. Since the docked compounds are virtual, they are either purchased or synthesized and then must be assayed in the laboratory. The initial VS process can be automated, so that millions of molecules can be docked sequentially. Advantages of this method include relatively low cost and rapid screening as compared to other methods. It is particularly useful to identify a small library of compounds when screening of larger libraries is not feasible. Disadvantages are a high false-positive rate and the fact that sometimes the virtual compounds may not be readily available.

Ligand-based virtual screening is a strategy that can be used when the structure of the protein target is not available but ligands that bind to that target have been described. The structure of the ligand(s) is described computationally to account for properties like size, polarity, H-bond donor and acceptor capabilities, and hydrophobicity. A model of the ligand, based on these descriptors, is then compared to the same descriptors of each member of a very large library of compounds in order to identify compounds that mimic those of the ligand. The source of the compound libraries from which the descriptors are generated may be real (actual compounds that have been previously synthesized), such as those found in ZINC, or they may be simulated (never previously synthesized), such as many of those generated in GDB-17. Hits are compounds that have similar properties to the known ligands but have a unique structure.

The success of this strategy, and the quality of the hits generated according to ligand-based VS methods, depends on the level of input. The simplest level would be one-dimensional descriptors of the small molecule such as molecular weight or lipophilicity, where no structural information is required; however, this is rarely used. A more common approach involves a two-dimensional model of a structure or substructure of compounds with known activity. Structures may be searched for descriptors such as number of aromatic bonds or the presence of functional groups such as alcohols or amines. Alternatively, where a limited number of compounds with known activity are available, **molecular fingerprints** may be used. These are a series of binary digits (bits) that are used to encode structural features of a molecule such as aromatic rings or other functional groups. In this type of search, a fingerprint is calculated for the template molecule and then used to search virtual libraries for compounds with a similar fingerprint. Fingerprints may be calculated by computational methods that correspond to certain structural features such as particular atoms or rings. A value called the **Tanimoto coefficient** is calculated that measures similarity between compounds. The overall goal is to identify hits that have features in common with the ligand model but have unique scaffolds holding those features in place. Highly similar compounds have a Tanimoto coefficient close to 1;

dissimilar compounds have a Tanimoto coefficient close to 0. This type of analysis can lead to the identification of structures with different backbones but with similar features, such as functional groups, and potentially similar biological activity.

Three-dimensional ligand-based virtual screening incorporates a three-dimensional model of the compounds that puts specific functional groups or properties, such as a hydrogen-bond donor or lipophilic group, in a specific orientation. This model is referred to as a pharmacophore and will be described in more detail in Chapter 3. Three-dimensional conformers of all library members are generated and compared to the three-dimensional model of the ligand. This type of effort requires more sophisticated calculations. If structural information on the target is available, a final step could be introduction of the target enzyme or receptor and docking of the three-dimensional conformers that have been identified.

One specific example of structure-based virtual screening is shown in **Figure 2.18** to illustrate this process. In this case, virtual screening was used to identify novel activators of peroxisome proliferator-activated receptors (PPARs), which are targets for disorders involving glucose and lipid metabolism. The screening began with several X-ray crystal structures of ligand–PPAR complexes found in the Brookhaven Protein Data Bank (PDB). Computational programs were used to derive three-dimensional models based on the bound conformation of the small molecules. Over 1 million (1,063,848) virtual compounds were compared to the known activators, which led to the identification of 14,311 screening hits. The hits were filtered to remove those that had unacceptable physicochemical properties, and 5898 virtual compounds remained.

The 5898 hit molecules were screened further for three-dimensional shape similarity and electrostatic similarity to compounds known to bind to the PPAR target, and the compounds that were most similar were prioritized for further advancement. By use of various software programs, those compounds that contained chemically labile groups were eliminated. To make sure the final compound set represented a wide range of structures, a computational diversity analysis was performed, which identified 305 unique compounds. Final refinement of those 305 compounds included removal of compounds that were highly similar in structure (two-dimensional similarity) to known PPAR-binding compounds as well as those with reported PPAR activity. Of the 21 remaining compounds, 10 were purchased and tested, and 5 were active in an assay for activation of PPAR activity.

Virtual screening of libraries, as well as HTS and FBS, are now widely used for identification of hits in modern drug discovery programs. All rely on the availability of a robust assay and the accessibility of high-quality small-molecule libraries (whether virtual or real). The identification of a high-quality hit is arguably one of the most important aspects of a successful drug discovery program.

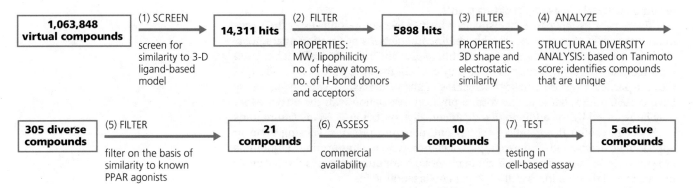

Figure 2.18 Virtual screening example used to identify five active compounds from a virtual library of >1 million compounds. Steps: (1) Screen for similarity to three-dimensional ligand-based model. (2) Filter for specific chemical properties. (3) Filter for similarity to compounds known to bind to target (those hits were kept); eliminate chemical labile compounds. (4) Filter for diverse structural classes (remove those too similar to known active compounds). (5) Filter to remove compounds similar to known PPAR-binding compounds. (6) Identify commercially available compounds. (7) Test in cell-based assay.

IDENTIFICATION OF HIGH-QUALITY HITS FROM SCREENING

The previous sections focused on sources of compounds and identification of hits by specific assays and screening methods. However, some of the screening methods described can suffer from high false-positive rates. In addition, the number of hits generated is often high, and for practical purposes all hits cannot be pursued. Therefore, it is important to identify high-quality hits as early as possible in the hit-to-lead process. These activities are especially important for hits identified from high-throughput screening and are defined as hit triage. The hit triage process helps to identify validated hits that are most likely to generate high-quality leads and includes the following components:

- elimination of false positives

- elimination of hits that are active via undesirable mechanisms

- evaluation of physical and pharmaceutical properties to identify those starting points most likely to generate high-quality leads

2.13 False positives and nuisance compounds need to be eliminated from primary hit lists

With the large numbers of compounds that are assayed by HTS and identified as active, there are inevitably some false positives and compounds that are undesirable. False positives include compounds that interfere with the assay detection method or that react with and/or deplete assay components. In addition, many compounds are indeed active against the target but work through undesirable mechanisms, such as formation of aggregates, redox activity, or promiscuous covalent reaction. One of the first priorities during the hit triage process is to identify and eliminate these compounds.

False positives are typically eliminated by the incorporation of control assays, independent re-assay of purified compound samples, and other protocols specific for the particular HTS. However, those active compounds that work through undesirable mechanisms are usually active across multiple assays and have come to be called **pan-assay interference compounds** (PAINS). Their promiscuous activity, through a variety of mechanisms, is considered artifactual. While a large number of specific compounds have been identified, a smaller subset of substructures is considered to contain the most frequent offenders. In practice, as a first step in hit triage, active hits identified by screening are often filtered through computational chemistry programs to eliminate these undesirable starting points.

There are a variety of mechanisms by which PAINS compounds exert their promiscuous activity. Some interfere with binding interactions by forming **aggregates**, which can then inhibit many enzymes or bind to proteins nonspecifically. It has been reported that compounds such as these may account for up to 95% of HTS hits, and they are particularly problematic in screening of plant extracts. These aggregates may be 100–1000 nm in diameter and form a physical association with the enzyme that may be reversed by the addition of a detergent such as Triton-B. Many compounds in this class exhibit detergentlike activity and denature proteins, causing them to appear to be inactivated. Some examples of common aggregate-forming compounds are shown in **Figure 2.19A** and include phenolic compounds such as the flavonols quercetin and rhamnetin, as well as polyphenolic tannic acid.

Another frequently found feature of PAINS compounds is **reactive functional groups** including peroxides, sulfonyl halides, primary alkyl halides, dicarbonyl compounds, epoxides, azides, α, β-unsaturated systems, and isocyanates, among others. These groups, and structural motifs such as rhodanines and hydroxyphenylhydrazones, can react nonspecifically with assay components by forming covalent bonds. **Redox-active compounds** are those that can generate free radicals under assay conditions and generate a redox cycle, thereby appearing to inhibit enzymes and/or proteins. This mechanism is especially prevalent when proteins being assayed contain active-site

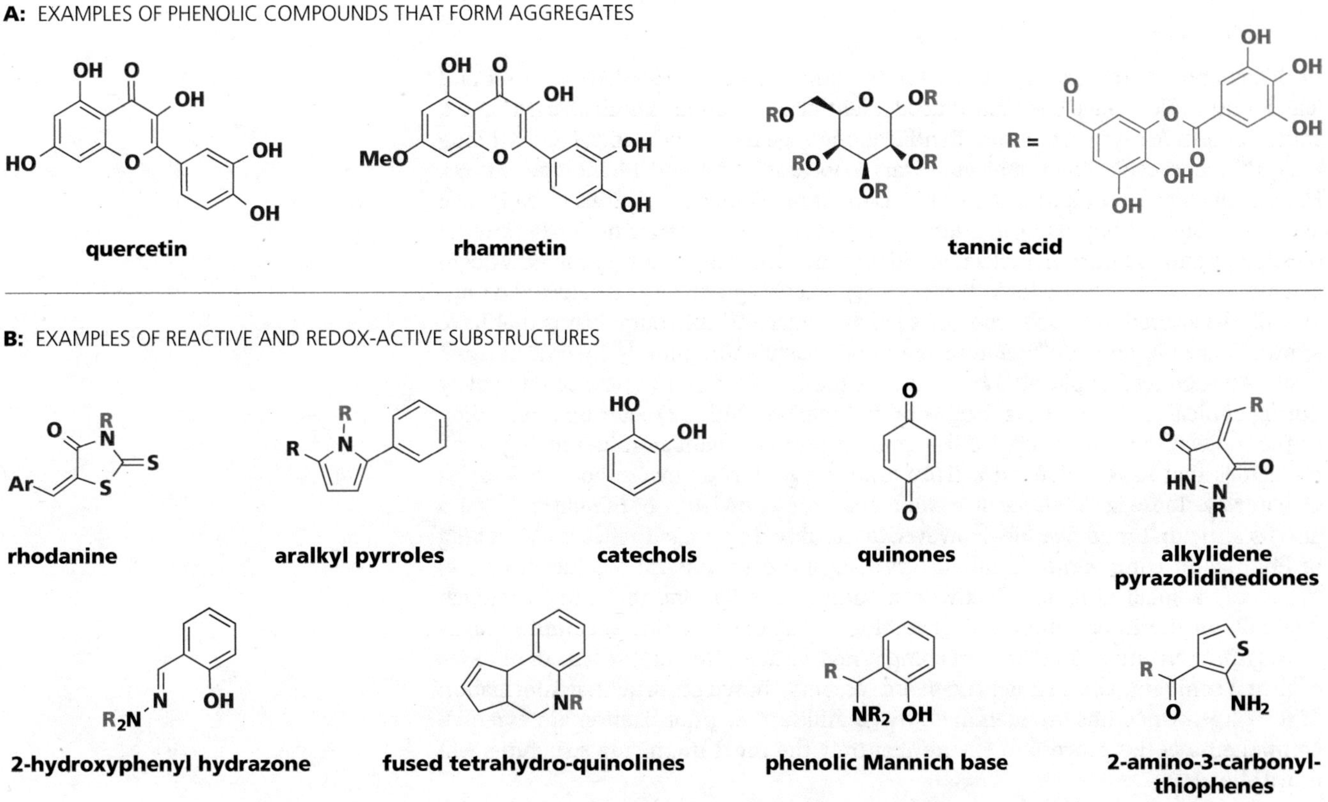

A: EXAMPLES OF PHENOLIC COMPOUNDS THAT FORM AGGREGATES

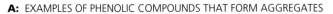

quercetin   rhamnetin   tannic acid

B: EXAMPLES OF REACTIVE AND REDOX-ACTIVE SUBSTRUCTURES

rhodanine   aralkyl pyrroles   catechols   quinones   alkylidene
                                                                           pyrazolidinediones

2-hydroxyphenyl hydrazone   fused tetrahydro-quinolines   phenolic Mannich base   2-amino-3-carbonyl-
                                                                                      thiophenes

Figure 2.19 Examples of PAINS compounds. A: Examples of phenolic compounds that form aggregates and cause false positives in HTS assays. B: Examples of reactive and redox-active substructures identified in HTS libraries.

cysteines or require reducing conditions. Examples of redox-active compounds include quinones and catechols (**Figure 2.19B**).

Triaging of hits must always be done with an awareness of the target class and the specific goals of the project in mind. For example, cysteine protease inhibitors require a reactive functional group, although those may be undesirable for other targets. The AIDS drug AZT (also known as zidovudine or ZDV) contains an azide functional group, and the anti-cancer drug ixabepilone contains an epoxide function; both are reactive functionalities that would be eliminated by some filters. There is also a growing appreciation that careful installation of reactive functionalities in certain cancer drugs can lead to very effective enzyme inhibitors. By some estimates, approximately 25% of known drugs would be eliminated by these filters.

2.14 Hits identified in screening campaigns need to be prioritized

Once undesirable compounds are eliminated, the process of hit prioritization takes place. These activities aim to identify the attributes and liabilities of the remaining compounds so that the most promising can be advanced further. Several characteristics are considered to identify druglike hits. The term **druglike** refers to "molecules that contain functional groups and/or have physical properties consistent with the majority of known drugs" (Walters & Murcko). This concept will be described in detail in Chapter 3, but certain parameters such as molecular weight, lipophilicity, number of rotatable bonds, and number of hydrogen-bonding groups fall into a specific range when drugs are evaluated in comparison to the larger chemical structure universe. Additional attributes evaluated often include lack of activity against other biological targets, patentability, and synthetic accessibility. Once high-quality hits and/or leads have been identified by any of the methods described in this chapter, there is still much work to be done to convert that lead to a drug. This process of lead optimization is described in Chapter 3.

SUMMARY

In this chapter, current practices used in the initial steps of drug discovery, hit and lead identification, have been introduced. Identification requires both an assay and a source of hits. Assays used for hit identification range from biochemical and binding assays for a specific macromolecular target to functional and phenotypic assays. Historically hits, leads, and drugs were based on previous observations of biological activity, either in humans or in animals. However, with a greater understanding of physiology and advances in molecular biology, modern drug discovery can now begin at a much earlier stage and look for bioactivity that was previously undetected. Drugs are still discovered in natural sources such as plants and microorganisms that have known bioactivity and from literature reports of bioactive compounds. In some unusual cases, serendipity has played a role, such as the observation of unexpected activity during clinical trials or after a drug is on the market. With a greater understanding of the molecular basis of disease has come a greater reliance on identifying small molecules that have a defined activity toward a particular macromolecular target or pathway. These small molecules can come from knowledge of the natural ligand and its structural modification. However, an unbiased approach relies on screening of libraries of compounds (synthetic, virtual, and even natural product libraries) to identify a small number of active compounds. The specific screening approach depends on the information and technology available and can encompass high-throughput screening of millions of compounds, virtual screening of tens of millions of virtual compounds, and fragment-based screening based on structural information of the target. Once hits are identified, triage and further prioritization are essential components of the process to ensure that only the most promising structures will move ahead.

CASE STUDY 1 EXAMPLE OF FRAGMENT-BASED SCREENING

In this article, a fragment-based drug discovery approach to the aspartic protease β-secretase (BACE-1) inhibitor is described. The approach led to the discovery of a potential Alzheimer's drug that advanced to clinical trials.

The approach used a combination of fragment-based NMR screening, X-ray crystallography, computational chemistry, and chemical modification of hits. Using ^{15}N-labeled BACE-1 protein, over 10,000 fragments were screened at concentrations of 100 µM–1 mM each, as mixtures of 12 each, based on ^{15}N heteronuclear single quantum coherence (HSQC) NMR. This NMR technique, which correlates nitrogen and hydrogen signals, is commonly used in FBDD. It allows observation of changes in the ^{15}N-labeled target (BACE-1 in this case) that occur when a compound binds. From this assay, nine structural classes of hit compounds were identified, binding with a K_d (dissociation constant) in the 30 µM–3 mM range. Of these classes, the authors focused on an isothiourea hit and prepared 204 analogs of this compound, leading to compound **1**, with a tighter binding profile (lower K_d) and low molecular weight, as preferred for druglike compounds. (**Figure 2.20**) This compound was optimized, in part, by studying X-ray structures of analogs. An X-ray structure of **1** co-crystallized with BACE-1 identified an important hydrogen-bonding network between the isothiourea portion and aspartates 32 and 228 in the active site of the enzyme.

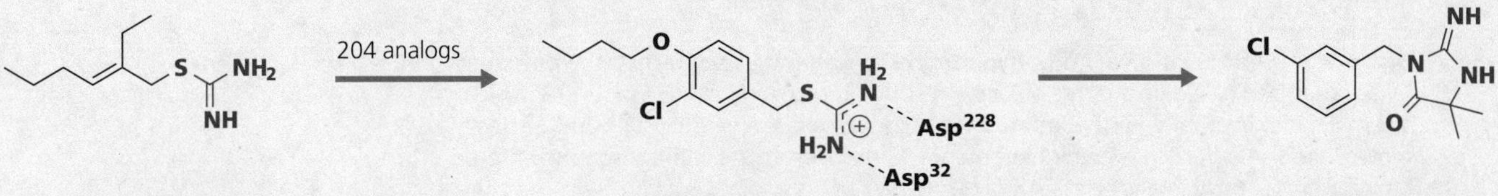

isothiourea hit
K_d = 550 µM
MW = 186

204 analogs →

compound 1
K_d = 15 µM
MW = 273

**compound 2
iminohydantoin**
K_d = 200 µM

Figure 2.20 Progression of initial isothiourea hit to analog 1. An isothiourea lead was identified by FBS, and evolved to Compound **1**, with a higher MW but tighter binding to the target. X-ray structure showed its interaction with key aspartic acid residues in the enzyme active site. Iminohydantoin compound **2** was designed to maintain interactions with the aspartic acids but improve stability. It has decreased binding compared to **1** but improved stability.

One liability of the isothiourea scaffold was its instability. Modification of that portion of the molecule, by comparison with other moieties with a similar pK_a (6–10) that maintained the hydrogen-bonding network, led to iminohyantoin **2** (see Figure 2.20). Although the binding of **2** (K_d = 200 µM) to the target enzyme was poorer than that of **1** (K_d = 15 µM), improved stability made this a more desirable lead compound.

Analysis of the binding site of the enzyme, where **2** was co-crystallized with BACE-1, identified binding pockets that could be occupied more efficiently by growing the hit at the site currently occupied by the *gem*-dimethyl groups, as seen in **Figure 2.21**. This ultimately provided **3**, with aromatic rings in place of the *gem*-dimethyl groups, as a lead. Attributes include low micromolar enzyme inhibition as well as appropriate lipophilicity (assessed by cLogP), a druglike quality. Further optimization can be seen in Figure 2.21. Addition of a 3-pyridyl group to one of the phenyls afforded additional binding interactions in a pocket of the enzyme, resulting in improved binding to the enzyme, as shown in the solved X-ray structure. An advanced analog in this series, verubecestat, entered phase III clinical trials as a drug to treat Alzheimer's disease.

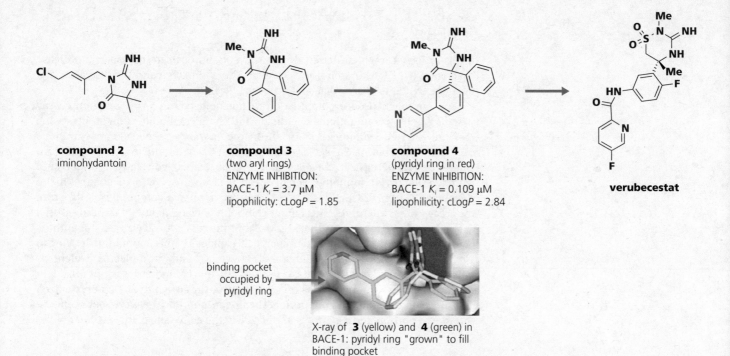

compound 2
iminohydantoin

compound 3
(two aryl rings)
ENZYME INHIBITION:
BACE-1 K_i = 3.7 μM
lipophilicity: cLog$P$ = 1.85

compound 4
(pyridyl ring in red)
ENZYME INHIBITION:
BACE-1 K_i = 0.109 μM
lipophilicity: cLog$P$ = 2.84

verubecestat

binding pocket
occupied by
pyridyl ring

X-ray of **3** (yellow) and **4** (green) in
BACE-1: pyridyl ring "grown" to fill
binding pocket

Figure 2.21 Optimization of iminohydantoin 2 to generate verubecestat. Compound
2 was optimized based on analysis of X-ray co-structures to generate Compound 3, which
had much higher affinity. Further optimization to incorporate an additional pyridine ring,
shown in red, **(4)** afforded even higher potency; Verubecestat, the final compound entered
clinical trials for Alzheimer's Disease. X-ray structures of Compound 3 and 4 are shown: the
pyridine ring fills an additional binding pocket. (From Wyss DF, Wang Y-S, Eaton HL et al.
[2012] *Top Curr Chem* 317:83–114. With permission from Springer.)

CASE STUDY 2 EXAMPLE OF VIRTUAL SCREENING

The authors in this study used structure-based virtual screening to identify potential
analgesic drugs. The goal was to identify novel compounds that alleviate chronic pain
by the same mechanism as Δ^9-tetrahydrocannabinol (THC), the active component of
marijuana. The molecular target for THC's analgesic activity, human glycine receptor
(hGlyR), is a chloride ion channel that affects neurotransmission in the brain stem and
spinal cord and has a role in pain regulation. Although an X-ray structure of the entire
ion channel was not available, the authors had previously determined the structure
of the α-subunit of the channel. It has been shown that THC binding at the receptor
requires a specific serine residue, Ser296, on the hGlyR α1 subunit. This portion of the
α-subunit was used for the structure-based virtual screening process.

The strategy for screening was to use FDA-approved drugs from the DrugBank
database, with an ultimate goal of repurposing any identified compounds. From this
database, 1549 drugs were screened at a specific site, the Ser296 site of the hGlyR α1
subunit.

The 1549 compounds screened were ranked on the basis of their predicted
binding energies of $K_d \leq 1$ μM. From the top 25 hits, 16 had activity when they were
screened both with and without lipids, and these 16 were further evaluated. These
compounds were also filtered for PAINS, and none were eliminated. As the goal was to
find structures distinct from THC, an additional filter used was calculation of Tanimoto
similarity to THC. All had low Tanimoto coefficients, indicating a lack of similarity to
THC, as shown in **Figure 2.22**.

Of the 16 identified hits, 13 were purchased and validated by phenotypic screening
in a cellular assay (*Xenopus laevis* oocytes expressing the target hGlyR-α1). Only one
of the compounds was a false positive, and seven had a greater effect than THC. An

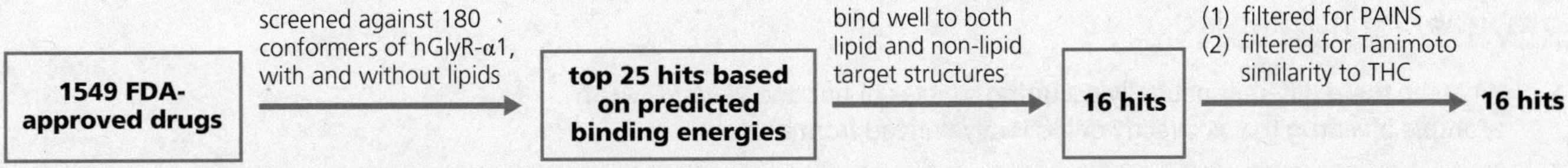

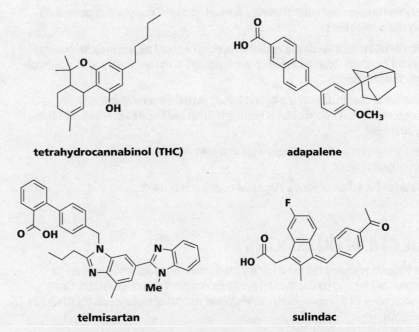

Figure 2.22 (process flowchart):

1549 FDA-approved drugs → screened against 180 conformers of hGlyR-α1, with and without lipids → **top 25 hits based on predicted binding energies** → bind well to both lipid and non-lipid target structures → 16 hits → (1) filtered for PAINS (2) filtered for Tanimoto similarity to THC → 16 hits

Figure 2.22 Process used in virtual screening for hits binding to hGlyR-α1. Screening of 1549 approved drugs from the DrugBank database against multiple conformers of the target gave 25 hits. Those 25 were narrowed to 16 hits that bound to both lipid and non-lipid models of the target. The top 16 hits were filtered to remove PAINS and those that were similar in structure to THC. None had PAINS or was too similar to THC, so all 16 remained as hits.

indication of selectivity was done by testing against oocytes expressing a nicotinic acetylcholine receptor subunit, α7 of nAChR. This is a receptor in the same structural family as hGlyR but with a different function. None of the compounds (including THC) had an effect on the nicotinic acetylcholine receptor. Several of the identified compounds shown in **Figure 2.23**, such as sulindac, have known analgesic effects, and this study suggests some insight into their mechanism of action.

tetrahydrocannabinol (THC)

adapalene

telmisartan

sulindac

Figure 2.23 Examples of hits identified by virtual screening for binding to hGlyR-α1 and natural ligand THC.

A novel aspect of this screening program was the incorporation of lipids into the drug target structure, so that the drugs were actually screened against multiple (180) conformations of the target with the rationale being that the membrane-bound receptors in biological systems have lipids present in their structure. Lipids included cholesterol and 1-palmitoyl-2-oleoylphosphatidylcholine (POPC). The presence of lipids in the modeling gives a more realistic model of the receptor and was found to reduce the number of hit compounds overall. **Figure 2.24** shows four representations of the receptor model and predicted improved binding for the drug hit adapalene in the lipid-based structure (A) versus the non-lipid structure (B). Conversely, another drug hit, telmisartan, showed better binding in the non-lipid structure (D) versus the lipid-based structure (C).

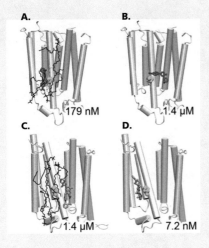

Figure 2.24 Hits docked into models of hGlyR with and without lipids. Transmembrane regions are shown as gray cylinders, and lipids are indicated in black in structures A and C. The drug hit adapalene is shown in magenta in structures A and B, and the drug hit telmisartan is shown in orange in structures C and D. The important binding residue serine 296 is shown in green. Numerical values shown represent predicted binding energies (K_d). Both drugs bind near serine 296 but with different orientations in the lipid-containing versus non-lipid-containing models. (From Wells MM, Tillman TS, Mowrey DD et al. [2015] *J Med Chem* 58:2958–2966. Copyright 2015 American Chemical Society).

REVIEW QUESTIONS

1.   What are three different naturally occurring sources of hits and leads? Give an example of a drug that is directly or indirectly derived from each.

2.   Explain the major differences between split-pool combinatorial synthesis and parallel synthesis.

3.   How does FBS differ from conventional HTS, and what are the benefits and limitations of each?

4.   Describe the pros and cons of using a phenotypic versus a biochemical assay.

5.   Explain the difference between a hit and a lead compound.

6.   What are the advantages of a drug discovery program that is based on clinical observations?

7.   Describe the pros and cons of using a natural ligand as the starting point for a drug discovery effort.

8.   When would structure-based virtual screening be most appropriate to apply to hit identification? What information is necessary? What are the disadvantages of using this strategy?

9.   Under what circumstances is a ligand-based virtual screening strategy appropriate? What information is required? What are the disadvantages of using this strategy?

10.   Name three categories of compounds that are often false positives in high-throughput screens.

11.   Give an explanation of how a Tanimoto coefficient is used.

APPLICATION QUESTIONS

1.   Atorvastatin is one of the most widely used cholesterol-lowering agents. Its design was inspired by the natural products compactin and lovastatin. Draw the structures of the three compounds. What structural features do they have in common?

2.   Research a drug whose structure is based on a natural ligand of (a) an enzyme substrate and (b) a receptor. Draw the natural ligand and the drug and compare the structures. Highlight the similar features.

3.   (a) The combinatorial, solid-phase synthesis of a benzodiazepine library was published in 1995 (Plunkett MJ & Ellman JA [1995] Solid-phase synthesis of structurally diverse 1,4-benzodiazepine derivatives using the Stille coupling reaction. *J Am Chem Soc* 117:3306–3307). (i) Design a library of 50–75 final products by choosing specific reagents to use at each step. (ii) In general terms, how would you design a library of more than of 5000 compounds?

   (b) Presume your library of 5000 compounds was synthesized in a split-pool synthesis and screened as a mixture. The mixture was active. How would you deconvolute the library to identify the active compound? In general terms, draw out the design of subsequent libraries that could be tested that would narrow down the identity of the active compound. Explain your reasoning.

4.   Use the synthetic sequence below and assume three substituents each at R^1, R^2, and R^3:

   (a) How many total reaction steps are required to synthesize 27 compounds by a split-pool method?

   (b) How many total reaction steps are required to synthesize 27 compounds by a parallel synthesis strategy?

5. Shown is the structure of a well-known natural product. What is this natural product and from where is it isolated? What medicinal properties have been attributed to it? If you found it to be active in a high-throughput screen, how would you evaluate it as far as it being a high-quality hit and why?

6. The compound shown was identified as a hit in a screen but is considered a poor-quality hit. Explain why. Design two analogs that, when tested, would determine whether the offending functional group was required for activity.

7. Modern phenotypic screening often relies on whole organisms such as zebrafish or flies. Research why these particular organisms have been so useful. Find a research paper that describes a high-throughput screen using one of these organisms to identify a small-molecule hit.

8. You have solved an X-ray structure of a kinase enzyme with an inhibitor bound to the active site. You also have developed a biochemical assay that detects the reaction products of the kinase reaction. Describe two hit identification methods that would be most appropriate for the information you have, briefly describe the strategy, and explain why you would use it.

9. The drug target Bcl-2 and related family members are proteins that regulate cell death through interaction with other protein partners. Their structures have been solved by both X-ray crystallography and NMR. Describe two hit identification methods that would be most appropriate for the information you have, briefly describe the strategy, and explain why you would use it. What types of assays could be used to evaluate hits? Is there any hit identification strategy you would not apply? Why not?

10. Use one of the online tools (for example, http://chemmine.ucr.edu/help/) for calculating a Tanimoto coefficient to compare two drug molecules that work at the same target; for example, sumatriptan and rizatriptan. Compare them to the natural ligand for the 5-HT receptor. How similar is each to 5-HT and to each other based on the Tanimoto coefficient? Is this result surprising?

FURTHER READING

High-throughput screening and library synthesis

Bleicher KR, Böhm H-J, Müller K & Alanine AI (2003) Hit and lead generation: beyond high-throughput screening. *Nat Rev Drug Discovery* 2:369–378.

Thompson LA & Ellman JA (1996) Synthesis and applications of small molecule libraries. *Chem Rev* 96:555–600.

Houghten RA (1985) General method for the rapid solid-phase synthesis of large numbers of peptides: Specificity of antigen–antibody interaction at the level of individual amino acids. *Proc Natl Acad Sci USA* 82:5131–5135.

Walters WP & Namchuk M (2003) Designing screens: how to make your hits a hit. *Nat Rev Drug Discovery* 2:259–266.

Murphy MM, Schullek JR, Gordon EM & Gallop MA (1995) Combinatorial organic synthesis of highly functionalized pyrrolidines: identification of a potent angiotensin converting enzyme inhibitor from a mercaptoacyl proline library. *J Am Chem Soc* 117:7029–7030.

Geseru GM & Masara GM (2009) The influence of lead discovery strategies on the properties of drug candidate. *Nat Rev Drug Discovery* 8:203–212.

Deng H, O'Keefe H, Davie CP et al. (2012) Discovery of highly potent and selective small molecule ADAMTS-5 inhibitors that inhibit human cartilage degradation via encoded library technology (ELT). *J Med Chem* 55:7061–7079.

Kleiner RE, Dumelin CE & Liu DR (2011) Small-molecule discovery from DNA-encoded chemical libraries. *Chem Soc Rev* 40:5707–5717.

Tan DS (2005) Diversity-oriented synthesis: exploring the intersections between chemistry and biology. *Nat Chem Biol* 1:74–84.

Fragment-based screening

Erlanson DA (2011) Introduction to fragment-based drug discovery. *Top Curr Chem* 317:1–32.

Erlanson DA, Wells JA & Braisted AC (2004) Tethering: fragment-based drug discovery. *Annu Rev Biophys Biomol Struct* 33:199–223.

Virtual screening

Sun H (2008) Pharmacophore-based virtual screening. *Curr Med Chem* 12:1018–1024.

Markt P, Petersen RK, Flindt EN et al. (2008) Discovery of novel PPAR ligands by a virtual screening approach based on pharmacophore modeling, 3D shape, and electrostatic similarity screening. *J Med Chem* 51:6303–6317.

Bajorath J (2002) Integration of virtual and high-throughput screening. *Nat Rev Drug Discovery* 1:882–894.

Identifying high-quality hits

McGovern SL, Helfand BT, Feng B & Shoichet BK (2003) A specific mechanism of nonspecific inhibition. *J Med Chem* 46:4265–4272.

Baell JB & Holloway GA (2010) New substructure filters for removal of pan assay interference compounds (PAINS) from screening libraries and for their exclusion in bioassays. *J Med Chem* 53:2719–2740.

Walters WP & Murcko M (2002) Prediction of drug-likeness. *Adv Drug Delivery Rev* 54:255–271.

Baell J & Walters MA (2014) Chemical con artists foil drug discovery. *Nature* 513:481–483.

List of publicly available resources

Databases of drugs: CMC (Comprehensive Medicinal Chemistry); MDDR (MACCS-II Drug Data Report); WDI (World Drug Index)

Examples of non-drugs: ACD (Available Chemical Directory)

Database of virtual compounds: ZINC (http://zinc.docking.org/)

Database of compounds and bioactivity: PubChem (pubchem.ncbi.nlm.nih.gov/); ChEMBL (https://www.ebi.ac.uk/chembl/)

Hit filtering: ADMET, false positives, etc. (http://www.cbligand.org/xielab/technology.php)

Case studies

Wyss DF, Wang Y-S, Eaton HL et al. (2011) Combining NMR and X-ray crystallography in fragment-based drug discovery: discovery of highly potent and selective BACE-1 inhibitors. *Top Curr Chem* 317:83–114.

Wells MM, Tillman TS, Mowrey DD et al. (2015) Ensemble-based virtual screening for cannabinoid-like potentiators of the human glycine receptor α1 for the treatment of pain. *J Med Chem* 58:2958–2966.

Lead optimization: drug–target interactions and the pharmacophore

3

LEARNING OBJECTIVES

- Identify properties evaluated and improved during lead optimization.
- Recognize the molecular interactions involved in drug–target binding.
- Describe some historical and current methods to evaluate structure–activity relationships.
- Understand how pharmacophores are identified and utilized.
- Learn the principles of ligand-based and structure-based drug design.

Once a bioactive lead has been identified, there is still a lengthy process involved in converting that lead to a drug used in humans. While there are notable exceptions where the initially discovered hit or lead becomes a drug, most modern drug discovery requires a process of **lead optimization**. Lead optimization involves chemical modification of the structure of a hit or lead compound through an iterative series of design, synthesis, and testing. This process eventually generates a clinical candidate, which, after further development and study, is appropriate for clinical trials in humans (**Figure 3.1**). This clinical candidate is a compound that exhibits desired potency, selectivity, efficacy, and physical and pharmaceutical properties, as well as an optimal safety profile. After testing in humans and clearing of regulatory requirements by the appropriate agency, the compound becomes an approved drug.

The multiparameter optimization of leads requires numerous compounds to be tested in a battery of assays, and the results of those assays inform the next round of design, synthesis, and testing. The process usually starts with testing in relatively simple *in vitro* assays and then, as compounds meet certain requirements, progresses to testing in increasingly complex secondary assays and eventually to evaluation in animal (*in vivo*) models of disease. The end result is a compound that fulfills all of the criteria required to become a clinical candidate that will eventually be tested in humans (**Figure 3.2**). However, lead optimization does not always begin with a primary assay and may begin at any point in the process where a liability in an advanced compound is uncovered and improvements in the molecule are required.

While the entire process of testing is outlined in Figure 3.2, the focus can be divided roughly into three main activities:

1. Testing for biological potency and efficacy is one key component. The lead compound is optimized by modification and then tested for biological activity in primary and secondary assays. An important aspect of this phase is the optimization of drug–target interactions involved in binding.

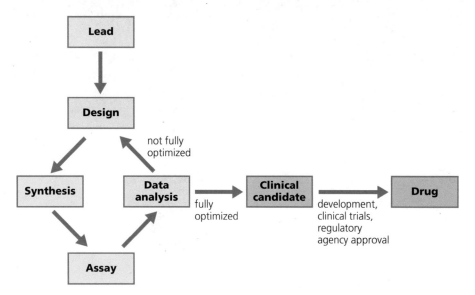

Figure 3.1 Iterative process of lead optimization, beginning with design of modified leads. After synthesis and assay, data are analyzed, and if acceptable, the modified lead becomes a clinical candidate. If unacceptable, further rounds of design, synthesis, assay, and analysis are undertaken until a fully optimized compound is generated. After further testing, clinical trials, and regulatory approval, the candidate becomes an approved drug.

2. A second component, often done in parallel, focuses on optimizing druglike properties. These druglike properties include **physical properties** such as solubility and lipophilicity that affect the ability of molecules to interact with biological systems. Also included are **pharmaceutical properties**, which are measured to predict or evaluate the effect of living systems on the small molecule. Success in these phases leads to compounds that are evaluated in animal models of disease.

3. The final component of drug development involves additional testing in animals, progression to human clinical trials, and eventually drug approval.

The first of these three components, understanding the molecular basis of biological activity, with an emphasis on drug–target interactions, is the focus of the remainder of this chapter. Chapter 4 describes medicinal chemistry strategies for optimizing biological, physical, and pharmaceutical properties, and Chapter 5 outlines the final stages of the drug development process.

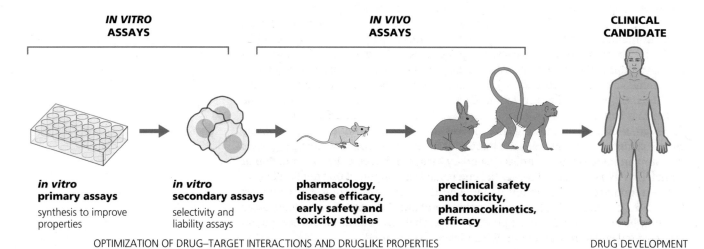

Figure 3.2 Progressive process of testing during lead optimization. Compounds are tested in primary assays, and those that pass a specified threshold advance to secondary and then *in vivo* (animal) testing during the lead optimization process. Compounds are optimized *in vivo* for toxicity, safety, pharmacokinetics, and efficacy to identify a compound appropriate for clinical trials. The optimized compounds become clinical candidates and are evaluated in a further battery of tests.

OPTIMIZATION OF DRUG–TARGET INTERACTIONS

In the early stages of lead optimization, measurement and optimization of biological activity are key activities. Additionally, assuring high affinity for the desired target and low affinity for other targets mitigates safety issues. In many cases, a biochemical assay is used, one that involves measuring the effects of a small molecule directly on a biochemical macromolecule. In other cases, a more complex system is used to measure a downstream event that is the result of the small molecule binding to a macromolecule. Regardless of the measurement, the overall goal is to optimize binding at the desired molecular target before moving on to more complicated secondary assays. To do so requires understanding of how the structure of the small molecule interacts with the biological target.

3.1   Optimization of binding depends on specific molecular interactions

Optimization of binding is directly related to improving potency and efficacy as well as selectivity. The affinity of a drug (D) for its protein target (P) can be measured by an equilibrium constant $K_{dissociation}$ (K_d), which compares the concentration of the drug–protein (D–P) complex to the concentrations of the individual drug (D) and protein (P) components and measures how readily the drug–protein complex dissociates.

$$D-P \rightleftharpoons D+P \quad \text{and} \quad K_d = \frac{[D][P]}{[D-P]} \tag{3.1}$$

On the basis of this equation, the smaller the K_d, the tighter the binding. Typical K_d values for drug–protein interactions are in the range 10^{-7}–10^{-9} M.

This equilibrium constant is directly proportional to the Gibbs free energy of binding (ΔG) according to Equation 3.2, where R is the gas constant and T is the absolute temperature.

$$\Delta G = -RT \ln K_d \tag{3.2}$$

ΔG is also a function of the binding enthalpy (ΔH) and the binding entropy ΔS:

$$\Delta G = \Delta H - T\Delta S \tag{3.3}$$

Therefore, for an interaction between a drug and its biological target to occur, two properties must be considered and optimized. **Enthalpy** (ΔH) involves the energetics of the drug–target system and is related to the specific interactions between the compound and the target. More energetically favorable interactions result in tighter binding, and therefore the interaction is likely to occur. The **entropy** term (ΔS) involves the disorder of the system. This term usually opposes the enthalpy term, since greater disorder is more favorable, but order is required to make specific interactions between the small molecule and target. One goal of medicinal chemistry activities is to maximize the enthalpy (that is, stronger and more binding interactions) and minimize the entropy terms.

Drugs typically bind to their biological target through noncovalent forces, mimicking the interactions observed in proteins that dictate their secondary structure. Therefore, understanding the possible interactions of functional groups present in amino acids and proteins is critical to understanding drug–protein interactions. These interactions include electrostatic, hydrogen-bonding, hydrophobic, dipole, and cation-π interactions, among others, and are energetically favorable. Any gain in enthalpy through the formation of new interactions between the drug and the target usually comes with an entropic penalty. This compensation is based on the specific geometric requirements of most binding interactions, which result in an ordered state of the complex. Energy is often required to orient the drug and protein target to optimal orientations, and once the complex is formed, rotational and translational freedom is limited compared to the individual components in an unbound state, and this process is entropically disfavored.

The process of a drug binding to its protein target is a complex set of events. The small molecule drug, surrounded by a shell of water molecules, must undergo conformational rearrangements, breaking any interactions it has with the surrounding water molecules to find its way into a binding site of the protein and make new and more energetically favorable interactions. This process is called **desolvation**. Similarly, solvent molecules occupy the vacant target binding site itself and must be displaced by the drug for drug–target binding to occur. When both the drug and binding site are relatively nonpolar, this is usually a favorable process. However, when either (or both) is highly polar, and therefore interacts favorably with water, this process is energetically unfavorable and can be offset only if the new interactions between drug and protein target are so favorable that they overcome the desolvation penalty.

3.2 Specific interactions contribute to the overall binding of drugs to their targets

The vast majority of drugs bind to particular amino acids (and sometimes metals) that comprise their target through a combination of specific binding interactions of varying strengths. Sometimes the interactions are covalent; however, most are noncovalent and depend on particular functional groups. These are described below and are illustrated in **Table 3.1**.

The strongest noncovalent forces occur between two ions and are termed **electrostatic (ionic) interactions**. These occur between oppositely charged species such as a carboxylate anion and an ammonium cation. The strength is approximately 5–10 kcal/mol and decreases in proportion to the square of the distance between the two atoms. Amino acid side chains containing acids (such as glutamic acid or aspartic acid) or amino groups (such as lysine or arginine) often participate in electrostatic interactions with drug molecules containing complementary functional groups. **Dipole–dipole interactions** occur between functional groups that have permanent dipoles, such as carbonyl groups and carbon–halogen moieties. The partial positive charge on one atom is attracted to the partial negative charge on the other. The presence of amide carbonyl groups in protein backbones offers abundant opportunities for this type of interaction in drug–protein complexes. An important subclass of dipole–dipole interactions is **hydrogen-bonding interactions**. Classical H-bonding interactions take place between a hydrogen donor that is covalently bound to an electronegative atom such as oxygen or nitrogen (N–H, O–H) and an electronegative atom acceptor such as oxygen, nitrogen, or fluorine. Optimal hydrogen bonds have specific geometries (often linear) and bond lengths (~2.4–3.0 Å). The energy of a hydrogen bond can be extremely high, but ΔG usually ranges from 2 to 5 kcal/mol. The amide function of each amino acid in target proteins offers H-bond donors and acceptors, as do many functionalized amino acid side chains; therefore, this interaction is frequently observed in protein–drug complexes. Weak hydrogen-bonding interactions have also been observed between many unconventional donor/acceptor pairs. Examples include C/N–H ··· π systems, C–H ··· O/N, and S–H ··· O/N. These weak interactions may not have the same geometric constraints as classical H-bonds, but nonetheless they can contribute to drug–target binding.

Ion–dipole interactions are observed between a charged species and a polar functional group. Common examples are a metal cation or protonated amine interacting with the oxygen atom of a carbonyl. These interactions are estimated to be between 0.5 and 2.0 kcal/mol in energy. Certain drug targets contain metals in their active sites, and these interactions are particularly important in those cases. Positively charged ions may also interact with π systems, and these **cation–π interactions** occur between the π system of an aromatic ring and a cation. The aromatic amino acids phenylalanine and tryptophan can contribute the π system; the cation may be either a metal or a protonated amine. The strength of these interactions is estimated to be between 0.2

Table3.1   Typical non-covalent binding interactions between drug and target.

Binding interaction	Example	Target residue, fragment or atom	Energy (kcal/mol)
ion–ion (electrostatic, ionic)		cation: Lys, Arg anion: Asp, Glu	5–10
dipole–dipole		backbone carbonyls	2–5
hydrogen bonding	 amide backbone side chains	backbone amide; Ser, Thr, Tyr (OH); Lys, Arg, His (NH)	2–5
ion–dipole			0.5–2.0
cation–π		cation: Lys, Arg π donor: Phe, Trp, Tyr	0.2–2.5
π–π	 sandwich T-shaped parallel displaced	Phe, Tyr, Trp, His	0.5–1.0
van der Waals		Ala, Val, Leu,Ile	0.5–1.0

and 2.5 kcal/mol. Another important class of interactions is π–π **interactions**. These occur between π systems in aromatic groups, are frequently observed in drug–protein complexes, and are also the basis for interactions between nucleobases in DNA and RNA. They occur with various geometries, termed sandwich, T-shaped (or edge-to-face), and parallel displaced. The weakest noncovalent interactions (0.5–1.0 kcal/ mol) are **hydrophobic interactions** or **van der Waals forces**. These occur between nonpolar groups and involve temporary dipoles. The most common examples of these in drug–protein complexes occur between nonpolar alkyl groups in the drug and alkyl amino acid side chains in the protein. While these are weak interactions, they are strong contributors to drug–protein binding. In addition to enthalpic considerations,

because they displace water from unfavorable interactions with nonpolar areas within the protein and drug–solvent shell (desolvation), these interactions are also entropically favorable. As many more high-resolution co-structures of small molecules bound to drug targets are being solved, some other types of interactions have been observed, including halogen bonding, orthogonal multipolar interactions, and interactions between the sulfur of a methionine and carbonyls or aryl rings.

Most interactions between drugs and their targets involve noncovalent interactions. However, there are several instances where **covalent binding** occurs and a formal bond is formed between the protein and the drug. This interaction is the strongest type of binding (50–150 kcal/mol). Irreversible enzyme inhibitors, such as penicillin G, bind through covalent interactions, usually between a nucleophilic amino acid residue such as serine and an electrophilic site on the drug (**Figure 3.3A**). Another example of covalent binding occurs in the anti-tumor nitrogen mustards, which covalently modify nucleophilic sites on DNA.

Most drugs rely on a combination of various binding interactions to contribute to their potency and efficacy. These attributes are a direct result of **biomolecular recognition** or specific binding interactions between the drug and target macromolecule. The asthma drug salbutamol, a member of the family of β-agonists that bind at β-adrenoceptors, is an illustrative example (see **Figure 3.3B**).

Binding interactions of salbutamol include an ionic interaction between the protonated amine and the carboxylate of an aspartic acid (Asp), a π–π interaction between the aromatic ring and a phenylalanine (Phe), van der Waals (hydrophobic) interaction between the aromatic ring and a valine isopropyl group (Val), and hydrogen-bonding interactions between the hydroxyls and two serine hydroxyls (Ser).

Stereochemistry also plays an important role in drug–receptor binding interactions. In a set of enantiomers, each contains identical functional groups that are capable of forming the same interaction with a specific residue of a protein target; however, their three-dimensional orientation is different. Therefore, their overall binding will differ. This effect was recognized in the 1930s when different effects of enantiomeric phenethylamines on adrenergic activity was observed.

Enantiomers of a drug often vary in potency. However, there may also be differences in rates of metabolism due to differences in affinity for metabolic enzymes, as well as differences in toxicity that each displays. The more active enantiomer is called the **eutomer** and the less active enantiomer is the **distomer**. The ratio of activity of eutomer to distomer is the **eudismic ratio**, which gives an indication of stereoselectivity of the drug-target interaction. For example, citalopram, a selective serotonin reuptake inhibitor, has a eudismic ratio of 167, with the *S*-enantiomer being the active isomer. Citalopram is marketed as a racemic mixture (Celexa), and (*S*)-citalopram is marketed as escitalopram (Lexapro); both are used to treat anxiety and depression (**Figure 3.4**). Methylphenidate, a widely used medication for attention deficit hyperactivity disorder (ADHD), is a racemic mixture of *R,R*- and *S,S*-enantiomers and also has a high eudismic ratio. The more active *R,R*-enantiomer is also marketed.

Figure 3.3 Examples of drugs binding through covalent and noncovalent interactions. A: A covalent bond forms between the carbonyl of penicillin G (blue) and a serine of the target enzyme (ENZ, black). B: Salbutamol (blue) binds through H-bonding, π–π, ionic, and van der Waals interactions to its target (black).

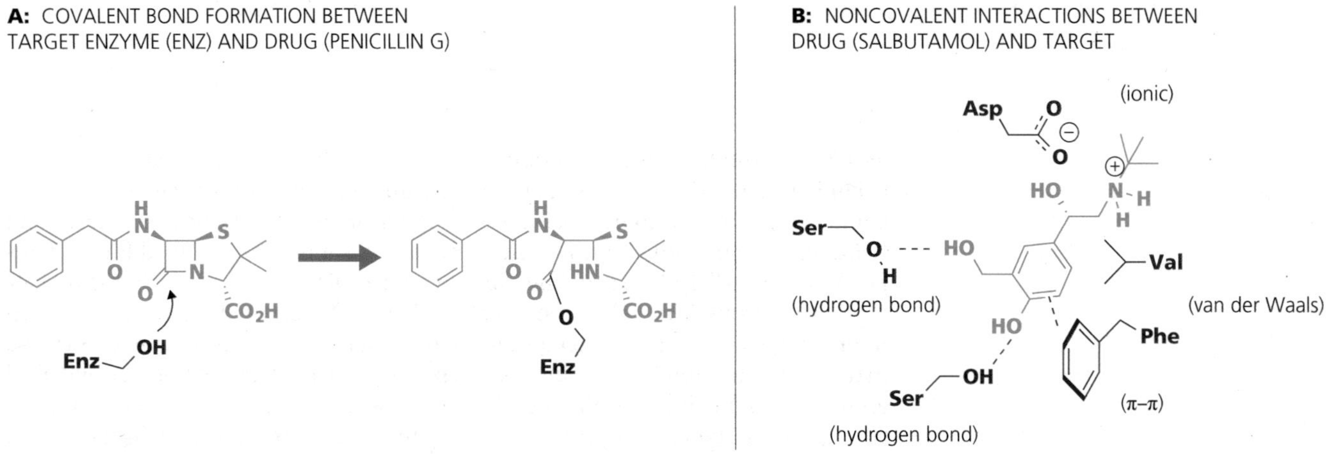

A: COVALENT BOND FORMATION BETWEEN TARGET ENZYME (ENZ) AND DRUG (PENICILLIN G)

B: NONCOVALENT INTERACTIONS BETWEEN DRUG (SALBUTAMOL) AND TARGET

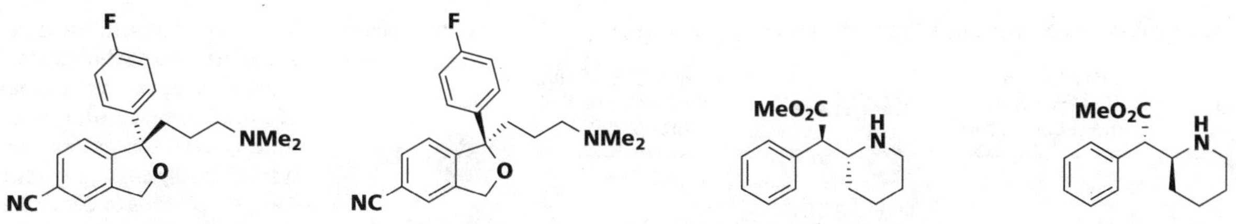

Figure 3.4 Enantiomers of citalopram and methylphenidate. (S)-Citalopram is marketed as escitalopram and is 167 times more active than the R-enantiomer. Methylphenidate also exhibits a high eudismic ratio and is marketed as both the racemate and the R,R-isomer.

TOOLS USED TO DEVELOP STRUCTURE–ACTIVITY RELATIONSHIPS

As described in the previous section, the ability of a drug to bind to its target is dependent on its various structural features. Medicinal chemists employ multiple tools to understand how molecules bind to a target, as well as to design novel compounds based on the data generated in the iterative cycle in Figure 3.1. A key element of the design process is the development of **structure–activity relationships** (SAR); that is, the effect of a change in the structure of the molecule on its biological activity. This process is an important underpinning of medicinal chemistry. Tools that incorporate SAR include pharmacophore modeling, commonly used in ligand-based drug design, and structure-based drug design, which relies on knowledge of the structures of a lead bound to the macromolecular target.

The relationship between structure and activity was recognized even before our current understanding of protein structures and was addressed in the mid-1900s by investigation of structure–activity relationships of **congeners**, compounds with similar core structures but varying functional group appendages. SAR studies are used throughout the lead optimization process. This entails modifying specific functional groups in the molecule and measuring activity of the new analog to determine whether that moiety is involved in binding to the target or, more broadly, what effect that change in structure has on activity. For example, if a lead molecule contains a hydrogen-bond donor, a molecule is designed in which that hydrogen-bond donor is removed while the other features of the molecule are maintained. When tested, if the molecule is considerably less active, the hydrogen-bond donor is deemed to be a critical feature of the structure. If the molecule maintains its activity, that hydrogen-bond donor is not an essential feature. In the specific case of salbutamol (see Figure 3.3), removal of the aromatic hydroxyl group removes that particular hydrogen bond and also decreases its activity as a bronchodilator.

While this concept seems simple, replacing one moiety without modifying another aspect of the molecule can be challenging. A hypothetical example is shown in **Figure 3.5**. Replacing the hydroxyl group in a potential hydrogen-bond donor, such as an alcohol, with a methoxy group will remove the H-bonding donor capacity, but it also changes the size and polarity of that particular feature. If the new molecule is less active, one conclusion is that the H-bond is important; however, the possibility that the new methyl group is too large to fit into the binding pocket cannot be ruled out. If it is similarly or more active, one conclusion might be that the H-bond is not important for binding but the oxygen acts as an H-bond acceptor. Replacing the alcohol with a secondary amine would maintain H-bond-donor and -acceptor features. If either was important for binding, activity of the secondary amine should be maintained or perhaps improved. To further corroborate the SAR data, the secondary amine could be changed to a tertiary amine, which removes the H-bond-donating capability. Inactivity of this analog would confirm the importance of the H-bond-donating feature. Equivalent or improved activity would indicate the importance of the H-bond accepting capabilities. In either case, further optimization may include design and synthesis of more amine analogs with various alkyl or acyl (R′) groups to probe the size of the binding pocket and perhaps optimize van der Waals interactions.

Hypothetical example (Hypothesis: lead with H-bonding group (OH) required for binding to target)

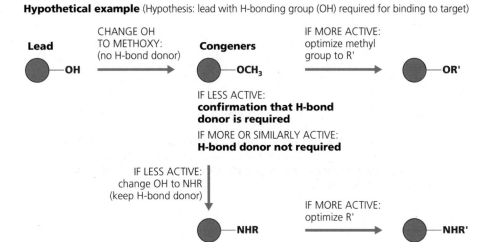

Figure 3.5 Hypothetical example showing lead optimization by synthesizing various congeners of a lead compound. This example shows how the logical process of systematically changing a structure (OH group) leads to conclusions about essential binding interactions.

   While the hypothetical example in Figure 3.5 shows a simple modification of one group, typically several different functional groups of the lead are modified to optimize each part of the compound. Furthermore, corroborating data need to be accumulated to support the conclusions based on each cycle of design, synthesis, testing, and analysis.

3.3   Historical methods for quantifying structure–activity relationships were based on physicochemical parameters

To streamline the process of drug discovery, starting in the mid-1900s, methods were developed to quantify structure–activity relationships. The earliest **quantitative structure–activity relationship** (QSAR) models were two-dimensional and relied on either properties of fragments of the molecules or properties of the entire molecule. The goal of two-dimensional QSAR was to develop a mathematical relationship between the structures and activities of a series of compounds. This model could then be used to guide future design of new compounds in the series. In general, the biological activity was defined as a function of the physicochemical properties of the drug, with certain specific **physicochemical parameters** correlating with biological activity. The most common parameters quantified were electronic characteristics, lipophilicity, and size of certain functional groups.

   Historically, **electronic properties** have been quantified in a number of ways. One of the most widely used was the Hammett equation, which was developed to study organic reactions and their mechanisms. Louis Hammett quantified the electronic properties of a series of functional groups by studying the ionization of substituted benzoic acids. He measured a series of constants (σ_X) that describe the effects of electron-donating or electron-withdrawing substituents (X) on the dissociation constant (K_X) compared to that of benzoic acid (K_H). The σ_X constants are equal to $\log K_X - \log K_H$, with electron-withdrawing groups having a σ value greater than zero and electron-donating groups having a σ value less than zero. In order to extend the application to instances where Hammett coefficients, σ, failed to explain reactivity, C. Gardner Swain and Elmer Lupton modified Hammett's σ parameter to include additional parameters: the field parameter includes inductive and pure field effects, and the resonance parameter includes electron-donating and electron-withdrawing effects.

   The importance of considering **lipophilicity**, the affinity of a molecule for lipids or nonpolar media, in SAR models came from the appreciation that drugs need to cross cell membranes in order to pass between the gut, blood, and tissues containing the

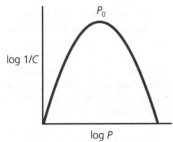

Figure 3.6 Relationship between drug concentration (log 1/C) and lipophilicity (log$P$) for a series of compounds where bioactivity correlates to lipophilicity. At low log$P$ (nonlipophilic compound), a high concentration is required for activity; at the optimal log$P$, a low concentration of drug is required for activity; at high log P (very lipophilic), a high concentration is required for activity.

macromolecular targets. If a molecule was not lipophilic enough, it would not cross the membrane, but if it were too lipophilic, it would get trapped in membranes and never reach the biological target. A pioneer of QSAR, Corwin Hansch, proposed that a lipophilicity parameter should be incorporated into QSAR analyses. This property could be measured by partitioning the molecule between 1-octanol (which is lipidlike) and water. The partition coefficient, P, is usually defined as the concentration of the compound in 1-octanol divided by its concentration in water. If a compound is equally soluble in both, then log$P = 0$. If it is more soluble in water than in 1-octanol (hydrophilic), then log$P$ is less than zero, and if it is more soluble in 1-octanol than in water (lipophilic), then log$P$ is greater than zero. The more lipophilic the drug is, the higher the value of log$P$. According to Hansch, lipophilicity of a drug relates to biological activity by Equation 3.4, where C is the concentration of a compound required to achieve a defined biological activity and k, k', and k'' are constants.

$$\log 1/C = -k(\log P)^2 + k'(\log P) + k'' \tag{3.4}$$

According to this equation, there is a parabolic relationship between the reciprocal of concentration of compound at which biological activity is observed and lipophilicity (**Figure 3.6**). For nonlipophilic compounds (those with low log$P$), a high concentration (C) would be required for activity; compounds that have an optimal log P require the lowest concentration of compound for activity; and compounds that are very lipophilic (a high log$P$), need a high concentration for activity.

Hansch also measured lipophilicity substituent constants, π, for various atoms and functional groups. Like the Hammett constants, the substituent (X) constant π is equal to logP_X – logP_H, where H refers to the unsubstituted case. The π constants are both additive and constitutive, meaning that π values for groups within a molecule can be added to give the overall lipophilicity or log$P$. However, the effect depends on the particular molecule, and only similar compounds should be compared to each other.

Finally, several methods have been developed to measure the size of various substituents on a lead molecule. Robert Taft measured the rates of hydrolysis of esters with varying alkyl substituents, RCO_2R', compared to the corresponding acetate esters, CH_3CO_2R'. Since the steric bulk of R will influence the rate of hydrolysis of the ester, this value, the steric parameter E_S, can be used as a surrogate measurement of size. Another set of parameters is the Verloop parameters that are calculated by the program STERIMOL. These values are based on bond angles, van der Waals radii, bond lengths, and possible conformers of various substituents to give five values. **Figure 3.7** exemplifies these parameters for a carboxylic acid substituent on a benzene ring: L = length of substituent along the bond axis from the parent (that is, the benzene ring in Figure 3.7) and B_1–B_4 = width of substituent perpendicular to the bond axis in four directions. One other example of a parameter that reflects size is the molar refractivity (MR), which is based on molecular weight, density, and index of refraction. This parameter gives an indication of the molar volume of a substituent as well as its polarizability.

In order to correlate these parameters with biological activity, a number of mathematical equations were developed. The Hansch analysis, among the earliest developed, can be used for a congeneric series. This is a linear multiple regression analysis that relates bioactivity as the dependent variable to physicochemical properties as independent variables. The general form of the **Hansch equation** is as follows:

$$\text{Hansch equation:}\quad \log 1/C = -a\pi^2 + b\pi + \sigma + cE_s + d \tag{3.5}$$

Within a given series of compounds, a number of analogs are tested for biological activity, where C is the concentration at which some given specified activity is observed and the calculated physicochemical parameters π, σ, and E_s (described above) are taken from sources in the literature. Regression coefficients a, b, c, and d are derived from a training set of known compounds. The reciprocal of concentration reflects the fact that a lower dose correlates to an inherently more potent drug. Once

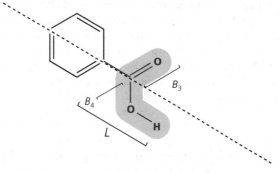

L = length extending from parent
B₃ and **B₄** = width extending from plane

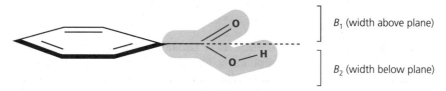

B_1 (width above plane)

B_2 (width below plane)

B₁ and **B₂** = width extending above/below plane

Figure 3.7 Illustration of Verloop parameters for a substituent (CO₂H) on a benzene ring. L = length of substituent (red) extending from the parent; B_1–B_4 = width of substituent extending within the plane (B_3 and B_4) and extending above and below the plane of the parent (B_1 and B_2).

the coefficients are known, the equation can be solved for hypothetical compounds to give predicted biological activity. Therefore, the medicinal chemist can predict whether or not a proposed compound may have activity without going to the trouble of synthesizing and testing it. However, for any given series of compounds, a large number of analogs have to be synthesized and tested for activity in order to develop a highly predictive equation.

Another classical two-dimensional QSAR method is the **Free–Wilson method** or **additivity method**. This method assesses the occurrence of additive substituent effects and estimates their magnitude. Unlike the Hansch method, this equation does not take into account any properties of the molecules or fragments, but it tries to directly relate the effects of changes in structure to changes in biological activity. The general form of the equation is as follows:

Free–Wilson or additivity equation: $BA = \Sigma a_i X_i + \mu$ (3.6)

In this case, BA is biological activity, a_i is the magnitude of the effect of a given substituent, and μ is average activity of the parent molecule. X is given a value of one if substituent i is present and zero if not. As in a Hansch analysis, a series of congeners needs to be prepared and tested for biological activity. These are then analyzed to determine values of a for various substituents, as well as a value for the average activity. Those values are then used to predict bioactivity for compounds in the same series that have not yet been synthesized and tested.

Development of either a Hansch equation or Free–Wilson analysis requires the synthesis and testing of a fairly large number of compounds as a basis set. Once the equation is established, predictions of activity of newly designed compounds can be made. As an alternative to these methods, in the 1970s John Topliss developed a flow diagram (**Topliss decision tree**) that begins with the biological analysis of a single compound, as seen in **Figure 3.8**. Bioactivity of a compound containing a substituted benzene (active or inactive) determines which is the next analog to prepare. The scheme was designed on the basis of electronic and lipophilic characteristics of the substituents and relied on Hansch principles.

For example, if a compound bearing an aromatic ring has biological activity, synthesis of the 4-chloro analog is undertaken, and that analog will be either less, equally, or more active than the parent compound. The specific data determine which analog to prepare next: if the 4-chloro analog is more active, then the 3,4-dichloro

Figure 3.8 Original Topliss scheme for aromatic substituents. A substituted derivative (4-Cl) of an aromatic parent compound (A) is prepared and tested. The results of testing (L = less active; E = equally active; M = more active) determine the next analog to prepare. In this manner, an efficient, systematic process for evaluating SAR and lead optimization is pursued.

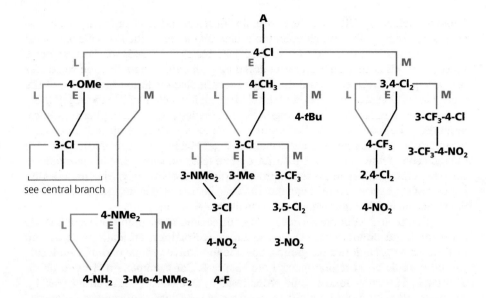

analog should be made; if the 4-chloro analog is less active, then the 4-methoxy analog is prepared next. The Topliss decision tree allows medicinal chemists to make rational decisions about which analogs to make on the basis of smaller numbers of congeners compared to Hansch and Free-Wilson methods, and it avoids the need to develop complex equations that describe biological activity.

Today these historical methods as described are used infrequently, but they have been modified and updated for the modern computational era. For example, Hansch analysis is the foundation for fragment-based QSAR, which uses molecular fingerprints, or fragments, to carry out two-dimensional QSAR assessment based on a partial-least-squares analysis. Likewise, the concept of ligand efficiency, which will be described later, is essentially a progression of Free–Wilson analysis. The basis of the Topliss scheme is still used to decide on the synthesis of analogs with aromatic substituents; indeed, there is some concern about an overall bias toward *p*-chlorophenyl substituents in many libraries due to the historical widespread application of Topliss schemes.

3.4 Ligand- and structure-based drug design are modern strategies that rely on knowledge of the pharmacophore

The classical two-dimensional QSAR method for drug design is a very time-consuming process. Many analogs have to be synthesized and tested for activity in a congeneric series in order to develop an appropriate equation. This can take years, depending on how many compounds are made. The initial process is essentially one of trial and error, with all imaginable changes being tried before a useful equation can be derived that accurately predicts active compounds prior to synthesis. Furthermore, while classical two-dimensional QSAR was used to relate biological activity to overall electronic and steric characteristics of the small molecule, it did not address biomolecular recognition.

With advances in computational abilities, medicinal chemists have come to use the important tool of three-dimensional QSAR for rational drug design. Two general strategies are employed. **Ligand-based drug design** depends on analysis of low-energy conformers of compounds that are known to bind to a specific target. **Structure-based drug design** relies on a known structure of the macromolecular drug target and is applied when a structure of the macromolecular target, or a closely related homolog, is available. All of these methods rely on a linchpin concept in medicinal chemistry: the pharmacophore.

In any series of active compounds, there are key binding interactions with the target that are made by specific functional groups of the molecule (Sections 3.1 and 3.2). The target has a defined three-dimensional structure, as do the important functional groups of the drug. The **pharmacophore** is defined by the International Union of Pure and

Applied Chemistry (IUPAC) as "the ensemble of steric and electronic features that is necessary to ensure the optimal supramolecular interactions with a specific biological target structure and to trigger (or to block) its biological response." Further notes specify that this is an abstract concept accounting for common interaction capacities of a group of molecules toward the target macromolecule. Much of the rest of the molecule is either scaffolding to hold the pharmacophoric elements in the appropriate three-dimensional orientation or fragments that modify physical and pharmaceutical properties. The goal during the lead optimization process is to develop and understand the pharmacophoric elements and to make changes that improve specific properties of the molecule. Knowledge of the pharmacophore tells you what parts of the molecule can be optimized to retain or even improve binding and, conversely, what moieties are not part of the pharmacophore and therefore can be modified to improve physical and pharmaceutical properties while binding to the target is retained.

Typical pharmacophores involve at least three binding elements that can include hydrogen-bond donors or acceptors, hydrophobic regions, aromatic regions, and positive or negative ionizable groups. Specific functional groups within a molecule will fill the role of these pharmacophore elements. For example, an H-bond donor element in a pharmacophore could be achieved by an alcohol (**ROH**), amine (**RNH₂**), or amide (**RCONH₂**). When a pharmacophore is described, the specific functional group (such as alcohol, amine, or amide) is less important than the element (H-bond donor) it presents.

3.5   Pharmacophore models are widely used in ligand-based drug design

Multiple methods to develop a pharmacophore model have evolved. One of the earliest appearances of the term pharmacophore was in a study by Lemont Kier on the use of molecular orbital calculations of the preferred conformations of three compounds (acetylcholine, muscarine, and muscarone) that bind potently to the muscarinic acetylcholine receptor. By identifying the compounds' low-energy conformations and comparing similarities of their structures and placement of functional groups, a pharmacophore model was derived. As seen in **Figure 3.9**, the three pharmacophoric elements identified were a positive ionizable group, presented by the quaternary amine in all three structures (red); an H-bond acceptor, presented by the carbonyls in acetylcholine and muscarone and by the oxygen atom of the alcohol in muscarine (blue); and a second H-bond acceptor, represented by the ester oxygen in acetylcholine and by the ring oxygens in muscarine and muscarone (green).

Overlaying these three structures provided the distance constraints between the pharmacophoric elements. Based on the model, any compound that fit these constraints should bind to the target. The concept of using a three-dimensional model to describe how small molecules interact with a target is central to ligand-based drug design. In these cases, the model developed from compounds known to bind to the

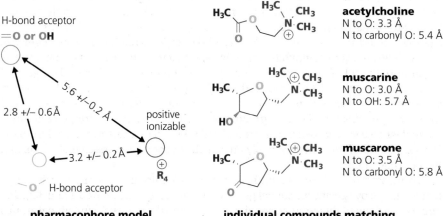

pharmacophore model   **individual compounds matching pharmacophore model**

Figure 3.9 Early example of pharmacophore model based on compounds that bind to acetylcholine receptor (acetylcholine, muscarine, and muscarone). The model on the left shows distances between pharmacophore elements in angstroms. Three groups are defined: blue and green = hydrogen-bond acceptors; red = positive ionizable group. Three molecules on the right show specific functional groups that present the pharmacophoric elements highlighted and the distances between them.

target (ligands) is used to predict whether or not novel analogs will bind. The structure of the binding pocket of the target may not be known.

The **active-analog approach**, pioneered by Garland Marshall in the late 1970s, used the three-dimensional arrangement of the low-energy conformers of multiple active compounds to find the minimal recognition elements. To apply the active analog approach, a set of both active molecules that exhibit a wide range of potencies and inactive analogs is accumulated. After the common pharmacophore elements are identified, conformers of each ligand are generated computationally. The conformers are then superimposed on each other so that the common pharmacophore elements are matched. Many times these will be superimposed on a rigid active ligand that will necessarily have those elements in a fixed three-dimensional conformation.

A three-dimensional pharmacophore model can then be proposed and used in the design of new compounds. Applying this approach to a target macromolecule led to the concept of **receptor-excluded volume** (binding pocket area occupied by the drug) and **receptor-essential area** (binding pocket area occupied by the macromolecule target). The receptor-excluded volume is generated from the superimposition of all active compounds that contain the pharmacophore in their lowest energy conformation. A volume map is then generated from inactive compounds that also contain the pharmacophore. The assumption is that these inactive compounds, despite containing pharmacophoric elements, do not bind tightly because their volume extends into the area that is occupied by the target (receptor-essential area). This comparison between the volume of active analogs and the volume of inactive analogs provides a rough three-dimensional map of the size and shape of a binding pocket within a protein target and provides the boundaries beyond which active small-molecule binders cannot extend (**Figure 3.10**).

As an example, Victor Hruby and co-workers developed a pharmacophore model for selective δ-opioid agonists based on cyclic analogs of enkephalins such as [(2S,3R)-TMT[1]]DPDPE (**Figure 3.11A**). The pharmacophore elements, in Figure 3.11, were defined as an aromatic and an OH group (red, substituted tyrosine in [(2S,3R)-TMT[1]]DPDPE), a positive ionizable group (blue, primary amine), and a second aromatic group (green, phenylalanine aryl ring). The model was developed by use of rigid analogs with selectivity for the δ-opioid receptor, such as oxymorphindole, which contains the same pharmacophoric elements and allowed imposing distance constraints within the pharmacophore. The model developed (**Figure 3.11B**) contains four pharmacophoric elements and shows the spatial relationships between them.

Today, with the development of computational chemistry, pharmacophore modeling is often done by use of specific software programs. In these programs, a number of active and inactive ligands are modeled, and low-energy conformers are determined and aligned to identify common proposed points of interaction with a target. For example, scientists at GlaxoSmithKline used a commercial software program to develop a pharmacophore model for ligands binding to one of the serotonin receptors (5-HT_{2c}). The pharmacophore model was based on compounds with high affinity and selectivity for the 5-HT_{2c} receptor; the three structures in **Figure 3.12** (**1–3**) are representatives of those compounds. These efforts resulted in a pharmacophore model in which the features are shown as spheres (green = H-bond acceptor; red = positive ionizable group; blue = hydrophobic group; and yellow = aromatic

Figure 3.10 Marshall's active-analog model for determining a pharmacophore. The combined volume of all active compounds that have the correct pharmacophore (region shaded pink) is the receptor-excluded volume. Any compound that adheres to the pharmacophore but is inactive is presumed to extend into the receptor-essential area (dotted lines), and this defines the receptor essential volume.

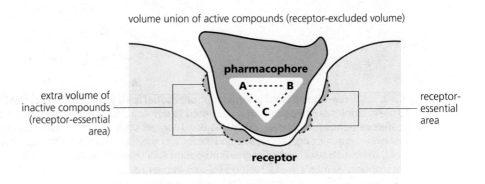

A: EXAMPLES OF COMPOUNDS USED TO DEVELOP PHARMACOPHORE MODEL FOR δ-OPIOID AGONIST

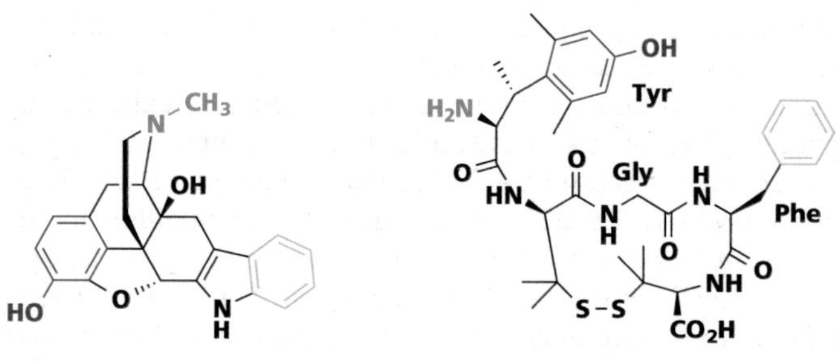

oxymorphindole

[(2S,3R)-TMT¹]DPDPE

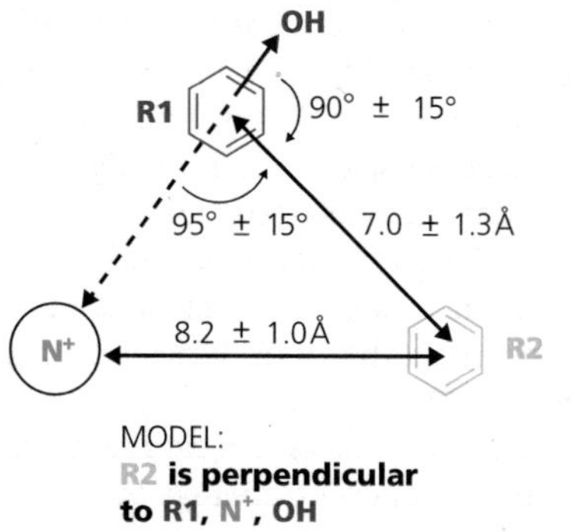

Figure 3.11 Hruby's δ-opioid agonist model for determining a pharmacophore. A: Two compounds, oxymorphindole and [(2S,3R)-TMT¹] DPDPE, used to develop the model. B: Pharmacophore model contains four pharmacophore elements: red = aromatic group (R1) and OH, blue = positive ionizable group, green = aromatic group (R2). Distances in angstroms between groups are defined, with the R2 group perpendicular to both R1, OH, and the positive ionizable group.

B: PHARMACOPHORE MODEL FOR δ-OPIOID AGONIST

OH

R1   90° ± 15°

95° ± 15°   7.0 ± 1.3Å

N⁺   8.2 ± 1.0Å   R2

MODEL:
R2 is perpendicular to R1, N⁺, OH

A: COMPOUNDS **1, 2,** AND **3** USED TO DEVELOP PHARMACOPHORE MODEL

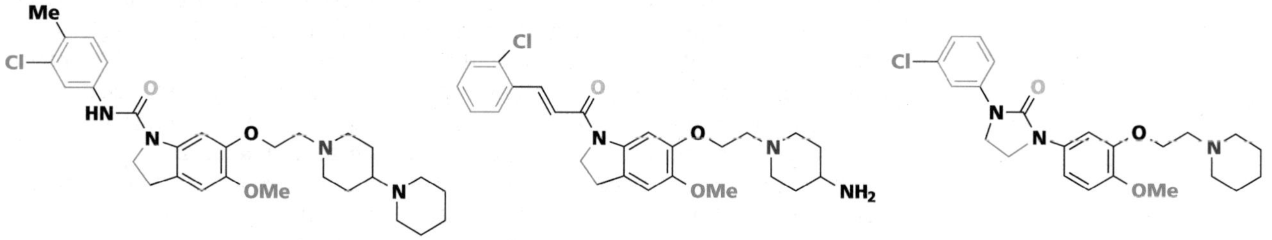

1   **2**   **3**

B: PHARMACOPHORE MODEL AND COMPOUND **4,** DESIGNED ON THE BASIS OF THIS MODEL

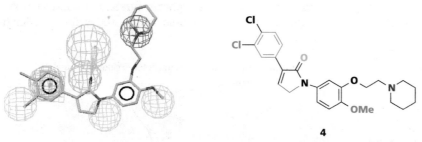

4

Figure 3.12 Three-dimensional pharmacophore model for ligands binding at the 5-HT₂c receptor. A: Analogs **1, 2,** and **3** are examples of compounds that were used to develop a pharmacophore model. B: Pharmacophore model, where the features are shown as spheres: green = H-bond acceptor, red = positive ionizable group, blue = hydrophobic groups, and yellow = aromatic ring. The volume and location of the sphere indicates the optimal position of the pharmacophoric element. The structure of newly designed compound **4,** developed on the basis of this model, is shown on the right. Common pharmacophore elements in all structures colored as pharmacophore model. (From Micheli F, Pasquarello A, Tedesco G et al. [2006] *Bioorg Med Chem Lett* 16:3906–3912. With permission from Elsevier.)

ring). The volume and location of the spheres define the optimal region in space where each of the elements must be located. A new compound (**4**) was designed on the basis of the model by ligand-based drug design; it is shown superimposed on the three-dimensional pharmacophore model.

Another example of the value of pharmacophore models is in virtual screening, as can be seen by the example of a pharmacophore model developed for a binding site on the GABA$_A$ receptor. Compounds such as benzodiazepines bind at this receptor and exhibit bioactivities including anti-anxiety, muscle relaxation, and sedation. In the early 1990s, James Cook reported a model that was based on 136 benzodiazepines, β-carbolines, pyridodiindoles, pyrazoloquinolines, and several other scaffolds that bound to the benzodiazepine site on the GABA$_A$ receptor. Later, as seen in **Figure 3.13**, Tommy Liljefors and co-workers applied the model to include a different class of compounds, the flavones.

In these models, features of both the small molecule and the target are described to characterize the pharmacophore: H1 and H2 represent sites on the receptor that contribute hydrogen-bond donors (X–H from receptor), L1–L3 and L$_{Di}$ are lipophilic sites on the small molecule, S1–S3 are regions of negative steric interaction (corresponding to receptor essential area), and A2 is a hydrogen-bond acceptor site on the receptor.

In a new search for compounds binding at the GABA$_A$ receptor, Liljefors went further and used virtual screening based on this unified pharmacophore model and identified a 4-quinolone ($K_i = 122$ nM) as a potential lead for binding at the benzodiazepine receptor. This quinolone, which is a close analog of a flavone yet binds somewhat differently, fits the same pharmacophore model (**Figure 3.14A**). Lead optimization (**Figure 3.14B**) by extension of the ester side chain was based on the strategy to fill the L2 pocket, with a propyl group found to be the optimal length. Chain-branching (isopropyl) and ring-chain transformation at this position (cyclopentyl) led to analogs that were less active than the propyl analog, possibly due to steric interactions with the S1 and S2 sites. Optimization of the H1 binding

Figure 3.13 Pharmacophore models for the benzodiazepine site on the GABA$_A$ receptor. A: Cook's pharmacophore model (with diazepam, CGS-9896, and a diazadiindole overlaid), where H1 and H2 are H-bond donor sites and A2 is an H-bond acceptor site on the receptor; L1–L3 and L$_{Di}$ are lipophilic sites on the small molecule, and S1–S3 are areas where steric interaction is unfavorable (receptor essential area). (From Clayton T, Chen JL, Ernst M et al. [2007] *Curr Med Chem* 14:2755–2775. With permission from Bentham Science Publishers.) **B:** Cook's GABA$_A$ receptor pharmacophore (rotated 180° counterclockwise) with a flavone mapped onto the model. H2/A3 is either a donor or acceptor and corresponds to H2 in Cook's model. (From Kahnberg P, Lager E, Rosenberg C et al. [2002] *J Med Chem* 45:4188–4201. With permission from American Chemical Society.)

A: COOK'S PHARMACOPHORE MODEL FOR THE BENZODIAZEPINE SITE ON THE GABA$_A$ RECEPTOR

B: FLAVONE OCCUPYING PHARMACOPHORE MODEL

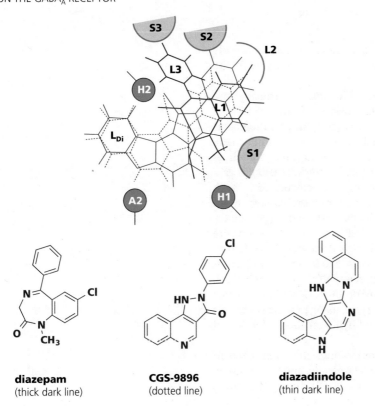

diazepam
(thick dark line)

CGS-9896
(dotted line)

diazadiindole
(thin dark line)

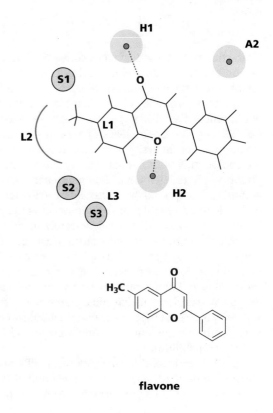

flavone

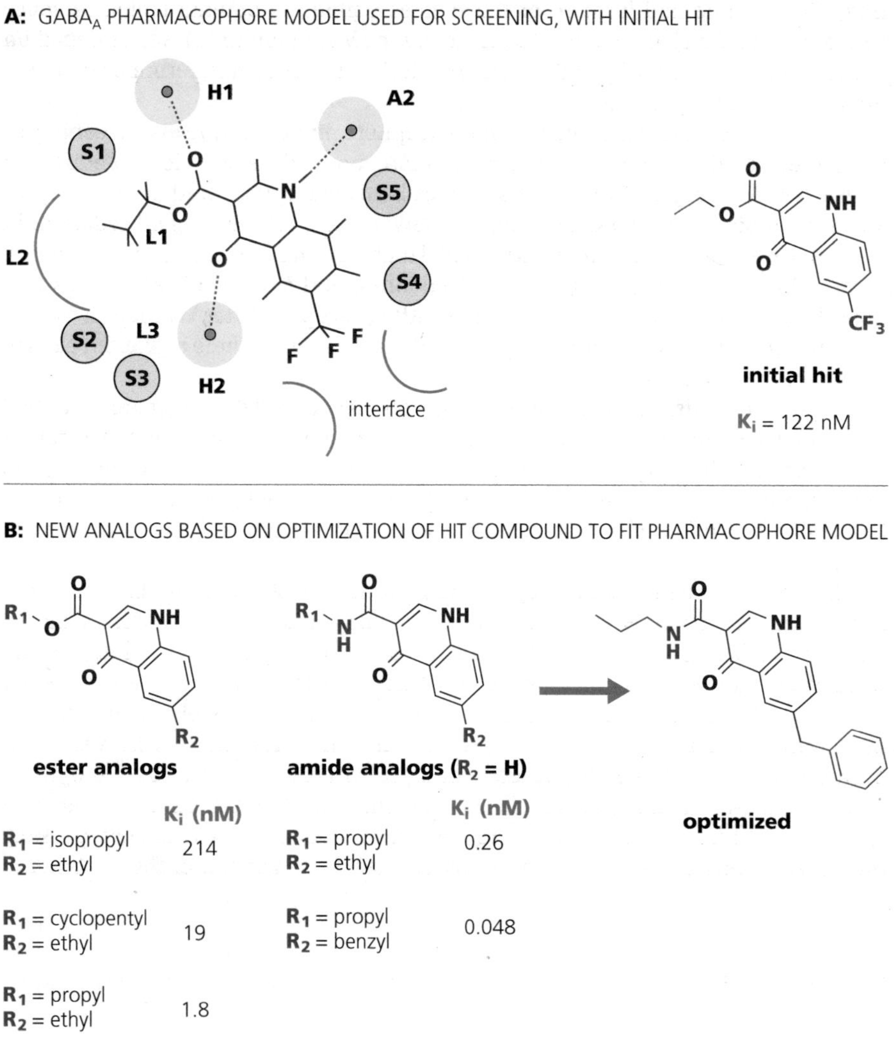

A: GABA$_A$ PHARMACOPHORE MODEL USED FOR SCREENING, WITH INITIAL HIT

initial hit

K_i = 122 nM

B: NEW ANALOGS BASED ON OPTIMIZATION OF HIT COMPOUND TO FIT PHARMACOPHORE MODEL

ester analogs

amide analogs (R_2 = H)

optimized

	K_i (nM)
R_1 = isopropyl R_2 = ethyl	214
R_1 = cyclopentyl R_2 = ethyl	19
R_1 = propyl R_2 = ethyl	1.8

	K_i (nM)
R_1 = propyl R_2 = ethyl	0.26
R_1 = propyl R_2 = benzyl	0.048

Figure 3.14 Use of a pharmacophore model in virtual screening and lead optimization. A: The initial hit was discovered by virtual screening of a compound library to fit the pharmacophore model shown in **Figure 3.13**, with addition of a lipophilic interface region. B: Optimization of R_1 and R_2 groups and the ester linkage was done by fitting the model so that R_1 (propyl) fills the L2 pocket and R_2 occupies the lipophilic interface region. The corresponding amides improved the H1 interaction, and an optimized lead was generated by combining all changes. Lower K_i values indicate improved binding to the receptor. (From Lager E, Andersson P, Nilsson J et al. [2006] *J Med Chem* 49:2526–2533. With permission from American Chemical Society.)

interaction was accomplished by converting the ester to an amide, where the amide carbonyl oxygen is more electron rich. By changing the R_2 group to a benzyl to fill the lipophilic interface region, an optimized lead was identified.

Another example of a valuable computational tool for pharmacophore development, based on regression analysis and three-dimensional QSAR, is the use of CoMFA (comparative molecular field analysis) and CoMSIA (comparative molecular similarity index analysis) programs. In this type of analysis, low-energy conformers for compounds with similar activity are generated and superimposed, matching pharmacophore elements. The computer establishes a three-dimensional grid around the compounds and two fields, electrostatic and steric, are calculated for each molecule in every grid point by approaching the grid with atomic probes such as an ion or a carbon atom. The calculations rely on Lennard-Jones and Coulomb potentials. A data table is generated, and a partial-least-squares analysis is done to determine the minimal set of grid points that explains the measured biological activity. Two different three-dimensional structures are generated: one of the steric field, to show where it is desirable and undesirable to have steric bulk, and a second of the electronic field, to show where electron-rich and electron-poor areas are optimal. CoMSIA calculates similarity indices at the intersections of the surrounding grid, using properties such as size, electrostatic potential, hydrophobic properties, and hydrogen-bond donor and acceptor capabilities.

CoMFA and CoMSIA analyses of 27 different 4-quinolones that were used in Liljefors' initial study provided a view of optimal steric, electrostatic, and hydrophobic interactions for binding to the brain GABA$_A$ receptor (**Figure 3.15**). The CoMFA steric

Figure 3.15 CoMFA analysis of with compound 5 shown. A: Example of CoMFA steric (left) and electrostatic (right) plots determined from 27 compounds, overlaid with structure of Compound **5**. In the steric plot (left), occupation of the green area is favorable, while occupation of the yellow area is unfavorable. In the electrostatic plot (right), the red area is most favorable for electron-rich substituents and the blue area is favorable for electron-poor substituents. (From Guarav A, Yadav MR, Giridhar R et al. [2011] *Med Chem Res* 20:192–199. With permission from Springer.) B: Structures of **5** and **6**, which have differing activity at the brain GABA$_A$ receptor.

A: CoMFA PLOTS WITH COMPOUND 5:
LEFT = STERIC PLOT (YELLOW UNFAVORABLE, GREEN FAVORABLE);
RIGHT = ELECTROSTATIC PLOT (BLUE = ELECTRON-POOR, RED = ELECTRON-RICH)

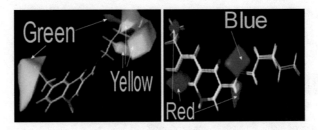

B: EXAMPLES OF COMPOUNDS WITH DIFFERING ACTIVITY

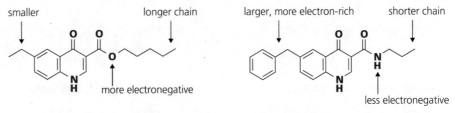

compound 5: less active   **compound 6: more active**

plot (left) in Figure 3.15A shows areas where steric bulk results in an increase in activity (green) and areas where steric bulk decreases activity (yellow). The electrostatic plot (right) shows areas in blue where more electropositivity (or less electronegativity) favors potency and shows areas where more negative charge, such as the electron-rich aryl ring, favors activity in red. Compound **5** (see Figure 3.15B) is overlaid in both plots. The utility of this approach can be seen in comparing the less active **5** to the more active **6** (optimized lead from Figure 3.14). The differences in potency can be explained by examining the CoMFA plots:

1. The benzyl substituent on the aryl ring of **6** is both larger (occupying more of the green area of the steric plot) and more electron-rich (red in the electrostatic plot); both are favorable.

2. The propyl chain of the amide in **6** is shorter than the corresponding pentyl group in **5** and therefore removes the unfavorable occupation of the yellow region in the steric plot seen for **5**.

3. The amide nitrogen in **6** is less electronegative than the ester oxygen in **5**, optimizing the blue region seen in the electrostatic plot.

The CoMSIA plot generated for the same pharmacophore overlaid with **6**, shown in **Figure 3.16A**, is similar to the CoMFA plot for steric interactions, with the addition of a second unfavorable (yellow) area (left). The electrostatic plot (center) bears some similarity to the CoMFA plot, but there is less electron density (red) in the aromatic rings. An additional plot for hydrophilic and hydrophobic areas (right) shows areas that favor hydrophilic groups in white and areas that favor hydrophobic groups in yellow. In comparing **6** (more active) to **7** (less active) (**Figure 3.16B**), it is seen that the methyl group of **7** occupies the new unfavorable region.

The availability of a pharmacophore model, in theory, allows a medicinal chemist to design new analogs, and if those analogs adhere to the pharmacophore model, theoretically they will be active. These models are the mainstay of medicinal chemistry and allow one to maintain and optimize potency and efficacy by understanding the structural features involved in binding to the macromolecular target. At the same time, optimizing physical and pharmaceutical properties while maintaining potency is possible by modifying the scaffold or other areas of the molecule that are independent of the pharmacophore.

A: CoMSIA PLOTS WITH COMPOUND 6 OVERLAID: STERIC PLOT (LEFT: YELLOW UNFAVORABLE, GREEN FAVORABLE); ELECTROSTATIC PLOT (CENTER: BLUE = ELECTRON-POOR, RED = ELECTRON-RICH), HYDROPHOBIC PLOT (RIGHT: WHITE = HYDROPHILIC, YELLOW = HYDROPHOBIC)

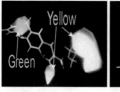 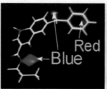 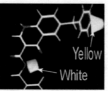

steric plot
yellow unfavorable, green favorable

electrostatic plot
blue = electron-poor, red = electron-rich

hydrophobic plot
white = hydrophilic, yellow = hydrophobic

Figure 3.16 CoMSIA analysis of 6.
A: CoMSIA steric (left), electrostatic (center) and hydrophobic (right) plots with **6** overlaid. The methyl of **7** would have an unfavorable steric interaction (yellow region in steric plot). (From Guarav A, Yadav MR, Giridhar R et al. [2011] *Med Chem Res* 20:192–199. With permission from Springer.) B: Structures of **6** and **7**, which have differing activity at the brain GABA_A receptor.

B: EXAMPLES OF COMPOUNDS WITH DIFFERING ACTIVITY

compound 6: more active   **compound 7: less active**

3.6   Structure-based drug design is based on the structure of the drug target

The preceding section describes how pharmacophores are developed from knowledge of ligands and active molecules and how they are used in ligand-based drug design. However, with the advent of methods to determine the structures of macromolecules such as X-ray crystallography, NMR, and cryo-electron microscopy, structure-based drug design (SBDD) is now a common strategy. For example, a compound bound to the target can be visualized based on an X-ray crystal structure that has been solved. Often the structure is solved when the small molecule is bound to a macromolecular target, as this provides the most reliable data. However, sometimes only the macromolecule structure is determined and the small molecule is docked into the site. In other cases a structure of a related protein is known, and it can be used to make a model of the protein of interest (a **homology model**) for docking purposes. The availability of a three-dimensional view of the small molecule bound to the macromolecular target allows observation of specific binding interactions, so that it is immediately apparent which functional groups are necessary for binding, and identification of a pharmacophore is expedited. SBDD also provides an opportunity to incorporate additional elements into a pharmacophore model based on the structure of the target and to design improved compounds that may not have been apparent without the availability of the structure. SBDD is frequently used for the design of enzyme inhibitors or other proteins that are amenable to structure elucidation, and a number of such examples are described in later chapters.

One of the earliest examples of the power of SBDD was the development of the human immunodeficiency virus (HIV) protease inhibitors in the 1990s. The antiviral drugs for acquired immunodeficiency syndrome (AIDS) and HIV infection that target HIV protease were all optimized by structure-based drug design. X-ray structures of the protein itself and many co-crystal structures of inhibitors bound to the protein were solved. For example the HIV protease inhibitor ritonavir was optimized from lead A-74704, shown in **Figure 3.17A**.

Compound A-74704 exhibited an IC_{50} of 3 nM against the protease enzyme, and an X-ray structure was solved with it bound to the active site. Two particular binding interactions observed were hydrogen bonds from two NH groups of the molecule to backbone carbonyls of glycines on the enzyme; however, this interaction did not have the optimal geometry for a hydrogen bond. Analogs, including A-77003 (**Figure 3.17B**), were designed that contained an additional central carbon and allowed a more optimal geometry for H-bonding; the new analogs were 10–50 times more potent. The drug

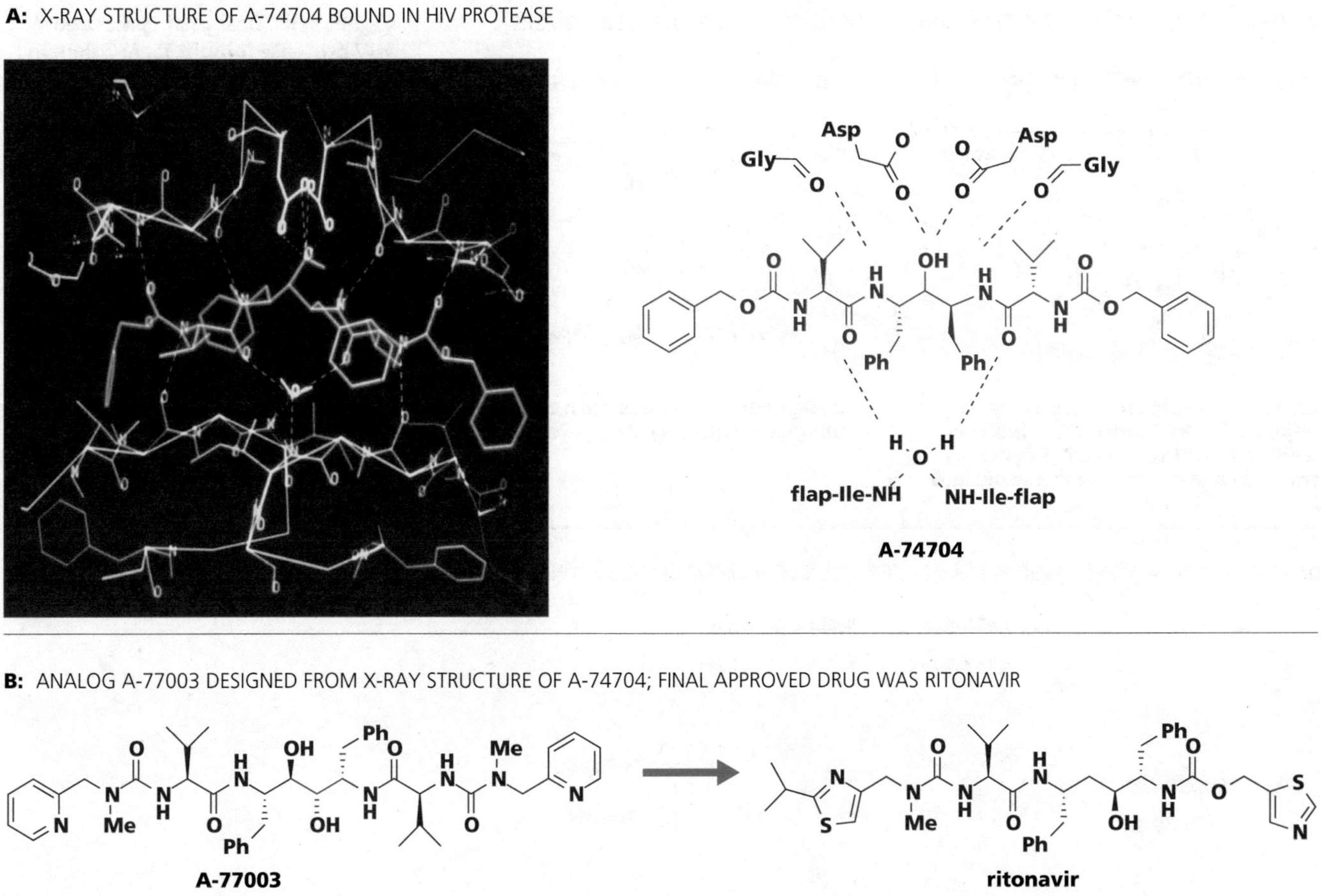

A: X-RAY STRUCTURE OF A-74704 BOUND IN HIV PROTEASE

A-74704

B: ANALOG A-77003 DESIGNED FROM X-RAY STRUCTURE OF A-74704; FINAL APPROVED DRUG WAS RITONAVIR

A-77003   **ritonavir**

Figure 3.17 Structure-based drug design of HIV protease inhibitor ritonavir. A: X-ray structure of A-74704 (pink) bound in the enzyme active site (side chains of enzyme in yellow, outline of backbone in blue, aspartic acid side chains and structural water in white) and depiction of A-74704 hydrogen-bond interactions (dashed lines) with protein and structural water (shown in black). B: Structures of A-77003 optimized for binding by inserting additional substituted carbon atom (in red) and ritonavir, the drug developed from these leads. (From Greer J, Erickson JW, Baldwin JJ & Varney MD [1994] *J Med Chem* 37:1035–1054. With permission from American Chemical Society.)

ultimately developed from this series was the AIDS/ HIV drug ritonavir. The availability of the X-ray structure allowed visualization of the unoptimized H-bonds and the realization that by changing their geometry, potency could be improved.

Another example of the use of SBDD in the design of HIV protease inhibitors was the development of a series of symmetric cyclic ureas that progressed to clinical trials. Published X-ray crystal structures showed that most HIV protease inhibitors made contacts with the enzyme mediated through a structural water molecule (as seen in Figure 3.17A). That is, a water molecule was an integral part of the inhibitory structure and made hydrogen bonds to the inhibitor and the enzyme flap region. Taking this observation into consideration, scientists at Dupont–Merck designed scaffolds that incorporated a carbonyl oxygen into the inhibitor molecule to mimic the H-bond accepting properties of the water molecule, rather than relying on the presence of a structural water in the enzyme (**Figure 3.18A**). In theory, this approach is entropically favored. Structure-based drug design and molecule modeling were used to design molecules such as DMP323 (**Figure 3.18B**).

DMP323 exhibited potent inhibition of the enzyme ($IC_{50} = 57$ nM), and X-ray crystallographic studies proved that the molecule bound to the enzyme as predicted, with the carbonyl oxygen displacing the structural water molecule. Hydrogen bonds between that oxygen and the backbone NH of two isoleucines (Ile50 and Ile50′) in the flap are observed, as well as H-bonds between the compound's alcohols and aspartate residues (Asp25 and Asp25′) in the active site. Additional binding interactions include H-bonds to the backbone NH groups of Asp 29/29′ and 30/30′ as well as hydrophobic interactions in the S1/S1′ and S2/S2′ lipophilic pockets.

These HIV protease inhibitor examples are examples of the power of structure-based drug design, which is now a common practice. This is especially true for the design of enzyme inhibitors, since these drug targets are more amenable to crystallization than membrane-bound receptors.

A: DESIGN OF CYCLIC UREA BASED ON X-RAY STRUCTURES OF HIV PROTEASE INHIBITORS

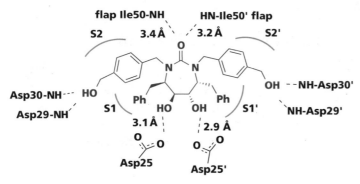

observed common interactions of peptidelike HIV protease inhibitors (red): all bind to flap of enzyme through a structural water molecule

designed cyclic ureas with carbonyl oxygen displacing structural water

Figure 3.18 Design of cyclic urea HIV protease inhibitors. A: Common binding interactions in peptidelike inhibitors include H-bonds to central alcohol and H-bonds to Iles in flap via a structural water molecule; design is based on use of a carbonyl oxygen to replace a structural water. B: Depiction of observed binding interactions, based on co-crystal structure of analog DMP323 bound to HIV protease, showing the carbonyl makes the same H-bond interactions previously made by structural water, and OHs making H-bonds to Asp residues. (S1, S2, S1′, and S2′ are lipophilic pockets on the enzyme).

B: BINDING INTERACTIONS OBSERVED IN X-RAY STRUCTURE OF INHIBITOR DMP323 BOUND IN ENZYME

observed binding interactions in X-ray structure of DMP323

SUMMARY

While Chapter 2 described hit and lead identification strategies, this chapter highlighted some of the properties that are important during the lead optimization process. Biological, physical, and pharmaceutical properties are all evaluated and optimized in order to identify a viable drug candidate starting from very simple primary assays, advancing to more complex secondary assays, and eventually moving to *in vivo* assays. Biological properties such as potency, efficacy, and selectivity of a small molecule are optimized by taking into account its specific binding interactions with the protein target and by development of a pharmacophore model.

Ligand- and structure-based design are modern tools that take into account the three-dimensional conformation of the small molecule and are used to design and optimize improved analogs. Ligand-based design is used to develop models around a series that binds to the same binding site of a target; the structure of the target does not need to be known. In contrast, structure-based drug design requires knowledge of the macromolecular target, and therefore is not applicable to all drug discovery projects.

Knowledge of the pharmacophore is necessary for the lead optimization process. It provides insight into which elements are required for binding to the biological target, and therefore which can be further optimized to improve potency and selectivity. At the same time, knowledge of the pharmacophore provides information about which aspects of the molecule can be modified in order to optimize physical and pharmaceutical properties without affecting target binding.

CASE STUDY 1 EXAMPLE OF THE USE OF A PHARMACOPHORE MODEL IN VIRTUAL SCREENING

Scientists at Schering-Plough reported a novel series of compounds that act to block the cannabinoid (CB1) receptor as potential anti-obesity drugs. One drug that was previously developed in this family is rimonabant, although it was removed from the market due to undesirable side effects. A combination of pharmacophore modeling and virtual screening was used to find lead compounds. The pharmacophore model was based on known ligands for the CB1 receptor and included eight compounds (**Figure 3.19**) with reported activity as antagonists (blockers) and inverse agonists (compounds that bind but with activity opposite to the natural ligand).

After a three-dimensional model of each compound was generated and low-energy conformers of each were found, pharmocophore models were generated by use of the Catalyst/HipHop commercial pharmacophore-generating program. Hydrogen-bond acceptor (HBA), aromatic ring (AR), and hydrophobic (HPO) features were incorporated, and eight different pharmacophore models were generated. Each model was mapped with all eight compounds, and the one pharmacophore that best fit rimonabant was chosen (**Figure 3.20**).

Virtual screening of an in-house virtual library of approximately 500,000 compounds to identify those that adhered to the pharmacophore model was carried out and provided ~22,000 hits. Those hits were filtered for molecular weight and sample availability, as well as other criteria. Remaining compounds met at least three of the following criteria: MW $\leq$ 500, calculated log$P$ $\leq$ 5, number of HBA $\leq$ 10, number of HBD $\leq$ 3, and number of rotatable bonds $\leq$ 10. This filtering step narrowed the pool

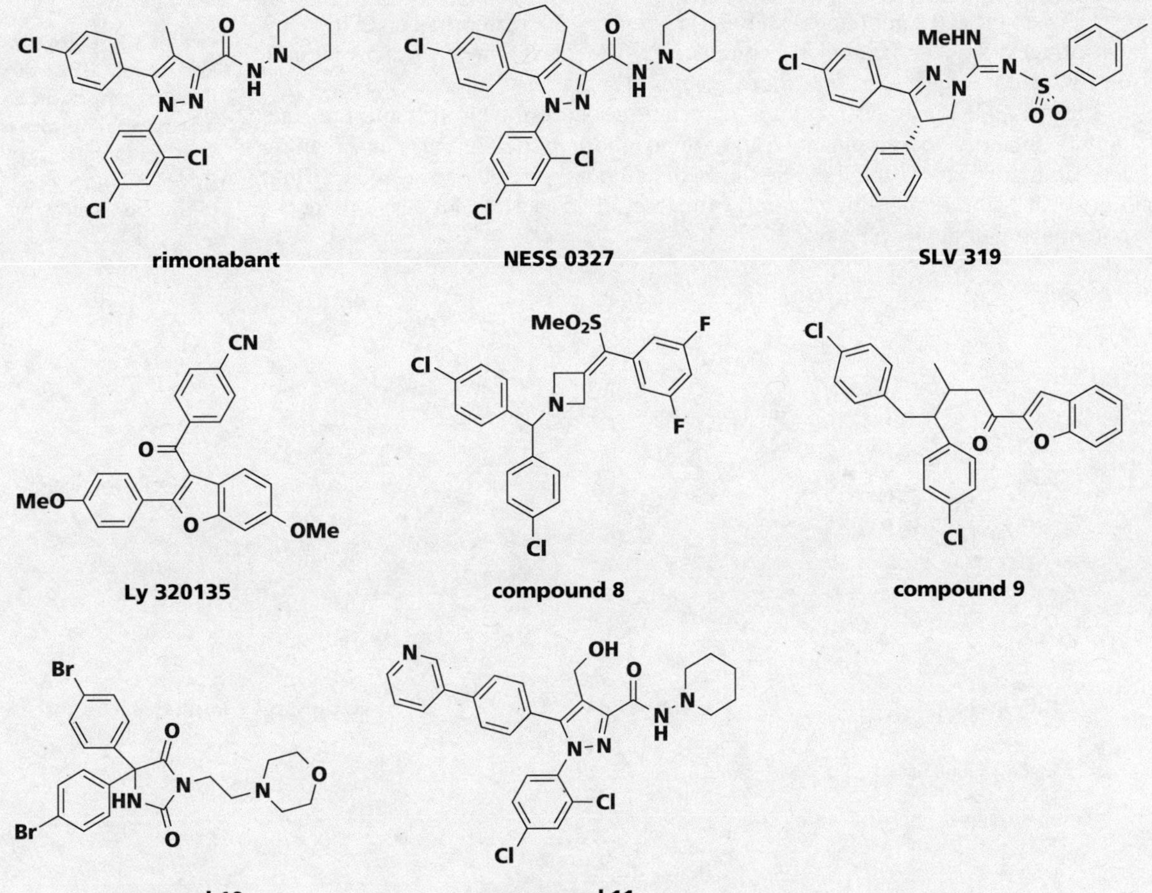

Figure 3.19 Structures of compounds used to develop the pharmacophore model for CB1.

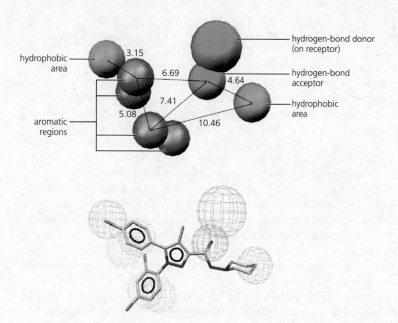

Figure 3.20 CB1 pharmacophore model. Brown spheres = aromatic ring (AR), cyan spheres = hydrophobic area (HPO), and small green sphere = hydrogen-bond acceptor (HBA). Large green sphere = hydrogen-bond donor (HBD) on receptor. Lower part of figure shows rimonabant superimposed onto pharmacophore model. (From Wang H, Duffy RA, Boykow GC et al. [2008] *J Med Chem* 51:2439–2446. With permission from American Chemical Society.)

of hits to 7247 compounds. Further filtering was carried out by developing a model of probability of activity, leading to 2100 compounds. Those compounds were then clustered on the basis of similarity to afford 420 groups, and the compound with the highest predicted activity in each group was selected for testing in a CB1 binding assay. Five of the 420 compounds exhibited greater than 50% inhibition at 0.1 μM. The most attractive was the azetidinone, compound E, which exhibited selectivity for CB1 over CB2 and was a novel scaffold for cannabinoid antagonists (**Figure 3.21**).

This example illustrates a number of techniques described in this and previous chapters, including development of a pharmacophore model and virtual screening based on that model. Using these methods, the authors were able to screen a virtual library of 500,000 compounds to identify a novel scaffold as a lead for development of a potential treatment for obesity.

Figure 3.21 Structures of rimonabant and novel CB1 antagonist compound E, with compound E superimposed on pharmacophore model. (From Wang H, Duffy RA, Boykow GC et al. [2008] *J Med Chem* 51:2439–2446. With permission from American Chemical Society.)

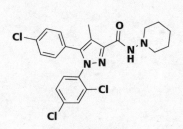

Rimonabant

CB1 K_i = 2.4 nM
CB2 K_i = 560 nM
MW = 464
clog$P$ = 6.5
HBD = 1
HBA = 4
rotatable bonds = 4

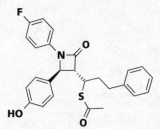

compound E

CB1 K_i = 52.8 nM
CB2 K_i = 282 nM
MW = 450
clog$P$ = 5.5
HBD = 1
HBA = 4
rotatable bonds = 8

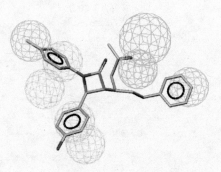

compound E in pharmacophore

CASE STUDY 2   EXAMPLE OF THE USE OF STRUCTURE-BASED DRUG DESIGN

Phosphodiesterases (PDEs) are a class of enzymes that hydrolyze the phosphodiester bonds of nucleotides, usually cGMP or cAMP. Numerous isoforms exist, and several are clinically significant, with PDE3 inhibitors having activity as cardiovascular drugs and the erectile dysfunction drugs, such as sildenafil, acting at PDE5. The isoform PDE10A is expressed in the striatum of the brain, and inhibition is a new target for the treatment of schizophrenia, based on the goal of raising cGMP levels in the striatum. Authors in this study used SBDD to identify a clinical candidate with high selectivity for inhibition of PDE10A. The internal compound library at Pfizer was screened for PDE10A inhibitors, and the triarylimidazole **10** was identified as a hit. The compound exhibited an IC_{50} of 35 nM and >100× selectivity over other PDEs. Co-crystallization of the lead with PDE10A suggested two reasons for the selectivity. First, all PDEs have a conserved glutamine Gln-726. In all previously solved co-structures, this side chain formed a hydrogen bond to inhibitors. However in this case, rather than forming an H-bond, the amine of Gln-726 is positioned above the aromatic ring of the imidazole, forming a cation–π interaction. It is hypothesized that this difference in the specific binding interaction contributes to selectivity. Second, all PDEs have a hydrophobic cleft near the entrance to the active site, but the PDE10A cleft is deeper and has a specific lipophilic pocket known as the selectivity pocket. In this case, the thiophene of **10** occupies that unique selectivity pocket of PDE10A (**Figure 3.22**).

The nature of the selectivity pocket is unique in PDE10A, due to the presence of a small amino acid (glycine) at position 725, next to the conserved Gln-726. All other PDEs have a larger amino acid at that same position, which blocks this pocket. Consequently, this pocket is deeper in PDE10A than in other PDEs. Another observation in the X-ray structure highlighted additional differences: PDE10A contains a Tyr at position 693 in that pocket that may be able to form a hydrogen bond to an inhibitor, while other subtypes do not offer the same H-bonding opportunities.

On the basis of this structural analysis of the hit-enzyme co-crystal, the authors pursued a second round of screening based on compounds that could fit into that lipophilic selectivity pocket and also hydrogen-bond to Tyr-693 in the pocket. Other factors for choosing compounds included early incorporation of druglike physicochemical properties, such as MW < 400, moderate lipophilicity, and minimal number of hydrogen-bond donors. These factors were considered in order to identify compounds likely to cross the lipophilic blood–brain barrier. On the basis of these factors, pyrazole **11** was identified as a hit and analog **12** was the optimized

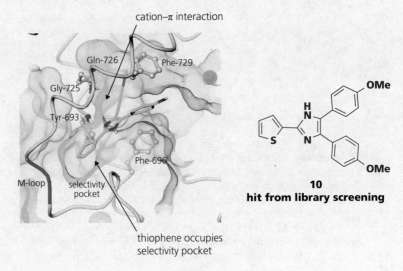

Figure 3.22 Library hit compound 10 co-crystallized with enzyme PDE10A. Important interactions with enzyme include Gln-726 to imidazole cation–π interaction and hydrophobic interactions from occupation of the selectivity pocket with the thiophene moiety. (From Verhoest PR, Chapin DS, Corman M et al. [2009] *J Med Chem* 52:5188–5196. With permission from American Chemical Society.)

cation–π interaction

Gln-726   Phe-729

Gly-725

Tyr-693

Phe-696

M-loop   selectivity pocket

thiophene occupies selectivity pocket

10
hit from library screening

lead, and X-ray analysis of a co-structure confirmed that the quinoline fits into the selectivity pocket and a hydrogen bond between the quinoline nitrogen and Tyr-693 is observed. This compound has greater selectivity for the PDE10A isoform of the enzyme compared to the thiophene hit compound **10**, presumably due to the larger quinoline group that extends farther into the pocket than the original thiophene, as well as the ability to form a hydrogen bond in that pocket. **Figure 3.23** shows the X-ray co-structure, with **11** in orange and **12** in green. Key binding interactions of **12** are the hydrogen bond to Tyr-693 and the cation–π interaction between Gln-726 and the aryl ring. The pyridyl nitrogen also forms a hydrogen bond to a water molecule (top of Figure 3.23) that binds to the backbone of the enzyme. Inhibition is improved from $IC_{50} = 35$ nM for the original compound **10** to $IC_{50} = 0.42$ nM, with >1000× selectivity over other PDEs for **12**.

Although **12** was promising on several levels, such as selectivity and binding affinity, results *in vivo* were not adequate. One secondary assay measured an increase in levels of cyclic guanosine monophosphate (cGMP) as a downstream result of PDE10A inhibition. While **12** did raise cGMP levels in the striatum of mice by 350% at a dose of 10 mg/kg, it had only modest brain penetration, which meant that it was not reaching its target *in vivo*.

SAR analysis was combined with SBDD for further optimization. For example, replacing the nitrogen of the pyridine with carbon, as well as incorporating other aryl groups, led to compounds with reduced activity, confirming the importance of the H-bond to the bridging water molecule. Other heterocycles as substitutes for the pyrazole were investigated, including an isoxazole and a pyrazine, which both had decreased potency. Replacement of the quinoline weakened the important H-bond to Tyr-693 and led to diminished potency. One successful strategy replaced the NH of the pyrazole ring with a methyl group, thereby removing one H-bond donor and increasing lipophilicity; this led to the clinical candidate PF-2545920 (**Figure 3.24**).

Overall, PF-2545920 maintained the best *in vivo* properties and became the first PDE10A inhibitor to enter clinical trials as a potential treatment for schizophrenia.

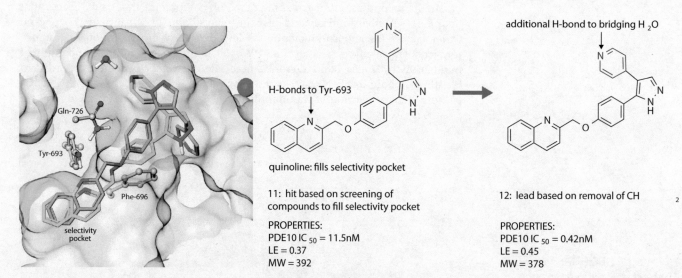

H-bonds to Tyr-693

quinoline: fills selectivity pocket

11: hit based on screening of compounds to fill selectivity pocket

PROPERTIES:
PDE10 IC$_{50}$ = 11.5nM
LE = 0.37
MW = 392

additional H-bond to bridging H$_2$O

12: lead based on removal of CH$_2$

PROPERTIES:
PDE10 IC$_{50}$ = 0.42nM
LE = 0.45
MW = 378

Gln-726
Tyr-693
Phe-696
selectivity pocket

Figure 3.23 X-ray co-structure of 11 and 12 bound to PDE10 showing specific interactions. Structures of hit compound **11**, discovered by virtual screening for compounds that fill the selectivity pocket and make a H-bond to Tyr-693, and optimized lead compound **12**. X-ray structure of **11** (orange) and **12** (green) show occupation of the selectivity pocket by the quinoline, as well as a H-bond to Tyr-693. Also evident are cation–π interaction between Gln-726 and the aryl ring. In the case of **12**, a H-bond between the terminal pyridine and a structural water is also observed. (From Verhoest PR, Chapin DS, Corman M et al. [2009] *J Med Chem* 52:5188–5196. With permission from American Chemical Society.)

Figure 3.24 SAR analysis of lead compound 12, showing optimization to give the clinical candidate PF-2545920.

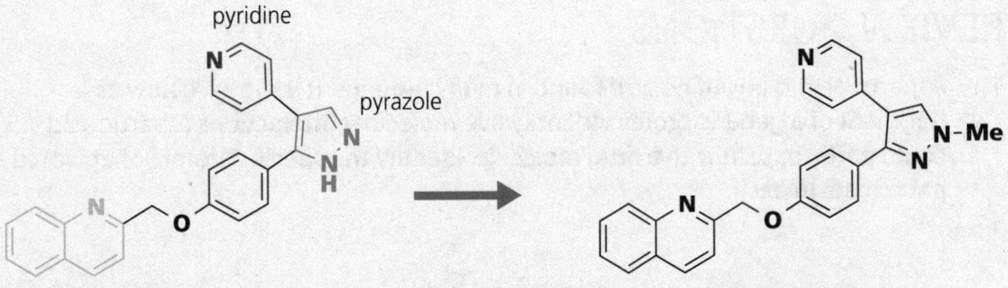

12: quinoline

PF-2545920 clinical candidate

REGIONS OF LEAD **12** SELECTED FOR OPTIMIZATION:
red: pyridine ring
blue: pyrazole
green: quinoline

SAR:

1. 4-pyridine optimal: removal of N, or movement to other positions, gave less active compounds

2. pyrazole: changing NH to N-methyl optimal (improves brain penetration)

3. quinoline (as shown) optimal: other bicyclic heterocycles less active

REVIEW QUESTIONS

1. Aspartic acid is an amino acid found in many proteins. It is drawn below as a fragment of a generic protein. Identify five molecular interactions aspartic acid could participate in with a drug molecule. Identify the specific atom(s) that would participate in each.

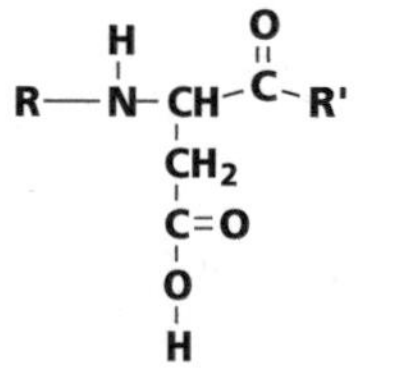

2. If aspartic acid itself were a drug candidate, explain whether desolvation would be an energetically favorable or unfavorable process.

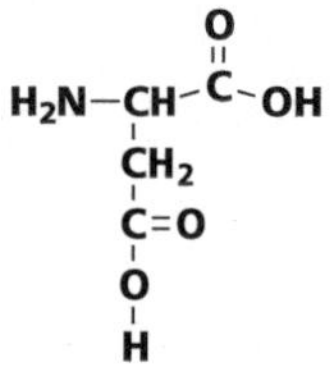

3. List some of the properties that were incorporated in early, historical QSAR models and some of the parameters used to reflect that property.

4. Explain the difference between receptor-excluded volume and receptor-essential area.

5. Define the concept of a pharmacophore.

6. What is required for structure-based drug design?

7. What properties are optimized during the lead optimization process?

8. How does the equilibrium dissociation constant of a drug–target interaction relate to the Gibbs free energy of binding?

9. What is a eudismic ratio?

10. Explain why hydrophobic interactions, despite being weak interactions, are strong contributors to drug–protein binding.

APPLICATION QUESTIONS

1. The three molecules shown here are all potent antagonists at the 5-HT$_6$ receptor.

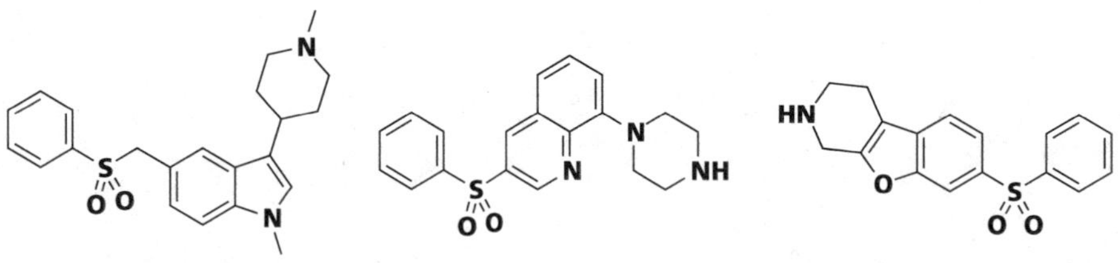

Design a pharmacophore for 5-HT$_6$ antagonism that is consistent with the three structures, and map the pharmacophore onto each compound (that is, identify which part of each molecule represents each pharmacophoric element).

2. Using the three 5-HT$_6$ antagonists in Application Question 1, design three different molecules that test your pharmacophore hypothesis. Explain your design and what you will conclude if testing shows your new compound to (a) maintain or improve activity or (b) lose activity.

3. Pioglitazone is a drug used to treat diabetes. It contains an asymmetric center on the thiadiazinedione ring (indicated by *), yet the racemate is used clinically. Research why the racemic mixture of pioglitazone is used rather than an enantiomerically pure form.

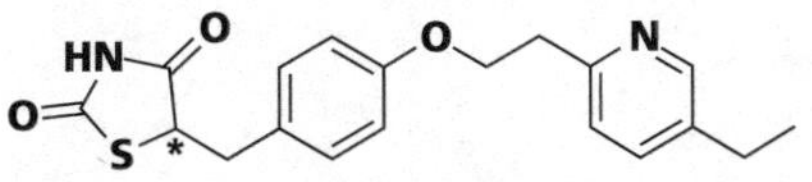

4. A pharmacophore model for monoamine oxidase A inhibitors is shown. It consists of an H-bond donor (D1, blue), two hydrophobic groups (H2, H4 green), and a π-stacking interaction (R6, orange). The three compounds shown beneath adhere to this pharmacophore. Map the features of this pharmacophore onto each structure. (Figure adapted from Shelke SM, Bhosale SH, Dash RC et al. [2001] *Bioorg Med Chem Lett* 21:2419–2424. With permission from Elsevier.)

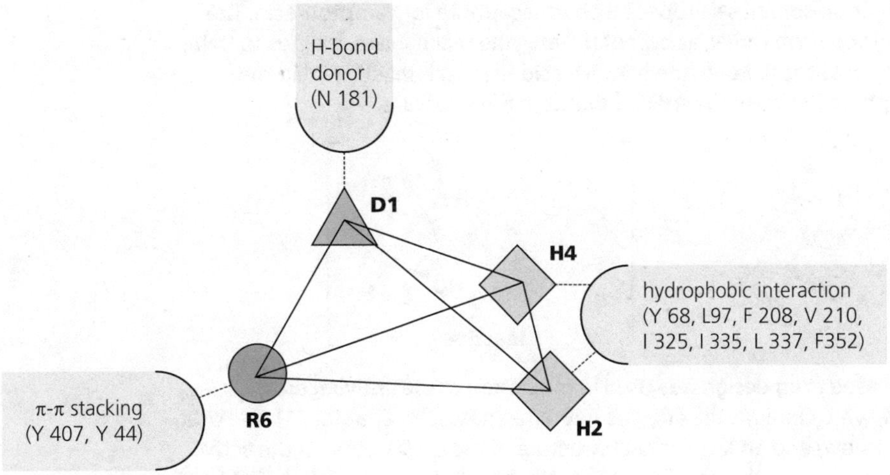

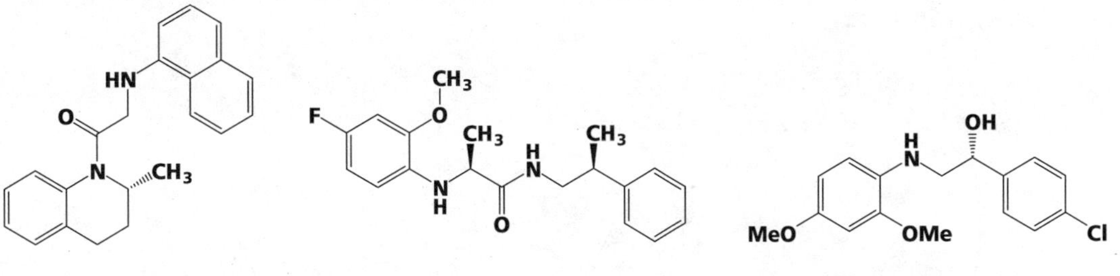

5. Structures of the selective estrogen receptor modulators raloxifene and lasofoxifene are shown. Draw a pharmacophore that is consistent with both structures. Identify the features of each molecule that correspond to each pharmacophoric element (map or label it).

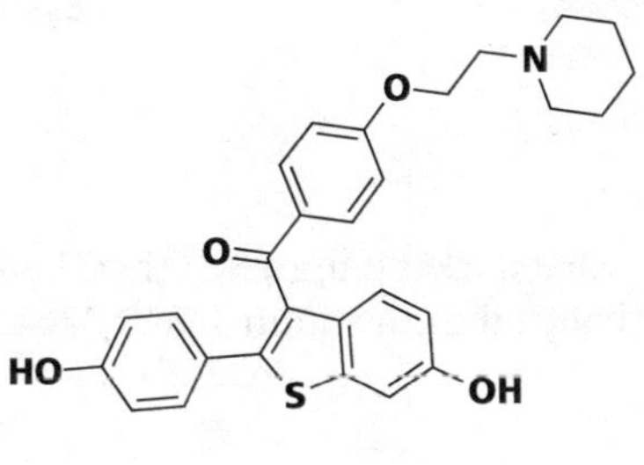

raloxifene

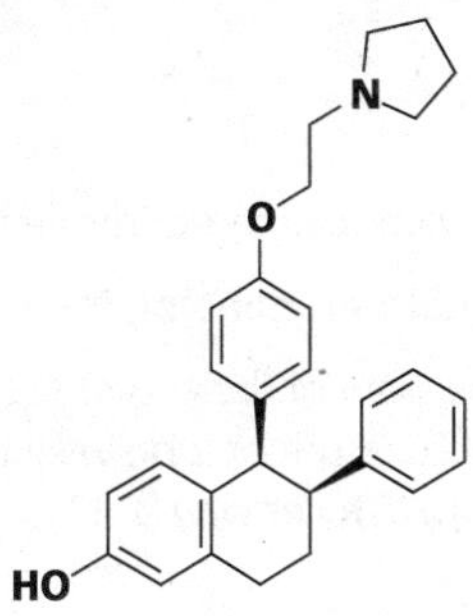

lasofoxifene

6. Identify five types of molecular interactions that the given fragment can make with a protein target. Identify which atoms or moieties are involved in each type of interactions.

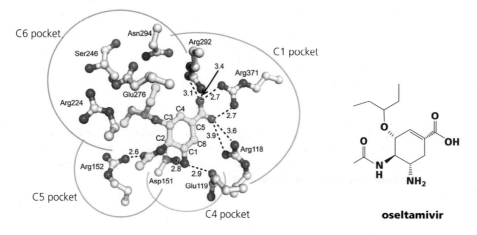

7. Research the structure of biotin and the molecular interactions it makes with streptavidin or avidin. What is its binding constant (K_d)? What are biotin and streptavidin or avidin binding partners used for?

8. Research a drug that works by making a covalent bond to its target. What is the structure of the drug, and what bond is made?

9. Camptothecin is a potent anti-cancer drug whose mechanism is inhibition of the enzyme topoisomerase. Propose a pharmacophore for camptothecin. The information you have is that, as part of the enzyme mechanism, it binds to DNA; the open form of the lactone (the hydroxy acid shown) is inactive. Map the pharmacophore points to the specific points in the structure.

10. Structure-based drug design was used in the design of the antiviral drug oseltamivir, which inhibits the enzyme neuraminidase (see Chapter 11). The drug structure (yellow) and an X-ray crystal structure of the drug bound in the active site of the enzyme are shown. (Figure from Naumov P, Yasuda N, Rabeh WM & Bernstein J [2013] *Chem Commun* 49:1948–1950. With permission from Royal Society of Chemistry.)

(a) Identify a key ionic binding interaction.

(b) Identify a hydrogen-bonding interaction.

(c) Based on the view of the active site, in what pocket is the alkyl ether? Looking at the X-ray structure, might it be wise to change the ether from 3-pentyl to a larger alkyl group? Why or why not?

FURTHER READING

Binding interactions

Smith AJT, Zhang X, Leach AG & Houk KN (2009) Beyond picomolar affinities: quantitative aspects of noncovalent and covalent binding of drugs to proteins. *J Med Chem* 52:225–233.

Ferenczy GG & Keseru GM (2010) Thermodynamics guided lead discovery and optimization. *Drug Discovery Today* 15:919–932.

Friere E (2008) Do enthalpy and entropy distinguish first in class from best in class? *Drug Discovery Today* 13:869–874.

Bissantz C, Kuhn B & Stahl M (2010) A medicinal chemist's guide to molecular interactions. *J Med Chem* 53:5061–5084.

Quantitative structure–activity relationship

Hansch C & Fujita T (1964) ρ–σ–π analysis. A method for the correlation of biological activity and chemical structure. *J Am Chem Soc* 86:1616–1626.

Free SM & Wilson JW (1964) A mathematical contribution to structure–activity studies. *J Med Chem* 7:395–9.

Topliss JG (1972) Utilization of operational schemes for analog synthesis in drug design. *J Med Chem* 15:1006–1111.

Cherkasov A, Muratov EN, Fourches D et al. (2014) QSAR modeling: Where have you been? Where are you going to? *J Med Chem* 47:4977–5010.

Pharmacophore

Leach AR, Gillet VJ, Lewis RA & Taylor R (2010) Three-dimensional pharmacophore methods in drug discovery. *J Med Chem* 53:539–558.

Marshall G, Barry CD, Bosshard HE et al. (1979) The conformation parameter in drug design: the active analog approach. *ACS Symp Ser: Comput-Assisted Drug Des* 112:205–226.

Tebib S, Bourguignon J-J & Wermuth C-J (1987) The active analog approach applied to the pharmacophore identification of benzodiazepine ligands. *J Comput-Aided Drug Des* 1:153–170.

Huang Q, He X, Ma C et al. (2000) Pharmacophore/receptor models for GABA$_A$/Bz subtypes (α1β3γ2, α5β3γ2, and α6β3γ2) via a comprehensive ligand-mapping approach. *J Med Chem* 43:71–95.

Lager E, Andersson P, Nilsson J et al. (2006) 4-Quinolone derivatives: high-affinity ligands at the benzodiazepine site of brain GABA$_A$ receptors. Synthesis, pharmacology, and pharmacophore modeling. *J Med Chem* 49:2526–2533.

Guarav A, Yadav MR, Giridhar R et al. (2011) 3D-QSAR studies of 4-quinolone derivatives as high-affinity ligands at the benzodiazepine site of brain GABA$_A$ receptors. *Med Chem Res* 20:192–199.

Structure-based drug discovery

Lounnas V, Ritschel T, Kelder J et al. (2013) Current progress in structure-based rational drug design marks a new mindset in drug discovery. *Comput Struct Biotechnol J* 5:e20130211.

Erickson J, Neidhart DJ & VanDrie J et al. (1990) Design, activity, and 2.8 A crystal structure of a C2 symmetric inhibitor complexed to HIV-1 protease. *Science* 249: 527–533.

Yamazaki T, Hinck AP & Wang Y-X et al. (1996) Three-dimensional solution structure of the HIV-1 protease complexed with DMP323, a novel cyclic urea-type inhibitor, determined by nuclear magnetic resonance spectroscopy. *Protein Science* 5: 495–506.

Visualizing noncovalent interactions

Johnson ER, Keinan S, Mori-Sánchez P et al. (2010) Revealing noncovalent interactions. *J Am Chem Soc* 132:6498–6506.

Contreras-García J, Johnson ER, Keinan S et al. (2011) NCIPLOT: a program for plotting noncovalent interaction regions. *J Chem Theory Comput* 7:625–632.

Caste studies

Wang H, Duffy RA, Boykow GC et al. (2008) Identification of novel cannabinoid CB1 receptor antagonists by using virtual screening with a pharmacophore model. *J Med Chem* 51:2439–2446.

Verhoest PR, Chapin DS, Corman M et al. (2009) Discovery of a novel class of phosphodiesterase 10A inhibitors and identification of clinical candidate 2-[4-(1-methyl-4-pyridin-4-yl-1H-pyrazol-3-yl)-phenoxymethyl]-quinoline (PF-2545920) for the treatment of schizophrenia. *J Med Chem* 52:5188–5196.

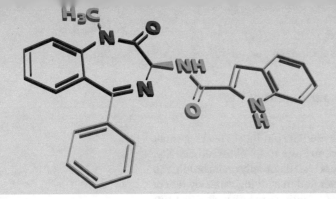

Lead optimization: properties optimized and medicinal chemistry strategies

4

LEARNING OBJECTIVES

- Understand the specific properties that are targeted during lead optimization.
- Become familiar with lead optimization assays and their target values.
- Apply the common rules used during lead optimization.
- Learn multiple strategies that are applied during the lead optimization process.
- Recognize when specific medicinal chemistry strategies should be applied.

The process of lead optimization to obtain a clinical candidate requires multi-parameter optimization of potency, selectivity, and physical and pharmaceutical properties, as well as safety. As described in Chapter 3, understanding the pharmacophore and optimization of binding is one key step in this process. It allows the medicinal chemist to maintain or improve potency and selectivity, and therefore safety, by focusing on the pharmacophoric elements that are essential for biological activity. At the same time, physical and pharmaceutical properties are optimized by maintaining the pharmacophoric features and modifying the portions of the molecule that are not essential to binding. These **druglike properties** are the necessary features for a compound to become a drug and include chemical and metabolic stability, solubility, lipophilicity, and safety, among others. The characteristics of a drug, including binding affinity, biological activity, and the aforementioned druglike properties, are interrelated, and modification of one often affects the others. The challenge for the medicinal chemist is to optimize all of the properties despite their interdependency.

PROPERTIES EVALUATED DURING LEAD OPTIMIZATION

This section describes some of the important biological, physical, and pharmaceutical properties that are evaluated and refined during the lead optimization process. On the basis of target goals for each of these parameters, medicinal chemists employ a number of strategies during the iterative optimization process to eventually generate a clinical candidate. These properties and the target values are described in the following sections, and some specific medicinal chemistry strategies follow. While some of these are categorized according to the property improved, in many cases more than one property is affected, and therefore this division should not be considered absolute.

4.1   Biological activity is optimized as a component of the lead optimization process

Chapter 3 described the molecular interactions that mediate binding between a small molecule and its biological target and how they contribute to its observed activity. However, the biological activity of a small molecule is based not only on its binding to the target but also on other attributes. The data generated in a biological assay reflect the aggregated effects of all these traits. The lead optimization process uses data from increasingly stringent biological assays to inform the iterative rounds of design and synthesis, with the understanding that target binding combined with a number of other properties contribute to the observed effects.

In a typical drug discovery program, primary assays that measure potency and sometimes selectivity toward a biological target are first utilized. These *in vitro* assays are relatively simple; they may be the same assays used during the original hit identification process, and many times (but not always) they measure the activity of the molecule toward a specific biological target. As described in Chapter 2, they can range from assays that quantify the activity of a compound on an isolated protein to a phenotypic screen that measures the effect of a small molecule on a particular cellular phenomenon. Secondary assays are then incorporated to measure potency and efficacy of the molecule in a more complex testing system that often reflects a downstream effect of interference with the primary target. For example, if a primary assay measures the ability of a compound to inhibit an enzyme, a secondary assay could measure the amount of the same enzyme's substrate and product in cells. An effective enzyme inhibitor in a secondary assay would result in accumulated substrate and reduced product levels compared to controls. These assays are more rigorous than primary assays since they require that the small molecule permeate the cell, be stable, reach the specific target, and interact with it, as does the natural substrate. Furthermore, the molecule should not interfere with other biochemical processes that might also be ongoing in the cell. Finally, *in vivo* assays are utilized to evaluate the effects of the compound in animals. *In vivo* assays are considerably more rigorous and relevant compared to primary and secondary assays. The use of a whole animal requires that the compound be absorbed, not be rapidly metabolized and excreted, reach the site of action at appropriate and sustained concentrations, and interact with the specific target to produce a measurable effect that is relevant to the disease, without causing significant side effects. Throughout the progression from primary and secondary *in vitro* to *in vivo* assays, the criteria for advancement become more stringent, and the compounds become further optimized. The three common components evaluated in optimization of biological activity are potency, efficacy, and selectivity.

Potency is the concentration of a compound that is required to achieve the desired effect. In contrast, **affinity** of a molecule, usually measured as a K_d or K_i, reflects its ability to bind to its target. As was defined in Chapter 3, K_d is the dissociation constant of a drug from a drug-target complex. The inhibition constant, K_i, for an enzyme (E) is the equilibrium dissociation constant of an enzyme inhibitor complex where $K_i = [E][I]/[E-I]$. Potency of hits and leads (usually measured as IC_{50} or EC_{50}) at the beginning of the lead optimization process can be in the 1–10 μM range in primary assays, and it is not unusual for hits and early leads to be inactive in secondary and *in vivo* assays. Values targeted during the lead optimization stage and common for clinical candidates are <10 nM in an isolated biochemical assay (primary assay); <100 nM in a cellular assay (secondary assay); and ≤50 mg/kg in an animal model of disease (*in vivo* assay). One common value calculated when a compound is active in *in vivo* models is the **minimum effective dose** (MED), which is the lowest dose that produces a statistically significant desirable effect. ED_{50} refers to the dose that produces 50% of the maximal response.

Efficacy refers to the degree of effect of the compound and is usually measured as a percentage compared to a standard (100%) and technically refers to receptor agonists. However, it is often applied to other systems. For example, complete inhibition of the activity of an enzyme (no substrate is turned over) is considered 100% efficacious. The target efficacy value is determined by the specific disease: in cancer drug discovery, 100% inhibition of tumor growth is required, while in some neuropsychiatric disorders, complete inhibition of neurotransmitter signaling is not desirable and target efficacies may be only 50%.

Selectivity for a specific target, with minimal activity against other biological targets, is an important criterion for the safety of the drug candidate. Usually, compounds will be tested for selectivity against related targets or those that are essential to avoid in a primary assay. Primary, secondary, and *in vivo* assays are also used to detect off-target effects, and ratios of >10–50 fold in favor of the desired target are expected.

4.2   Physical and pharmaceutical properties are optimized in parallel with biological properties

The biological activity of a small molecule is based not only on its binding to the target but also on its physical properties. One barrier to drugs reaching their target is the cell membrane: either cellular membranes they must traverse to reach intracellular targets or those that the compounds must pass through in the GI tract to enter circulation. Therefore, appropriate physical properties based on lipophilicity and aqueous solubility are required for membrane permeability. Furthermore, if a molecule is highly polar, it will prefer to be in an aqueous solution and therefore will never reach nonpolar sites of biological targets, since the desolvation penalty will be high. These properties, in addition to biological activity, must also be optimized during the lead optimization process and are often specifically measured in primary and/or secondary assays. The method by which drugs are eventually administered to humans (oral, intravenous, transdermal, etc.) may require specific physical properties and also must be considered during this stage.

Lipophilicity refers to the affinity of a compound for a lipophilic environment. It relates to a compound's ability to move from an aqueous medium, when first administered, through lipophilic membranes, to be absorbed into the aqueous environment of blood circulation, and then through additional membranes, in order to reach its protein target. While an optimized lead needs to have sufficient lipophilicity, compounds that are highly lipophilic also tend to have higher levels of target promiscuity, leading to safety issues. Compounds that are too hydrophilic (low lipophilicity) will not cross the biological membranes.

Lipophilicity can be measured experimentally by a number of methods, but one of the most common is by partitioning a compound between 1-octanol and water and measuring the concentration of the drug in each layer. As described in Chapter 3, the partition coefficient, P, is the concentration of compound in 1-octanol divided by the concentration in water, and log$P$ is the value most commonly reported. A more useful value for acidic or basic compounds is log$D$, the logarithm of the apparent partition coefficient at a specified pH, which uses a buffered system as the aqueous layer. This important variation eliminates the effects of the test compound's acidity or basicity on the aqueous solution and therefore takes into account the ionization state of the molecule being measured. Log$D$ values always include the pH at which they were measured: for example, log $D_{7.4}$ indicates that the measurement was taken at pH 7.4. As an alternative to experimental methods, calculated log$P$ values (referred to according to the specific program used, such as cLog$P$, aLog$P$, or xLog$P$) are available in chemical drawing programs and in cheminformatics and computational chemistry software.

In order to optimize lipophilicity, a careful analysis of the functional groups in a hit or lead molecule is required. For compounds that contain a large number of polar functionalities (low log$P$), elimination, replacement, or incorporation of additional hydrophobic or lipophilic groups (such as halogens or alkyl groups) is considered. For those compounds whose log$P$ value is too high, introduction of heteroatoms is a frequent strategy.

Lipophilicity is an important characteristic of drugs that passively cross the blood–brain barrier (BBB). Rather than the typical log$P$ value of 2–4 for orally available drugs, molecules that cross the BBB fall in a slightly higher range of 3–5.

Solubility is another important characteristic of drugs, and it is influenced by the lipophilicity of the molecule. Drugs will be in an aqueous environment in the body and should have acceptable aqueous solubility. This characteristic, like lipophilicity, is related to a compound's ability to be absorbed into the bloodstream and cross biological membranes. A compound must be in solution in order to be permeable. In addition, the aqueous solubility of a compound will also allow it to be easily formulated for delivery to animals and humans such that consistent levels are absorbed. Solubility depends on the specific functional groups within the molecule as well as the physical characteristics of the solid. Features that increase aqueous solubility include the presence of hydrogen-bonding and ionizable groups. Both kinetic and thermodynamic solubility are usually measured at physiological pH, and typical values are in the range 5–100 μM.

Permeability is a property that relies on both solubility and lipophilicity of a compound. In order to reach the desired target organ, compounds need to be lipophilic enough to permeate a cell membrane but hydrophilic enough to be soluble. Permeability of a lead compound can be measured in primary assays such as a parallel artificial membrane permeability assay (PAMPA) that measures the rate of passage through an artificial membrane. A common secondary assay is the Caco-2 assay, which measures rate of transit through a monolayer of epithelial cells. Permeability is measured as a rate and is characterized by comparison to reference standards. High or medium permeability is preferred, and having highly permeable compounds with low or moderate solubility can sometimes still be acceptable. For instance, all other things being equal, to achieve a projected dose of 1 mg/kg, a compound with medium permeability will require aqueous solubility of about 50 μM, whereas a compound with high permeability might require solubility of only about 10 μM.

Pharmaceutical properties are evaluated by absorption, distribution, metabolism, and elimination (ADME) studies, which are discussed in more detail in Chapter 5. While these evaluations become increasingly detailed as a lead is optimized to a clinical candidate, early indications of some of these properties are an important component of the lead optimization phase of drug discovery. For example, a prediction of *in vivo* metabolic stability may come from an *in vitro* assay based on incubation with liver microsomes that contain active metabolic enzymes. Although a compound may exhibit suitable chemical stability in pH 7.4 buffer, it may be rapidly degraded in the presence of metabolic enzymes in liver microsomes.

Another desirable pharmaceutical property is oral bioavailability, which is measured in early *in vivo* models. **Oral bioavailability** is the concentration of drug in the blood after oral dosing, as compared to the concentration after intravenous dosing. High oral bioavailability allows a low dose to be administered, thereby reducing the risk of off-target effects that might occur if high doses of compound were required. A low dose also translates to other benefits such as simpler formulation development, easier dosing regiment for the patient, and ultimately, lower cost of the drug substance. A highly permeable, soluble, and metabolically stable compound will most likely have high oral bioavailability.

These biological, physical, and pharmaceutical properties are interrelated. For example, a compound that is highly potent in secondary cell-based biological assays will, by necessity, be permeable and soluble. Conversely, if a compound is highly potent in primary biochemical assays but not in secondary cellular biological assays, poor physical and pharmaceutical properties may be the culprit. While each specific project or disease therapy has specific requirements for biological, physical, and pharmaceutical properties, **Table 4.1** summarizes the characteristics and values that are generally targeted. Most of these properties are measured routinely throughout the iterative design, synthesis and assay process, with *in vivo* assays being implemented on fewer compounds at the latter stages.

OPTIMIZATION OF LEAD PROPERTIES

Modifying the lead structure optimizes the specific properties outlined in Table 4.1. The data generated in the assays described above are analyzed, and new compounds are designed that are predicted to have improved properties. In the following sections, tools and strategies that have been developed to aid the medicinal chemist are described.

Table 4.1 Summary of some properties and measurements evaluated during lead optimization.

Biological properties	
affinity	tendency of a small molecule to associate with its target
	measured in primary binding assays
	target values: K_d or K_i < 10 nM
	impacts potency, safety, and eventual dose of final drug substance
potency	concentration or dose at which a compound elicits a specific effect
	measured in primary, secondary, and *in vivo* assays
	target values for primary and secondary assays: IC_{50} and EC_{50} < 10 nM in isolated system; <1 μM in cell-based system[a]
	target values for *in vivo* assays: ED_{50} or EC_{50} < 50 mg/kg
	minimum effective dose (MED) <50 mg/kg (lowest dose possible is desirable)
	related to eventual dose and safety of compounds in humans
efficacy	degree of a given biological response (technically refers to receptor agonists)
	measured in primary, secondary, and *in vivo* assays reported as a percentage, usually compared to a control
	target value is determined by specific indication and protein target
	reflects the physiological effect of the compound
selectivity	ratio of magnitude of desired effect compared to undesired effect
	usually calculated as a ratio of potency and/or affinity in primary, secondary, and *in vivo* assays
	target values are usually >10 but may be as low as 2 for some life-threatening diseases
	reflects the safety of the drug
Physical and pharmaceutical properties	
aqueous solubility	amount of compound that dissolves in an aqueous solution, under either kinetic or thermodynamic conditions
	measured in primary (kinetic) and secondary (thermodynamic) assays; values of >10 μM are targeted
	related to a compound's ability to cross biological membranes, to be absorbed after administration, and to be formulated for delivery to animals and humans
lipophilicity	affinity of a compound for lipophilic environment
	measured in primary and secondary assays by various measurements such as partition coefficients
	target values are 2–4 for log*P* or log*D*
	reflects the ability of a compound to cross biological membranes, its safety, and its ability to be formulated
permeability	rate at which a compound transits across a membrane
	measured in various primary or secondary assays such as PAMPA (primary) or Caco-2 (secondary)
	high or medium permeability is preferred
	reflects ability of the drug to reach the bloodstream or the target organ

(Continued)

Table 4.1   Summary of some properties and measurements evaluated during lead optimization (*Continued*).

metabolic stability	ability of compound to withstand metabolic transformation by liver enzymes
	measured in primary or secondary assays, such as liver microsomes, to detect half-life of compound
	$T_{1/2} > 60$ min is ideal, although very long $T_{1/2}$ may be unsafe
	contributes to drug achieving concentrations at the site of action that are essential for efficacy at the lowest dose possible
oral bioavailability	concentration of drug in the blood via oral route, compared to concentration achieved with intravenous administration
	measured in animal models; values of >50% are preferred
	when preferred human dosing regimen is via oral route, high oral bioavailability ensures consistent drug concentrations are achieved at lowest possible doses
state (solid, liquid)	physical state of compound
	measured via melting point or differential scanning calorimetry (DSC)
	crystalline, nonhygroscopic, stable samples preferred
	will affect solubility, stability, and reproducibility of drug sample

[a]IC_{50} = concentration that reduces response by 50%; EC_{50} = concentration that causes 50% of maximal response; ED_{50} = median dose that causes 50% of maximal response.

4.3   Rules and metrics have been developed to aid the lead optimization process

A number of metrics have been developed and are used by medicinal chemists as a guide during the optimization process. Applying these metrics and rules, specific properties (biological, physical, and pharmaceutical) are identified that need to be improved during the iterative design, synthesis, and testing cycle, and newly designed analogs aim to improve on these metrics. These metrics and rules are not steadfast, but they provide a tool that helps simplify a complex, multidimensional set of interdependent properties.

Several different metrics are used in order to assess the value of specific atoms or fragments of a compound. These include ligand efficiency and lipophilic ligand efficiency, which evaluate atoms' or a fragment's contribution to affinity and potency and to lipophilicity, respectively. **Ligand efficiency** (LE) assesses and compares compounds on the basis of how efficiently they bind (affinity). This metric is a ratio of the molecular weight of a molecule compared to its affinity and is defined as the free energy of binding of a ligand averaged for each non-hydrogen or heavy atom (HAC = heavy atom count). The term used for the binding parameter is ideally K_d or K_i, but EC_{50} or IC_{50} values can also be substituted. If it is assumed that an oral drug candidate should have MW ≤ 500 and K_d or K_i (or EC_{50} or IC_{50}) <10 nM, then an LE of ≥ 0.3 is considered a desirable number.

$$LE = -\Delta G / HAC \cong -RT \ln K_d \text{ (or } IC_{50} \text{ or } EC_{50}) / HAC \qquad (4.1)$$

For $T = 300$ K, this equation can be simplified to

$$LE = -1.37 / HAC \times \log K_d \text{ (or } pIC_{50}) \text{ (where } pIC_{50} = -\log IC_{50})$$

This concept allows for evaluation and comparison of hits and leads on the basis of their efficiency of binding, and it sets a goal (≥ 0.3) or direction (greater LE) for medicinal chemistry efforts. Ligand efficiency refers to the whole molecule, whereas the idea of group efficiency (GE) refers to specific functional groups within the molecule. Within a series of similar analogs, the value of individual groups can be assessed by comparing changes in free energy of binding that occur when a functional group is changed. In this case, HAC refers to the heavy atom count of the individual group.

As an example of how to use ligand efficiency metrics, consider two compounds, A and B, that both have IC_{50} values of 10 nM. Compound A contains 30 non-hydrogen atoms, but compound B has 40 non-hydrogen atoms. Using the equation $LE = -RT \ln IC_{50}/HAC$, and $\ln IC_{50} = -18.4$, the calculated LE values (at 298 K) for compounds A and B would be calculated as follows:

compound A:

$$LE = -(0.00198 \, \text{kcal/deg} \cdot \text{mol})(298 \, \text{K})(-18.4)/30 \, \text{atoms} = 0.36$$

compound B:

$$LE = -(0.00198 \, \text{kcal/deg} \cdot \text{mol})(298 \, \text{K})(-18.4)/40 \, \text{atoms} = 0.27$$

In this example, even though both compounds have identical potency, the efficiency with which they achieve that potency differs. Compound A requires fewer atoms (and has a higher LE, 0.36) than compound B to exhibit the same potency. During the optimization process, efficiency is considered carefully and monitored, and modifications that improve potency and maintain or even improve efficiency are preferred.

Ligand lipophilic efficiency (LLE) or lipophilic ligand efficiency (LipE) is a gauge of how the lipophilicity of a compound contributes to its potency. It is defined as activity minus log$P$ (either experimental or calculated, clog P) and can be used as an assessment of the molecule's affinity for its target versus its general affinity for a lipophilic environment.

$$LLE = LipE = pIC_{50} - \log P \tag{4.2}$$

For compounds that will be administered via oral dosing, an LLE of 5_7 is targeted. An example of the use of LLE in the optimization of a series of HIV nonnucleoside reverse transcriptase inhibitors is shown in **Figure 4.1**. An early compound (**1**) exhibited potency of 0.66 μM (IC_{50}) and had a clog$P$ of 4.3 and therefore an LLE of 1.9. Substituting cyano groups for the chlorines and an oxygen for the methylene led to **2** (lersivirine), with a lower clog$P$ of 2.1 and greater potency ($IC_{50} = 0.12$ μM), and therefore an improved LLE of 4.9. Maintaining a high LE and optimal LLE often helps guide the optimization process.

In addition to metrics that focus on optimizing each fragment for contributions to potency and lipophilicity, rules have been developed for optimization of the pharmaceutical property of oral availability. In order for a drug to be orally available, it needs to survive the acidic environment of the gastrointestinal tract, be able to penetrate membranes (either through passive or active transport), and survive the metabolic machinery of the liver. Some of the general factors that can decrease oral bioavailability include export by transporter enzymes and first-pass metabolism.

In 1997, Christopher Lipinski and co-workers at Pfizer proposed a set of rules that predict the likelihood of a compound being orally bioavailable. The **Lipinski rules**, known as the **rule of five** (Ro5), are based on observations of common features of compounds that had progressed to phase II clinical trials and were dosed orally. A modified version, proposed by Miles Congreve and co-workers at Astex, applies to the smaller molecular weight hits identified in fragment-based drug discovery and is called the **rule of three**. Another set of rules was proposed in 2002 by Daniel Veber and co-workers at GlaxoSmithKline to predict oral availability. The **Veber rules** incorporate molecular flexibility and polar surface area and take into account the unexpected oral bioavailability of certain larger molecular weight drugs. Both sets of rules are summarized in **Table 4.2**. While these correlations are termed rules, there are a significant number of

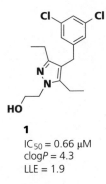

1

$IC_{50} = 0.66$ μM
clog$P = 4.3$
LLE = 1.9

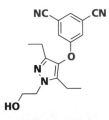

2 (lersivirine)

$IC_{50} = 0.12$ μM
clog$P = 2.1$
LLE = 4.9

Figure 4.1 Optimization of LLE in a series of reverse transcriptase inhibitors. Compound 1 exhibited an LLE = 1.9; to improve the LLE, the linkage to the aryl ring was replaced with the more polar oxygen atom, and the substituents on aryl ring were replaced with nitriles to give Compound 2 (changes are shown in red). These changes decreased clog$P$, increased potency and improved the LLE to 4.9.

Table 4.2   Rules for optimization of oral bioavailability.

Lipinski rules: rule of five[a]
A compound must have no more than five hydrogen-bond donors (counted by the number of NH and OH groups).
There must be no more than 10 hydrogen-bond acceptors (counted by the number of N and O atoms).
The molecular weight must be under 500 daltons.
The $\log P$ (partition coefficient; lipophilicity) must be no more than 5.
Variation of Lipinski rules: rule of three[b]
A compound should have no more than three hydrogen-bond donors.
There should be no more than three hydrogen-bond acceptors.
The molecular weight should be under 300 daltons
The $\log P$ should be no more than 3.
Veber rules
A compound should have no more than 10 rotatable bonds.
The hydrogen-bond count (donors and acceptors) should be no more than 12, or polar surface area (PSA) should be no more than 140 $(\text{Å})^2$.

[a]All of the components of the rules are multiples of five.
[b]Used most often in fragment-based screening and hit triage.

drugs that deviate from them, such as Lipitor, at one time the world's best-selling drug. Therefore, they are typically used as guidelines to consider during the optimization process. Drug discovery scientists are still trying to understand what physical properties of drugs are most important to consider during the optimization process and which accurately predict oral bioavailability and drug development success.

SPECIFIC STRATEGIES TO ADDRESS DEFICIENCIES IN LEAD STRUCTURES

The overall goal of lead optimization is to take a promising lead and progress it to a druglike clinical candidate. While the rules and metrics described above can be used as target values, the following sections describe specific medicinal chemical strategies that are applied to improve physical and pharmaceutical properties of drug candidates. The improvements in properties typically also result in improvements to potency, and therefore these strategies cannot be considered in isolation.

4.4   Lipophilicity is optimized so that a drug can reach its target

Lipophilicity is one of the most important physical characteristics of a drug candidate. If a drug is too lipophilic, it will not be soluble, or it may compartmentalize into lipid membranes, never reaching its target tissue or organ. Lipophilic compounds are known to bind indiscriminately to proteins, thereby preventing them from reaching their targets. Furthermore, highly lipophilic compounds are often more rapidly metabolized than less lipophilic compounds, decreasing their bioavailability. Conversely, compounds that are not lipophilic enough may not cross cell membranes and may be so highly solvated that binding to the target protein is not a favorable process. Therefore, the appropriate balance between hydrophobicity and hydrophilicity is essential.

Aurora kinase inhibitor

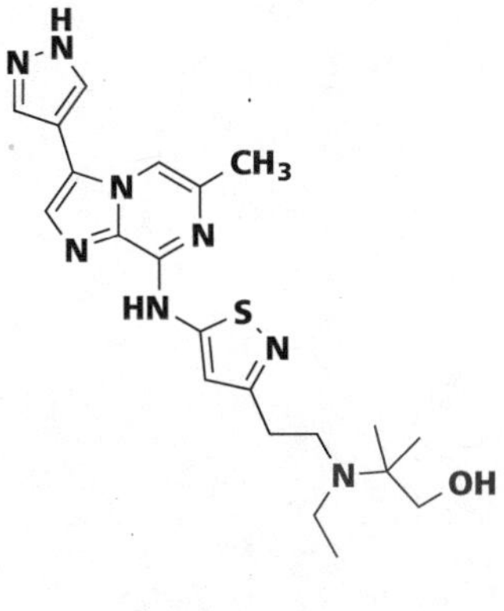

SCH 1473759

Figure 4.2 Optimization of solubility by incorporating polar functional groups. To improve the aqueous solubility of an aurora kinase inhibitor, the azepine was replaced with an acyclic alcohol moiety (changes are shown in red) resulting in SCH 1473759 that displayed 500 × greater solubility than the original Aurora kinase inhibitor.

4.5   Leads need to be optimized for solubility in aqueous media

Small-molecule binding sites on a protein target are often lipophilic, and therefore potent hits and leads may likewise be lipophilic, and they often suffer from poor or low aqueous solubility. However, high solubility is a prerequisite for both *in vitro* and *in vivo* activity, so improving solubility may be a significant effort during the optimization stage. The two most important factors affecting aqueous solubility in the context of medicinal chemistry are the polarity of the molecule and the crystal lattice energy of the solid crystal form; thus, the most commonly applied strategies to improve solubility are the introduction of polar solubilizing groups and disruption of crystal packing.

Adding aqueous solubilizing groups, a common method to improve solubility, typically involves adding polar functional groups such as alcohols, amines, or acids to sites of the molecule that are not required for binding to the target. In addition to adding hydrophilicity, some of these functional groups also offer the opportunity to make salts of the molecule that may further increase solubility. In the example shown in **Figure 4.2**, replacing the azepine ring (seven-membered ring) in an Aurora kinase inhibitor with the more polar acyclic alcohol (shown in red) improved solubility by almost 500-fold. An X-ray co-crystal structure of SCH 1473759 bound to Aurora A kinase showed that the alcohol group extended out of the binding pocket, and into a solvent-accessible site.

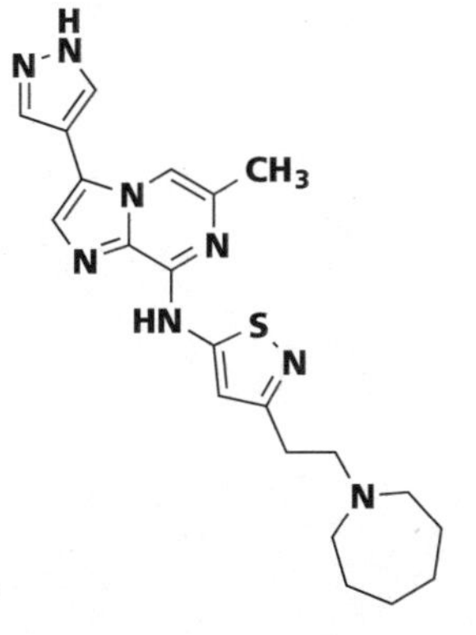

A second strategy to improve solubility is disruption of crystal packing. This approach is most often applied when there is evidence of high crystal lattice energy, such as a high melting point and/or small-molecule X-ray crystal structure showing numerous intermolecular interactions. By incorporation of functional groups that disrupt those interactions, lower melting points and higher water solubility are obtained.

This strategy was successfully applied to a series of inhibitors of B-Raf^{V600E} kinase that showed potential as anti-cancer agents. The small-molecule X-ray structure of the original compound showed a head-to-tail arrangement and four hydrogen bonds between two molecules. (**Figure 4.3**) In addition, π-stacking and hydrogen bonds were also observed with molecules above and below the plane of the dimers. These interactions combined to afford high crystal packing lattice energy. Replacement of one aryl fluorine with a larger chlorine atom interfered with the dimer interface, and substitution of the methoxy group with a cyclopropane disrupted the π-stacking between planes of the dimer (analog B, changes are in red). By designing a molecule that disrupted some of these interactions, a >10-fold improvement in aqueous solubility was observed along with >50° decrease in melting point.

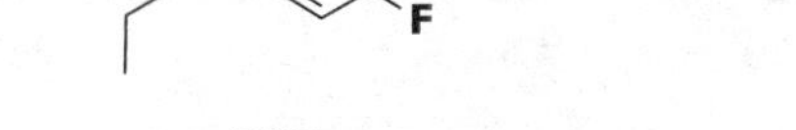

Figure 4.3 Optimization of solubility by disruption of crystal lattice. Inhibitor A self-associates through hydrogen bonds (shown as dashed lines) and π-stacking between planes. Incorporation of the larger chlorine atom and a cyclopropyl group (shown in red) disrupts hydrogen bonding and π-stacking and leads to higher aqueous solubility in analog B.

B-Raf^{V600E} kinase inhibitor A: strong crystal lattice
AQUEOUS SOLUBILITY:
9 µg/mL at pH 6.5, 7.4

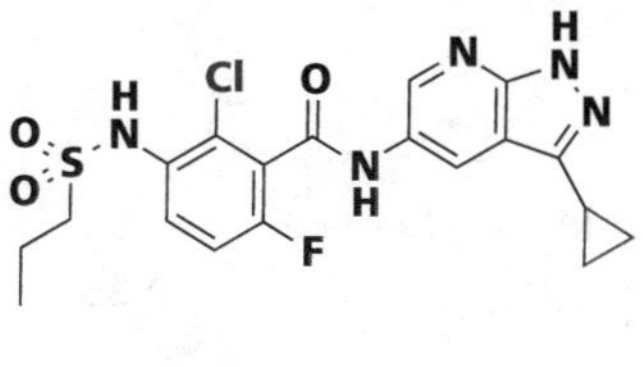

analog B: disrupted crystal lattice
AQUEOUS SOLUBILITY:
127 µg/mL at pH 6.5, 7.4

4.6   Optimization of metabolic stability is a necessary component of lead optimization

One of the most frequent causes of poor bioavailability is rapid metabolism of the lead molecule, typically through oxidative processes. The process of metabolism will be described fully in Chapter 5; however, a common early strategy is to identify the metabolically labile positions and minimize the potential to be oxidized by metabolic enzymes. Standard strategies include reducing lipophilicity (more lipophilic compounds are more likely to be metabolized), inverting stereochemistry (metabolic processes may be stereoselective), modifying the steric environment of the metabolic site, manipulating electronic characteristics, and introducing conformational constraints. For example, introduction of fluorine is a common method to improve metabolism. Its small size may not drastically change the conformation of the active molecule. In some examples, direct replacement of a metabolically labile hydrogen atom or methyl group with a fluorine atom or trifluoromethyl group, respectively, physically blocks metabolism. Alternatively, introduction of a fluorine atom or another electron-withdrawing group on an aromatic ring deactivates the entire ring toward oxidative metabolism and will often improve metabolic stability.

The introduction of deuterium in order to block metabolism is a similar strategy. In these cases, due to the deuterium isotope effect, cleavage of a C–D bond may be 10 × slower than cleavage of the corresponding C–H bond, slowing drug metabolism and increasing metabolic stability. Recently, the first deuterium-containing drug was approved. Deutetrabenazine replaces six hydrogen atoms in a previously known drug, tetrabenazine, with deuterium atoms. This change results in significantly longer half-life of the drug and active metabolites.

Increasing steric hindrance at or near the site of metabolism is another frequently applied approach. In the example shown in **Figure 4.4**, the *N*-methylpiperazine of a potential allergy medication was found to be rapidly metabolized, particularly through demethylation (red). On the other hand, the sterically encumbered and conformationally constrained bicyclic piperazines are typically considerably more stable to metabolism. When these moieties were incorporated into the parent molecule, stability toward metabolism was significantly improved. Within the same series, reducing the lipophilicity by replacement of the piperazine with a smaller aminopyrrolidine or aminoazetidine also produced a stabilizing effect, as measured by the percent of compound remaining after incubation with rat liver microsomes (RLM).

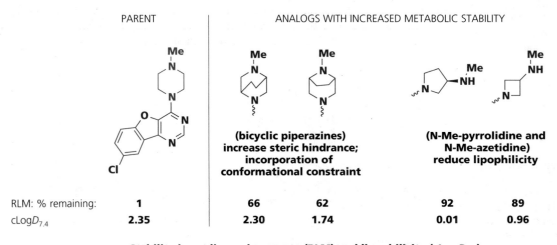

	PARENT	ANALOGS WITH INCREASED METABOLIC STABILITY			
		(bicyclic piperazines) increase steric hindrance; incorporation of conformational constraint		(N-Me-pyrrolidine and N-Me-azetidine) reduce lipophilicity	
RLM: % remaining:	1	66	62	92	89
cLog$D_{7.4}$	2.35	2.30	1.74	0.01	0.96

Stability in rat liver microsomes (RLM) and lipophilicity (cLog$D_{7.4}$)

Figure 4.4 Optimization of metabolic stability by increasing steric bulk, introducing conformational constraint and modifying lipophilicity. The parent compound (left) is rapidly metabolized at the *N*-methylpiperazine group (shown in red), with only 1% remaining after incubation with rat liver microsomes (RLM). Replacement of the piperazine with conformationally constrained and more sterically hindered bicyclic piperazines, or decreasing ring size (to five or four membered rings) to reduce lipophilicity (right) improved metabolic stability as evidenced by the increased % remaining.

4.7   Targeting strategies and the use of prodrugs improve drug properties

When physical properties of a drug are nonoptimal, a prodrug strategy can sometimes be applied to solve the problem. A **prodrug** is a molecule, typically inactive, that when metabolized within the body affords the active drug molecule. This approach is used to solve issues of poor permeability and/or solubility and thereby improve oral bioavailability. However, it can also be applied to affect distribution of the drug and improve safety, among other characteristics. It has been estimated that between 5% and 7% of all approved drugs are actually prodrugs. In general, however, prodrug strategies are applied only when other strategies have been unsuccessful. The reasons for this are based on several factors, including a relatively poor understanding and predictability of the biological processes and phenomena that can be exploited for prodrug design and the additional complications during the drug development process that prodrugs can encounter due to the fact that two molecules, the prodrug and the active drug, need to be studied and characterized. A schematic of the use of a prodrug with a masked functional group is shown in Figure 4.5.

One of the functional groups most frequently masked in a prodrug is a carboxylic acid. The charged, polar nature of the acid can severely impede its permeability, thereby making these drug candidates ineffective since they never reach their intended biological target. In these instances, the acid can be masked as a hydrolyzable group such as an ester, amide, carbonate, or other acid derivative that is less polar and more permeable, and usually inactive. Once absorbed, the derivative is cleaved by physiological enzymes to reveal the active acid moiety and the by-product, which is often a biologically inert molecule.

The influenza drug oseltamivir is one example of a prodrug (Figure 4.6A). It is administered as an ethyl ester and, once absorbed, is cleaved by physiological esterases to generate the carboxylic acid, the active molecule. By use of an ethyl ester prodrug rather than the acid, the oral bioavailability of the active molecule improves from 5% to over 80%. A second example is the anti-cancer drug irinotecan. The active drug SN-38 (Figure 4.6B) is highly insoluble and therefore is difficult to formulate. By incorporation of a water-solubilizing prodrug, the dipiperadinocarbamate, the solubility and formulation problem was solved.

In the first two examples in Figure 4.6, the prodrug was designed for cleavage by nonspecific esterases or other physiological enzymes. However, an alternate strategy incorporates a prodrug moiety that is specifically recognized by transporters or enzymes in or near certain cells or organs in the body, thereby accumulating and/or releasing the active molecule only at the site of action. In this manner, the drug can be targeted and may be more efficacious and less toxic. This strategy has been most often applied to central nervous system (CNS) and cancer targets due to the unique

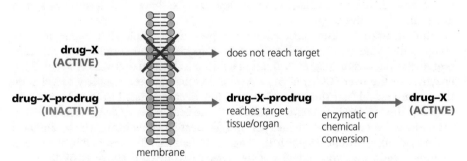

Figure 4.5 Schematic of prodrug crossing biological barrier that the active drug cannot. The active agent (drug-X, where X indicates a group required for activity but that also contributes to poor permeability) cannot cross the membrane, so no drug reaches its target. The prodrug, where X is masked by a hydrolyzable functional group, can cross the membrane by virtue of improved properties. Biotransformation inside the barrier affords the active drug.

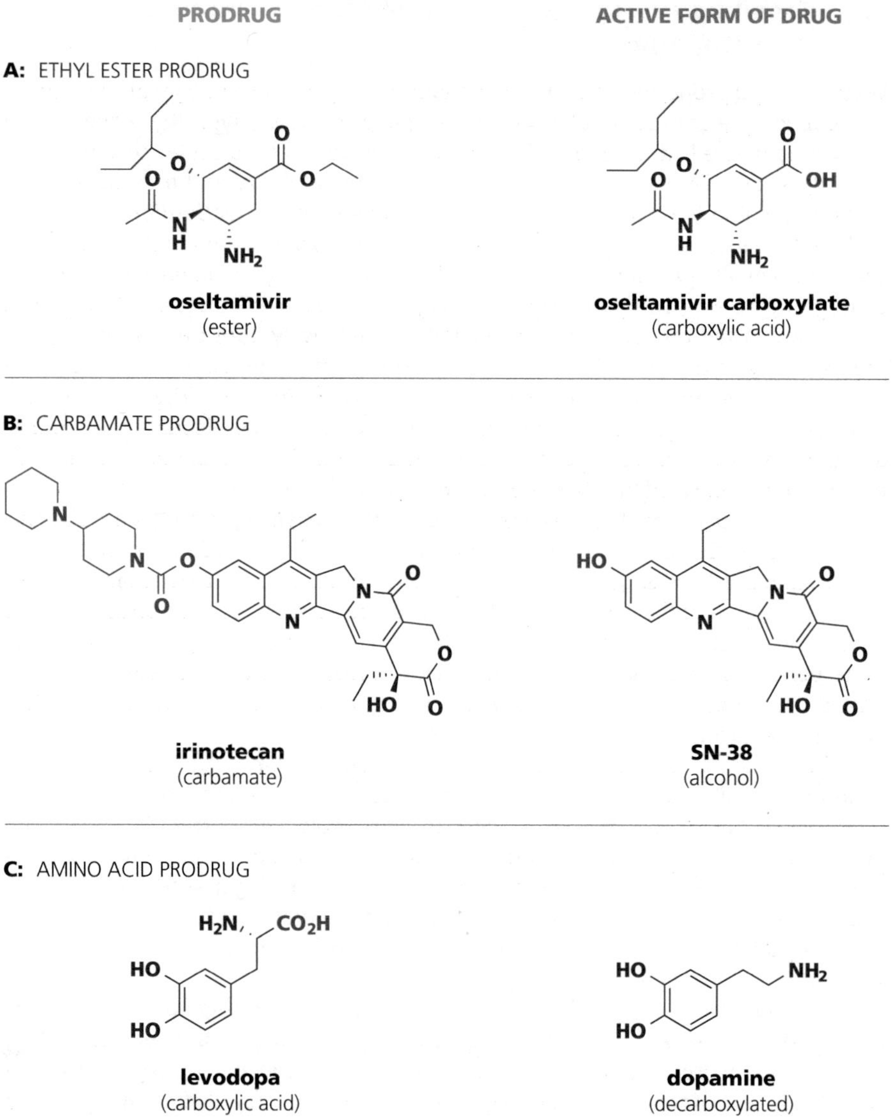

PRODRUG ACTIVE FORM OF DRUG

A: ETHYL ESTER PRODRUG

oseltamivir
(ester)

oseltamivir carboxylate
(carboxylic acid)

B: CARBAMATE PRODRUG

irinotecan
(carbamate)

SN-38
(alcohol)

C: AMINO ACID PRODRUG

levodopa
(carboxylic acid)

dopamine
(decarboxylated)

Figure 4.6 Prodrug examples. A: The ethyl ester in oseltamivir is cleaved to generate the active carboxylic acid, and provides a significant increase in bioavailability compared to the acid. B: The prodrug carbamate in irinotecan shows improved solubility. C: Levopoda is recognized by a CNS-specific transporter, and accumulates in the brain, where it is decarboxylated to generate the active dopamine. Prodrug functional groups in red.

features of the blood–brain barrier and the tumor environment, respectively. The drug levodopa, used for Parkinson's disease, is one such example (**Figure 4.6C**). It is a substrate for a brain-specific transporter called large neutral amino acid transporter (LAT1) and therefore accumulates in the brain. Once there, it is decarboxylated to dopamine, the active drug.

The anti-cancer drug capecitabine is a prodrug example that highlights how complex the route to the active moiety can be. Capecitabine undergoes three different biotransformations to generate 5-fluorouracil, an established anti-cancer agent. First, enzymes in the liver (CES1, CES2) cleave the carbamate ester moiety to generate the carbamic acid (not shown), which is rapidly decarboxylated to form 5'-deoxy-5-fluorocytidine (5'-dFCyd). Enzymes called cytidine deaminases (CDA) that are located primarily in liver and tumor tissues perform the next bioconversion, which generates 5'-deoxy-5-fluorouridine (5'-dFUrd). Finally, an enzyme that is highly expressed in tumor cells, deoxythymidine phosphorylase (dThdPase), converts 5'-dFUrd to the active substance, 5-fluorouracil (5-FU), as shown in **Figure 4.7**. In this way, the cytotoxic 5-FU is released selectively in tumor cells, thereby significantly reducing its exposure to normal cells and improving the therapeutic window of this drug. In addition, the oral bioavailability of the molecule is improved and reaches almost 100%.

A recent approach to targeting takes advantage of the high specificity of antibodies to recognize specific molecules on the surface of certain cell types. This approach has

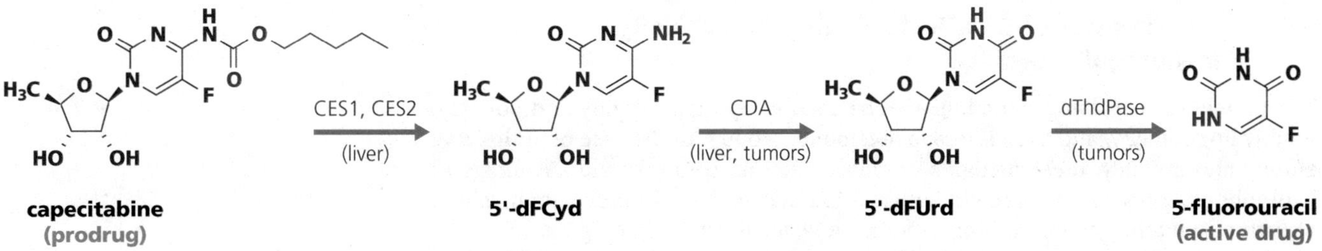

Figure 4.7 Transformation of capecitabine to the active form, 5-fluorouracil. Hydrolysis of the carbamate by enzymes CES1 and CES2 and decarboxylation gives the amine 5′-dFCyd; oxidation by CDA gives 5′-dFUrd; and then cleavage of the base from the carbohydrate ring gives the active drug, 5-fluorouracil.

been successfully applied to cancer therapies. It allows highly toxic molecules to be targeted to tumor cells while reducing exposure of normal cells, thereby improving the safety profile of the drug. Maytansine is a natural product that is highly potent in anti-cancer assays. Unfortunately, the drug also exhibited unacceptable toxicity in clinical trials and was never advanced. To alleviate the toxicity, an analog (mertansine) of the molecule was linked to an antibody called trastuzumab, which recognizes specific proteins on certain metastatic breast cancer cells and is an effective drug on its own (**Figure 4.8**). The antibody directs the cytotoxic agent to the metastatic breast cancer cells, where it is released and preferentially absorbed by the cancer cell. The conjugate, trastuzumab–mertansine, was approved in 2013 for the treatment of certain types of breast cancer.

MEDICINAL CHEMISTRY STRATEGIES APPLIED DURING LEAD OPTIMIZATION

Optimizing affinity of a small molecule against a biological target requires optimization of the size, orientation, and polarity of the functional groups that interact at the binding site. As described in Chapter 3, a majority of the molecular interactions (for example, H-bonding, dipole–dipole, π–cation, and electrostatic interactions) that contribute to binding energy have a specific geometry that provides an optimal interaction. In addition, hydrophobic interactions are optimized by adjusting the size and shape of the substituent. However, a drug candidate requires not only high affinity but also high potency and excellent physical and pharmaceutical properties. The lead optimization process requires all of these parameters to be optimized in parallel, but improving one often results in worsening of another. A series of medicinal chemistry strategies have been developed that can be applied under certain circumstances to address various liabilities of an early lead during the optimization process. They aim to maintain or improve potency while addressing weaknesses in specific physical or pharmaceutical properties.

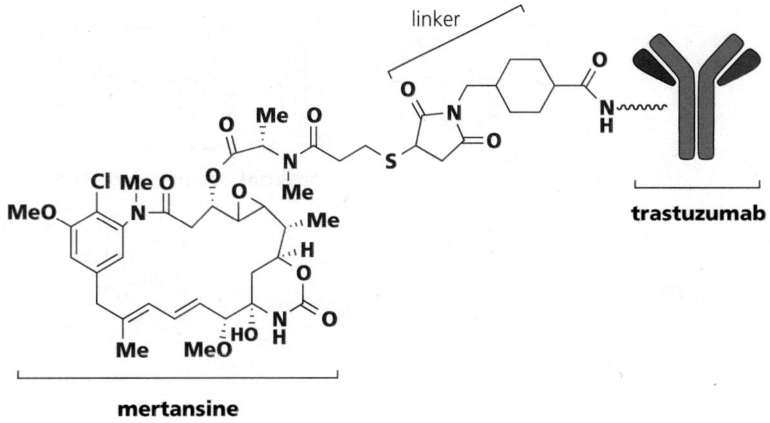

Figure 4.8 Structure of trastuzumab–mertansine, an antibody conjugate used to treat cancer. The active drug (mertansine) is connected through a linker to the antibody (trastuzumab), which selectively delivers the drug to cancer cells.

4.8   Increasing steric bulk affects binding, lipophilicity, and metabolic stability

The strategy of increasing steric bulk can be used to optimize affinity and potency, modify lipophilicity, and even improve metabolic stability. In the case of optimizing affinity and potency, these methods are most often used to take full advantage of hydrophobic sites on the protein target. Methods include homologation, chain branching, and ring–chain transformations, which are illustrated in **Figure 4.9**.

Homologation is the sequential addition or subtraction of methylene (CH_2) units to an alkyl chain. This change may affect binding to the target and will always have an effect on lipophilicity. In the hypothetical example shown in Figure 4.9, a methyl group in lead A is changed to an ethyl, propyl, or butyl group. If the butyl analog is the most active, it may be further modified. Increasing steric bulk can affect metabolic stability by hindering access to the metabolic site. The addition of alkyl branching points to an alkyl chain is termed **chain branching**. As with homologation, this will affect lipophilicity and may affect target binding. In the example shown starting from the newly optimized lead B, branching at different positions may provide a new compound with optimized activity (lead C). The third type of direct change to alkyl groups involves **ring–chain transformations**. In this type of transformation, the size of a ring may be increased or decreased or a chain may be converted to a ring and vice versa. As shown in the hypothetical example in Figure 4.9, a ring in lead C may be broken open or a chain may be closed to give a new ring. These modifications have an

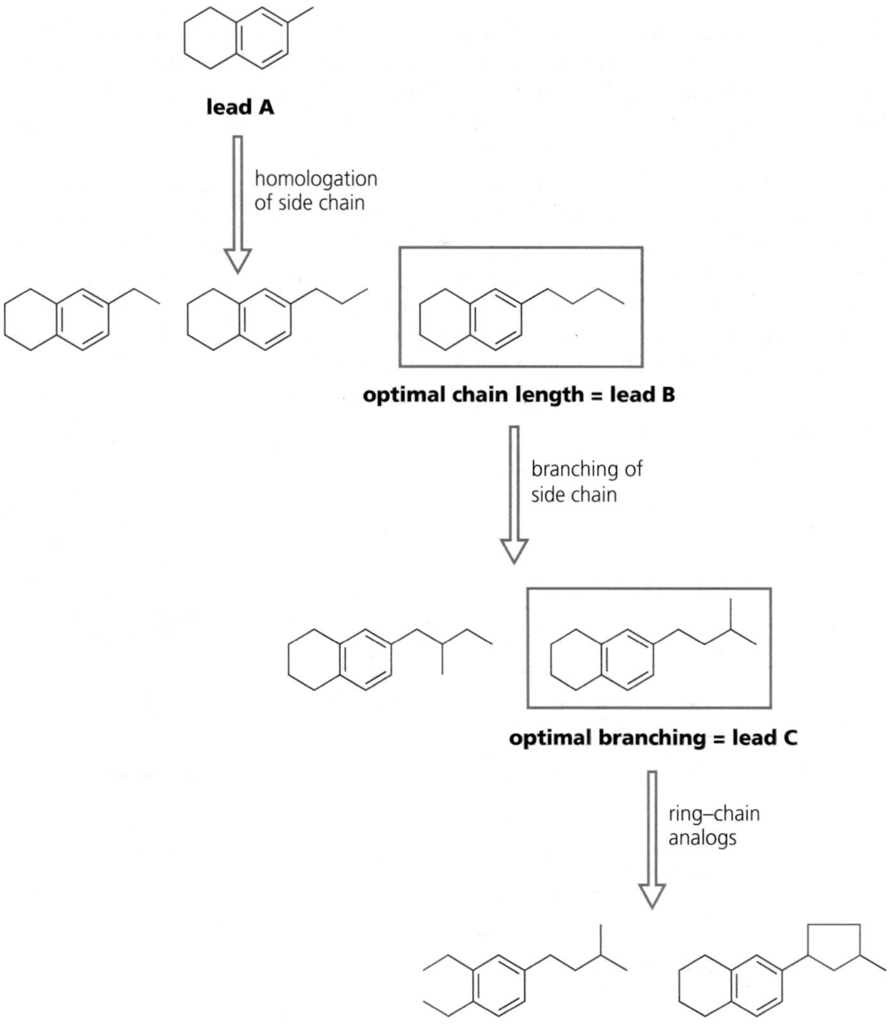

Figure 4.9 Theoretical example of lead modification, showing homologation, chain branching, and ring–chain transformations. Lead A is homologated from a methyl to ethyl, propyl, and butyl analogs (in red). If the homologated butyl analog (lead B, boxed) exhibits improved activity, in a second round of optimization, branch points are added to the butyl chain (red). If the branched analog lead C exhibits improved potency, further optimization may include either cleaving a ring (red, left) or forming a ring (red, right).

effect on the entropy of the system that will impact affinity, in addition to an effect on metabolic stability.

4.9 Bioisosteres are used as substitutions for specific functional groups

Bioisosteres (or **isosteres**) have been defined by Alfred Burger as "compounds or groups that possess near-equal molecular shapes and volumes, approximately the same distribution of electrons, and which exhibit similar physical properties." The strategy of replacing a function group with a bioisostere is frequently applied when the goal is to maintain the affinity of a molecule but change its pharmaceutical properties. Over time, their importance in medicinal chemistry has grown and their characterization has evolved. Today, the definition of a bioisostere is even broader, and replacing one functional group with a bioisostere may result in changes in size, electronics, liphophilicity, and other physical and pharmaceutical properties, however the overall goal is to maintain the optimal properties of the original molecule but decrease its liabilities.

Classical isosteres were originally defined by Grimm's hydride displacement law as "atoms that bond to one to four hydrogens to reach similarity to an inert gas." By this definition, O, NH, and CH_2 would be isosteric with each other. This view was later expanded by Erlenmeyer to include atoms, ions, and molecules with identical peripheral layers of electrons, rather than just number of bonds. In this case Cl, SH, and PH_2 would be isosteric, since all have seven peripheral electrons. Classical bioisosteres can be categorized as monovalent, divalent, trivalent, tetravalent, or ring equivalents, as shown in **Table 4.3**.

Table 4.3 Examples of classical bioisosteres, where each entry in a row is a distinct isostere of the parent.

	Functional group	Classical bioisosteres			
monovalent	—CH_3	—NH_2	—OH	—F	—Cl
	—Cl	—PH_2	—SH		
	—Br	—$CH(CH_3)_2$			
	—I	—$C(CH_3)_3$			
	—H	—F	—D		
divalent	—CH_2—	—NH—	—O—	—S—	—Se—
	—C=C—	—C=N—	C=O	C=S	
trivalent	—C=	—N=			
	—P=	—As=			
tetravalent	—C—	—Si—			
ring equivalents	—CH=CH—	—S—	example: benzene thiophene		
	—CH=	—N=	example: benzene pyridine		

| X = O IC_{50} = 140 nM | R = H IC_{50} = 4.3 nM | X = CH; R = H **antergan** | R = H **uracil** |
| X = NH IC_{50} = 160 nM | R = F IC_{50} = 6.9 nM | X = N; R = OCH$_3$ **mepyramine** | R = F **5-fluorouracil** |
| X = S IC_{50} = 17 nM |

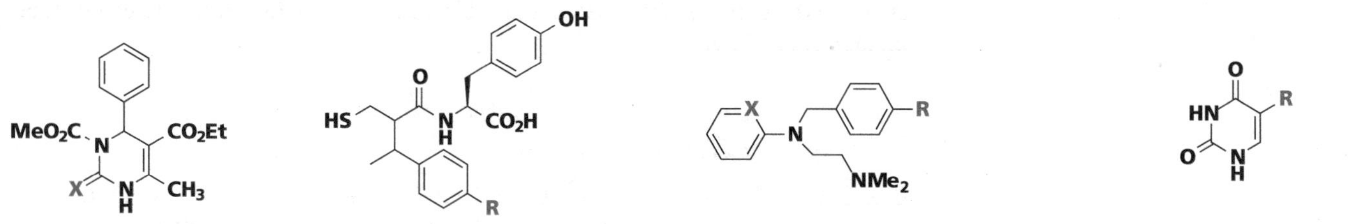

calcium channel blockers   **ACE/NEP inhibitors**   **antihistamines**

Several examples of the use of classical bioisosteres are shown in **Figure 4.10**. For instance, in a series of calcium channel blockers, the divalent isosteres NH and S were used to replace the O and led to improved activity in the thiocarbonyl analog. One widely used isosteric replacement is that of fluorine for hydrogen. In a series of angiotensin-converting enzyme/neutral endopeptidase (ACE/NEP) inhibitors, replacement of hydrogen with a fluorine atom resulted in a slight decrease in activity. The antihistamine mepyramine is a derivative of the earlier drug antergan, with the main difference being an isosteric replacement of a CH in the phenyl ring with a nitrogen atom. Another example is 5-fluorouracil, a commonly used anti-tumor agent. 5-Fluorouracil is still recognized by the enzyme thymidylate synthase, whose natural substrate is uracil, thereby illustrating the value of a fluorine atom as an isostere. These examples highlight how classical isosteres can be used to generate new molecules with equivalent and even sometimes improved potency compared to the parent.

Nonclassical bioisosteres do not necessarily have the same number of valence electrons or the same number of atoms, but they still result in similar biological activity. Substitution may have effects on parameters such as size, hydrogen-bonding ability, lipophilicity, and stability. Some examples of nonclassical bioisosteres are summarized in **Table 4.4**.

In some of these examples, it is relatively easy to see the similarity; for example, a carbonyl and a sulfonyl group are similar in both size and electronic structure. However, the use of dicyanomethylene as a replacement for oxygen is less obvious, and one needs to consider the nitriles as similar to the oxygen lone pairs. Both the carboxylic acid and hydroxy isosteres, while they may not be identical in size, have similar pK_a values for the acidic hydrogens. For example, the widely used carboxylic acid bioisostere 1*H*-tetrazole has a pK_a of ~4.5, and the corresponding acetic acid pK_a is 4.75.

There are numerous examples of the application of nonclassical bioisosteres. An early example was the use of an N-cyano group as a sulfur replacement for a problematic thiourea in the development of histamine blockers. The early clinical candidate, metiamide, although active, caused the undesirable side effect of granulocytopenia. The N-cyano analog, cimetidine, was equally active but without the side effects, and it became the first histamine blocker approved to treat gastric ulcers (**Figure 4.11**).

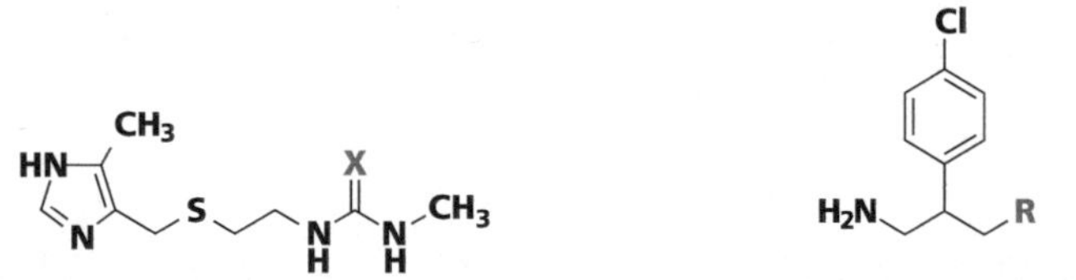

Figure 4.10 Examples of lead modification using classical bioisosteres. Isosteric replacement of a carbonyl oxygen with an N-H or S, resulted in calcium channel blockers with equivalent or improved potency. Isosteric replacement of a hydrogen atom with a fluorine results in equivalent activity in a set of ACE/NEP inhibitors. Mepyramine, based on the drug Antergan, includes an isosteric replacement of a CH within an aromatic ring with a nitrogen atom. The anti-cancer drug 5-FU is still recognized by the enzyme thymidylate synthase, whose natural substrate is uracil (isosteric replacement of H with F).

blockers of histamine receptor

X = S **(metiamide)** ED_{50} = 1.6 μmol/kg
X = N–CN **(cimetidine)** ED_{50} = 1.4 μmol/kg

R = CO$_2$H **(baclofen: activates GABA$_B$ receptor)**

INHIBITORS OF BACLOFEN BINDING:

R = PO$_3$H$_2$ **(phaclofen)** IC_{50} = 118 μM
R = SO$_3$H **(saclofen)** IC_{50} = 8 μM

Figure 4.11 Examples of lead modification using nonclassical bioisosteres. The thioamide in metiamide, which was suspected of causing toxicity, was replaced with the isosteric N-cyano group to afford cimetidine, the first histamine blocker approved to treat gastric ulcers. Baclofen, a carboxylic acid, activates GABA$_B$ receptors. Isosteric replacement with phosphonate (phaclofen) or sulfonate (saclofen) generated compounds that competed with baclofen for binding.

Table 4.4 Examples of nonclassical bioisosteres.

Functional group	Non-classical bioisosteres			

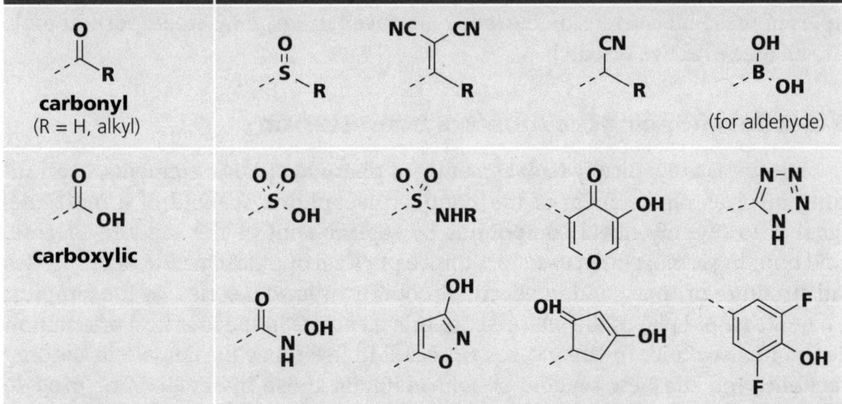

Carboxylic acids are often important binding elements in leads, and there are many examples of bioisosteric replacements that contain ionizable hydrogens ($pK_a \cong 1$–8) or H-bonding donor or acceptor capabilities. By incorporation of a carboxylic acid isostere, the same binding interactions to the target are usually maintained but the physical and pharmaceutical properties of the molecule, such as lipophilicity, permeability or metabolic stability, can be modified. By isosteric replacement of the carboxylic acid in the GABA$_B$ activator baclofen, both new analogs, the phosphonic acid (phaclofen) and sulfonic acid (saclofen), bind to the receptor but act as blockers.

The specific classification of isosteres has become less important as this strategy is finding broad use, and new examples of bioisosteric replacements are being reported. A recent successful example is the use of boronic acid, replacing an aldehyde functional group in the proteasome inhibitor bortezomib.

Peptide mimetics can be considered a special class of bioisosteres. While peptides or segments of proteins exert a biological effect as ligands for receptors or as substrates for enzymes, they are often not suitable as drugs due to their physical properties and susceptibility to hydrolysis. To address these limitations, peptide mimetics have evolved. These include functional groups that are designed to mimic the peptide bond's polarity, H-bonding capabilities, and other features but exhibit improved stability. Examples, some of which are shown in **Figure 4.12**, include alkenes

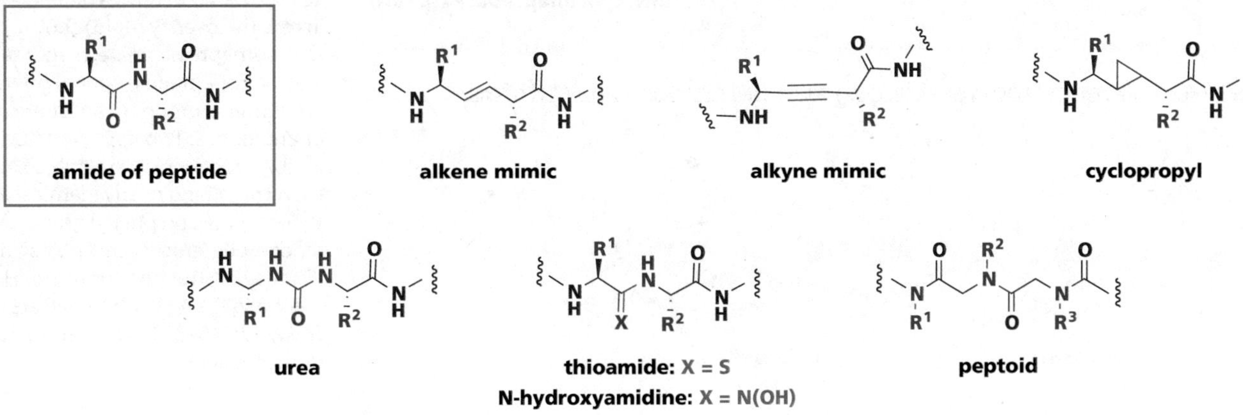

Figure 4.12 Examples of peptide mimetics. Replacement of an amide bond (red) in a peptide (boxed) with various isosteres can result in similar potency and improved properties particularly metabolic stability. Alkene and alkyne isosteres mimic the planar features of a peptide bone; a cyclopropane isostere orients the side chains (R^1, R^2: purple) in an orientation similar to the amide bond; ureas, thioamides, N-hydroxy amidine, and peptoids provide similar H-bonding capacity. In each case, the amide replacement is shown in red.

and alkynes that mimic the planar features of the peptide bond; cyclopropanes that correctly orient the amino acid side chains; ureas, thioamides, N-hydroxyamidine, and peptoids that maintain some hydrogen-bonding features. While there are few examples of these bioisosteres in currently approved drugs, they are important tools and are an area of active research.

4.10 Scaffold hopping is a subset of bioisosterism

While bioisoteres are typically replacements for pharmacophoric elements, **scaffold hopping** involves replacement of the nonpharmacophoric scaffold of a molecule. The goal is to identify novel compounds by replacement of the scaffold or core. Scaffold hopping is most often used to improve physical or pharmaceutical properties of lead structure or to expand intellectual property around a series. In the simplest case, a new scaffold places the pharmacophoric elements in the identical orientation as the original scaffold. In some cases the scaffold itself may participate in binding interactions, and the new scaffold should maintain those interactions or provide additional binding over the original scaffold.

Scaffold hopping can be considered a subset of bioisosterism and often involves traditional strategies such as isosteric replacements within rings and chains. Typical changes to a lead may include replacing one heterocycle with another, and addition of rings or groups to reduce conformational flexibility. Some examples of drugs with different scaffolds but similar bioactivity are shown in **Figure 4.13**. An older example of drugs with similar activity but different scaffolds is seen in the antihistamines pheniramine and the more rigid cyproheptadine. In the overlay, it can be seen that the pharmacophoric elements, the two aryl rings and the amine are held in the same position (scaffold differences highlighted in red). The cyclooxygenase (COX) inhibitors celecoxib and rofecoxib have different heterocyclic scaffolds (red), but very similar functional groups on their periphery. While the two drugs have similar potencies, their pharmacokinetic profiles are different.

Computational methods have been developed to classify bioactive compounds on the basis of their scaffolds, and virtual screening programs use these methods to

A: STRUCTURES OF ANTIHISTAMINES WITH DIFFERENT SCAFFOLDS

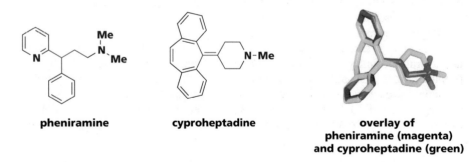

pheniramine   **cyproheptadine**   **overlay of pheniramine (magenta) and cyproheptadine (green)**

B: STRUCTURES OF CYCLOOXYGENASE (COX) INHIBITORS CELECOXIB AND ROFECOXIB

celecoxib   **rofecoxib**

Figure 4.13 Examples of pairs of compounds with the same bioactivity but different scaffolds. A: Two antihistamines, pheniramine and cyproheptadine, contain the same pharmacophoric features (two aryl groups and a positive ionization group), on distinct scaffolds, with key scaffold differences highlighted in red. The overlay (right) shows that both (pheniramine, magenta and cyproheptadine, green) orient the terminal groups in an identical orientation. B: Two approved COX inhibitors, celecoxib and rofecoxib each containing nearly identical aryl sulfonamide and phenyl groups, but different heterocyclic scaffolds (in red). (Overlay of structures from Sun H, Tawa G & Wallqvist A [2010] *Drug Discovery Today* 17:310–324. With permission from Elsevier.)

identify compounds that are predicted to be similar enough in properties to be active but have scaffolds that are different enough to be novel. Scaffold hopping during lead optimization involves synthesis and testing of designed compounds that maintain the pharmacophoric elements of a lead but have replaced the scaffold, or core, of the structure with different structures. If a screening program had been used to identify the original hits, scaffold hopping may involve a return to the original active hits to identify those with different scaffolds.

4.11 Incorporation of fluorine may affect potency and pharmaceutical properties

One of the most powerful strategies in medicinal chemistry is the use of fluorine to modify the properties of a lead molecule. Despite its small size, introduction of a fluorine atom into a molecule can drastically change its potency, physical properties, and pharmaceutical properties. Recent advances in synthetic methods have made fluorine-containing drug candidates more accessible, and there has been a corresponding increase in the percentage of drug molecules containing fluorine. Currently, approximately 25% of drugs contain a fluorine atom. Fluorine is a relatively small atom, with a van der Waals radius of 1.47 Å. It is larger than hydrogen (1.2 Å) and smaller than oxygen and nitrogen ($\sim$1.5 Å) or carbon (1.7 Å). A trifluoromethyl group is estimated to be between the size of an isopropyl group and a *tert*-butyl group. The other defining characteristic of fluorine is its strong electronegativity. For example, introduction of one fluorine atom into acetic acid reduces the pK_a from 4.7 (CH_3CO_2H) to 2.6 for CH_2FCO_2H; the pK_a of CF_3CO_2H is 0.23. In addition, fluorine can act as a hydrogen-bond acceptor. These characteristics can influence the properties of lead molecules in a variety of ways. The electronic effects of fluorine on neighboring acid or base moieties can tune and optimize their acidity or basicity. Due to its ability to form hydrogen bonds and participate in dipole–dipole interactions, introduction of a fluorine atom can improve affinity by making additional molecular interactions with the target protein, without significantly changing the steric environment. For example, in a series of thrombin inhibitors (**Figure 4.14**), addition of a fluorine atom at the 4-position of a benzyl group (X) in the parent compound resulted in a greater than 5-fold increase in potency. An X-ray structure of the molecule bound to thrombin revealed that the fluorine atom was in close proximity to a backbone carbonyl unit, suggesting a new hydrogen bond between the small molecule and target (F $\cdots$ H–Cα–CO) and/or a new dipole interaction between the fluorine atom and the backbone carbonyl carbon (F $\cdots$ C=O).

The incorporation of a fluorine atom can also have a profound effect on the physical and pharmaceutical properties of a lead molecule. Typically, lipophilicity increases with the addition of a fluorine atom, which often improves permeability and brain penetration. Fluorination is a strategy frequently employed to improve metabolic stability. By replacing a metabolically labile hydrogen (either aromatic or aliphatic) with a similarly sized fluorine atom, metabolism is blocked. Additionally, fluorination of an aromatic ring deactivates the ring toward oxidative metabolism. This effect is nicely demonstrated in the example of ezetimibe (Zetia), a cholesterol absorption

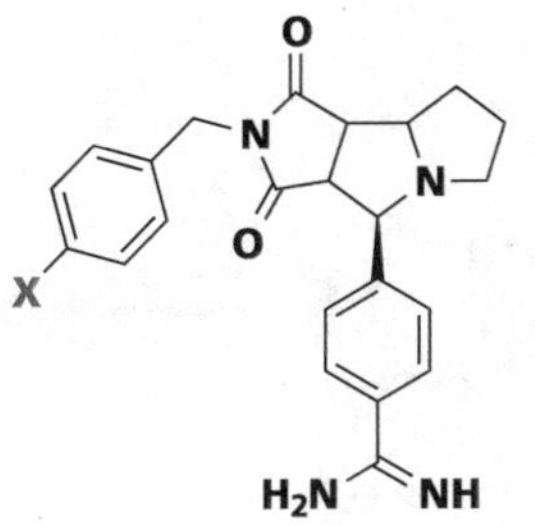

Figure 4.14 Improved binding due to fluorine substitution on thrombin inhibitor. Introduction of a para-fluorine substituent in a thrombin inhibitor improved binding to the enzyme by 5-fold (change shown in red).

substituent	thrombin inhibition
X = H	K_i = 0.31 µM
X = F	K_i = 0.057 µM

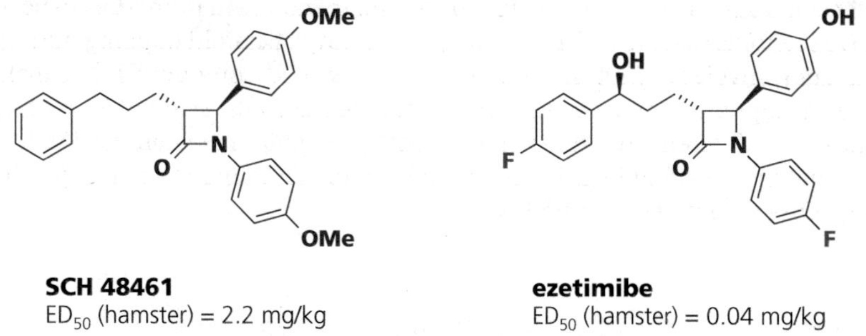

SCH 48461
ED$_{50}$ (hamster) = 2.2 mg/kg

ezetimibe
ED$_{50}$ (hamster) = 0.04 mg/kg

Figure 4.15 Effect of fluorine substitution on *in vivo* activity of cholesterol absorption inhibitors. An early lead, SCH 48461, was optimized in part by addition of two fluorines (shown in red) and led to ezetimibe, marketed as a cholesterol-lowering drug. The ED$_{50}$ in a hamster model of disease improved from 2.2 to 0.04 mg/kg and reflected the improved metabolic stability imparted by the fluorine atoms.

inhibitor, as seen in **Figure 4.15**. The parent compound, SCH 48461, exhibited moderate oral bioavailability, as evidenced by the effective dose in a hamster model of disease (ED$_{50}$) of 2.2 mg/kg. The eventual drug, ezetimibe, contains two fluorine atoms that were incorporated to minimize metabolism and has an effective dose of 0.04 mg/kg, a greater than 50-fold improvement.

Another benefit of the incorporation of fluorine is that molecules containing a fluorine atom can be rapidly converted into imaging agents for positron emission tomography (PET) by incorporation of the radioactive isotope of fluorine (^{18}F).

4.12 Transition-state mimetics are common features of enzyme inhibitors

One strategy that has been particularly valuable in the development of enzyme inhibitors is the use of **transition-state mimetics**. Since an enzyme stabilizes the transition state of the reaction it catalyzes, effective inhibitors can be developed by mimicking the transition state with a stabilized structure. Inhibitors of proteases, enzymes that catalyze the hydrolysis of a peptide bond, are one such example where this approach has been particularly successful. During hydrolysis of the substrate peptide, an sp^2 carbonyl is attacked by a nucleophile (usually derived from either serine or cysteine or threonine; or a water molecule) and generates an sp^3-hybridized tetrahedral intermediate, which then collapses to generate the hydrolysis products. This process, when the nucleophile is part of the enzyme, is outlined in abbreviated form in **Figure 4.16**.

On the basis of this hydrolysis mechanism, a stable sp^3-hybridized mimic of the tetrahedral intermediate is predicted to bind tightly to and inhibit the protease. A number of examples of transition-state mimetics of proteases have been developed and are shown in **Figure 4.17**. Hydroxyethylenes, dihydroxyethylenes, statines, hydroxyethylamines, phosphinates and silanediols not only contain the tetrahedral carbon mimetic but also display a hydroxyl group that may mimic the alkoxide that is present in the transition state. Other examples, such as reduced amides maintain all the features of the transition state, except the hydroxyl group.

These peptidelike transition-state mimetics resemble the extended conformation of the substrate peptide and are incorporated into a larger scaffold that is based on the natural substrate. Hydroxyethylene and hydroxyethylamine were incorporated into

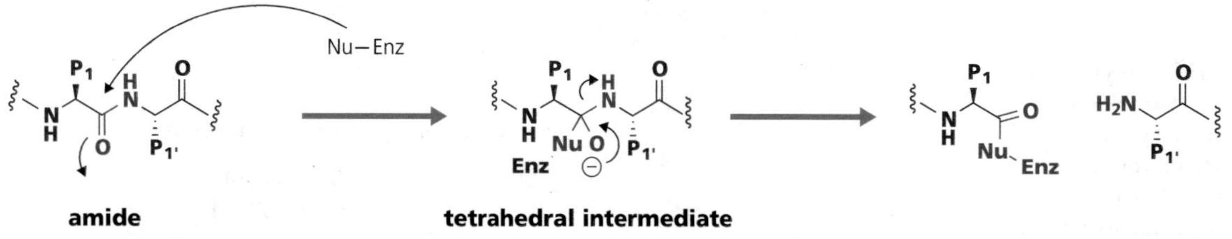

Figure 4.16 Abbreviated mechanism for enzyme-catalyzed amide-bond hydrolysis based on cysteine, serine or threonine nucleophile, showing tetrahedral intermediate. A nucleophile in the enzyme (e.g. O$^-$ derived from serine or threonine or S$^-$ derived from cysteine) attacks the carbonyl of the amide bond to generate a tetrahedral intermediate, which then collapses to generate the cleaved peptide fragments.

amide   **tetrahedral intermediate**

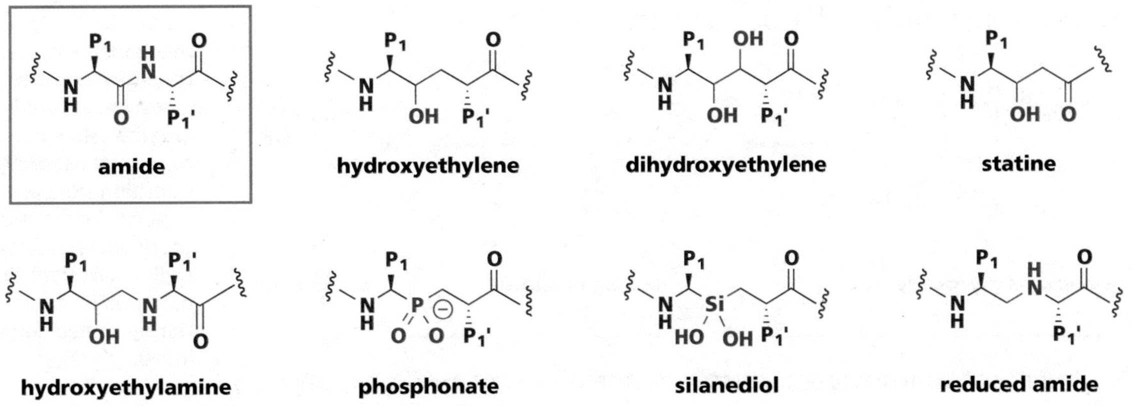

Figure 4.17 Cleaved amide bond and examples of amide-bond hydrolysis transition-state analogs. P_1 and $P_{1'}$ are the amino acid side chains on either side of the cleaved (scissile) bond (red, boxed), and the specific transition-state mimetic is shown in red. Hydroxyethylenes, dihydroxyethylenes, statines, hydroxyethylamines, phosphinates, and silanediols contain a hydroxyl group at the sp³ center that may mimic the alkoxide present in the transition state. Reduced amides maintain all the features of the transition state, except the hydroxyl group.

the HIV protease inhibitors indinavir and amprenavir, respectively (**Figure 4.18**), and are examples of the successful application of this strategy.

Another example of transition-state mimics is found in the influenza drugs zanamivir (Relenza) and oseltamivir (Tamiflu). The viral surface glycoprotein neuraminidase (HB-Enz) is a glycohydrolase enzyme that relies on acid-base catalysis to cleave terminal sialic acid residues from sialic acid glycoconjugates on the virus and host cell surfaces, allowing for release of viral particles (**Figure 4.19**). The reaction proceeds through a planar intermediate prior to addition of water, which generates sialic acid. The unsaturated rings in zanamivir and oseltamivir mimic the sialosyl cation in which the anomeric carbon transitions from an sp³-hybridized carbon to an sp² carbon.

The use of transition-state mimetics is a powerful strategy for the design of enzyme inhibitors. In theory, if the transition state of an enzymatic reaction is understood, inhibitors can be designed. The current challenge in this area is the design of transition-state mimetics of multicomponent enzymatic reactions and those that involve high-valency intermediates; for example, intermediates in phosphate transfer reactions catalyzed by kinases that are not easily mimicked by traditional organic functional groups. Chapter 7 provides additional details on transition-state mimetic strategies as applied to drugs and drug design.

4.13 Conformational constraints can be used to improve binding to the drug target

The goal of introducing conformational constraints into an active molecule is to maintain the enthalpic effects contributed by the binding interactions but reduce the entropic effects. The overall result is an increase in binding energy, since the molecule does not require energy to rotate into an active conformation. This strategy is frequently applied by incorporating rings into acyclic structures. For example, the natural ligand for the metabotropic glutamate receptors (mGluR) is the excitatory amino acid glutamic acid. A number of cyclic analogs of this flexible molecule have been developed that bind tightly to the receptor. LY354740 (eglumegad), which progressed to clinical trials as a potential anti-anxiety drug, uses a rigid bicyclic

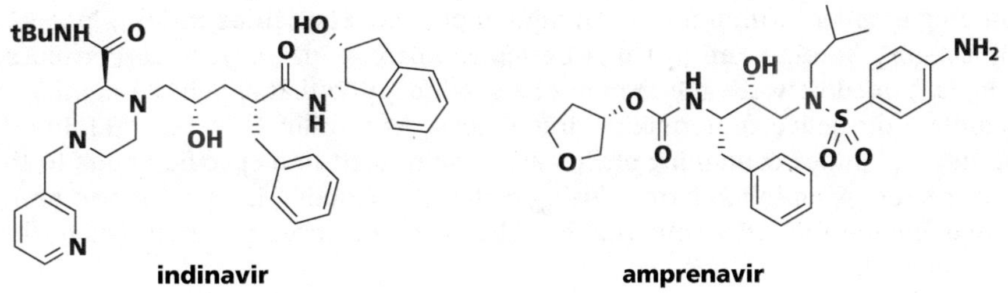

Figure 4.18 Examples of HIV protease inhibitors that contain transition-state mimetics (shown in red). Indinavir contains a hydroxyethylene moiety in place of the amide bond, and amprenavir contains a hydroxyethyl amine group.

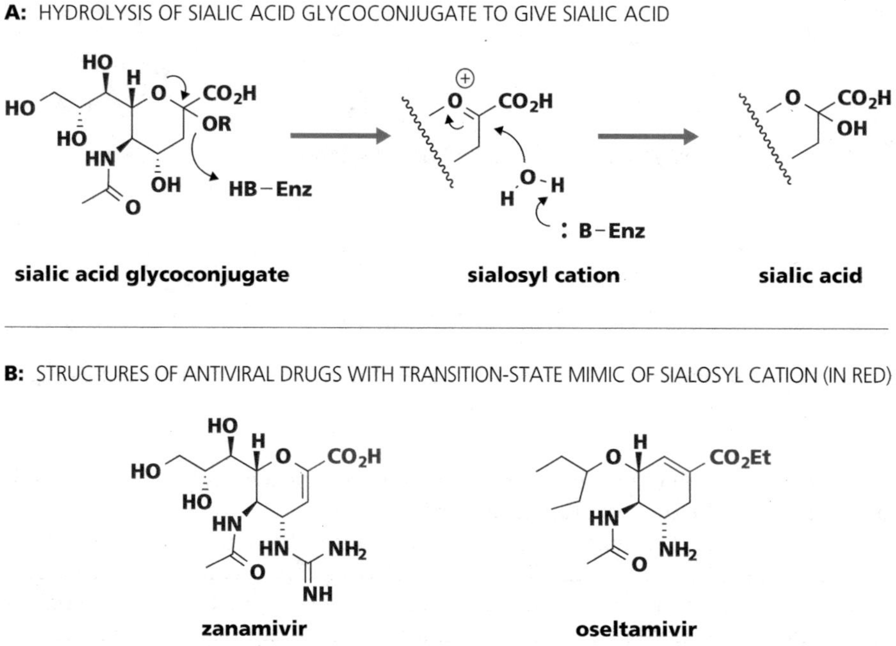

A: HYDROLYSIS OF SIALIC ACID GLYCOCONJUGATE TO GIVE SIALIC ACID

sialic acid glycoconjugate   sialosyl cation   sialic acid

B: STRUCTURES OF ANTIVIRAL DRUGS WITH TRANSITION-STATE MIMIC OF SIALOSYL CATION (IN RED)

zanamivir   oseltamivir

Figure 4.19 Glycohydrolase mechanism and examples of transition-state mimics. A: Sialic acid glycoconjugate is hydrolyzed by the enzyme using acid-base chemistry, to generate a sialosyl cation in the transition state, which eventually generates sialic acid. B: Structures of antiviral agents zanamivir and oseltamivir. Transition-state mimetic moieties (here mimicking the planar transition state intermediate) are shown in red.

scaffold to constrain the amine and carboxylic acid binding elements into specific orientations, as shown in **Figure 4.20A**. In another example, a series of macrocyclic analogs of a hexapeptide inhibitor of the hepatitis C viral protease HCV NS3 were shown to be 26–50 times more potent than the acyclic analog. The macrocyclic ring (red) introduces a conformational constraint compared to the flexible linear peptide.

The final example in Figure 4.20A shows a kinase inhibitor that was identified by high-throughput screening as a potential cancer drug. Its common aniline–pyrimidine scaffold core was reported in multiple patent applications covering kinase inhibitors. In this case, macrocyclic analogs were designed (SB1317/TG02, red highlights constraining atoms) that would maintain binding interactions as well as improve patentability. Docking of each inhibitor into a kinase model shows they both adopt nearly identical conformations (**Figure 4.20B**) and detects hydrogen bonds to the backbone of the binding pocket, with an additional ionic interaction between the macrocycle nitrogen and an aspartic acid. SB1317/TG02 is in clinical trials for several different types of cancer.

In addition to incorporating a ring into a linear structure to constrain its conformation, other strategies include incorporating unsaturation (alkenes and alkynes) into an alkyl chain, incorporating steric bulk to restrict rotation and/or favor one conformation, and designing intramolecular H-bond pairs into molecules. By pre-organizing the small molecule into the active conformation, considerable increases in affinity and potency and permeability can be realized.

The strategy of constraining conformation has also been applied to larger structural motifs, for example, secondary structures of peptides, such as α-helices and β-turns. In these cases, a linear peptide fragment that is known to exert some desirable biological activity is constrained so that it mimics the conformation of the binding fragment within the larger, natural peptide. **Stapled peptides**, pioneered by Gregory Verdine, are just one example, where a macrocyclic carbon-based ring is formed between the termini of a small peptide that allows the peptide to maintain the active conformation and increase its stability (**Figure 4.21**). In one strategy, peptides containing olefins are incorporated into specific points in the linear peptide, and then a ring closing metathesis reaction is used to form a ring that maintains the active conformation. The use of this strategy is discussed further in Chapter 8.

A: EXAMPLES OF CONSTRAINED, CYCLIC ANALOGS

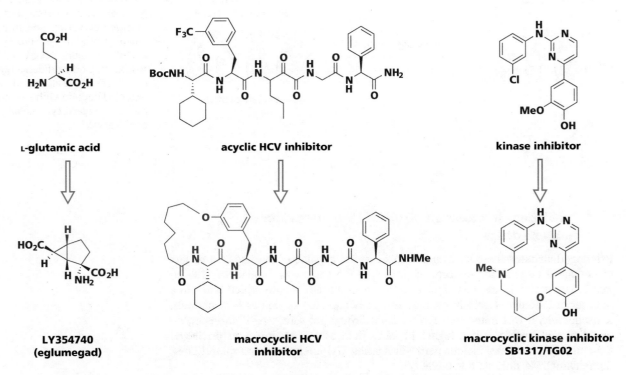

L-glutamic acid   acyclic HCV inhibitor   kinase inhibitor

**LY354740
(eglumegad)**   **macrocyclic HCV
inhibitor**   **macrocyclic kinase inhibitor
SB1317/TG02**

B: X-RAY STRUCTURES OF KINASE INHIBITOR AND MACROCYCLIC ANALOG

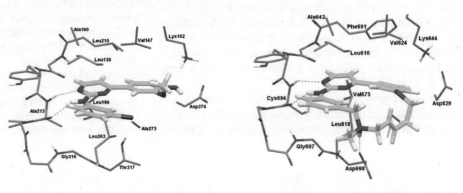

kinase inhibitor (green) docked in binding
pocket of Aurora A kinase: two H-bonds to
side chain are dotted lines

macrocyclic kinase inhibitor (green) docked
in binding pocket of cyclin-dependent
kinase: two H-bonds to side chain are
dotted lines as is an additional ionic
interaction between ring nitrogen and an

**Figure 4.20 Examples of experimental drugs incorporating conformational
constraints.** A: Examples of constrained cyclic analogs and original linear
analogs: eglumegad contains a rigid bicyclic core and mimics l-glutamic acid; the
linear peptide HCV protease inhibitor was constrained by incorporation of a
macrocycle which improved potency; and a macrocyclic kinase inhibitor, based on
a common kinase inhibitor core afforded SB1317/TG02 that had improved
patentability and entered clinical trials. (Conformational constraints are shown in
red). B: Structures of kinase acyclic inhibitor (left) docked into ATP pocket in X-ray
of Aurora kinase, and macrocyclic analog (right) docked into ATP pocket in X-ray
of cyclin dependent kinase 2 (CDK2). (Docked X-ray structures from Poulsen A,
William A, Blanchard S et al. [2013] *J Mol Model* 19:119–130. With permission from
Springer.)

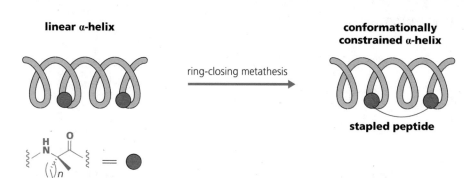

Figure 4.21 Diagram showing general structure of stapled peptides. Incorporation of alkene-containing amino acids (red balls) into a peptide strand (pink alpha helix) is a strategy to form stapled peptides. Ring-closing metathesis of the alkenes affords a stapled peptide, with an alkene-containing macrocycle linking the two amino acids.

4.14 Privileged structures are structural templates found in multiple drugs

Privileged structures are structural motifs that are capable of binding to a variety of biological targets. The concept of privileged structure was defined in 1988 by Ben Evans at Merck, and first applied to the benzodiazepine core, which binds to a number of different G protein-coupled receptors (GPCRs) as well as ion channels. Subsequently, it was noted that certain high-throughput screening libraries based on privileged structures had higher hit rates than others. Examples of privileged structures (**Figure 4.22**) include benzodiazepines, arylpiperazines, spiropiperidines, diphenylmethyls, purines, and biphenyls.

The benzodiazepine structure is found in compounds such as devazepide that bind to the cholecystokinin (CCK) receptor (Figure 4.22), in anti-anxiety drugs such as Valium that bind to ion channels, and in compounds that bind to other G protein-coupled receptors and enzymes. The spiropiperidine core is found in growth hormone secretagogues such as ibutamoren (Figure 4.22), as well as in compounds that bind to the melanocortin 4 (MC4) receptor. Buspirone contains the same core and binds to the serotonin receptor. The biphenyl core is found in the anti-hypertensive drug losartan, as well as in a number of other drugs.

Why privileged structures are privileged is not well understood. Some suggest that the structures have an optimized balance of conformational bias to adopt various geometries and excellent drug and pharmaceutical properties. Medicinal chemists

Figure 4.22 Examples of privileged structures and drugs containing those substructures (shown in red). Some common examples of privileged structures are given on the top row in the figure. Specific examples of drugs that contain those priviliged structures (in red) include: devazepide, with a benzodiazepine; ibutamoren, with a spiropiperidine, and losartan, with a biphenyl structure.

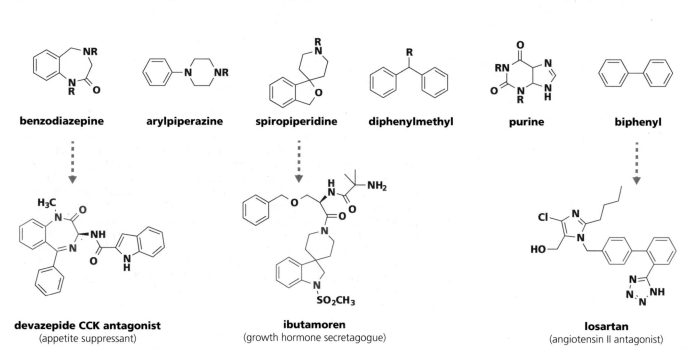

benzodiazepine   arylpiperazine   spiropiperidine   diphenylmethyl   purine   biphenyl

devazepide CCK antagonist
(appetite suppressant)

ibutamoren
(growth hormone secretagogue)

losartan
(angiotensin II antagonist)

often prioritize hits and early leads that contain these functional groups over other hits and look to incorporate them into new structures during lead optimization programs.

SUMMARY

The process of lead optimization is an arduous process, where many changes to the original lead may be necessary in order to prepare a compound with all of the properties appropriate for clinical development. Chemists have developed many strategies that are commonly used in this process in order to optimize biological, physical, and pharmaceutical properties. These include bioisosteric replacement, incorporation of fluorine atoms at key positions, transition state mimetics, conformational constraint and use of privileged structures. Optimal binding to the target must be achieved, while other properties such as lipophilicity, metabolic stability, and solubility are optimized. In some instances, it may be necessary to use a prodrug or targeting agent that, while not active itself at the target, will be converted in a living system to the active drug.

CASE STUDY 1 LEAD OPTIMIZATION OF LOSARTAN

An example of the optimization of a lead, using a number of the strategies outlined above, can be found in the development of the anti-hypertensive drug losartan. The initial lead was reported in the patent literature as an angiotensin receptor II (AII) antagonist (blocker). Chemists at DuPont Merck used a combination of molecular modeling and medicinal chemistry strategies to make hundreds of analogs of the initial lead, ultimately resulting in the first AII receptor antagonist to be approved, losartan. As outlined in **Figure 4.23**, the initial leads, which were the only reported non-peptide AII antagonists at the time, were modified on the basis of molecular modeling done by aligning it with the natural peptide substrate. It was predicted that an acidic group in the para position of the benzene ring (shown in red) could mimic a tyrosine hydroxyl of the substrate, and, once prepared, the resulting compound exhibited improved binding over the original compound by 100-fold ($IC_{50} = 1.2\ \mu M$ vs. 150 μM). Further optimization of the position of the acid moiety, by inserting an additional aryl ring (shown in blue), constrained the acid into a specific position and led to a compound with potency in the submicromolar range ($IC_{50} = 0.14\ \mu M$).

Figure 4.23 Losartan leads and modifications. Initial lead was optimized on the basis of molecular modeling by adding an acid group at the para position of the aryl ring (red) which provided a >100-fold improvement in potency. Further optimization by inserting an extra aryl group between the phenyl moiety and the acid improved binding by constraining the acidic group into a specific position (red).

DEVELOPMENT OF LOSARTAN:
initial leads and modifications

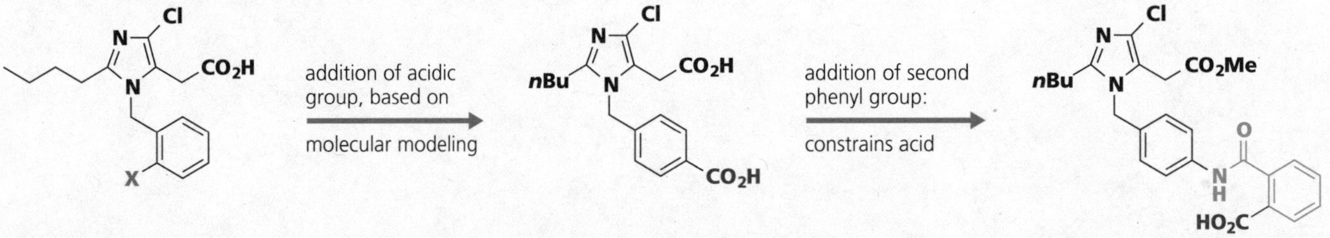

INITIAL LEADS:
X = H, Cl, NO_2
IC_{50} = 150 μM (**for X = H**)

addition of acid to para position
IC_{50} = 1.2 μM

addition of second phenyl group
IC_{50} = 0.14 μM

Optimization of the hydrophobic R^2 position in a simplified imidazole scaffold involved homologation, branching, and ring–chain transformations (**Figure 4.24** orange). For example, in the amide-linked series, the R^2 position was varied to H, methyl, ethyl, propyl, butyl, pentyl, hexyl, heptyl, isopropyl (branched), phenylethyl, benzyl, and cyclohexylmethyl (ring–chain). The conclusion was that the R^2 butyl group was optimal.

The amide linker (blue) was replaced with CO (ketone), O, S, OCH_2, *trans*-C=C, and NHCONH (carbamate), as well as eliminated (biphenyl). The amide, ketone, and O- and S-linked compounds, as well as the biphenyl analog, had similar potencies in a binding assay (not shown). In the series with the privileged biphenyl scaffold (Figure 4.22, right), when the R^2 butyl group was maintained, changes in the size of the substituent at the R^5 position affected potency by about 10-fold. A summary of the SAR results is shown in **Figure 4.25A**.

The changes to this point had optimized receptor-binding activity (IC_{50}), but the analogs did not have acceptable oral availability. The most promising were those in the biphenyl series. The position of the carboxylic acid was found to affect oral activity, with the 2-isomer (ortho) being optimal. A variety of bioisosteres that maintained the same pK_a (5–6) as the acid were prepared, including substituted triazoles and tetrazoles. The optimized tetrazole (losartan, **Figure 4.25B**) was almost ten times more potent than the acid ($IC_{50} = 0.019\ \mu M$ vs. 0.23 μM) and showed efficacy at doses of less than 1mg/kg, while the acid required ~3mg/kg to see the same effects. Losartan contains the bioisosteric tetrazole and the privileged biphenyl moiety.

Some of the medicinal chemistry strategies employed in this drug development program included the use of homologation, bioisosteres, and privileged structure (biphenyl).

AMIDE SERIES

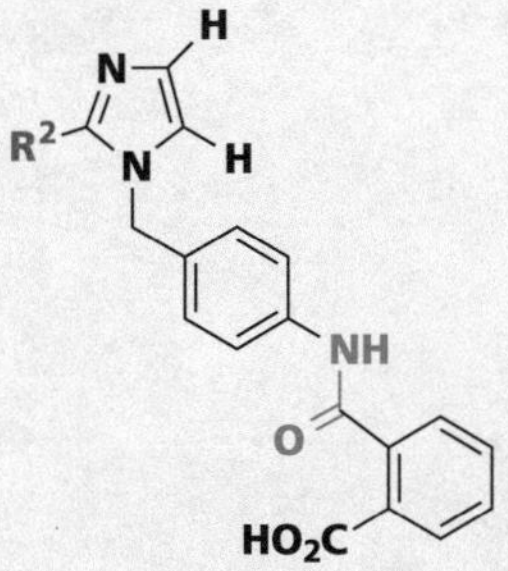

R^2	IC$_{50}$ (μM)
H	100
CH$_3$	100
CH$_3$CH$_2$	8.5
CH$_3$(CH$_2$)$_2$	3.7
CH$_3$(CH$_2$)$_3$	*0.62*
CH$_3$(CH$_2$)$_4$	0.24
CH$_3$(CH$_2$)$_5$	0.35
CH$_3$(CH$_2$)$_6$	1.1
PhCH$_2$CH$_2$	9.4
4-CH$_3$OPhCH$_2$	2.5
cyclohexyl-CH$_2$	2.8
(CH$_3$)$_2$CH	12

optimization of R^2 in amide series

BIPHENYL SERIES

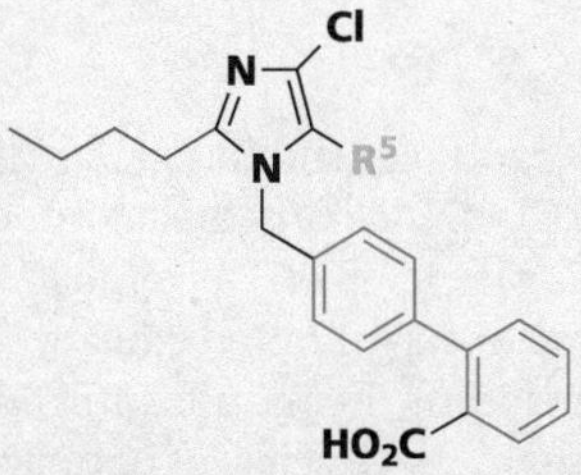

R^5	IC$_{50}$ (μM)
CH$_2$OH	0.23
CH$_2$OCH$_3$	0.099
CH$_2$NH$_2$	3.2
CH$_2$NHCO$_2$ Et	0.20
CH$_2$NHCO$_2$ adamantyl	0.6

optimization of R^5 in biphenyl series

Figure 4.24 Examples of compounds prepared during the losartan optimization process in amide and biphenyl series. Strategies used for lead optimization in the amide series (left) included homologation, branching, and ring–chain transformations for optimization of the R^2 group (orange). The biphenyl series (right) resulted from incorporation of a privileged scaffold (biphenyl, blue) that eliminated the amide and use of bioisosteres to investigate the the R^5 group (green).

A: SUMMARY OF SAR

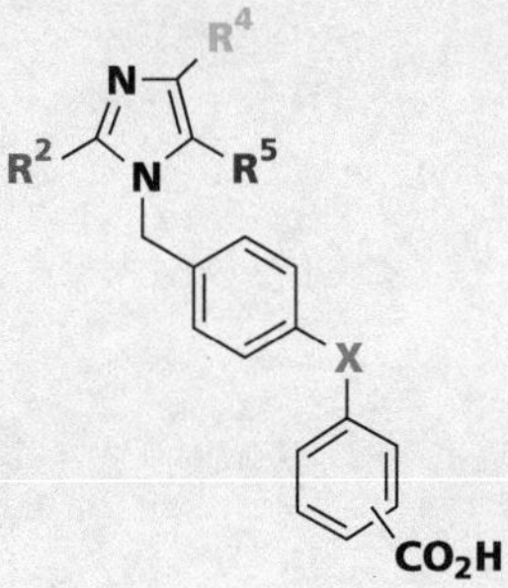

R^2: butyl group is optimal;
bioisosteres and homologation:
S-ethyl or S-propyl lower potency
ethyl, hexyl, and phenyl (ring–chain substitution) lower potency

R^4: Cl, H, CH$_2$OH, or CH$_2$OAc had similar potency

R^5: ester, Cl, CH$_2$OH, or CH$_2$OAc had similar potency

X: series included X = single bond, CO, O, S, OCH$_2$, CH=CH (*trans*) and NHCONH (bioisosteres) with the optimal linkage being 0–1 atoms in length

B: COMPARISON OF POTENCY AND IN VIVO ACTIVITY OF ACID AND TETRAZOLE SERIES

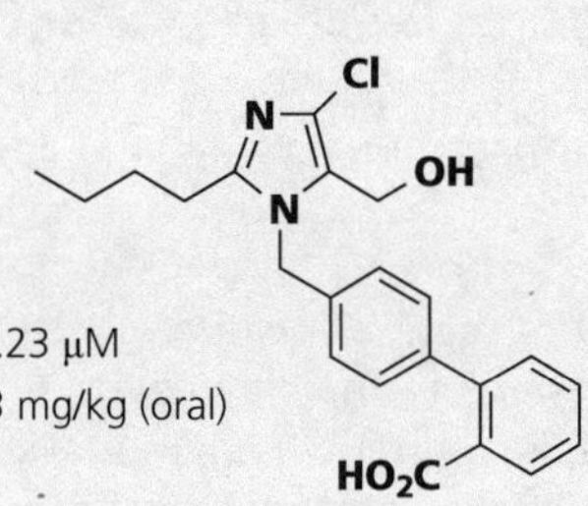

IC$_{50}$ = 0.23 μM
ED$_{30}$ = 3 mg/kg (oral)

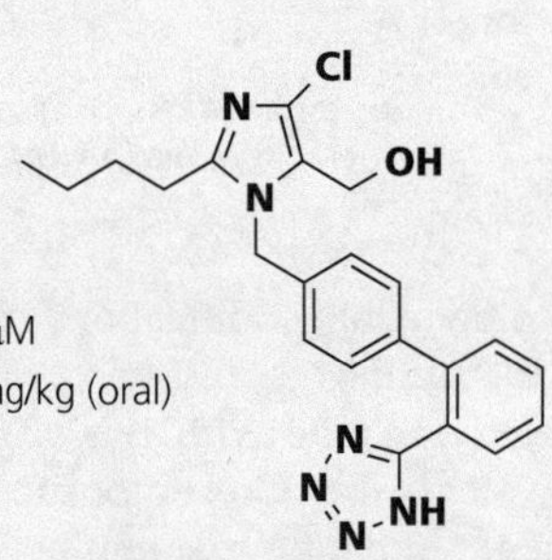

IC$_{50}$ = 0.019 μM
ED$_{30}$ = 0.80 mg/kg (oral)

losartan

Figure 4.25 Summary of lead optimization to convert initial lead compounds to the optimized drug losartan. A: Summary of SAR: the R^2 group was optimized to butyl. The R^4 position tolerated a variety of groups, as did the R^5 position; linkage (X) between the two aryl groups was best with zero or one atoms. B: Comparison of potency and ED$_{50}$ of acid and tetrazole series. Incorporation of the tetrazole bioisostere improved both *in vitro* and *in vivo* potency.

CASE STUDY 2 DISCOVERY AND STRATEGIES USED IN DEVELOPMENT OF CIMETIDINE TO TREAT GASTRIC ULCERS

An early example of the use of rational drug design strategies is seen in the development of anti-ulcer drugs based on blocking the action of histamine. In the 1960s, the only drugs available to treat gastric ulcers, as opposed to surgery, were antacids and anti-cholinergic drugs. Antacids have limited efficacy, and anti-cholinergic drugs have a number of side effects, including dry mouth, blurred vision, and urinary retention. At that time, it was understood that release of both acetylcholine and histamine contributed to gastric acid secretion. Histamine has a number of roles in the body, including increasing heart rate, causing allergy symptoms, and stimulating gastric acid secretion. Initiation of a specific biological response depends on histamine binding at its target, the histamine receptor, of which two subtypes were identified: H_1 and H_2. At Smith, Kline & French in England, a group including pharmacologist Sir James Black and chemist Robin Ganellin began working on finding an antihistamine drug with target selectivity for the H_2 receptor, which is found on gastric parietal cells and is responsible for the gastric acid secretion effects. Drug design was based on the natural ligand histamine, which binds and activates the receptor (**Figure 4.26A**). A number of medicinal chemistry strategies were used to modify the structure so that it would still bind at the H_2 receptor and block binding of histamine but not cause activation itself. This type of drug is known as a receptor antagonist.

A: NATURAL LIGAND AND EARLY LEAD STRUCTURES IN THE DEVELOPMENT OF CIMETIDINE

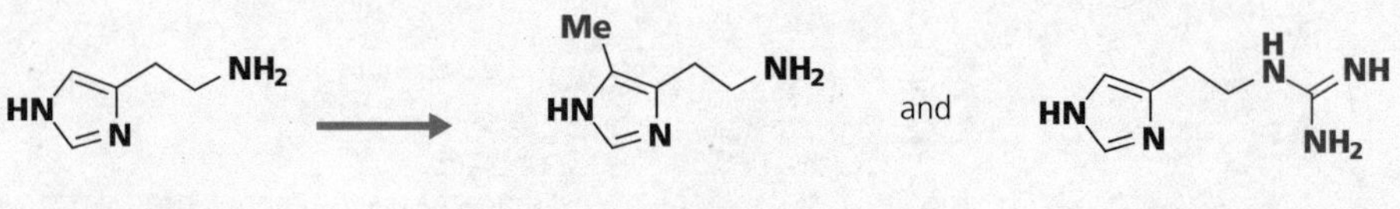

histamine
(natural ligand)

4-methylhistamine
(selective for H_2 receptor)

and

amidine
(weak antagonist)

B: CONSIDERATION OF IMIDAZOLE pK_a AND EQUILIBIRIUM OF TAUTOMERS AND CATION IN THE DEVELOPMENT OF CIMETIDINE

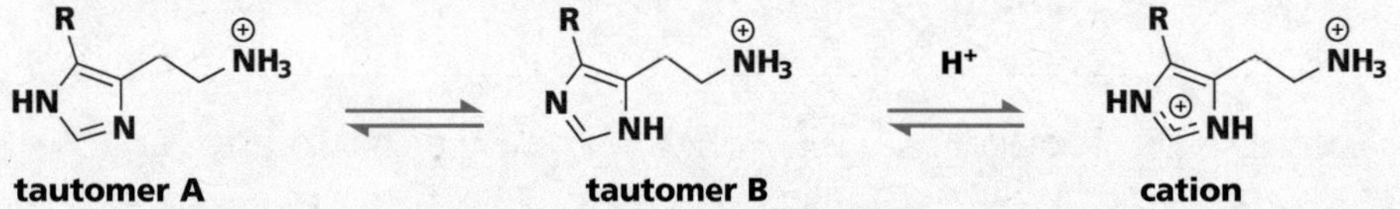

tautomer A

tautomer B

H^+

cation

histamine (R = H) favors tautomer A (imidazole pK_a = 5.9)
4- methyl histamine (R = Me) favors tautomer B (imidazole pK_a = 7.4)

Figure 4.26 Design of an antihistamine drug with target selectivity for H_2 receptor. A: Structures of histamine and early leads in cimetidine development. B: Tautomers of histamine at physiological pH of 7.4. Tautomer A is the most prevalent, and both A and B are in equilibrium with the cation.

Chemical modifications of the natural ligand structure included substitutions on the imidazole and homologation and substitutions in the side chain. A clue to selectivity came with the synthesis of 4-methylhistamine, which was a selective activator of the H_2 receptor subtype. However this methyl group affected the imidazole ring pK_a and tautomer equilibrium, shifting the pK_a from 5.9 for histamine to 7.4. This change shifts the equilibrium of the three ring species, which are two tautomers and a cation. With the 4-methyl in place, equilibrium shifts from tautomer A (preferred for histamine) to tautomer B (see **Figure 4.26B**). It was assumed that tautomer A was preferred for optimal binding, and these characteristics were one consideration in the development of further analogs.

After more than four years and the synthesis of about 200 analogs with and without a 4-methyl group, burimamide was the first H_2-selective antagonist identified (**Figure 4.27**). Medicinal chemistry strategies to develop burimamide included

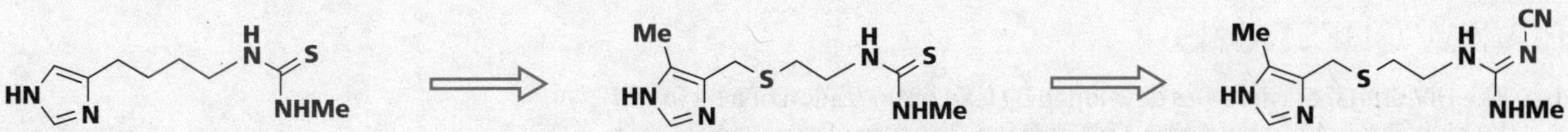

**burimamide
(first clinical candidate)**

ring pK_a = 7.25, favors tautomer B

CHANGES FROM HISTAMINE:
homologation of side-chain
bioisosteric replacement of **NH$_2$**

**ED$_{50}$ = 6.1 μmol/kg
(not orally available)**

**metiamide
(second clinical candidate)**

ring pK_a = 6.8, favors tautomer A

CHANGES FROM BURIMAMIDE:
bioisostere **S** for **CH$_2$** and addition
of 4-methyl group

**ED$_{50}$ = 1.6 μmol/kg
(orally available, but
caused granulocytopenia)**

**cimetidine
(approved 1976)**

CHANGES FROM METIAMIDE:
bioisostere **N–CN** for **S**

ED$_{50}$ = 1.4 μmol/kg

**(orally available, no
granulocytopenia)**

**Figure 4.27 Structures of clinical
candidates and cimetidine. Changes
are shown in red.** Burimamide was
the first clinical candidate, although
not orally available. Introduction of
a 4-methyl group and a bioisostere
(sulfur) in the side chain led to
metiamide. Metiamide had improved
potency and oral availability, but was
found to cause granulocytopenia.
Substituting the N-cyano isostere
for sulfur led to cimetidine, with
similar potency and oral availability of
metiamide, but no granulocytopenia.

homologation of the side chain and use of a thioamidine isostere for the primary
amine of histamine.

During this period, compounds were assayed by measuring the gastric pH of rats
infused with histamine both before and after dosing. While burimamide was effective
enough to proceed to human trials, it suffered from a lack of oral bioavailability
and would require intravenous dosing. This was in part due to the imidazole pK_a of
7.25 and preference for tautomer B, rather than tautomer A preferred by histamine.
Modification of the structure by addition of a 4-methyl group was balanced
electronically by using sulfur as a CH$_2$ bioisostere in the side chain, resulting in the
first orally available clinical candidate, metiamide, with a lower imidazole pK_a and
preference for the desired tautomer A. Metiamide was extremely effective, eliminating
gastric ulcers within three weeks of dosing.

Unfortunately, in clinic trials, patients taking metiamide developed
granulocytopenia, a lowering of white blood cells that are important in the immune
system. This side effect was attributed to the thiourea moiety, so bioisosteres for
the thiourea sulfur were investigated. While substitution of either oxygen or NH for
the sulfur atom in the thioamide decreased activity by about 20-fold, use of either
N-cyano or N-nitro moieties maintained activity. The N-cyano analog of metiamide is
cimetidine, which is orally active and had no granulocytopenia side effects. Cimetidine
was approved as a drug in 1976, approximately 12 years after initiation of the drug
discovery effort. Within 10 years of marketing, it had sales of $1 billion and became the
number one prescribed drug worldwide.

Some of the medicinal chemistry strategies employed in the cimetidine
development program included design based on the natural ligand, use of bioisosteres,
and chain homologation.

REVIEW QUESTIONS

1. The HIV drug maraviroc was developed by lead optimization of a hit found by high-throughput screening. Compare the structure of maraviroc to that of the original hit and identify three strategies that were applied during lead optimization and incorporated into the drug molecule.

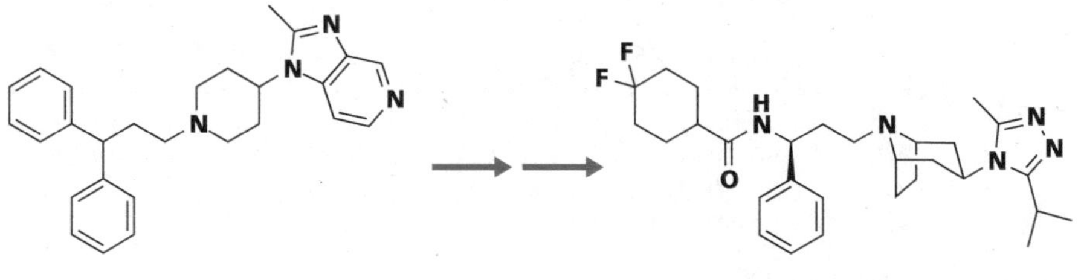

hit from HTS   **maraviroc anti HIV agent**

2. Each of the drugs shown contains a different privileged structure. Circle and identify that portion of each molecule. (Structures adapted from Constantino L & Barlacco D [2006] Privileged structures as leads in medicinal chemistry. *Curr Med Chem* 13:65–85.)

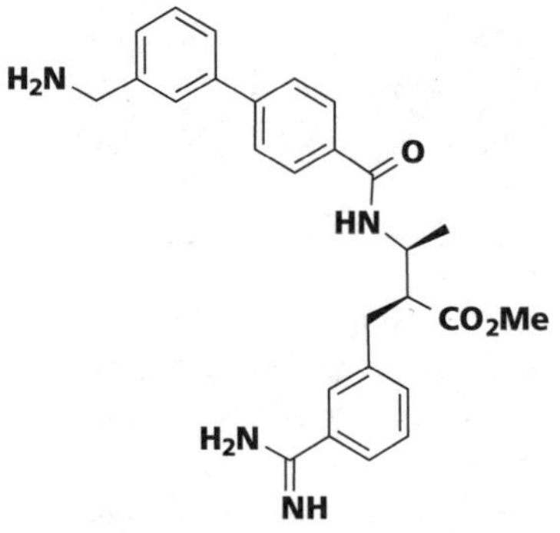

factor Xa inhibitor 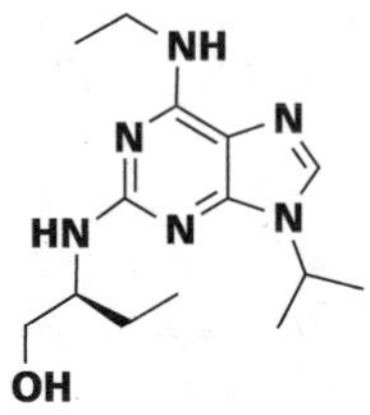   **roscovitine CDK inhibitor** 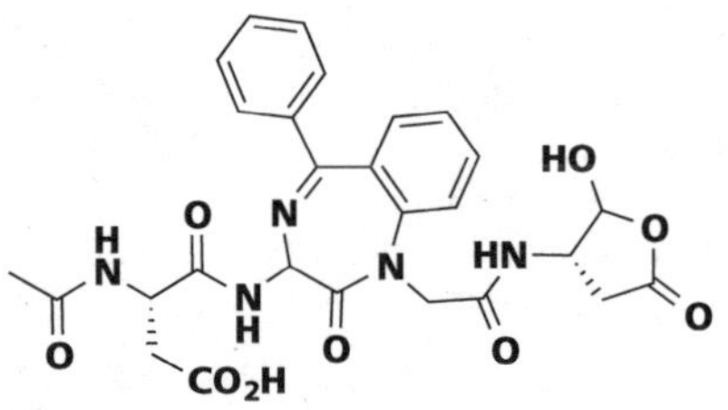   **caspase inhibitor**

3. Explain the difference between a prodrug approach and a targeting approach.

4. The compound shown, daltroban, is a thromboxane antagonist. Design two new compounds, each containing one fluorine atom. Explain what changes the incorporation of the fluorine atom should impart onto the new analog compared to daltroban.

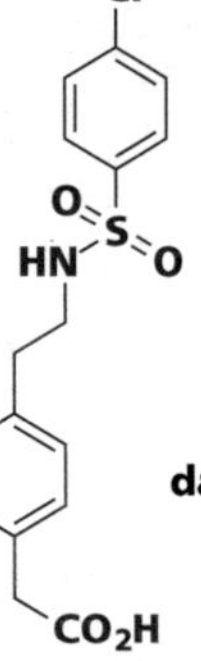

daltroban

5. What important features should an acid isostere have in order to mimic a carboxylic acid?

6. Fluoxetine, shown below, is a highly prescribed antidepressant. It is a selective serotonin reuptake inhibitor and acts on serotonin transporters in the brain. It contains a CF_3 functional group. What properties might the CF_3 impart on this molecule that are important for its effects as a drug of this class?

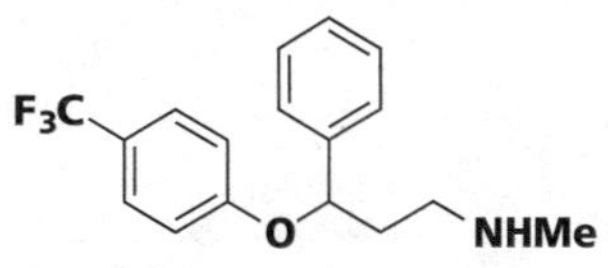

fluoxetine

7. Explain why lipophilicity is an important property for a drug candidate.

8. Explain why solubility is an important property for a drug candidate.

9. What are some reasons a prodrug strategy might be adopted (for example, what problems of the original active compound could be solved with a prodrug)?

10. Explain the difference between primary and secondary assays and some of the reasons a compound may be active in a primary assay but inactive, or much less potent, in a secondary assay.

APPLICATION QUESTIONS

1. AVPI is a tetrapeptide that mimics activity of the protein Smac. The Smac protein binds and inhibits the protein XIAP. Therefore AVPI is a potential starting point (hit) for a drug discovery effort targeting inhibitors of the protein XIAP. Identify two groups that could be replaced with isosteres and design two different molecules that incorporate two isosteric replacements.

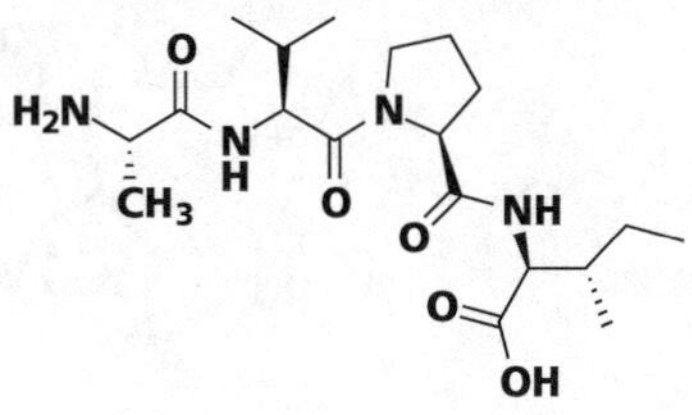

AVPI

2. Using the same AVPI peptide, assume that the pharmacophoric elements are those in red. Design two different molecules that incorporate conformational constraints. The molecule is drawn in a way that is suggestive of the active conformation.

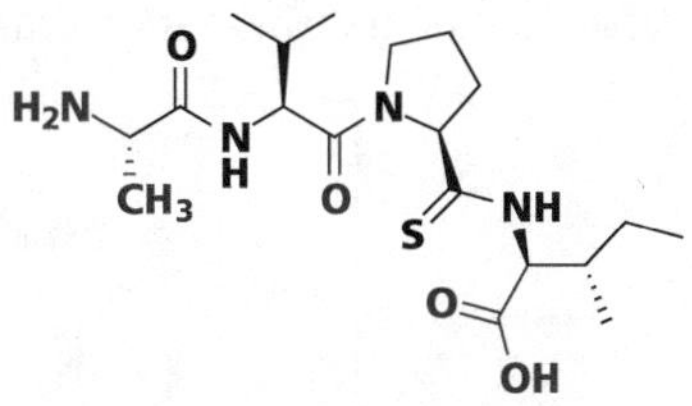

3. Design two different peptide-bond isosteres for the peptide substrate AVPI.

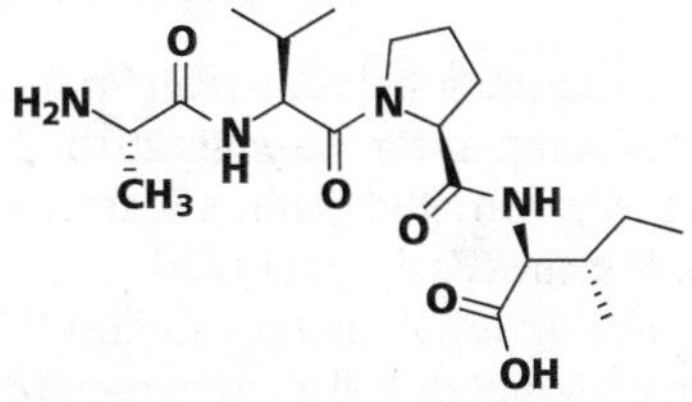

4. Phenytoin is an anticonvulsant drug. It is metabolized to generate a product that is hydroxylated on one of the phenyl rings. Design two analogs of phenytoin that would reduce the metabolism at this position and explain your rationale.

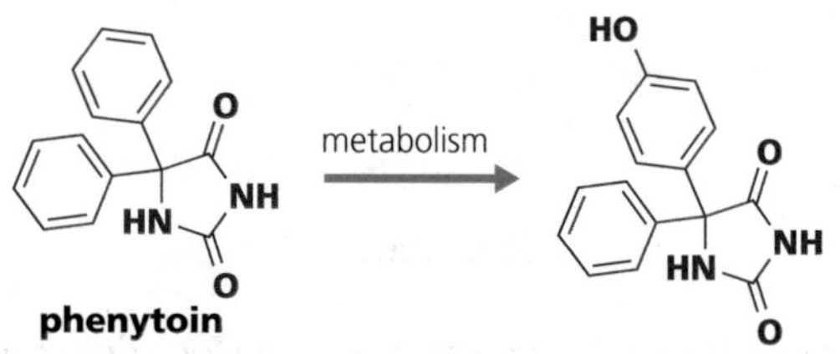

phenytoin → metabolism

5. Pubchem is a publically available database, sponsored by the National Center for Biotechnology Information: https://pubchem.ncbi.nlm.nih.gov. Perform a compound search for the three orally available drugs Valium, aspirin, and saquinavir. For each compound, compare the information in Pubchem to the values in Table 4.2 to determine whether each of the three compounds adheres to Lipinski's rule of five. Similarly, use the values to evaluate whether each of the three complies with the Veber rules.

6. Silicon is isosteric with carbon. It has been used in several drug candidates and some research compounds, but to date, no approved drugs have resulted. What similarities and differences will a silicon-containing compound have compared to the carbon analog? Research a drug for which the silicon analog has been prepared and compare the properties.

7. Paclitaxel, a natural product, is an important anti-cancer drug, but it has poor solubility. Design two new analogs that you predict would be more soluble than paclitaxel itself and rationalize your designs.

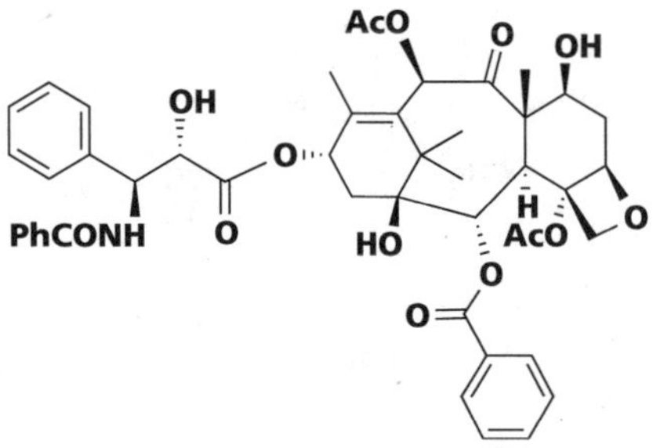

8. The structure shows a portion of one of the peptide substrates of an enzyme thought to contribute to the progression of Alzheimer's disease and the transition state through which it proceeds to generate the peptide cleavage products. An inhibitor of this protease has the potential to treat Alzheimer's disease. Design two peptide mimetics based on the transition state drawn.

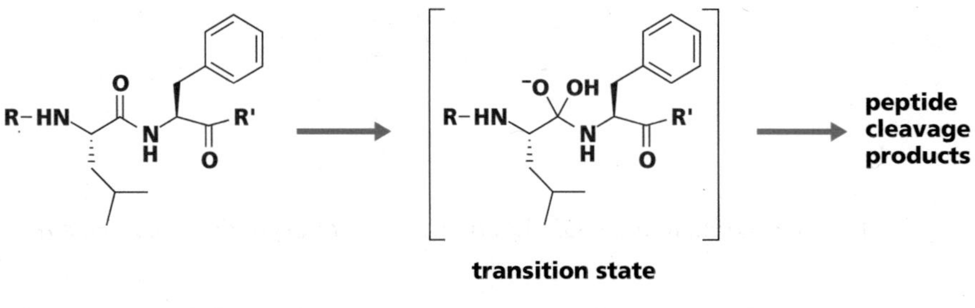

transition state

9. A literature search for "conformational constraint" in the Journal of Medicinal Chemistry gives over 30 examples for the years 2016–2017. One article describes a series of conformationally restricted gamma-secretase inhibitors that were evaluated as potential Alzheimer's drugs (J. Med. Chem. 2017, 60, 2383–2400). Identify the two different conformational constraints that were introduced to the lead compound. These compounds will need to penetrate the blood-brain barrier, so describe the effect of modifications on the cLogP.

10. The -SF$_5$ moiety is related to the -CF$_3$ group, and has been incorporated into drug candidates as a CF$_3$ substitution. Research the properties or this group compared to the CF$_3$ group—size, lipophilicity, electronic character in the context of a drug discovery project.

FURTHER READING

Optimization of physical and pharmaceutical properties

Lipinski CA, Lombardo F, Dominy BW & Feeney PJ (1997) Experimental and computational approaches to estimate solubility and permeability in drug discovery and development settings. *Adv Drug Delivery Rev* 23:4–25.

Veber DF, Johnson SR, Cheng H-Y et al. (2002) Molecular properties that influence the oral bioavailability of drug candidates. *J Med Chem* 45:2615–2623.

Hopkins AL, Keseru GM, Leeson PD et al. (2014) The role of ligand efficiency measures in drug discovery. *Nat Rev Drug Discovery* 13:105–121.

Bembenek SD, Tounge BA & Reynolds CH (2009) Ligand efficiency and fragment-based drug discovery. *Drug Discovery Today* 14:278–283.

Wenglowsky S, Moreno D, Rudolph J et al. (2012) Pyrazolopyridine inhibitors of B-RafV600E. Part 4: An increase in aqueous solubility via the disruption of crystal packing. *Bioorg Med Chem Lett* 22:912–915.

Bioisosteres, peptidomimetics, and scaffold hopping

Patani GA & LaVoie EJ (1996) Bioisosterism: A rational approach in drug design. *Chem Rev* 96:3147–3176.

Meanwell NA (2011) Synopsis of some recent tactical application of bioisosteres in drug design. *J Med Chem* 54:2529–2591.

Bursavich MG & Rich DH (2002) Designing non-peptide peptidomimetics in the 21st century: inhibitors targeting conformational ensembles. *J Med Chem* 45:541–558.

Eguchi M & Kahn M (2002) Design, synthesis, and application of peptide secondary structure mimetics. *Mini Rev Med Chem* 2:447–462.

Langdon SR, Ertl P & Brown N (2010) Bioisosteric replacement and scaffold hopping in lead generation and optimization. *Mol Inf* 29:66–385.

Böhm H-J, Flohr A & Stahl M (2004) Scaffold hopping. *Drug Discovery Today: Technol* 1:217–224.

Sun H, Tawa G & Wallqvist A (2010) Classification of scaffold hopping approaches. *Drug Discovery Today* 17:310–324.

Metabolic stability

St Jean DJ Jr & Fotsch C (2012) Mitigating heterocycle metabolism. *J Med Chem* 55:6002–6020.

Kerekes AD, Esposite SJ, Doll RJ et al. (2011) Aurora kinase inhibitors based on the imidazo[1,2-*a*]pyrazine core: fluorine and deuterium incorporation improve oral absorption and exposure. *J Med Chem* 54:201–210.

Fluorine

Gillis EP, Eastman KJ, Hill MD et al. (2015) Applications of fluorine in medicinal chemistry. *J Med Chem* 58:8315–8359.

Losartan

Duncia JV, Chiu AT, Carini DJ et al. (1990) The discovery of potent nonpeptide angiotensin II receptor antagonists: a new class of potent antihypertensives. *J Med Chem* 33:1312–1329.

Larsen RD, King AO, Chen CY et al. (1994) Efficient synthesis of losartan, a nonpeptide angiotensin II receptor antagonist. *J Org Chem* 59:6391–6394.

Cimetidine

Black JW, Durant GJ, Emmett JC & Ganellin CR (1974) Sulfur-methylene isosterism in the development of metiamide, a new histamine H_2-receptor antagonist. *Nature* 248:65–67.

Durant GJ, Emmett JC, Ganellin CR et al. (1977) Cyanoguanidine–thiourea equivalence in the development of the histamine H_2-receptor antagonist, cimetidine. *J Med Chem* 20:901–906.

Tagamet: Discovery of histamine H_2 receptor antagonists. Commemorative booklet 1998. American Chemical Society.

Ganellin CR (1981) 1980 Award in medicinal chemistry. Medicinal chemistry and dynamic structure-activity analysis in the discovery of drugs acting at histamine H_2 receptors. *J Med Chem* 24:913–920.

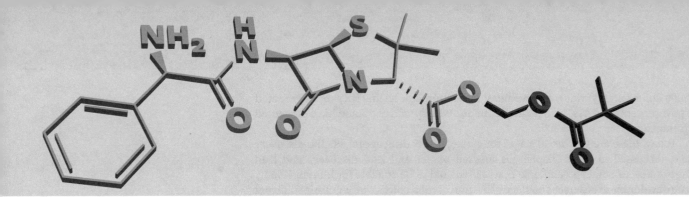

The process of developing a drug from an optimized lead

5

LEARNING OBJECTIVES

- Develop an understanding of the historical evolution of the drug approval process.
- Summarize the different types of patents important for drug discovery and development.
- Identify the characteristics of process chemistry synthesis.
- Become familiar with the pharmacokinetic parameters that are evaluated during the drug development stage.
- Understand some of the toxicity testing undertaken during the drug development stage.
- Summarize aspects of formulations that are critical for a drug development project.
- Learn the various phases of clinical trials and what is evaluated in each.

Historically, the process of new drug evaluation and approval has evolved so that drugs are proven to be both safe and effective in order to comply with increasing levels of regulatory oversight. In the United States, the first regulations imposed were decreed by the Pure Food and Drug Act of 1906, which required accurate labeling of medicines and listing of "addictive and/or dangerous" substances such as morphine, cannabis, and alcohol. The issue of safety was addressed further in 1938 with the passage of the Food, Drug, and Cosmetic Act. This law came about in response, in part, to a tragedy when approximately 100 people died in 1937 as a result of taking a diethylene glycol preparation of sulfanilamide, a drug used to treat streptococcal infections. Although there had been isolated reports of diethylene glycol's toxicity, it was not widely known at the time. The new act required testing of medicines in animals in order to prove safety. However, it was not necessary to prove efficacy of the drug until the Kefauver–Harris Amendment (Drug Efficacy Amendment) was added in 1962. This amendment required clinical trials establishing efficacy in humans and mandated reporting serious side effects of a drug even after its approval and marketing. It also increased the power of the U.S. Food and Drug Administration (FDA) by requiring that it approve a drug before the drug can be marketed. This amendment was enacted partly in response to the thalidomide tragedy. Thalidomide was widely prescribed in the late 1950s in Europe and Canada as both a sedative and a treatment for morning sickness. Sadly, it was later realized to have caused serious birth defects in more than

10,000 children. It is widely believed that more thorough testing (perhaps mandated by government agencies) prior to thalidomide's widespread use could have prevented this tragedy.

Today, there are two broad stages for getting a new drug approved. The discovery stage, discussed in prior chapters, is focused on hit and lead discovery and lead optimization to obtain a candidate that is predicted to be suitable for human testing. **Drug development** is the second stage of the process and consists of acquiring sufficient data to support the approval of the drug. It differs from the discovery stage in that all efforts are focused on characterizing and testing the one (or few) molecules that have evolved from the discovery stage and that exhibits all of the appropriate pharmacological effects and desirable physical and pharmaceutical properties, while at the same time being predicted to be safe. In the simplest cases, these two processes occur sequentially; however most often some of the specific activities overlap, and data generated during the development stage can often impact the direction of the discovery stage. Activities during this stage are numerous. One early activity, which may begin in the discovery stage, is patenting, which will give the developer exclusivity when marketing a drug. Process chemistry development concentrates on developing an efficient, safe, and cost-effective method to prepare pure drug substances in large quantities. Pharmacokinetic studies evaluate how the body handles the drug. Toxicology studies evaluate the safety of the drug in multiple species. Formulation development creates and tests combinations of the drug molecule and excipients and identifies the final form of the drug (capsule, tablet, injection, etc.) that will be used in patients.

Results of these studies, plus a plan for clinical evaluation, are required in order to file documents with regulatory agencies, such as an Investigational New Drug Application (IND) required by the US FDA. In the United States, 30 days must pass after the submission before human (clinical) trials can be initiated. Clinical trials consist of four phases and the first three take approximately 3–7 years for completion. During Phase I, Phase II, and Phase III clinical trials, the drug is tested for safety and efficacy, as well as for its potential to interfere with other drugs. It is also compared to other medications for the same disorder. In the United States, at the end of these three trials, a New Drug Application (NDA) is filed for review by the FDA. This review may take 1–2 years before final approval of the drug. An outline of the entire discovery and development process is shown in **Figure 5.1**.

In an industrial setting, the discovery stage typically lasts 1–3 years, and the development stage continues for many years beyond that. The odds of a compound proceeding from hit and lead discovery to an approved drug have been approximated at about 10,000 to 1. According to some estimates, the process of drug discovery and development for one drug takes an average of 12 years, and costs up to \$2.3 billion.

Figure 5.1 Overview of the drug discovery and development process. The discovery stage includes hit discovery, hit to lead activities and lead optimization and results in the identification of a clinical candidate. This process usually takes between 1-3 years. The development stage focuses on the most promising compound(s). Several clinical candidates are evaluated in extensive toxicity studies, efficient chemical synthesis and formulations are developed, and an IND is filed to advance even fewer drug candidates to clinical trial, from which only one may become an approved drug.

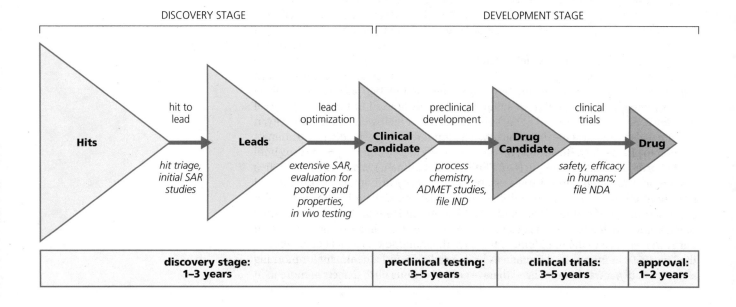

DISCOVERY STAGE   DEVELOPMENT STAGE

| hit to lead | lead optimization | preclinical development | clinical trials |

Hits   **Leads**   **Clinical Candidate**   **Drug Candidate**   **Drug**

hit triage, initial SAR studies

extensive SAR, evaluation for potency and properties, in vivo testing

process chemistry, ADMET studies, file IND

safety, efficacy in humans; file NDA

| **discovery stage: 1–3 years** | **preclinical testing: 3–5 years** | **clinical trials: 3–5 years** | **approval: 1–2 years** |

PATENTING AND DRUG DISCOVERY AND DEVELOPMENT

For all practical purposes, only commercial organizations have the capacity and resources necessary to complete the entire drug development process. Therefore, given the very high cost of drug development, protecting intellectual property through **patenting** is a high priority and often is a prerequisite for the molecule being advanced through clinical trials. A patent, according to the U.S. Patent and Trademark Office (USPTO) is an intellectual property right granted by the Government of the United States of America to an inventor "to exclude others from making, using, offering for sale, or selling the invention throughout the United States or importing the invention into the United States" for a limited time in exchange for public disclosure of the invention when the patent is granted. In other words, it allows the holder (or licensee) of the patent the exclusive right to sell a drug for a specified purpose in the country where the patent is held. This right allows the patent holder (or its licensee) the opportunity to recoup the investment made in the lengthy and expensive drug discovery and development process, as well as to make a profit. In some cases a patent is held by one organization (such as a university) and is licensed by a commercial entity (licensee) to complete the drug development process. After a patent expires, the drug can be sold by anyone, once studies showing bioequivalence of the product have been performed and regulatory agencies approve the application. Drugs that are sold by commercial organizations other than the original patentor or licensee, after patent expiration, are termed generic versions of the drug.

Producing and marketing **generic drugs** is a very active and lucrative business, in which many companies specialize. Generic firms do not need to support drug discovery research efforts, and therefore their costs of developing a generic drug are much less than those of the pharmaceutical firms, who develop new drugs.

The patenting process usually takes between 2 and 5 years and is concurrent with drug discovery and early preclinical development stages. In the United States, the process starts by submitting some version of a patent application to the USPTO. The application contains claims of the invention that are reviewed by an examiner. Over the course of several years, the examiner's office will often request changes or even reject certain claims, based on his or her analysis of the literature and other patents. Eventually a patent may be awarded, but it is often very different from the application originally submitted. Today, in the case where multiple patents are filed on the same subject matter, virtually all countries recognize the first to file as the inventor, as opposed to the individual(s) who were the first to invent. Once a patent is conferred, the government office is not responsible for enforcing the patent; that responsibility falls to the patent holder.

5.1 Three versions of patents are commonly filed during the drug discovery process

In the context of drug discovery and development, the most comprehensive kind of patent is termed a **composition of matter patent**. This protects the specific compounds claimed in the patent. In order to be patentable, a compound must be novel (not previously disclosed to the public), have proven utility, and "not be obvious to one skilled in the art." In other words, if similar compounds have been previously described as having the same or related utility, it would be obvious to one skilled in the art that the new compounds should have the same activity and therefore would not be patentable. The patent can cover a specific chemical entity and/or structurally related series with multiple modifications specified. The patent will also include a description of syntheses of the compounds claimed, physical data that characterize them, and usually preliminary data, (i.e. biological data) that support the utility of the compound(s).

A second type of patent important for drug discovery and development is a **method of use patent**. These patents are filed on known compounds for which a new, unobvious use has been discovered. For example, in Chapter 2, clinical observation was one of the lead sources described, with minoxidil as an example. Upjohn originally patented this compound as a blood pressure drug. When clinical observations showed minoxidil's ability to promote hair growth, they filed and were awarded a method of use patent for it as a hair-growth promoter. The granting of this new patent extended the time that Upjohn could exclusively market minoxidil as a hair-growth promoter.

A third type of patent is commonly referred to as a **process patent**. These patents usually describe the synthesis that will be used to manufacture the drug, as well as other possible syntheses. These syntheses can differ significantly from the one that may have been included in the original composition of matter patent. Process patents prevent others from using the protocols described in the owner's patent and are an additional method to strengthen the intellectual property estate surrounding a drug. A process patent can prevent anyone except the patent holder from manufacturing the compound by the same methods claimed, regardless of who holds the patent for use of the compound.

The lifetime of United States and most international patents is 20 years from the time of the application. This may seem like a long time until you consider that the average time to bring a drug to market is 12 years. This leaves only about 8 years for an organization to try to recover the enormous investment that was expended during the discovery and development stages. Deciding when to file patent applications, how to structure the application, and in what countries to file is a complex, strategic process. Applications that cover a large number of compounds (real and virtual) are often weaker than those that cover just a few compounds. However, patenting usually occurs early in the drug discovery and development process, well before the exact drug candidate is identified, so including multiple potential drug candidates is necessary. There is careful consideration as to when to file and what to file. Factors involved in the decision include the timing for exclusivity and when any product might be marketed, as well as the competitive landscape. In addition, fees to file and maintain patents can be very significant, and therefore cost is also a factor.

PROCESS CHEMISTRY RESEARCH

Process chemistry research involves the development of a process to synthesize multikilogram quantities of a drug candidate for animal testing and eventually for human testing. The synthetic protocols developed during this process are typically very different from the synthesis used to prepare the molecule during lead optimization, when only small quantities are necessary. The criteria for acceptable synthetic procedures require the process to be safe, efficient, highly reproducible, and consistent in yield and impurity profile. It should also be cost-effective and capable of generating kilogram quantities of drug candidate product with a minimal number of operations. Furthermore, there is now considerable effort to incorporate principles of green chemistry into these processes. **Green chemistry** focuses on the design of chemical products and processes that reduce waste, conserve energy, and replace hazardous substances. At the latter stages of the drug development process and postmarketing, the production of drugs is monitored and regulated by government authorities, who ensure that a set of standards called current Good Manufacturing Practices (cGMP) protocols are followed.

An excellent example of the differences between an early medicinal chemistry synthesis and a production-scale process can be highlighted by work on the anti-diabetic drug sitagliptin (Januvia). The original synthesis, first reported in 2005, was convergent, where each half of the molecule was synthesized and the halves (red and blue) were coupled to give the final product (**Figure 5.2**). Although fairly efficient, and acceptable for the production of gram quantities, this route required 19 steps and proceeded in 17% overall yield. Several reagents that are incompatible with a kilogram-scale synthesis due to safety issues were involved, one of which was diazomethane, used in the Arndt–Eistert homologation step. Chirality of the β-amino acid product originated from an α-amino acid that required four steps to prepare via alkylation of a valine-derived Schöllkopf reagent. The synthesis also relied on several expensive reagents, like 1-ethyl-[3-(3-dimethylamino)propyl]carbodiimide (EDC) used to couple the two halves and silver benzoate, as well as multiple chromatographic steps.

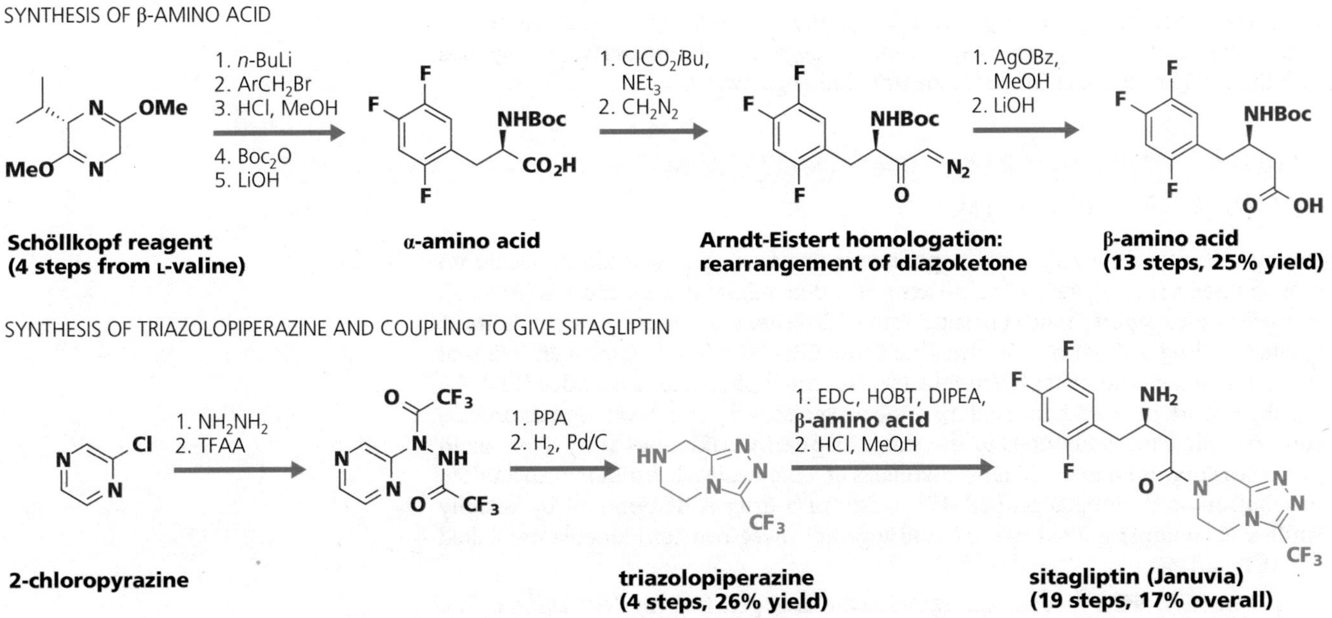

SYNTHESIS OF β-AMINO ACID

Schöllkopf reagent
(4 steps from L-valine)

α-amino acid

Arndt-Eistert homologation:
rearrangement of diazoketone

β-amino acid
(13 steps, 25% yield)

SYNTHESIS OF TRIAZOLOPIPERAZINE AND COUPLING TO GIVE SITAGLIPTIN

2-chloropyrazine

triazolopiperazine
(4 steps, 26% yield)

sitagliptin (Januvia)
(19 steps, 17% overall)

Figure 5.2 Originally reported synthesis of sitagliptin. Top: Outline of synthesis of the β-amino acid component in nine steps from a valine-derived Schöllkopf reagent. Alkylation and release of the chiral auxiliary followed by N-protection and ester hydrolysis, afforded the N-protected α-amino acid. Arndt–Eistert homologation, involving conversion to the acid chloride and reaction with diazomethane, followed by treatment with silver benzoate, and hydrolysis yielded the β-amino acid (red). Bottom: Outline of the synthesis of triazolopiperazine and final coupling steps. Substitution of 2-chloropyrazine with hydrazine and N-acylation is followed by acid-catalyzed cyclization with polyphosphoric acid (PPA) and reduction to give the triazolopiperazine (blue). Amide formation between the β-amino acid (red) and triazolopiperazine (blue), followed by N-deprotection, afforded sitagliptin (Januvia). The sequence entails 19 steps and proceeds in 17% overall yield.

In contrast, a process synthesis (**Figure 5.3**) reported in 2009 proceeds in four linear steps (the first three occurring in one pot) starting from the aryl acetic acid and the triazolopiperazine and 65% overall yield. Homologation of the aryl acetic acid by use of Meldrum's acid, was followed by amide coupling with the triazolopiperazine (prepared separately) and conversion to the crystalline enamine amide, in a one-pot process for the three steps. Hydrogenation with an asymmetric rhodium catalyst introduced the chirality in the final step with 95% enantiomeric excess. This extremely efficient process eliminated hazardous reagents and minimized both expensive coupling reagents and chromatography.

This example highlights some common strategies used in developing a process chemistry synthesis. These include using a minimal number of steps, employing

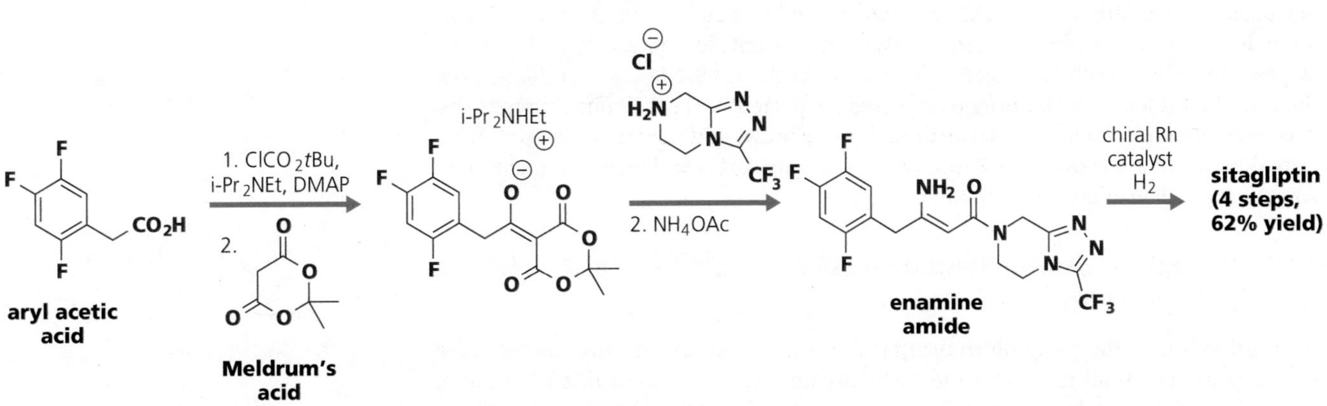

aryl acetic
acid

Meldrum's
acid

enamine
amide

sitagliptin
(4 steps,
62% yield)

Figure 5.3 Process chemistry synthesis of sitagliptin. Acylation of Meldrum's acid is followed by coupling with the triazolopiperazine to give an enamine amide, and then reduction of the enamine by use of a chiral rhodium catalyst affords sitagliptin. This sequence entails 4 linear steps and proceeds in 65% overall yield.

inexpensive reagents, avoiding chromatography by utilizing crystallization for purification, and avoiding especially hazardous reagents. This process was recognized with the 2006 Presidential Green Chemistry Challenge Award.

CHARACTERIZATION OF PHARMACOKINETIC PROPERTIES OF LEADS

During the drug discovery stage, experiments focus on effects of the molecule on protein targets (usually using *in vitro* assays) and in animal disease models (*in vivo*). However, unless appropriate concentrations of drug are present in the target tissue or organ, the drug will not be effective. The correlation between drug concentration at the site of action and effect (often efficacy) is termed **pharmacodynamics** (PD). An equally important consideration during the drug discovery and development process concerns what the body does to the drug, or **pharmacokinetics** (PK). Four main processes contribute to the pharmacokinetics of a molecule: absorption, distribution, metabolism, and elimination (**ADME**). Safety of a drug is determined by **toxicity studies** in multiple animal species, and together these five components are called **ADMET** studies.

- **Absorption** is the mechanism by which the drug gets into the bloodstream. The specific route of administration directly affects this parameter.

- **Distribution** is the process through which the drug is distributed from the bloodstream to various compartments of the body, including tissues, brain, and other organs. This parameter is important to evaluate whether the drug reaches the specific organ or tissue that is targeted.

- **Metabolism** is the chemical modification of a substance in the body. This process typically occurs in the liver and generates more polar derivatives of the drug, called **metabolites**, often through oxidation or conjugation with small, polar molecules. Metabolism is one aspect of the body's sophisticated and efficient method to remove toxic and/or foreign substances, termed **xenobiotics**.

- **Elimination**, or excretion, is the second part of the body's detoxification process. The intact drug or its metabolites are removed from the bloodstream, usually in urine or feces but also through other fluids such as sweat or tears and even exhalation.

The pharmacokinetics of a drug involves a series of complex processes, but specific measurements corresponding to each of these are evaluated in both primary and secondary *in vitro* assays as well as *in vivo* assays. *In vitro* assays are incorporated early in the course of drug discovery and medicinal chemistry activities and are used to predict *in vivo* ADME results. For example, lipophilicity, permeability, and solubility measurements are used to predict absorption, and tests in isolated liver microsomes are used to evaluate how quickly molecules are metabolized *in vivo*. Studies in animals are more complex and usually start with rodents and progress to dogs and/or primates. These animal studies, grouped under the umbrella term of PK studies, measure blood levels of the drug over a specific period of time, determine how the drug is metabolized, where it is distributed in the body, and how it is excreted. Data from these analyses allow comparison across several species and give an indication of what doses will be effective in humans.

5.2   Absorption is one determinant of how much drug reaches its biological target

Absorption is the process by which drugs pass through membranes, most often those in the gastrointestinal tract, into the bloodstream. For the sake of this discussion, absorption of drugs administered orally (po or *per os*, by mouth) will be described. When a drug is ingested, it first passes through the highly acidic environment of the stomach (pH = 1–2.5). Only acidic drugs that have the appropriate balance of solubility and lipophilicity can be absorbed at this site. Acid-sensitive compounds will decompose here, and basic drugs, because they will be protonated in the acidic environment, will not be absorbed due to their charged nature. However, since the residence time in the stomach is only 20–60 minutes, there is relatively little absorption. The second phase of absorption occurs in the small intestine, where the pH gradient moves from a partially acidic environment (pH ~ 5) to a neutral one (pH ~ 7) as the distance from the stomach increases. Most drugs are absorbed as they pass through the small intestine, due to its large surface area and the 4–6 hour transit time. The large intestine (pH 8–8.5) has a smaller surface area, and absorption here is less efficient. Upon absorption into the intestines, the drug passes through the portal vein into the liver (called the first pass) and then into general circulation, where it can be carried to the target tissue. The overall process is outlined in **Figure 5.4**.

Drugs delivered via other routes of administration, such as intravenous (iv), intramuscular (im), and transdermal (through the skin) delivery, enter circulation without first passing through the intestines and liver. Many routes of administration are possible, and each has its own absorption characteristics. Others include inhalation, sublingual (under the tongue), intraperitoneal (ip), rectal, and buccal (through the mucous membranes in the mouth) delivery.

As described in Chapter 4, three characteristics of a molecule are known to dramatically influence absorption: its solubility, lipophilicity, and permeability. Molecules must be soluble in their aqueous environment for absorption to occur, and polar molecules and those that contain charged functional groups favor excellent solubility. They must also be sufficiently lipophilic that they can pass through a cellular membrane, be it cellular membranes in the stomach and intestines that allow drugs to get into the bloodstream or, once in the bloodstream, the specific cell membrane that may contain the pharmacological target of the drugs. The permeability of a

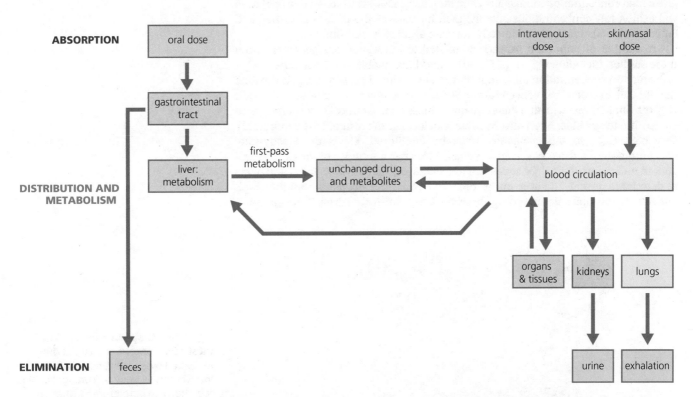

Figure 5.4 General process of absorption, distribution, metabolism, and elimination of drugs. An orally dosed drug passes through the gastrointestinal tract where it may either be directly eliminated in the feces or pass through the liver. In the liver, the drug can be metabolized (called first-pass metabolism), and metabolite and any unmodified drug enter into general circulation. An intravenously administered drug or one administered through the skin or nasal passage enters directly into general circulation (avoiding first-pass metabolism). Once in circulation by any route, the drug is distributed to various organs and tissues. Elimination of drugs occurs by metabolism in the liver to more polar derivatives and then excretion in urine and feces as well as other routes.

compound depends on both of these characteristics. Drugs permeate through cell membranes through two main routes. Most drugs rely on **passive diffusion**, driven by a concentration gradient, as a mechanism to enter cells. Molecules that are lipophilic, like the lipid membrane, or lipid-soluble are most effectively transported through the passive route, whereas charged molecules are not passively diffused. A second mechanism by which molecules can cross cell membranes is called **active transport**. This mechanism relies on protein transporters that recognize specific molecules, often biomolecules such as amino acids or carbohydrates, and transports them across the lipid bilayer. This process is often difficult to predict; therefore, most drug discovery programs work on the assumption that molecules will be absorbed by passive diffusion.

In vitro assays to characterize solubility, lipophilicity, and permeability are used to predict absorption. To get a more complete assessment in an animal, **PK studies** are performed. They evaluate the concentration of the drug in plasma over a specific time frame after administration of the compound at a certain dose (or doses). Since the dose administered is rarely reflective of the compound concentration in circulation due to all of the processes outlined above, PK studies allow one to more fully understand the behavior of the compound. They are an important bridge between the *in vitro* ADME assays described in Chapter 4 and the results of studies in animal models of disease. By understanding the concentration of drug in circulation and other parameters after dosing, the behavior of the compound in animal models of disease becomes more interpretable, since one can then relate effects observed to a plasma concentration. As an example of the design of a single-dose PK study, animals are given one dose of a compound by the preferred route of administration. Concentrations (C) of the drug are measured at various time points (t) over an extended period of time, often 24 hours, and then plotted versus time. A typical PK graph is shown in **Figure 5.5**, plotting plasma concentration versus time in hours. An intravenous (iv) dose will give a high concentration immediately and then decrease over time. An oral (po) dose will exhibit low concentrations initially, then increase as the drug is absorbed and enters the bloodstream, and ultimately decrease again as it is eliminated.

A number of important parameters related to absorption are generated from these studies, including C_{max}, t_{max}, C_{ss}, AUC, and bioavailability, among others. C_{max} is the highest concentration the compound achieves after dosing, and t_{max} is the time that it takes to reach that concentration. Some *in vivo* effects require that a certain C_{max} threshold is reached, and therefore this value is often a critical determinant for a compound to advance. Alternatively, some toxicities are the result of the compound's very high C_{max}, so this parameter must be monitored. C_{ss} is the steady-state concentration of a drug, observed at equilibrium after a number of doses. This will give an indication of the drug concentration after a multiple-dose regimen and helps to determine dosing. The **area under the curve** (AUC) is calculated from the graph and reflects the total amount of drug absorbed or exposure of the drug. **Bioavailability**

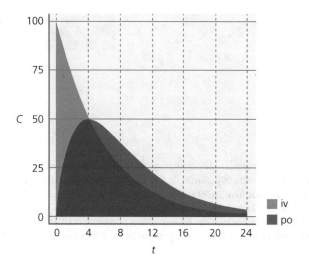

Figure 5.5 Graph of a theoretical PK study. Concentration (*C*) of drug measured over time (*t*, hours) after intravenous (iv, shown in orange) or oral (po, shown in purple) administration. Various parameters are calculated from this graph: C_{max} is the peak concentration reached, t_{max} is the time required to reach C_{max}, AUC reflects overall exposure of the compound, and bioavailability is calculated as the ratio AUC_{oral}/AUC_{iv}.

(or fraction absorbed, F or FA) is also derived from a PK study and reflects the fraction of the molecule absorbed after a specific route of administration compared to what is theoretically possible. It is calculated by comparing the AUC when the drug is dosed by the preferred route (usually orally), to the AUC for intravenous dosing (considered 100% absorbed). Oral bioavailability is equal to AUC_{oral} divided by $AUC_{iv} \times 100$. High oral bioavailability values are >70%, with >50% preferred. Compounds with oral bioavailability of less than 50% may advance, but they often require additional formulation efforts due to their poor absorption characteristics.

Many different factors influence a drug's PK properties. Some of these factors are intrinsic to the specific molecule and therefore cannot be changed. Others, however, such as formulations, can be modified to optimize parameters such as C_{max}, exposure, and bioavailability. High bioavailability is an important goal for any drug discovery project for a number of reasons including the following:

- Safety: the PK performance of a drug that exhibits excellent oral bioavailability is often less variable than those with poorer bioavailability. Therefore, unexpectedly high or low drug concentrations, which can result in over- or underdosing, respectively, rarely occur. In addition, the lower doses that are possible when bioavailability is high may minimize off-target effects.

- Cost: Highly bioavailable drugs minimize the amount of active ingredient required in each drug substance, be it a tablet, capsule, or iv solution. The amount of active drug ingredient required will influence the cost of the materials of the drug as well as the cost to manufacture the drug.

- Compliance: smaller doses (for example, tablet, pill sizes) taken less frequently are preferred by patients and improve compliance.

5.3   Distribution determines which tissues accumulate drugs

The body has various compartments into which a drug can distribute. The blood is considered the first compartment; the second compartment is the rest of the body. Once in the bloodstream, drugs can further distribute to specific tissues within the body. The distribution may not be uniform and is influenced by characteristics of the drug and of the specific tissue. For example, drugs that accumulate in fat tissue are typically lipophilic. Differences in pH between blood and specific cells will also influence where drugs concentrate. Drugs can also build up in certain organs, such as the brain, for example, where central nervous system (CNS) drugs need to accumulate to be efficacious. Additional factors determining distribution include the ability of molecules to bind to plasma proteins or to be recognized by transport mechanisms.

Drugs in circulation reversibly bind to **plasma proteins** such as albumin to various degrees, and this phenomenon affects not only their distribution but also their *in vivo* potency. The unbound drug molecules are in equilibrium with plasma protein-bound drug molecules, and as the unbound molecules migrate into tissues, the equilibrium between bound and unbound drug in plasma is reestablished. Therefore, drugs that are highly bound to plasma proteins usually are not widely distributed or only slowly distributed. Furthermore, when they are evaluated *in vivo*, highly bound drugs may not be as potent as molecules that are less tightly bound because only the unbound molecule is available to bind to the target. On the other hand, highly bound drugs can act as a reservoir for free drug and therefore provide long-lasting concentrations of drug in plasma. The effects of a drug's binding to plasma protein are complex and difficult to predict; however, high plasma protein binding is often a valid explanation for lack of *in vivo* effects despite potent *in vitro* activity. Assays to determine the extent of protein binding are often performed during lead optimization and can be done in plasma, tissue, or blood by dialysis, ultrafiltration, or ultracentrifugation methods. These secondary assays determine the **fraction unbound** (f_u) of compound and are often used to rank compounds. When the f_u value is low, it can be used to rationalize the unexpectedly poor behavior of a potent compound in *in vivo* animal models. An alternative way to assess the effects of plasma protein binding is to include serum in the original *in vitro* assay and determine if there is a shift in potency with and without serum.

A second determinant of drug distribution is the activity of transporter proteins, found in specific types of cells that recognize and transport distinct small molecules. When a small molecule is recognized by a transporter protein, it can be taken up by cells expressing that transporter and accumulate in those cells. Since transporters are responsible for both influx and efflux of compounds, they can also play a role in keeping molecules out of specific tissues. The most well-known example of an efflux pump is the P-glycoprotein transporter (P-gp), which functions by rapidly transporting substrate molecules out of cells against a concentration gradient. P-gp is widely expressed in the intestine, and its activity is the reason some drugs are poorly absorbed despite good solubility and permeability. It is also present in the brain, where it protects the CNS from xenobiotics and therefore is a powerful barrier to drugs reaching the brain. Loperamide is an over-the-counter treatment for diarrhea that works though the same mechanism as morphine: both bind at the μ-opioid receptor. However, whereas morphine is brain-penetrant, loperamide is rapidly transported out of the brain by P-gp, making it safe and nonaddictive, in contrast to morphine (**Figure 5.6**). P-gp is also present in some cancer cells, where its expression or induction is a common mechanism of drug resistance caused by its transport of drugs out of the cancer cells. Assays to determine whether a compound is a substrate for an efflux pump are common during lead optimization.

The distribution of a drug affects its potency as well as its potential for toxicity. Certain drugs are highly effective and safe because they accumulate in the specific tissues where they need to act. For example, iodine concentrates almost exclusively in the thyroid gland, and therefore iodine and its derivatives are often used to treat thyroid disease. The apparent **volume of distribution** (V_d) is a value used to reflect the amount of drug that is distributed throughout the organism compared to the amount present in plasma; it is measured in a PK study. For molecules with high volumes of distribution, plasma levels will be low. Conversely, low volumes of distribution reflect high plasma concentrations. The specific disease targeted will dictate whether a high or low volume of distribution is desirable.

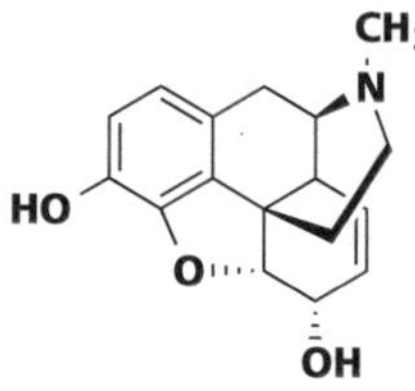

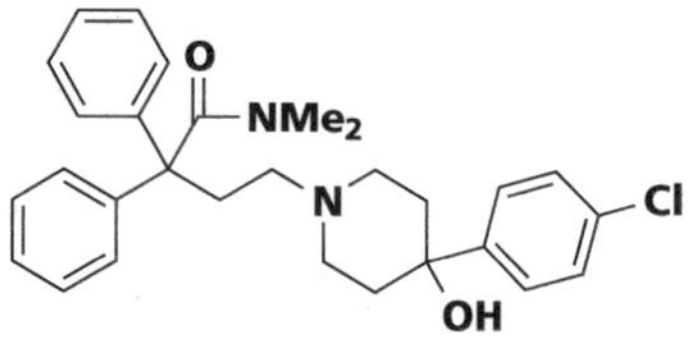

Figure 5.6 Structures of morphine and loperamide. Both bind at the μ-opioid receptor, but, in contrast to morphine, loperamide does not accumulate in the brain due to its efflux by the P-gp transporter, and therefore has no CNS effects.

5.4 Metabolism and elimination are the body's method for removing drugs

One mechanism by which the body detoxifies itself is through metabolism, also termed biotransformation. Metabolism chemically modifies the xenobiotic, typically in two phases, I and II, to generate more polar, water-soluble derivatives called metabolites. Metabolites are more efficiently eliminated than the parent. Specific enzymes in the liver carry out most of these reactions, although metabolism also occurs in other organs and tissues. The degree of metabolism of a drug candidate and the specific metabolites formed affect its potency, dosing schedule, and toxicity. Molecules that are rapidly metabolized are then rapidly eliminated and never attain appropriate blood levels to exhibit the desired effects. Conversely, when drugs are metabolized very slowly, their concentration in blood and tissues can build up to unsafe levels. The specific metabolites of drugs need to be identified and studied, as they often exhibit their own pharmacological effects. In some cases, the metabolites are inactive; in other cases they exert similar, beneficial effects as the parent; and in still other situations, the metabolites might exhibit some serious toxicity.

Phase I metabolic reactions usually occur in the liver and modify a functional group of the parent drug. Three of the most common phase I reactions are oxidation, reduction, and hydrolysis. Oxidation is carried out chiefly by cytochrome P-450 enzymes (CYPs), which are heme proteins associated with an NADPH–cytochrome P-450 reductase. There are many different CYP variants (known as isozymes), each denoted with a three-figure notation of number-letter-number. The CYP isozymes responsible for most drug metabolism are CYP 3A4, CYP 2D6, CYP 1A2, CYP 2C9, and CYP 2C19. Additional enzymes that play a role in oxidative metabolism include alcohol and aldehyde dehydrogenases, aldehyde oxidase, amine oxidases, and lipoxygenases. The most common oxidation reactions are hydroxylation, oxidation of alcohols, and epoxidation. **Table 5.1** shows some examples of typical oxidation processes.

Table 5.1   Oxidation substrates and products of phase I metabolism

Substrate	Product
arene	phenol
arene	benzylic alcohol → aldehyde → acid
alkene	allylic alcohol
carbonyl compound	α-hydroxy carbonyl
alkyl amine	unstable hemiaminal → aldehyde + amine
alkane	alcohol → ketone
alkene	epoxide
alcohol	aldehyde → carboxylic acid
amine heterocycle	N-oxide
thioether	sulfoxide → sulfone

Hydroxylation reactions can occur on arenes, at benzylic or allylic positions, at a position α to carbonyls, on carbons bearing a nitrogen, and even on unactivated alkyl groups. Epoxidation occurs on alkenes and also on arenes (not shown). Other oxidations include oxidation of alcohols, and direct oxidation of nitrogen or sulfur to generate N-oxides and sulfoxides or sulfones, respectively.

Often the first metabolite formed is also a substrate for the metabolizing enzyme and secondary reactions occur. For example, when a primary alcohol is formed, it can undergo subsequent oxidation to the aldehyde and then to the carboxylic acid. The hemiaminal, $RC(OH)NR_2'$, formed from oxidation at a carbon α to a nitrogen, decomposes to give a carbonyl product and an amine product (NHR_2'). Further reaction of the resulting carbonyl product is common. Some examples that follow this pathway are shown in **Figure 5.7**. Amphetamine undergoes oxidative deamination to give a ketone metabolite and ammonia. Propranolol, a β-adrenergic blocker, follows two pathways, based on the site of oxidation. Path A involves oxidation at the N-isopropyl site, followed by N-dealkylation to generate the dealkylated primary amine metabolite and acetone (not shown). An alternative pathway is oxidative deamination and further oxidation (path B), which ultimately gives a carboxylic acid.

Metabolic reductions (usually stereospecific) are carried out by α-keto reductases and flavin-independent NADPH–cytochrome P-450 reductases. Typical substrates are carbonyl and oxidized nitrogen compounds, as shown in **Table 5.2**.

Reductions can occur on aldehydes and ketones, including quinones. Nitrogens that are in an oxidized state, as in nitro, nitroso, or hydroxylamine

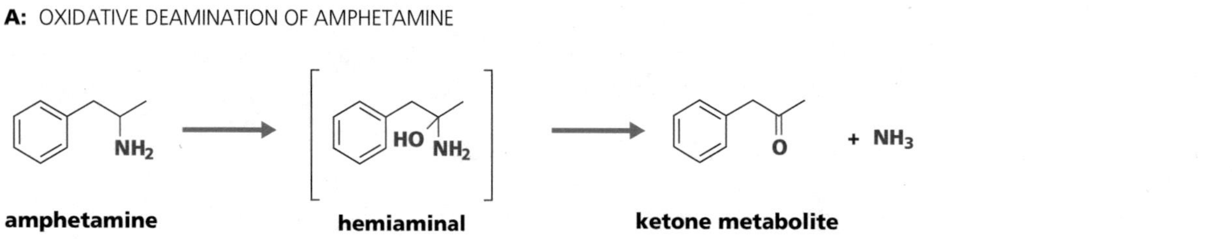

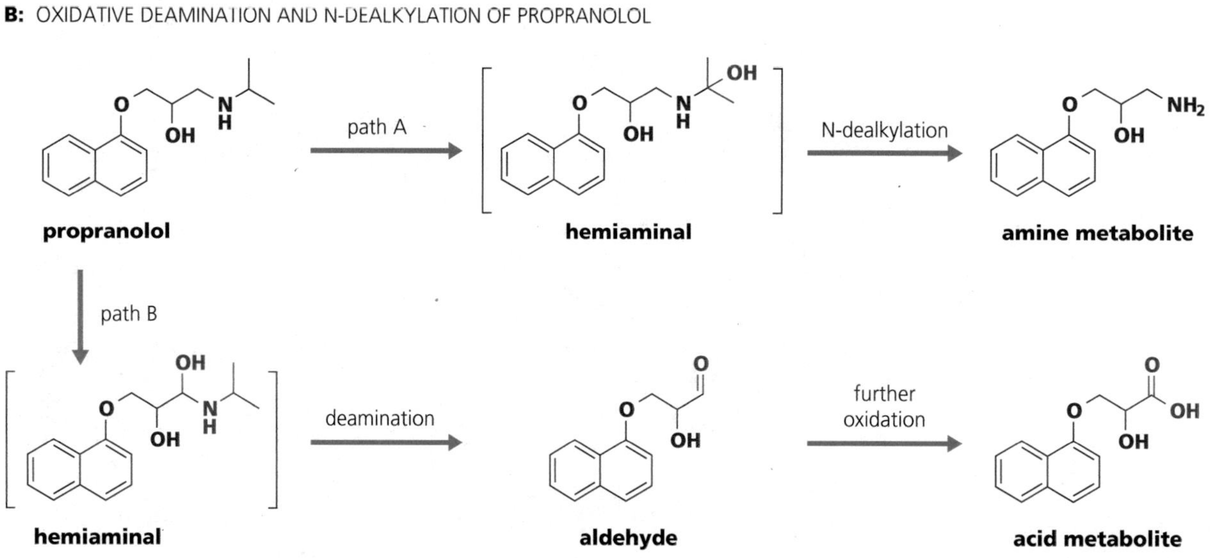

A: OXIDATIVE DEAMINATION OF AMPHETAMINE

B: OXIDATIVE DEAMINATION AND N-DEALKYLATION OF PROPRANOLOL

Figure 5.7 Oxidative N-dealkylation and deamination and of amine-containing drugs. Fragments introduced and metabolized are shown in red. A: Oxidative deamination of amphetamine gives a hemiaminal intermediate, which hydrolyzes to the ketone metabolite and ammonia. B: Propranolol is metabolized by two oxidative pathways to give intermediate hemiaminals. Path A begins with hydroxylation of the isopropyl group, which is then converted to the N-dealkylated metabolite. Path B begins with hydroxylation of the methylene adjacent to the nitrogen; deamination affords an aldehyde, which is further oxidized to an acid.

Table 5.2 Reduction substrates and products of phase I metabolism

Substrate	Product
ketone/aldehyde	chiral alcohol
quinone	hydroquinone
RNO$_2$ or RNO nitro/nitroso	RNHOH hydroxylamine
RNHOH hydroxylamine	RNH$_2$ amine
RN=NR azo	2 RNH$_2$ amine
RX haloalkane	RH alkane

groups, are deoxygenated to generate either hydroxylamines or amines. Azo bonds are cleaved to produce two primary amines, and haloalkanes are typically reduced to alkanes.

The stereoselectivity of the reduction of carbonyl groups may be species-dependent, as shown for the metabolism of naltrexone, an opioid antagonist (**Figure 5.8A**). Reduction of the ketone in chickens gives the *S*-alcohol, whereas reduction in either rabbits or humans gives the *R*-configuration at the carbinol. These results highlight an important caveat when animal data are used to predict human metabolism.

A third type of phase I transformation is a hydrolytic reaction, typically carried out on esters and amides by nonspecific esterases and amidases, respectively. The substrates may be aromatic or aliphatic, but hydrolysis may sometimes be highly chemospecific. For example, esterases hydrolyze the methyl ester (red) of cocaine in the presence of a benzoate ester (blue, **Figure 5.8B**). Hydrolysis may also be stereoselective for one enantiomer over another, such as the hydrolysis of the amide of prilocaine (**Figure 5.8C**). Both enantiomers of this local anesthetic are active, but only the amide (red) of the *R*-isomer is hydrolyzed to give the products toluidine and the *R*-carboxylic acid. *o*-Toluidine is toxic, so it is safest to administer only the *S*-isomer of prilocaine, which is not metabolized by this route.

Prodrugs, discussed in Chapter 4, are administered as inactive forms of the drug and are metabolized, usually through phase I processes, to generate the active species. Esters are a common form of prodrugs, and hydrolysis by an esterase to the corresponding acid provides the active form. Examples, shown in **Figure 5.9**, include the antibacterial drug pivampicillin, a prodrug of ampicillin, and the blood pressure drug enalapril, a prodrug of enalaprilat. Biotransformation or metabolism played an important role in the history of the nonsedating antihistamine terfenadine (Seldane). Upon administration, it is rapidly oxidatively metabolized in the liver to produce another active molecule, fexofenadine. At high doses, terfenadine is cardiotoxic but fexofenadine is not. This observation led to the decision to replace the allergy drug terfenadine with fexofenadine.

After phase I functional group transformations occur, there are further **phase II metabolic reactions**. The drug or metabolite is conjugated (connected) to some small endogenous molecule in order to expedite elimination or to reduce reactivity. These phase II reactions are carried out by various transferase enzymes. Some examples, illustrated in **Table 5.3**, are as follows:

- **Glucuronidation**. In this reaction, glucuronic acid is conjugated to alcohols, acids, and other nucleophilic groups. A functional group of the drug or metabolite attacks the anomeric carbon of UDP-glucuronic acid to give the glycoside, or conjugate, of the drug or one of its phase I metabolites.

- **Amino acid conjugation**. An amide is formed between an amino acid (usually L-glutamine in primates) to a carboxylic acid of the drug or one of its metabolites.

- **Glutathione conjugation**. The thiol group of glutathione, a tripeptide found in all tissues, attacks a variety of electrophiles, such as aldehydes and Michael acceptors of the drug or drug metabolite, to provide the thiol adduct.

- **N-acetylation**. Amines are often conjugated during phase II metabolism to generate the N-acetate derivatives.

Some examples of complete metabolic processes are shown in **Figure 5.10**. Metabolism of phenytoin, a drug to treat epilepsy, involves an oxidative phase I transformation where one of the aromatic rings is hydroxylated at the para position. Phase II conjugation of that metabolite by glucuronidation gives the final metabolite. In the second example, the antihistamine brompheniramine proceeds through four different metabolic reactions to generate the carboxylic acid. Two successive N-demethylations generate the primary amine; oxidative deamination of that metabolite generates the aldehyde, which is further oxidized to the carboxylic acid metabolite. Phase II conjugation of the acid to the amine of glycine gives an amide as the final metabolite. Finally, the

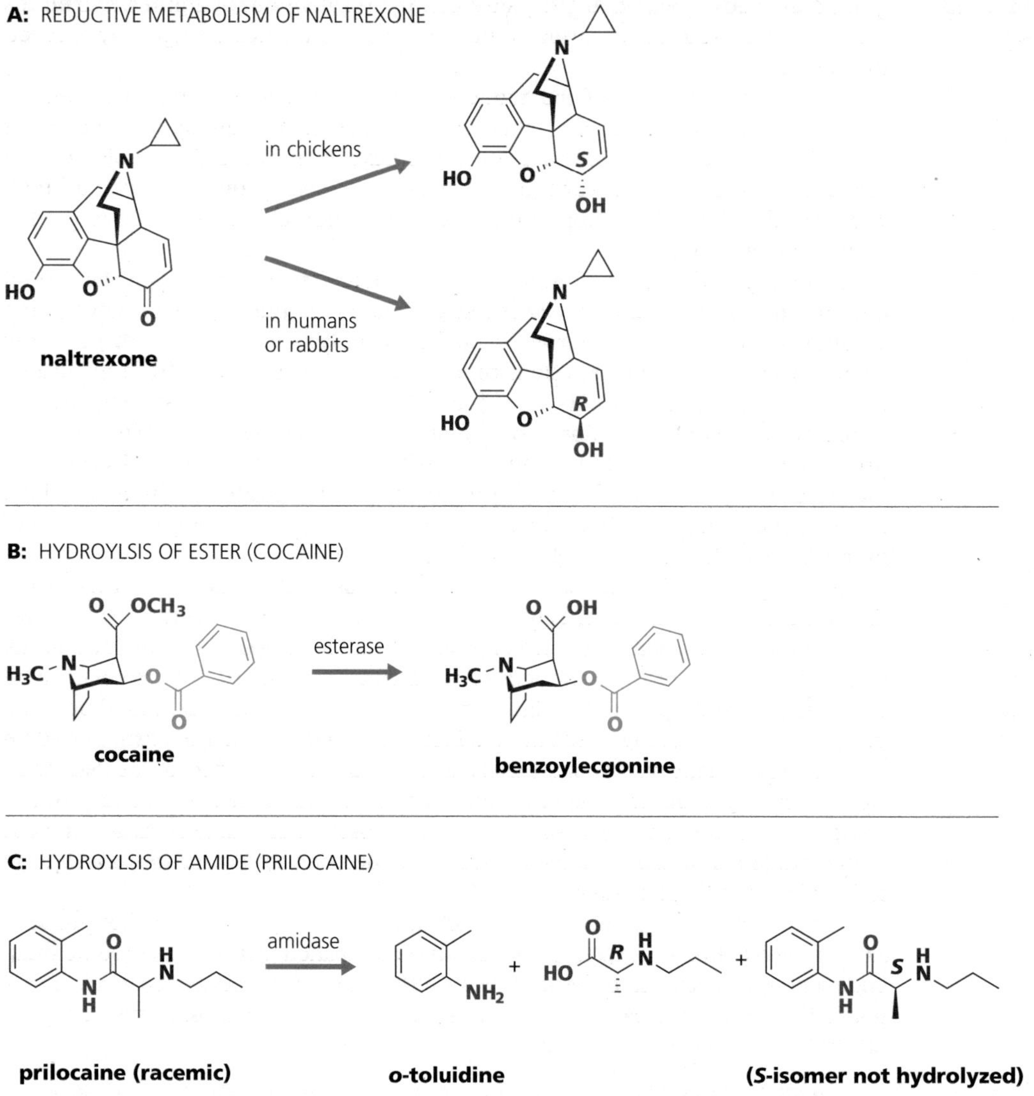

A: REDUCTIVE METABOLISM OF NALTREXONE

Figure 5.8 Examples of reductive and hydrolytic metabolism. A: Reduction of the ketone of naltrexone affords the S-alcohol in chickens but the R-alcohol in rabbits and humans. B: Hydrolysis of the methyl ester of cocaine (shown in red) occurs without hydrolysis of the benzoate ester (shown in blue). C: Hydrolysis of the amide of prilocaine (shown in red) is specific for the R-enantiomer.

B: HYDROYLSIS OF ESTER (COCAINE)

C: HYDROYLSIS OF AMIDE (PRILOCAINE)

alcohol of the analgesic morphine is oxidized to a ketone, generating an electrophilic enone (Michael acceptor). Conjugation to glutathione affords the final metabolite.

During lead optimization, the potential for compounds to be metabolized is evaluated in an assay that measures the stability of the compound in liver microsomes. A half-life is determined to indicate which compounds will be stable to metabolism and which are likely to be prone to rapid degradation. These assays report on phase I metabolic processes only. During the drug development stage, metabolites of the drug candidates are identified and quantified through sophisticated mass spectrometric analysis. Metabolites that are formed in significant quantities are synthesized and tested in the same battery of assays as the parent to evaluate whether they exhibit pharmacological activity and/or toxicity. Predicting the identity of metabolites from the parent structure relies on understanding the metabolic reactions and is fairly reliable. For example, alkyl chains and neutral or electron-rich aromatic groups are considered metabolic hot spots for hydroxylation. Hydroxyl groups and acids are often glucuronidated. Medicinal chemistry strategies are frequently applied in order to limit metabolism, either through introducing steric hindrance or blocking functional groups or isosteric replacement, as discussed in Chapter 4. Computational chemistry programs are available to predict both the sites and extent of metabolism; however,

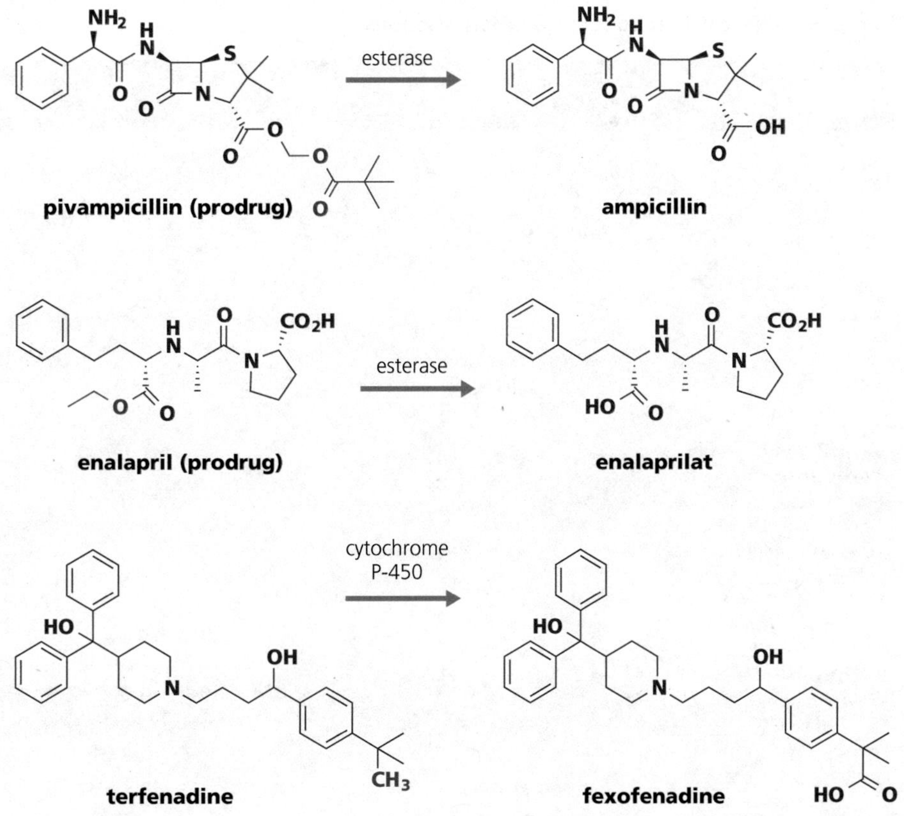

Figure 5.9 Examples of drugs generated by metabolism. The active forms of pivampicillin (ampicillin) and enalapril (enalaprilat) are formed by ester hydrolysis. Fexofenadine is a metabolite of terfenadine, formed by cytochrome P-450-mediated oxidation of a methyl group to a carboxylic acid.

pivampicillin (prodrug) →(esterase)→ ampicillin

enalapril (prodrug) →(esterase)→ enalaprilat

terfenadine →(cytochrome P-450)→ fexofenadine

predicting the extent of metabolism, in contrast to the identity of metabolites, is much less precise.

Key parameters that are extracted from PK studies that reflect metabolism include measurements of the clearance of a drug and its half-life. **Clearance** (CL) is the volume of plasma cleared of the drug per unit time and reflects not only metabolism but also excretion. High clearance rates indicate that the compound is rapidly eliminated from the body and may not have sufficient exposure for *in vivo* effects to be observed. The drug's **half-life** ($t_{1/2}$) is the time it takes for 50% of the drug to disappear from circulation. Like CL, $t_{1/2}$ informs the appropriate dosing schedule. Drugs with longer half-lives can be dosed less frequently than those with short half-lives. However, drugs with very long $t_{1/2}$ (>24 hours) may result in serious side effects.

The final step in the elimination of xenobiotics is **excretion**. Drug molecules are most often eliminated through urine or feces, but other routes are also known, for example, through saliva or exhalation. While some molecules are excreted unchanged, most are excreted as metabolites. Evaluating the route of excretion is done in animal models, by detecting the concentration or presence of the parent or metabolite in urine or feces.

DRUG TOXICITY DETERMINATION

According to Paracelsus, "All things are poison, and nothing is without poison; only the dose permits something not to be poisonous." This statement is particularly relevant to drug discovery and development, where identifying doses and conditions at which toxicity caused by a drug is observed, and understanding the nature and cause of the toxicity, is essential. As the overall goal of drug discovery and development is to identify molecules that are safe and effective, toxicity testing plays a major role during the development stage. The **therapeutic index** (TI), the ratio between the highest

Table 5.3 Phase II metabolic conjugation reactions

Phase II transformation	Reaction
Glucuronidation: Nucleophile present in drug adds to anomeric carbon of UDP-glucuronic acid	
Amino acid conjugation: amide forms between acid in a drug and amine group of glutamine	
Glutathione conjugation: thiol of glutathione adds to electrophile present in a drug	
N-acetylation: acetyl group is transferred to nitrogen atom of a drug	

tolerated dose (or exposure) and the minimally efficacious dose (or exposure), should be as high as possible. However, the specific disease will determine an appropriate TI. For non-life-threatening diseases, high TI values are required. For life-threatening disorders such as cancer, TI values of only 2 are sometimes acceptable.

5.5 Indications of toxicity are identified early in the drug discovery stage by *in vitro* assays

During lead optimization, there are a number of *in vitro* assays that are employed to give an early indication of potential toxicity. These assays are used so that the best leads for progression to animal testing for efficacy are identified. Some common assays include the following:

- **Cytotoxicity assays.** These assays involve treating cells with a small molecule for some period of time and then measuring specific biological readouts of cell viability to determine if the compound causes cell death. No mechanism can be inferred, but this assay provides an indication of potential toxicity. Predictive software, based on the presence of functional groups with reported toxicities,

A: METABOLISM OF PHENYTOIN BY OXIDATION AND CONJUGATION TO GLUCURONIC ACID

B: METABOLISM OF BROMPHENIRAMINE BY SUCCESSIVE OXIDATIONS AND CONJUGATION TO GLYCINE

C: METABOLISM OF MORPHINE BY OXIDATION AND CONJUGATION TO GLUTATHIONE

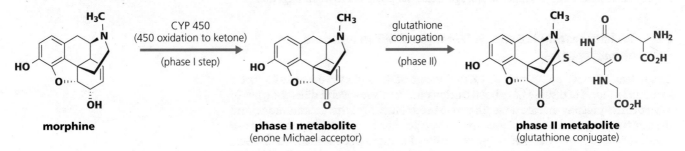

Figure 5.10 **Examples of drug metabolism showing both phase I and phase II metabolites.** A: Phenytoin undergoes phase I metabolism to a phenol and then phase II conjugation to the glucuronide. B: Brompheniramine is converted by four successive phase I reactions to the acid, and then phase II amino acid conjugation affords the final glycine conjugate metabolite. C: Phase I oxidation of morphine generates an α, β-unsaturated Michael acceptor, which reacts with glutathione in a phase II reaction to generate the glutathione adduct as the metabolite.

is also available and is often used in the earliest stages of hit identification to prioritize compounds for advancement.

- **Cytochrome P-450 Inhibition or Induction assays.** One important toxicity evaluated predicts the potential for **drug–drug interactions**. When one drug prevents the metabolism of another drug by inhibiting a cytochrome P-450 (CYP) enzyme, the second drug can reach dangerously high, toxic drug levels because it is not eliminated. For example, ingredients in grapefruit are known to inhibit certain CYP isozymes, and therefore patients are often told to avoid consuming the fruit while taking certain medications. Drug–drug interactions can also be exploited. The HIV protease inhibitor ritonavir is part of a multidrug regimen prescribed to AIDS patients. In addition to its desired pharmacological effect, ritonavir inhibits CYPs and therefore causes a desirable increase in blood levels of the other protease inhibitors, which typically have low bioavailability, in the drug cocktail. Alternatively, a molecule may induce a CYP enzyme, causing an overall increase in the amount of a particular CYP isoform and therefore its metabolizing ability. This induction can result in the rapid metabolism of a second drug, making that second drug ineffective. Another important reason for evaluating CYP inhibition or induction is the large genetic variability of CYP enzymes among the human population. Certain genetic determinants may influence how a particular drug is metabolized; therefore, knowing that a subpopulation may exhibit drastically different pharmacokinetics than the general population allows safer patient selection. Assays to assess drug–drug interactions are done early in the drug discovery process by determining the effects a molecule has on the ability of a specific CYP isozyme (for example, CYP 3A4, CYP 2D6, or CYP 2C9) to metabolize a specific substrate.

- **hERG Channel.** The human ether-à-go-go related gene (hERG) encodes an ion channel that transports potassium ions in heart muscle and is critical for coordinating the heart's beating. When its activity is compromised, a fatal condition called QT prolongation syndrome can result. Recently, several well-known examples of drugs (for example, Seldane), previously considered safe, were found to cause sudden death in some patients because the drug inhibited the hERG channel. Since then, testing the activity of molecules in *in vitro* assays for hERG activity is a routine part of the drug discovery and development process.

- **Genetic toxicity.** Genetic toxicity studies establish the mutagenic potential (whether or not it causes DNA damage) of a drug and therefore its potential to cause cancer. The **Ames test** is the gold standard for *in vitro* genetic toxicity testing. In this assay, a mutant form of the bacterium *Salmonella* is treated with the test agent. This specific mutant requires histidine in the growth medium in order to replicate. The mixture is then placed in a low-histidine medium. If there are no changes to the DNA, the bacteria will not grow. If the DNA has mutated, it replicates and suggests that the test agent has the potential to be mutagenic.

5.6   Toxicity testing is done with *in vivo* assays in multiple animal species

Once a lead has been optimized and PK studies and other studies to evaluate its effects in animal models of disease have been carried out, there are several different types of *in vivo* toxicity testing that are done. These are used to identify a therapeutic index, find the safest dosing levels, and uncover any unexpected effects of the compounds. These studies will also show effects of long-term dosing that may not be evident otherwise.

Acute toxicity studies are done in animals at increasing doses until toxicity is observed. Studies are generally begun in rodents and progress to dogs or rabbits. Acute testing begins with a single dose, and the animal is observed for signs of toxicity such as vomiting, diarrhea, weight loss, lethargy, or death over the course of 7–14 days after the dose. Blood levels of the drug are also monitored to determine at what drug concentration toxicity is observed. The relationship between toxicity and concentration of drug in the blood is termed **toxicokinetics** (TK).

Range-finding studies are then carried out in which several different doses (usually a high, medium, and lose dose) are administered daily over 2–4 weeks. These studies establish the range of doses that can be administered without significant toxicity, as well as the maximum tolerated dose (MTD), and they dictate the doses that will be used in subsequent subchronic and chronic toxicity testing.

Subchronic testing and **chronic testing** comprise the next level of *in vivo* toxicity testing and involves much longer duration of dosing. During subchronic testing the animals (either rodents or non-rodents) are dosed daily for three months and monitored for signs of toxicity, including weight loss or gain. After completion of the study, tissues are harvested and examined for histological changes compared to control animals. Chronic testing lasts for longer than three months, and should have at least the same duration as the proposed clinical trials. These are carried out in at least one rodent and at least one non-rodent species. Animals are monitored after dosing stops to identify effects that appear after long-term dosing. Chronic testing has two components: first is 6–12 months of observation, looking for signs of toxicity, and second is 12–24 months of observation for signs of carcinogenicity.

These acute and chronic toxicity studies are used to establish the no observed adverse effect level (NOAEL) of the drug. This value is the highest dose of the drug that can be administered without serious toxicity, and helps define the tolerable dose for clinical trials.

Reproductive toxicity determines whether the drug will have any effects on fertility, the ability to maintain a pregnancy, and the health of the progeny of patients. It is completed in three parts:

1. **Segment I testing** looks at fertility and reproductive performance in both male and female animals that are administered the drug.

2. **Segment II testing** evaluates embryonic toxicity (teratogenicity) during early pregnancy of mothers being dosed with the drug.

3. **Segment III testing** determines if there are any effects of the drug on the final stage of pregnancy, as well as delivery and lactation (milk production), when administered to a pregnant female or mother.

Most drug candidates that have unacceptable levels of toxicity, whether acute, chronic, or reproductive, will not proceed to clinical trials. In these cases, lead optimization is re-initiated in order to find an acceptable candidate. Depending on the therapeutic area, however, different levels of toxicity are acceptable. For example, several of the coxib anti-inflammatory drugs were withdrawn from the market after exhibiting cardiac liabilities. However, doxorubicin, an anti-cancer drug, is still in use despite its cardiotoxicity because its benefits outweigh the toxicity. In another example, thalidomide, the teratogenic sedative, has found new use to treat both leprosy and multiple myeloma and is now marketed with extensive warnings of its teratogenicity.

A summary of some important parameters that are commonly measured or calculated during ADMET studies is given in **Table 5.4**.

5.7 Formulation of the final drug product

The active drug substance is termed the **active pharmaceutical ingredient** (API); however, the medication itself contains additional components, and together these make up the pill, capsule, or liquid medication. The combination of the API and the other components, known as excipients, is the **formulation** of the drug. The specific formulation can affect the site and degree of absorption, half-life, bioavailability, and dosing schedule, among other factors. In addition, the formulation must be stable over long periods of time, inert to heat and humidity, and consistently deliver the same drug levels. Specific disease states and patient populations are additional factors considered during formulation development. In infant and pediatric patients, for example, liquid formulations for oral administration are preferred over capsules or pills.

Many of the factors that influence the specific formulation developed are related to the physical properties of the drug molecule: solid-state form (for example, the specific crystalline polymorph), particle size of solids, pK_a, solubility, and dissolution rates are key determinants. The bioavailability of compounds of low solubility and high permeability can be improved with formulations; however, it is difficult to improve PK characteristics through formulation of compounds with low permeability, regardless of their solubility.

While complex formulation science is beyond the scope of this text, the generation of salts of drugs that are acids or bases is an important component of formulation studies. The free acid or base of the API is often evaluated in the earliest stages of the drug discovery process, but evaluation of various salt forms can occur during lead optimization to identify products that have improved solubility, crystallinity, stability, and permeability. These characteristics will all affect exposure and bioavailability of the compound.

Table 5.4 Summary of pharmacokinetic and safety parameters and measurements

Absorption Parameters, Measurements and Relevance	
C_{max}, maximum concentration, and t_{max}, time to reach maximum concentration	peak plasma concentration of a drug after administration and the time it is reached
	measured in *in vivo* PK assays in concentration and time units; C_{max} values should be sufficient for activity depending on drug potency (C_{max} should exceed *in vitro* IC_{50})
	important to understand pharmacodynamics and toxicity effects; used to determine most appropriate dose and dosing schedule
C_{ss}, steady-state concentration	equilibrium concentration of drug after a number of doses (when the amount of drug absorbed/time = amount eliminated/time)
	measured in *in vivo* PK assays in concentration units; based on AUC taken over different times; dependent on dosing
	used to determine most appropriate dose and dosing schedule
AUC, area under the curve	integral of plasma concentration over a set time period
	measured in *in vivo* PK assays; values should be sufficient for activity depending on drug potency and pharmacodynamic requirements
	related to the required dose and frequency of dosing
F or FA, oral bioavailability	fraction of drug that reaches systemic circulation upon oral administration compared to an iv dose; equal to $AUC_{oral}/AUC_{iv} \times 100$
	measured in *in vivo* PK assays; greater than 20% is considered developable, albeit low, with >50% usually considered acceptable
	related to dose required and efficiency of absorption
Metabolism, Distribution, and Elimination Parameters, Measurements and Relevance	
Fraction of drug unbound (f_u); plasma protein binding	degree of binding to plasma proteins
	measured in secondary *in vitro* assays; fraction unbound (f_u) >99% usually undesirable, as is irreversible binding
	reflective of how much drug is available to bind to the target
V_d, distribution volume	volume (in liters or liters per kilogram) in which drug is distributed, if homogeneous distribution is assumed
	measured in *in vivo* PK studies; drug may be in plasma and/or tissue
	when V_d < 6 L, most of the drug is in blood or plasma; when V_d > 42 L, all of the drug is in tissue
	indicates how much drug is distributed outside of plasma; specific disease target dictates desirable values
CL; clearance	rate at which a drug is eliminated, calculated as dose/AUC or volume of plasma cleared of drug per unit time
	measured in *in vivo* PK assays; can also be predicted from *in vitro* ADME assay data
	one parameter that contributes to effective *in vivo* drug concentration; used to determine appropriate dose and dosing schedule
$t_{1/2}$, half-life of drug	time required to halve the plasma drug concentration
	measured in *in vivo* PK assays
	related to required dose and frequency of dosing

metabolic stability ($t_{1/2}$)	ability of compound to withstand metabolic transformation by liver enzymes
	measured in primary or secondary assays, such as liver microsomes, to detect half-life of compound
	$t_{1/2} > 60$ min is ideal, although very long $t_{1/2}$ may be unsafe
	related to achieving high compound concentrations (bioavailability) required for *in vivo* biological activity

Safety and Toxicity Parameters

cytochrome P-450 (CYP) inhibition or induction	ability of compound to inhibit or induce metabolism of specific compounds by specific CYP isoenzymes
	measured in primary assays; no/low inhibition preferred
	acceptable values are related to the differential between CYP affinity (K_i) and C_{max}
	Indication of potential to interfere with metabolism of other administered drugs and is a safety consideration
hERG, human ether-à-go-go gene, channel activity	potential of compounds to inhibit the hERG ion channel
	measured in primary and secondary assays as a concentration; inhibition of >10 μM usually acceptable, with 30-fold safety margin desirable
	reflection of safety of the compound
MTD, maximum tolerated dose	highest dose that is tolerated without significant toxicity
	measured in *in vivo* toxicity assays, higher doses are better
	indication of safety of the drug
LD_{50}, lethal dose	dose that is lethal to 50% of animals tested
	measured in *in vivo* toxicity assays; higher values are safer
	indication of safety of the drug
TI, therapeutic index	ratio between maximum tolerated dose (or exposure) and minimal efficacious dose (or exposure) = MTD/MED
	measured in animal efficacy and toxicity studies (*in vivo*)
	higher TI values are preferable, but the specific condition dictates a tolerable TI: for example, drugs to treat cancer often exhibit a TI between 2 and 10, while drugs that treat less serious disorders, childhood diseases, and chronic diseases require a much higher TI (>10)
	indication of safety of the drug

CLINICAL TRIALS IN HUMANS

After the 4–8 years it takes to complete the discovery and preclinical development studies, a clinical candidate is identified from the optimized leads. This compound will exhibit the best combination of potency, physical and pharmaceutical properties, and low toxicity. The preclinical data, including method of synthesis, formulation plan, and results of pharmacokinetic and toxicity studies in multiple animal species, as well as a plan for clinical trials, is submitted to the US FDA as an **Investigational New Drug Application** (IND). This proposal needs to be approved by the FDA and by an Institutional Review Board (IRB), where the trials will take place before proceeding with trials in humans. Testing of drugs in humans usually occurs in four phases, but only the first three are required for approval:

1. During **phase I clinical trials**, the drug is tested in a very small number of healthy volunteers (20–80) for a short duration, often in a hospital so subjects can be closely monitored, with the goal of uncovering unexpected toxic effects

and gathering data on pharmacokinetics in humans. Approximately 70% of the drugs that enter Phase I trials move onto Phase II studies.

2. If no unacceptable toxicity is observed, the efficacy of the drug in patients is then evaluated in **phase II clinical trials**. These studies involve a larger number of carefully selected subjects (~100–300), and they compare the efficacy of the drug candidate with either a placebo or a drug that is already proven to be effective. These studies can be **double-blind**, meaning that neither the patients nor the clinicians administering the drug are aware of which agent (drug candidate or comparator) is being given to each patient. At the same time, safety is continually monitored. These studies can last for a few months to several years, and only 33% of tested drugs move into the next phase.

3. If efficacy is observed in phase II, the program progresses to **phase III trials**. These studies are more complex and involve an even larger number of patients (~200 to >3000), often in different stages of the disease to study efficacy, different dosages, different patient populations, combinations with other drugs, tolerability, and safety. Only 25–30% of drugs successfully complete Phase III studies

4. Additional studies that further evaluate efficacy, safety, and optimal use after drug approval are termed **phase IV trials**.

Once the Phase I-III studies are completed, and the drug candidate shows statistically significant effects and acceptable toxicity, an extensive report is filed with the regulatory agency. This is called a **New Drug Application** (NDA) in the United States. This report contains not only data from the clinical trials on efficacy, safety, and PK but also all previously acquired data in animals, as well as specifics on how the drug will be manufactured after approval. Prior to 1992, the average time for the FDA to grant approval was 2–3 years, although this could be considerably shorter for drugs to treat a life-threatening disease. In 1992, the Prescription Drug User Fee Act (PDUFA) was passed, in which the applicant pays a fee to the FDA. It is estimated that the FDA receives approximately $100 million per year from applicants, part of which has been used to increase FDA staffing. Since then, the time for approval has shortened to about 6 months–2 years. Once approved, the drug can be marketed for a specific use, based on the regulatory agency's review and requirements.

After the drug is approved, additional studies are usually required that further evaluate efficacy, safety, and optimal use; these are termed phase IV, which includes **postmarketing surveillance**. The regulatory agency continues to monitor reports on side effects and any results from post-marketing studies, as well as results on new uses for the drug. Should new data arise, the regulatory agency can change the labeling of the drug, add new uses, add specific warnings, change the suggested dosing, or remove the drug from the market.

Once a molecule enters clinical trials, the probability that it will become an approved drug is approximated at only 11%. The entire process, from the earliest stages to drug approval, takes an average of 12–14 years, and costs are estimated to be well over $2 billion, according to FDA figures (https://www.fda.gov and https://clinicaltrials.gov). Out of the 5000–10,000 molecules that might be evaluated in the earliest stages of drug discovery project, chances are that only one will be approved and marketed.

SUMMARY

As described in the first five chapters of this text, the overall process of developing a drug is a complex and lengthy process. Hit and lead identification, followed by lead optimization, and then extensive testing are required to identify a viable clinical candidate. The optimization process requires a cycle of design, synthesis, testing, and data analysis to achieve the optimal balance of potency, properties, and low toxicity. This is all a part of the preclinical discovery process, which also includes the important process of patenting viable leads. As an optimized lead emerges from preclinical *in vivo* assays, attention turns toward complete understanding of that compound. Evaluation of the pharmacokinetics of the compound in several animal species determines whether the compound is suitable for further advancement and helps predict human dosages. Development of a process synthesis to produce kilogram quantities of a drug is an important activity during this phase, as is formulation of the drug substance to the eventual final form of the medicine. Extensive testing in animals to uncover any potential for toxicity is also done in preparation for human trials. For this final stage of development, a drug needs to pass three phases. Phase I clinical trials establish safety and dosing levels, as well as human pharmacokinetics. Phase II trials test efficacy, and then phase III trials, in larger populations, verify efficacy and particular aspects of safety. Even after many years are invested into a drug discovery program, there is still only about a 10% chance that a drug candidate will progress through all phases of clinical trials and receive approval.

CASE STUDY 1   DISCOVERY OF FLUOXETINE

Fluoxetine, an antidepressant, was the first of the selective serotonin reuptake inhibitors (SSRIs) approved, and, at that time, had a number of advantages over other drugs used to treat depression. Although fluoxetine was not approved until 1987, it was first reported as LY110140 in 1974 as a selective serotonin reuptake inhibitor. The tricyclic antidepressants (TCAs) used at that time, such as imipramine, were nonselective and inhibited the reuptake of serotonin (5-HT), norepinephrine (NE), and dopamine (DA). Although effective as antidepressants, the TCAs have cardiac and anti-cholinergic side effects.

Diphenhydramine is an antihistamine, but it also acts as a norepinephrine reuptake inhibitor. On the basis of its activity in animal models of depression, Bryan Molloy and Robert Rathbun at Eli Lilly began a medicinal chemistry program focused on phenoxyphenylpropylamines, with structures similar to diphenhydramine (Figure 5.11), aimed at retaining the therapeutic activity of TCAs but eliminating or reducing their side effects. These efforts first led to the discovery of nisoxetine (LY94939), which was as effective as TCAs in animal models of depression. However, *in vitro* testing showed that nisoxetine was a selective inhibitor of NE uptake rather than a pan-inhibitor of reuptake of multiple neurotransmitters. Realizing that subtle changes in structure could have profound effects on selectivity, they continued their investigations on this structural class in the hopes of identifying a selective 5-HT reuptake inhibitor, which many believed would retain the antidepressant effects of the TCAs but produce fewer side effects. Investigation of compounds with minor differences in this series led to the discovery of fluoxetine (Prozac), which was found to be a selective inhibitor of 5-HT reuptake. Initial results measured a K_i of 1.7×10^{-8} M for inhibition of reuptake of 5-HT, with 200–300-fold selectivity over NE and DA reuptake.

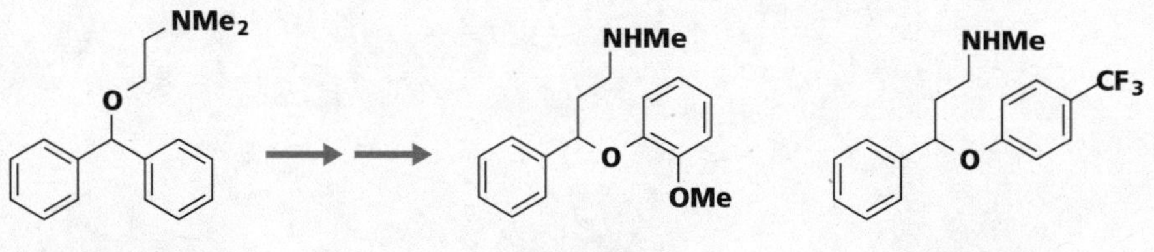

diphenhydramine
antihistamine,
NE reuptake
inhibitor

**nisoxetine
(LY94939)**
NE reuptake
inhibitor

**fluoxetine
(LY110140)**
5-HT reuptake
inhibitor

Figure 5.11 Structures of diphenhydramine, nisoxetine, and fluoxetine. Diphenhydramine was an antihistamine and also was an inhibitor of NE reuptake. Analogs based on diphenhydramine included nisoxetine, an NE reuptake inhibitor, and fluoxetine, a potent 5-HT reuptake inhibitor. Fluoxetine was the first 5-HT reuptake inhibitor approved to treat depression.

The initial synthesis of fluoxetine was described in the patent literature, and a number of process syntheses have been reported. Both the initial and subsequent process syntheses begin with 3-(dimethylamino)propiophenone, which is readily available by Mannich reaction of acetophenone, formaldehyde, and dimethylamine. The initial synthesis used diborane to reduce the ketone, followed by reaction with thionyl chloride to introduce the benzylic chloride, as seen in Figure 5.12. Williamson ether synthesis using the *p*-trifluoromethyl phenol was followed by von Braun N-demethylation using cyanogen bromide followed by treatment with KOH. Points identified in this route that would be incompatible with a process scale include the use of hazardous reagents such as thionyl chloride, cyanogen bromide, and diborane on a larger scale and the expense of the phenol reagent. In an improved process synthesis, the order of steps is revised. Diborane is replaced with sodium borohydride, and the demethylation is effected by the use of ethyl chloroformate and subsequent hydrolysis. An S_NAr reaction replaces the Williamson ether synthesis, using the less expensive *p*-trifluoromethyl chlorobenzene.

INITIAL SYNTHESIS

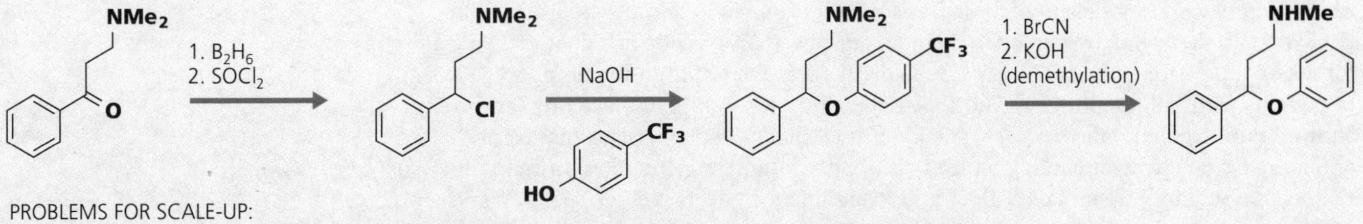

PROBLEMS FOR SCALE-UP:

1. hazardous on large scale: handling of diborane, thionyl chloride, and cyanogen bromide

2. high reagent cost: *p*-trifluoromethyl phenol

PROCESS SYNTHESIS

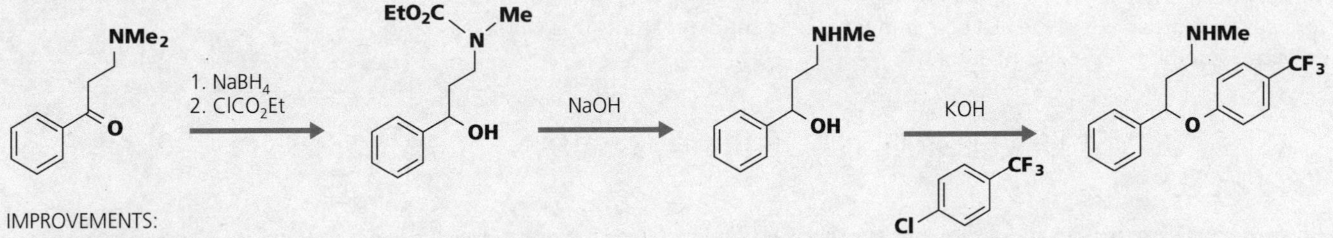

IMPROVEMENTS:

1. Safer reagents

2. low reagent cost: *p*-trifluoromethyl chlorobenzene

Figure 5.12 Comparison of initial and process syntheses of fluoxetine, both beginning with 3-(dimethylamino) propiophenone. The initial synthesis occurred over five steps and used materials that would be hazardous on a large scale. In addition, some of the reagents were also expensive. The process synthesis rearranges some of the order of reactions, avoids hazardous reagents and is more cost-effective.

A number of compounds with different substituents on the phenoxy ring were prepared, including F, Cl, Me, OMe, and CF_3 derivatives in ortho, meta, and para positions. Substitution in the ortho position generally led to selective NE reuptake inhibition, with the exception of the CF_3 analog, which showed some selectivity for 5-HT reuptake inhibition, although with low potency. The *p*-CF_3 analog (fluoxetine) had the optimal profile, with 17 nM K_i for 5-HT reuptake versus 2703 nM K_i for NE reuptake. Compounds with other substituents in the para position showed some selectivity for 5-HT over NE but with lower potency.

The primary amine analog of fluoxetine (norfluoxetine) has the same activity profile as the parent compound and is the major active metabolite. While both enantiomers of fluoxetine are equally active, the *S*-enantiomer of norfluoxetine is 14 times more potent than the *R*-enantiomer. Fluoxetine is metabolized by N-demethylation to norfluoxetine and then further oxidized to the acid, which is eliminated as the glucuronide conjugate, as seen in **Figure 5.13**.

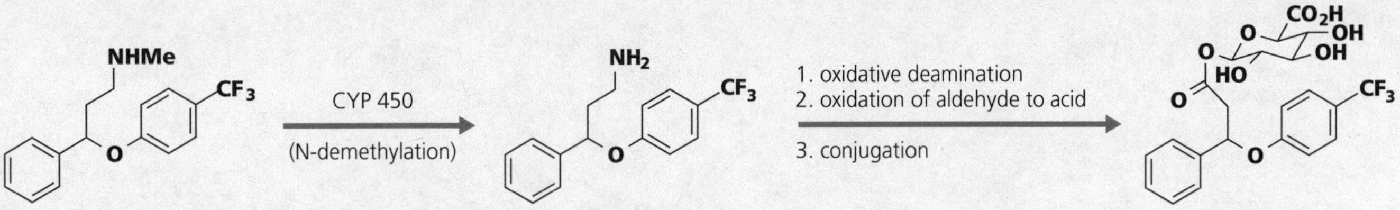

fluoxetine (LY110140)

norfluoxetine

glucuronide conjugate

Figure 5.13 Metabolism of fluoxetine and structures of metabolites. Fluoxetine is metabolized to norfluoxetine, which exhibits a similar activity profile. Norfluoxetine is further metabolized in Phase II reactions to generate the glucuronide conjugate.

Preclinical testing of fluoxetine in mouse and rat models showed efficacy in a wide range of behavioral models of both depression and obsessive–compulsive disorder. In clinical trials, fluoxetine was found to be more effective than placebo at a dose of 20 mg for major depression, melancholia, and mild depression. For example, in one study, 62% of patients with mild depression who took fluoxetine, versus 19% of those on placebo, showed improvement after 8 weeks. The older tricyclic antidepressants exhibited anticholinergic side effects including blurred vision, dry mouth, constipation, urinary retention, and memory dysfunction. Their anti-histaminergic effects include sedation and hypotension as well as reflex tachycardia. Fluoxetine was found to produce few of these side effects. The lack of motor and cognitive defects and the lack of cardiac effects were particularly noteworthy and distinguished fluoxetine from previous antidepressants, although at higher doses (80 mg) 24% of patients experienced nausea as a side effect.

After its introduction in 1987, fluoxetine became the leading antidepressant worldwide. It is used in the treatment of depression, obsessive–compulsive disorders, and panic disorder. It was the first of a number of new antidepressants that worked as selective serotonin reuptake inhibitors.

CASE STUDY 2 DEVELOPMENT OF RIVAROXABAN (XARELTO)

Rivaroxaban (Xarelto) is an anti-coagulant drug that was developed by scientists at Bayer AG in Germany. Older drugs to treat blood clots include heparin, which must be given intravenously, and warfarin, which requires regular blood monitoring due to its low therapeutic index. Rivaroxaban resulted from the search for an alternative that was safe and orally active. One proposed novel target was activated serine protease factor Xa (FXa), which plays a role in the blood coagulation cascade. This enzyme converts prothrombin to thrombin. Thrombin then converts fibrinogen to fibrin, activates platelets, and, through feedback activation of other coagulation factors, increases its own levels. By inhibiting FXa, coagulation would be inhibited, and blood clots would be prevented.

As a starting point to identify inhibitors of FXa, the initial hits 1 and 2 were discovered by high-throughput screening (HTS) of over 200,000 compounds (Figure 5.14).

INITIAL HITS FROM HTS AND OPTIMIZATION TO LEADS

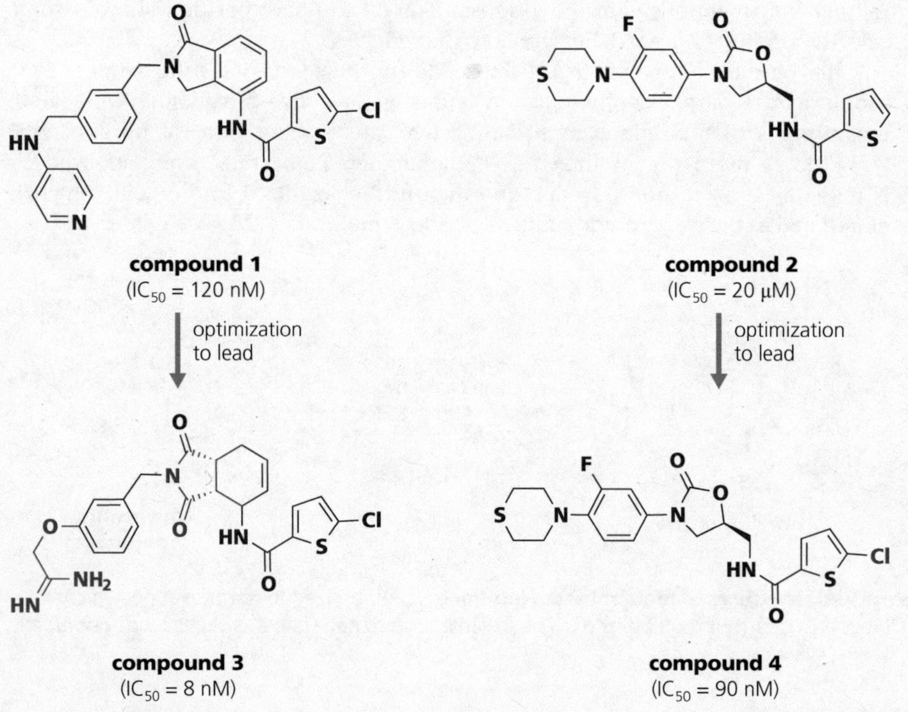

compound 1
(IC_{50} = 120 nM)

compound 2
(IC_{50} = 20 μM)

optimization to lead

optimization to lead

compound 3
(IC_{50} = 8 nM)

compound 4
(IC_{50} = 90 nM)

Figure 5.14 Structures of the hit and leads that led to the discovery of rivaroxaban. Compounds 1 and 2 were initial hits, and optimized to lead compounds 3 and 4. Changes are shown in red.

The assay used at the discovery stage detected cleavage products of fluorogenic substrates of FXa. Optimization of hit compound **1** led to **3**, which had improved potency, but the series exhibited poor pharmacokinetics due to low absorption.

The SAR developed during the investigation of hit **1** suggested that the 5-chlorothiophene-2-carboxamide was necessary for activity. On the basis of that information, the lower-potency hit **2** was re-examined. Optimization to lead compound **4** simply involved addition of the chloro group to the thiophene and afforded a nearly 200-fold improvement in potency.

Further optimization of **4** first involved replacement of the thiomorpholine group (Zone 1). Investigation of a number of different heterocycles led to morpholinone as the optimal group. The S-configuration at the oxazolidinone (indicated by *) was required for optimal activity, and in the S-isomers, replacement of the fluoro group of the aryl ring with hydrogen (Zone 2) doubled activity. These changes resulted in **5** (rivaroxaban). The lipophilic 5-chlorothiophene of **5** is responsible for low aqueous solubility (8 mg/L); however, investigation of other heterocycles and substituted thiophenes (Zone 3) gave a sharp decrease in potency. For example, introduction of an amino group at the 3-position of the thiophene resulted in a 10-fold loss of potency (IC_{50} = 8.5nM). The SAR studies are summarized in **Figure 5.15**.

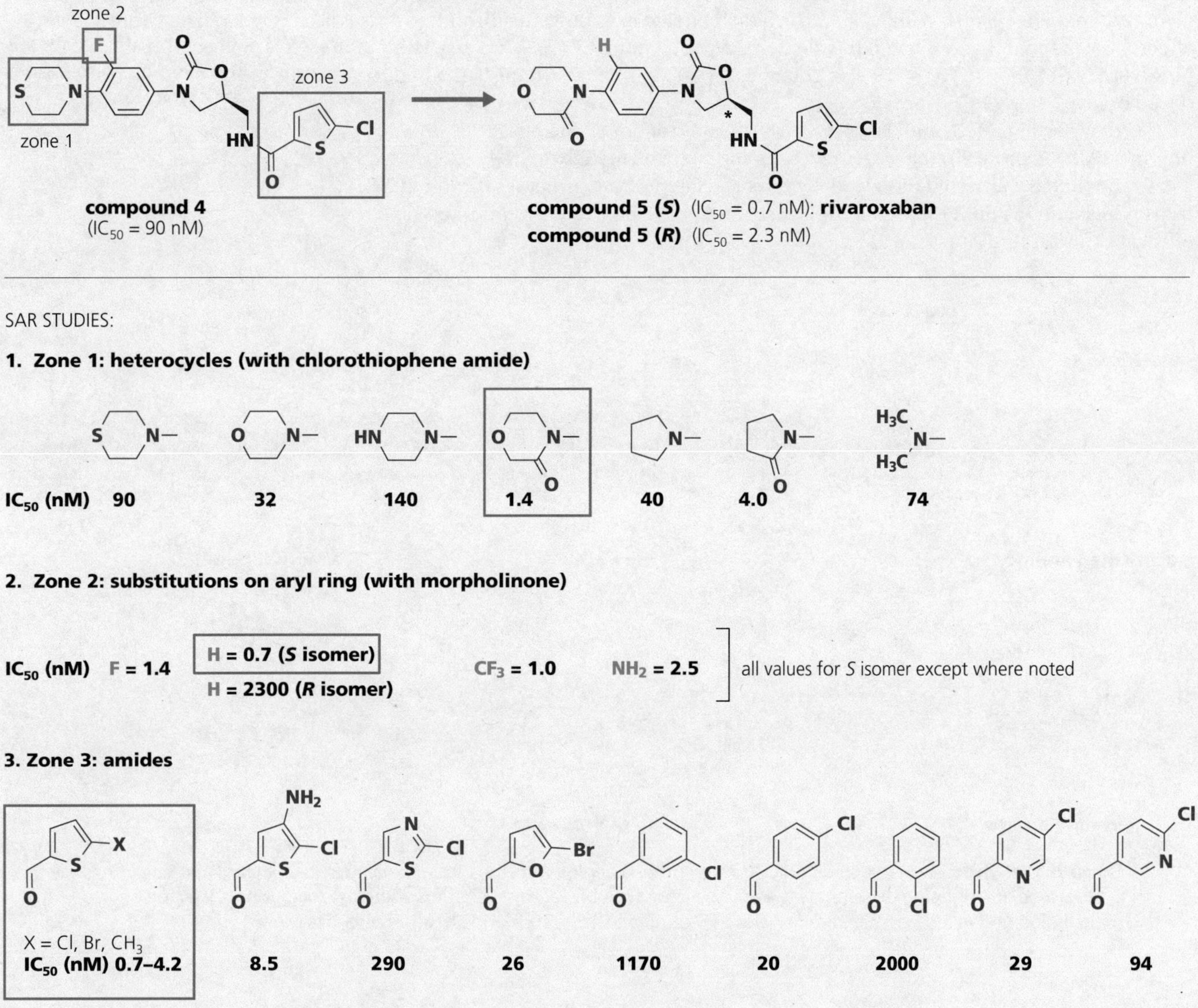

Figure 5.15 Summary of SAR studies from optimization of lead compound 4 to rivaroxaban. Zone 1 was optimized to the oxomorpholine. Zone 2 optimization led to the unsubstituted aryl ring (H) with the S-configuration at the stereogenic center. Zone 3 was found to be optimal with chlorothiophene.

Solution of the X-ray co-structure of rivaroxaban bound to FXa shows several key binding interactions, as seen in **Figure 5.16**, where rivaroxaban is shown in orange and the enzyme is shown in green. The molecule adopts an L-shape that is optimal for binding, with the chlorothiophene amide extending back into the binding site in the S1 pocket. The oxazolidinone ring is coplanar with the aryl ring; two hydrogen bonds to Gly219 are observed—one from the oxazolidinone carbonyl and another from the amide nitrogen. The morpholinone ring, which is orthogonal to the aryl ring, fits into the S4 pocket.

Compound **5** (rivaroxaban) is synthesized by the efficient route shown in **Figure 5.17**, where the substituted aniline adds to the chiral epoxide to give the amino alcohol oxazolidinone precursor. Cyclization with carbonyldiimidazole (CDI) is followed by cleavage of the phthalimide group to afford a primary amine, which is then coupled to the chlorothiophene.

In addition to the inhibition assay, further characterization of **5** included secondary *in vitro* assays that measured prolongation of prothrombin time in both rat and human plasma. This assay measures the inhibitor concentration required to double the time to fibrin formation, compared to no inhibitor being present. Compounds, all containing the oxomorpholine ring but with varying aryl substituents (X, Figure 5.18), were tested, with **5** and the F (**6**), CF_3, and NH_2 analogs giving comparable results. Testing *in vivo* in a rat model to examine anti-thrombotic effects showed that **5** and **6** had equivalent intravenous potency (ED_{50} = 1 mg/kg); however, rivaroxaban (**5**) was twice as potent as **6** (ED_{50} = 5 versus 10 mg/kg) when dosed orally.

Further testing of **5** and **6**, as well as the pyrrolidone analog **7**, for their pharmacokinetic profile in rats gave the results summarized in **Figure 5.18**.

Compound **5** was tested for selectivity against related serine proteases thrombin, trypsin, plasmin, FVIIa, FIXa, FXIa, urokinase, and activated protein C and had no effect at concentrations up to 20 μM.

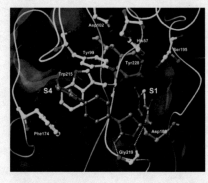

Figure 5.16   X-ray crystal co-structure of rivaroxaban (orange) bound to FXa. Rivaroxaban adopts an L-shape in the binding site. Hydrogen bonds to Gly219 from the oxazolidinone carbonyl and amide nitrogen are shown as dotted lines. The S4 pocket is filled by the morpholinone ring; the S1 pocket is filled by thiophene. (From Roehrig S, Straub A, Pohlmann J et al. [2005] *J Med Chem* 48:5900–5908. With permission from American Chemical Society.)

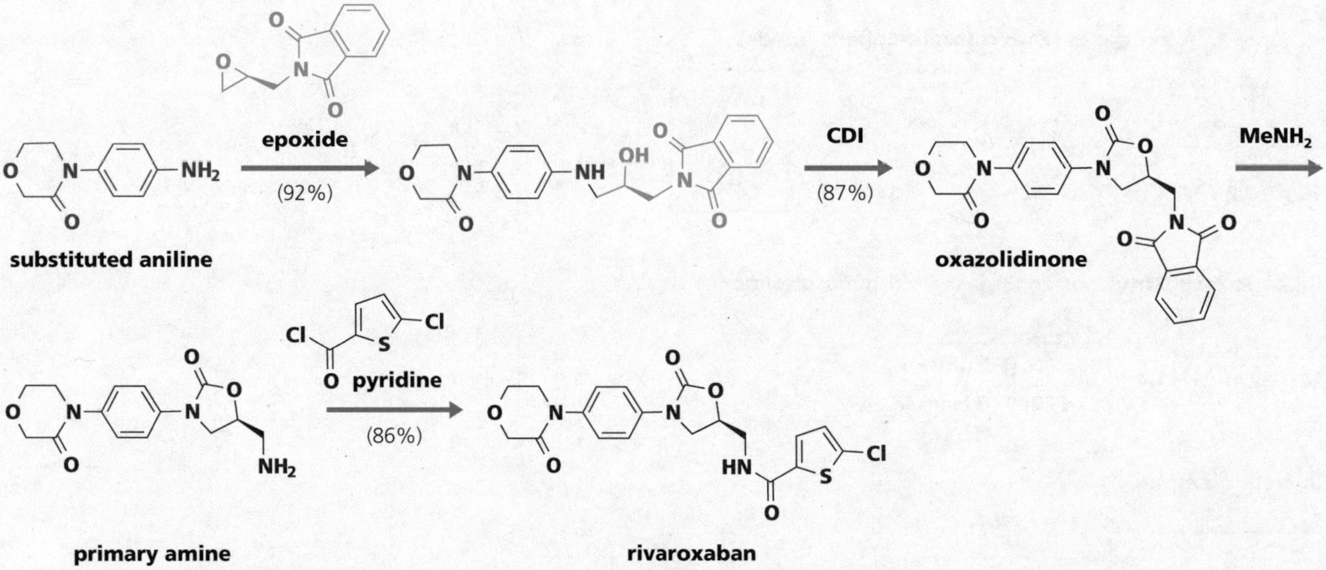

Figure 5.17   Synthesis of rivaroxaban (5). The synthesis begins with substituted aniline (shown in red) and epoxide (shown in blue). Epoxide opening to generate the amino alcohol is followed by formation of the oxazolidinone. Cleavage of the phthalimide generates a primary amine, which is coupled to an acid chloride to afford rivaroxaban.

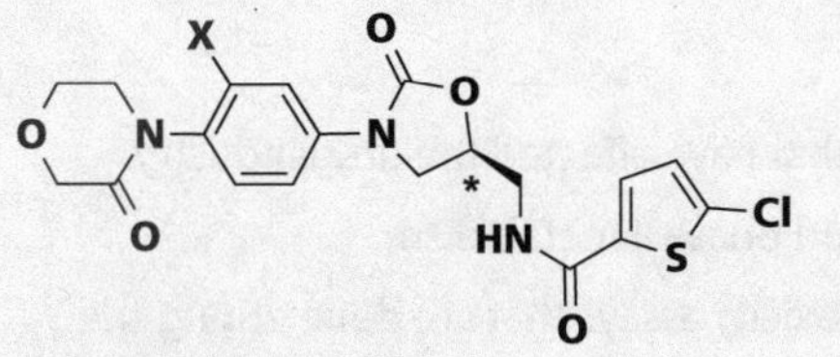

Figure 5.18 Summary of pharmacokinetic data of compounds 5, 6, and 7 in male Wistar rats. Compound 5 (rivaroxaban) had the best combination of low clearance, appropriate volume of distribution, acceptable half-life and plasma protein binding profile and high bioavailability compared to 6 and 7.

5: X = H (rivaroxaban)
6: X = F

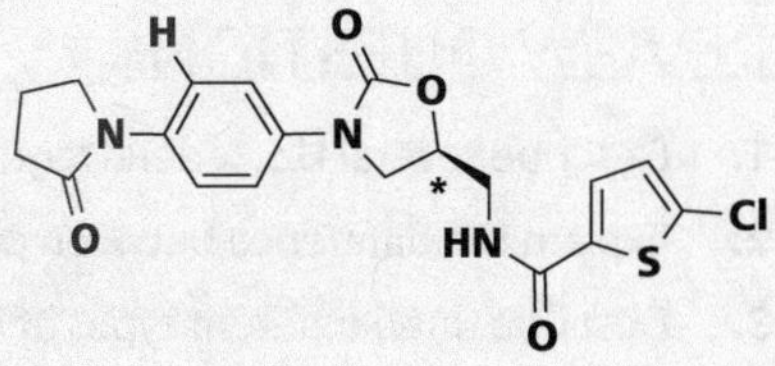

7

compound	CL [L·h⁻¹kg⁻¹]	V_ss [L·kg⁻¹]	t_1/2 [h]	bioavailability [h]	f_u [%]
5	0.4	0.3	0.9	60	1.3
6	1.09	0.32	0.3	n.d.	n.d.
7	0.17	0.21	1.1	65	0.2

f_u = fraction unbound in plasma

On the basis of its potency, effects in animal models, and pharmacokinetic profile, **5** entered clinical trials. In phase I trials, it was found to be well tolerated, with predictable pharmacokinetics. In phase II trials, over a range of 5–80 mg, it exhibited anticoagulant effects with no bleeding. It was examined for prevention of venous thromboembolism following surgery and was effective at a 10 mg dose. Rivaroxaban received FDA approval in 2008 for prevention of blood clots in surgical patients.

REVIEW QUESTIONS

1. Describe several U.S. federal regulations that have affected the drug industry.

2. Explain the difference between phase I and phase II metabolism.

3. Describe three different types of *in vitro* toxicity assays that are done during the early drug discovery stages and what they predict.

4. Give at least four characteristics of a process synthesis and explain why it may differ from the original synthesis of a drug candidate.

5. Describe the three types of testing done for reproductive toxicity.

6. Describe three types of patents that are used to protect drug and drug candidates.

7. What are some of the properties and characteristics of a molecule that can affect its distribution in the body?

8. Explain why a highly bioavailable drug is preferable to a poorly bioavailable drug.

9. Define pharmacokinetics, pharmacodynamics, and toxicokinetics.

10. Explain several reasons why a drug might have excellent potency in *in vitro* assays but poor activity in *in vivo* animal models.

APPLICATION QUESTIONS

1. In spite of toxicity screening in both preclinical and clinical trials, sometimes serious side effects do not become apparent until after a drug has been approved and marketed and has been taken by large numbers of patients. This was the case with several selective COX-2 inhibitors, such as rofecoxib and valdecoxib, that were in use as anti-inflammatory agents. Research these two drugs and identify the side effects that were discovered, leading to their voluntary removal from the market.

2. Two metabolic pathways for cimetidine involve S-oxidation to the sulfoxide and hydroxylation of the 5-methyl group on the imidazole ring. Draw structures of these two metabolites.

3. Studies on ^{14}C-labeled rivaroxaban (case study 2 in this chapter) led to the identification of the four metabolites (I–IV) shown. Classify each metabolic step (a–d) by reaction type as well as whether it represents phase I or phase II metabolism.

4. The metabolism of brompheniramine is shown in Figure 5.10B. Draw the reaction pathway of the first phase I reactions to generate the carboxylic acid metabolite.

5. Two metabolites of ephedrine are shown here (major and minor).

ephedrine   **major metabolite**   **minor metabolite**

(a) What type of phase I transformations lead to each metabolite? The diol (minor) metabolite is excreted as a glucuronide: draw that phase II metabolite.

(b) Using some of the strategies described in Chapter 4, design a molecule that could slow or modify the formation of each metabolite and explain the rationale of your design.

6. Green chemistry is "the design of chemical products and process that reduce or eliminate the generation of hazardous substances," according to the U.S. Environmental Protection Agency. The concepts of green chemistry are an important component of process chemistry research, and a number of processes for the synthesis of drugs have received the Presidential Green Chemistry Challenge Award. Research one of these award winners.

7. Formulation and final drug delivery form is an important consideration during the drug development stage. Consider what disease or circumstances would warrant a pill versus an intravenous formulation. What physical characteristics of the drug substance would be necessary for an intravenous formulation?

8. During your drug discovery program, you learn that the thiophene fragment of your lead is extensively metabolized, resulting in very poor oral bioavailability. Unfortunately, thiophene contributes to the potency of the molecule. On the basis of the concepts described in Chapter 4, design two new replacements or changes to the thiophene that would address the metabolism issue but would likely maintain potency.

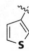

9. Developing new formulations of existing drugs has been one way to extend the patent life of certain drugs. These new formulations often benefit patients since they are often easier or more convenient to take. Research one of the particularly well-known examples of this successful strategy.

10. Many drugs progress to phase II clinical trials and then fail for a variety of reasons. Two examples are preladenant and darapladib. Research one of the two drugs:

(a) Identify its intended use and drug target.

(b) Summarize preclinical and phase I clinical data.

(c) Why did it fail in clinical trials?

FURTHER READING

Drug development costs

DiMasi JA, Grabowski HG & Hansen RW (2016) Innovation in the pharmaceutical industry: new estimates of R&D costs. *J Health Econ* 47:20–33.

Dickson MD & Gagnon JP (2004) Key factors in the rising cost of new drug discovery and development. *Nat Rev Drug Discovery* 3:417–429.

Sitagliptin synthesis

Kim D, Wang L, Beconi M et al. (2005) (2*R*)-4-Oxo-4-[3-trifluoromethyl)-5,6-dihydro[1,2,4]triazolo[4,3-*a*]pyrazin-7(8*H*)-yl]-1-(2,4,5-trifluorophenyl) butan-2-amine: a potent, orally active dipeptidyl peptidase IV inhibitor for the treatment of type 2 diabetes. *J Med Chem* 48:141–151.

Hansen KB, Hsiao Y, Xu F et al. (2009) Highly efficient asymmetric synthesis of sitagliptin. *J Am Chem Soc* 131:8798–8804.

Desai AA (2011) Sitagliptin manufacture: a compelling tale of green chemistry, process intensification, and industrial asymmetric catalysis. *Angew Chem, Int Ed* 50:1974–1976.

Pharmacokinetics and toxicity

Jang GR, Harris RZ & Lau DT (2002) Pharmacokinetics and its role in small molecule drug discovery research. *Med Res Rev* 21:382–396.

Parasuraman S (2011) Toxicological screening. *J Pharmacol Pharmaceut* 2:74–79.

Food and Drug Administration and clinical trials

Adams CD & Brantner VV (2003) New drug development: estimating entry from human clinical trials. Working Paper 262, Federal Trade Commission, Bureau of Economics. https://www.ftc.gov/reports/new-drug-development-estimating-entry-human-clinical-trials.

The Biopharmaceutics Classification System (BCS) Guidance. (2016) http://www.fda.gov/AboutFDA/CentersOffices/OfficeofMedical ProductsandTobacco/CDER/ucm128219.htm

The FDA's drug review process: ensuring drugs are safe and effective. (2014) http://www.fda.gov/drugs/resourcesforyou/consumers/ucm 143534.htm

Case studies

Wong DT, Bymaster FP & Engleman EA (1995) Prozac (Fluoxetine, Lilly 110140), the first selective serotonin uptake inhibitor and an antidepressant drug: twenty years since its first publication. *Life Sci* 57:411–441.

Wirth DD, Miller MS, Boini SK & Koenig TM (2000) Identification and comparison of impurities in fluoxetine hydrochloride synthesized by seven different routes. *Org Process Res Dev* 4:513–519.

Crnic Z & Kirin SI (1997) N-substituted derivatives of *N*-methyl-3-(*p*-trifluoromethylphenoxy)-3-phenylpropylamine and the procedure for their preparation. U.S. Patent 5,618,968.

Perzborn E, Roehrig S, Straub A et al. (2011) The discovery and development of rivaroxaban, an oral, direct factor Xa inhibitor. *Nat Rev Drug Discovery* 10:61–75.

Roehrig S, Straub A, Pohlmann J et al. (2005) Discovery of the novel antithrombotic agent 5-chloro-*N*-({(5*S*)-2-oxo-3-[4-(3-oxomorpholin-4-yl)phenyl]-1,3-oxazolidin-5-yl}methyl)thiophene-2-carboxamide (BAY 59-7939): an oral, direct factor Xa inhibitor. *J Med Chem* 48:5900–5908.

PART II
CLASSES OF DRUG TARGETS

Receptors, ion channels, and transporters as drug targets

6

LEARNING OBJECTIVES

- Describe the basic structural features of different classes of receptors, ion channels, and transporters.
- Understand the various ways small molecules can affect the activity of receptors, ion channels, and transporters.
- Become familiar with different types of assays used to categorize drug activity of G protein-coupled receptors, ion channels, nuclear receptors, and transporters.
- Develop a basic understanding of receptor theory.
- Learn examples of various drugs that act at G protein-coupled receptors, nuclear receptors, ion channels, and transporters.

Based on current knowledge, there are approximately 3000 genes in the human genome that code for proteins that are considered druggable; that is, capable of having their activity modulated by binding of druglike compounds. This number is expanding, however, as medicinal chemistry evolves to develop and optimize methods and strategies aimed at interfering with historically undruggable targets such as proteins that mediate physiological processes through protein–protein interactions. It has been estimated that between 600 and 1500 proteins are involved in disease processes, and the actual number of human targets of approved drugs has recently been estimated to be over 650. Target proteins that are unique to pathogens number almost 200. Of the approximately 1000 small-molecule drugs on the market, the vast majority bind to fewer, approximately 600 macromolecular targets. Some specific antitumor and antiviral agents, as well as a few small-molecule therapeutics that treat genetic disorders, bind to nucleic acids. Of the human proteins targeted by drugs, G protein-coupled receptors (GPCRs) account for 12%, ion channels 19%, and nuclear receptors 3%. Kinases, which have both receptor and enzyme functions, account for 10% of the protein targets, according to a 2016 report. Another way to assess these figures is to consider the proportion of drugs that act at each protein target type. This analysis takes into consideration that there are often multiple drugs that modulate the same protein target. The percentages are somewhat different when focusing on drugs: 33% of drugs target a G protein coupled receptor, approximately 24% act on enzymes (including kinases),18% act at ion channels, 16% at nuclear receptors, and 6% target **transporters**. This analysis shows that over two-thirds of drugs bind to receptors as defined in the broadest sense. These target classes (**Figure 6.1**), as well as some historically undruggable targets, will be described in this and the following two chapters.

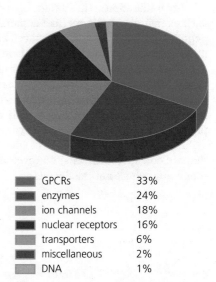

GPCRs	33%
enzymes	24%
ion channels	18%
nuclear receptors	16%
transporters	6%
miscellaneous	2%
DNA	1%

Figure 6.1 Distribution of macromolecular drug targets based on 2016 analysis. The majority of drugs bind to proteins, such as enzymes, GPCRs, ion channels, nuclear hormone receptors, and transporters, with a small percentage binding to nucleic acids.

In the most general sense, receptors, ion channels, and transporters are macromolecular protein complexes that propagate a signal or initiate subsequent events in response to some stimulus. The specific stimuli include binding of small molecules, hormones, or proteins as well as changes in electrical membrane potential. The effects initiated can be as diverse as activation or deactivation of other proteins, up- or down-regulation of gene expression, protein localization, or release and uptake of chemical messengers such as ions, small organic molecules, and even gases like nitric oxide. These macromolecules are a critical component of highly complex systems and are involved in physiological processes as diverse as neurotransmission, muscle contraction, and embryonic development. As such, they are frequent targets of drug discovery activities. Receptors can broadly include GPCRs, ion channels (ligand- and voltage-gated), transporters and nuclear receptors. Receptor tyrosine kinases have both receptor and enzyme functions and will be discussed in Chapter 7. Among drugs that act at these receptors, the majority target GPCRs, followed by ion channels and nuclear hormone receptors (in similar proportion), and transporters. While these drug targets are similar in that they are proteins involved in signal transduction, GPCRs, ion channels, nuclear receptors, and transporters are distinct classes of drug targets, with each having specific structural features and functioning via specific mechanisms.

G PROTEIN-COUPLED RECEPTORS AS DRUG TARGETS

G protein-coupled receptors (**GPCRs**) span the cell membrane and act to relay messages from outside the cell to the inside. They are typically linked to an **effector system** that is usually an enzyme or ion channel. Occupation of the receptor via binding of its ligand (usually a small molecule, protein, or lipid) results in activation or deactivation of the effector system, which in turn ultimately results in a change in concentration of a **second messenger**. This second messenger is often an ion or a small molecule. The second messenger then activates other enzymes or affects ion channels, resulting in a specific physiological effect (**Figure 6.2**). This entire process of an extracellular event (for example, binding of a small molecule) activating a membrane receptor and ultimately altering intracellular concentrations of specific molecules is termed **signal transduction**.

The initial stimuli (the natural ligands) are typically small endogenous molecules such as neurotransmitters (like dopamine and histamine), steroid hormones, small peptides, proteins, lipids, light, or even odorant molecules. The small molecule second messengers are compounds whose levels are changed by the action of enzymes or by the result of ion channels opening or closing (effector systems) after binding of the ligand to the receptor. A common messenger, cAMP, is formed by the action of the enzyme adenylate cyclase on adenosine triphosphate (ATP). Two other common messengers are diacylglycerol (DAG) and inositol trisphosphate (IP_3), formed by phospholipase C (PLC)-catalyzed hydrolysis of a diacylphosphate (**Figure 6.3**).

It is estimated, on the basis of DNA sequences, that there are nearly 800 proteins that are considered GPCRs; however, only about 550 are considered known. Those remaining, whose natural ligands are unknown, are termed **orphan GPCRs**.

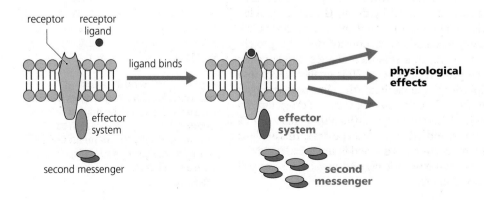

Figure 6.2 General scheme for ligand binding to GPCR and resultant signal. Unoccupied GPCR (green) is embedded in the plasma membrane (light pink); an effector system (gray) and second messengers (orange) sit in the inside of the cell. Binding of a ligand (red) at the extracellular ligand binding site results in a change in the effector system (now dark pink) and those changes, in the case illustrated, increase levels of second messengers. Changes in the concentration of second messengers result in physiological effects.

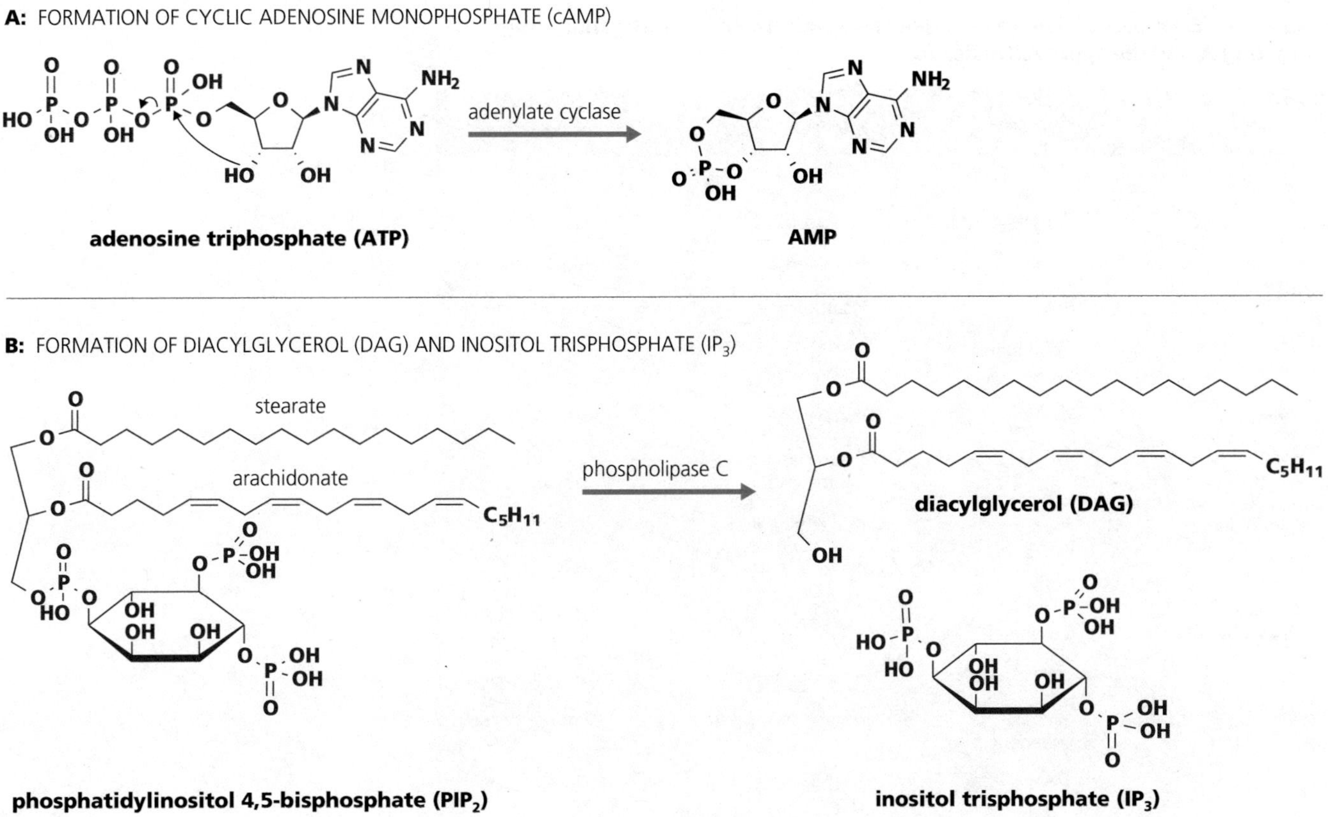

A: FORMATION OF CYCLIC ADENOSINE MONOPHOSPHATE (cAMP)

adenosine triphosphate (ATP)   adenylate cyclase   **AMP**

B: FORMATION OF DIACYLGLYCEROL (DAG) AND INOSITOL TRISPHOSPHATE (IP$_3$)

stearate

arachidonate

phospholipase C

diacylglycerol (DAG)

phosphatidylinositol 4,5-bisphosphate (PIP$_2$)   **inositol trisphosphate (IP$_3$)**

Figure 6.3 Formation of second messengers by effectors. A: Generation of cyclic AMP (cAMP) from adenylate cyclase catalyzed reaction of adenosine triphosphate (ATP). B: Generation of diacylglycerol (DAG) and IP$_3$ (phosphatidyl inositol trisphosphate) from phospholipase C-catalyzed hydrolysis of phosphatidyl inositol bisphosphate (PIP$_2$).

6.1 GPCRs are defined by structural features

GPCRs fall into at least six different classes based on sequence similarity and characteristics of their ligands. Most drugs on the market affect class A receptors, with some examples targeting class C. Several important GPCRs in terms of drug action are β adrenergic, opiate, serotonin, chemokine, angiotensin, histamine, and dopamine receptors. **Table 6.1** gives some examples of G protein-coupled receptors and their corresponding drugs and/or drug candidates. Of note, class B GPCRs have been quite resistant to drug discovery efforts, with no approved drugs targeting this group to date.

Structurally, GPCRs are characterized by seven membrane-spanning helical domains arranged in a semicircular fashion. Binding of ligands usually occurs within this transmembrane array of helices. In most cases, it is believed the intracellular portion of the protein associates with a G protein (GDP-binding protein) upon binding of a ligand. The G proteins are composed of an α(Gα), a β(Gβ), and a γ(Gγ) subunit, and multiple subtypes of each subunit exist. Binding of the natural ligand results in a conformational change of the receptor, followed by its translocation within the cell membrane and coupling to the G protein, as illustrated in **Figure 6.4**.

In this simplified model, the α subunit of the G protein releases a molecule of guanosine diphosphate (GDP). The unoccupied G protein now binds guanosine triphosphate (GTP), and then the Gα subunit dissociates. Upon interaction of the Gα subunit or the Gβγ subunit with their effector systems, the signaling cascade is propagated, and downstream proteins are activated or deactivated. Enzyme effector systems include adenylate and guanylate cyclase, phosphodiesterases, phospholipases A$_2$ and C, and phosphoinositide-3-kinases. Activation or inactivation of these enzymes results in changing levels of the second messengers, which then go on to elicit further biological responses, such as activating or deactivating transcription factors in the nucleus or changing the levels of phosphorylated proteins. This traditional view has been complicated by the fact that some GPCRs have been identified that do not bind G proteins and also that some cellular responses are not mediated by second-messenger levels.

Table 6.1   Examples of G protein-coupled receptors, their natural ligands, drugs targeting it, and the approved indication.

Natural ligand (agonist)	Receptor	Drug or ligand examples	Indication
Class A			
acetylcholine	muscarinic (M_{1-5})	pilocarpine	glaucoma
adenosine	A_1, A_{2A}, A_{2B}, A_3	tecadenoson[a]	atrial fibrillation
angiotensin II	A II	losartan, valsartan	hypertension
anandamide	cannabinoid (CB_1, CB_2)	Δ^9-tetrahydrocannabinol, rimonabant[a]	weight loss
chemokine	CCR5	maraviroc	AIDS
dopamine	D_{1a}, D_{1b}, D_{2-5}	chlorpromazine, haloperidol	psychosis
histamine	H_1, H_2, H_3	diphenhydramine (H_1)	allergy
		cimetidine (H_2)	gastric ulcers
adrenaline (epinephrine)	α_1 and α_2 adrenergic	clonidine	hypertension
		phenylephrine	nasal congestion
	β_1, β_2, β_3 adrenergic	propranolol (β_1)	hypertension
		albuterol (β_2)	asthma
enkephalin, endorphins	μ, δ, κ opioid	morphine (μ)	pain
		loperamide (μ)	diarrhea
serotonin (5-HT)	$5\text{-}HT_{1a-d}$, $5\text{-}HT_2$	sumatriptan	migraine
		buspirone	anxiety
	$5\text{-}HT_4$	tegaserod	irritable bowel
somatostatin	SSTR	pasireotide	Cushing's disease
sphingosine 1-phosphate	S1PR1–5	fingolimod	multiple sclerosis
vasopressin	V_1, V_2, V_3	conivaptan	hyponatremia
Class B			
calcitonin	CTR	b	
corticotropin-releasing factor	CRF_1	antalarmin[a]	antidepressant
glucagon	glucagon receptor	b	
glucagon-like peptide	GLPR	b	
growth hormone-releasing hormone	GHRHR	b	
parathyroid hormone	PTH1R, PTH2R	b	
secretin	secretin receptor	b	
Class C			
glutamate	metabotropic $GluR_{1-8}$	eglumegad[a]	anxiety
γ-aminobutyric acid	$GABA_B$	baclofen	alcoholism

[a]Compound is either in development, in clinical trials, or has been removed from the market.
[b]No reported ligands in advanced development.

Figure 6.4 GPCR mechanism. GPCRs (green), consisting of 7 membrane (pink) spanning domains are often associated with a GDP-bound form of a G protein (orange, 3 ovals). Upon ligand binding, the α subunit of the G protein releases GDP, binds GTP, and dissociates. The individual subunits of the G protein interact with effector systems to change the levels of second messengers, which then may change protein phosphorylation patterns and activate or deactivate transcription factors in the nucleus.

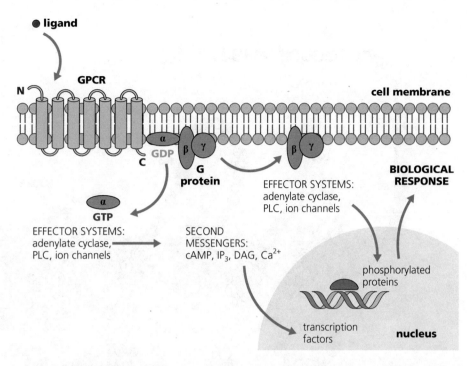

Figure 6.5 Binding sites in the major GPCR classes A, B, and C. Cylinders 1–7 (green) denote helical transmembrane domains (TMD) that all GPCR families have in common. Classes B and C contain large extracellular domains (ECD) (green ovals) compared to class A members. The ligand-binding domain (pink) is in the TMD for class A receptors, in both the ECD and TMD (linked) for class B receptors, and in the ECD in class C receptors. (Adapted from Congreve M, Langmead CJ, Mason JS & Marshall FH [2011] *J Med Chem* 54:4283–4311. With permission from American Chemical Society.)

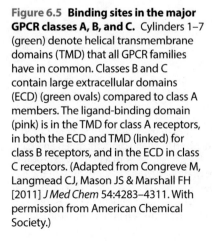

The ligand binding sites of GPCRs vary with the class of receptor. A model of each of the three major classes is shown in **Figure 6.5**, where the cylinders represent transmembrane domains (TMD) 1–7. In class A receptors, the natural ligand binds in the TMD region. In class B receptors, which contain a large extracellular domain (ECD), ligands bind by the "hot dog in a bun" model in both the ECD and TMD. In class C, which also has a large extracellular domain, the ligand binds only to the ECD by the "Venus flytrap" model.

An important advance in structural information came in 2000, when the first X-ray structure of a GPCR (rhodopsin) was solved. Prior to 2000, many computational homology models of various GPCRs had been developed on the basis of site-directed mutagenesis studies. Although very similar to most drug-targeted GPCRs, rhodopsin differs in that it binds its natural ligand 11-*cis*-retinal through covalent rather than noncovalent interactions. Since 2007, several additional structures of GPCRs have been reported. The β$_2$ adrenoceptor bound to the partial inverse agonist carazolol was the first noncovalent ligand-mediated GPCR structure published. More recently, structures of β$_1$ adrenoceptor, A$_{2A}$ adenosine receptor, and a chemokine receptor have been solved, all of which are class A GPCRs. Recently, a Class B GPCR, the calcitonin receptor, bound to a G protein and its natural ligand, calcitonin, was solved by cryo-electron microscopy. In addition, an X-ray structure of the smoothened receptor (SMO) has been solved, which is a class F GPCR, a small group of unique GPCRs. **Figure 6.6** shows a model of the β$_2$ adrenergic receptor, as well as an X-ray crystal structure of the receptor bound to carazolol, an inverse agonist. The transmembrane domains (TM1–TM7) are evident in the X-ray structure, as are the extracellular and intracellular loops.

While only a handful of GPCRs have succumbed to structure elucidation, many others have been cloned, expressed, and subjected to site-directed mutagenesis,

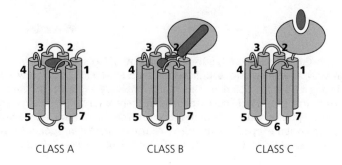

CLASS A   CLASS B   CLASS C

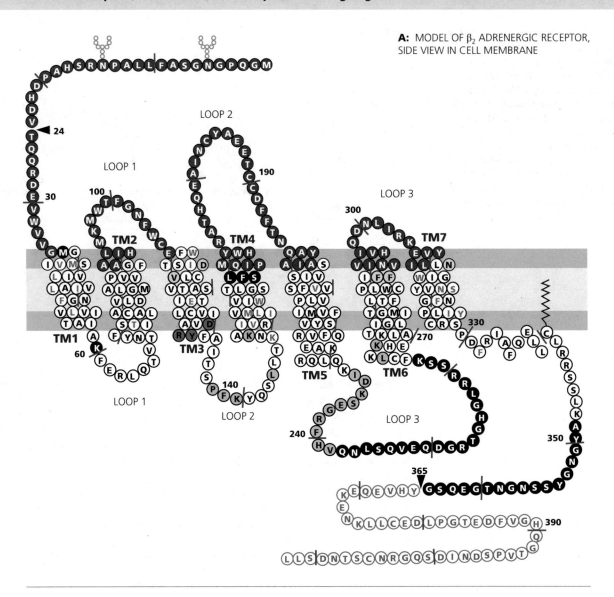

A: MODEL OF β₂ ADRENERGIC RECEPTOR, SIDE VIEW IN CELL MEMBRANE

B: X-RAY STRUCTURE OF β₂ ADRENERGIC RECEPTOR, SIDE VIEW IN CELL MEMBRANE, BOUND TO CARAZOLOL

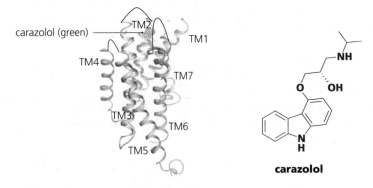

carazolol (green)

TM2
TM1
TM4
TM7
TM3
TM6
TM5

carazolol

Figure 6.6 Structure of β₂-adrenoceptor bound to carazolol. A: Model of the β₂-adrenoceptor in membrane (pink/gray) based on X-ray structure where each circle represents one amino acid. Yellow indicates residues involved in ligand binding; green and pink identify residues that bind to or are near an antibody fragment used for stabilization in the X-ray. Residues with a black background are disordered and were not used for model generation. Small blue Y-shapes indicate glycosylation sites. B: X-ray structure of the β₂-adrenoceptor bound to carazolol (structure on right), showing α-helices of transmembrane domains in yellow (TM1–TM7). Carazolol is in green at the top of the structure. Green in the helix corresponds to antibody-binding regions, as described for part A. (From Rasmussen SGF, Choi H-J, Rosenbaum DM et al. [2007] *Nature* 450:383–387. With permission from Macmillan Publishers Limited.)

allowing further understanding of the overall structure and function of the receptor based on amino acid sequences. Availability of high resolution structures as well as homology models provides some additional insight into drug design and medicinal chemistry strategies. However, structure-based drug design for GPCRs is not a very mature field because of the conformational flexibility of GPCRs and the poor understanding of the structural requirements for drugs that activate versus those that inactivate a receptor. Hit identification typically relies on ligand-based drug design derived from known small molecules or screening of focused libraries.

A particular challenge in GPCR-based drug discovery is the issue of selectivity. GPCRs are widely expressed throughout the body, and many different receptors respond to the same ligand. For example, there are currently six types of GPCRs that use 5-hydroxytryptamine (serotonin) as a ligand, and each of those includes multiple subtypes. Within just the 5-HT_1 GPCR are five subtypes: 5-HT_{1A}, 5-HT_{1B}, 5-HT_{1D}, 5-HT_{1E}, and 5-HT_{1F}. Other GPCRs have similarly large numbers of subtypes. Drug discovery activities often focus on optimizing selectivity on the basis of differences among the specific receptors and receptor subtypes. In addition, the location of the receptor in the body can also influence specificity.

Because GPCRs are membrane-bound proteins, testing often relies on cellular assays or membrane preparations where the particular receptor of interest is overexpressed. Prior to the availability of genetically engineered cells, specific tissue samples were utilized. Quantification of receptor binding activity is done through **competition binding assays** in which a labeled compound is incubated with a receptor preparation. The label is typically either a radiolabel (for example, ^{3}H or ^{125}I) or a fluorescent label. After incubation, the ligand–receptor complex is isolated and quantified. For radiolabeled ligands, quantification may be done by filtration and radioactivity counting or by scintillation proximity assay (SPA), among other methods. Fluorescent techniques include fluorescence polarization assays and FRET assays. Functional assays are based on detection of an event downstream from direct binding to the receptor. Activation of the G protein (a very early event) by detection of products of GDP/GTP exchange, second-messenger levels, and even further downstream events such as translocation or transcription can all be measured as part of a functional assay for GPCR activity. A frequently used technology involves detecting changes in the level of Ca^{2+} through the use of fluorescent or chemiluminescent dyes that are responsive to Ca^{2+} concentrations.

6.2   Ligands bind to GPCRs and may activate or inactivate a receptor

Ligands, typically small molecules, can bind to GPCRs and either activate or inactivate a receptor, and drugs acting at these receptors are broadly classified as either agonists (activators) or antagonists (blockers). An **agonist**, like the natural ligand, binds at the receptor and the binding results in a physiological response. A **partial agonist** binds to the receptor but gives less than a full response in relation to some defined response by a full agonist or the natural ligand, regardless of increasing concentration. An **antagonist** (or a **neutral antagonist**) binds to the receptor and prevents the natural ligand from eliciting a response. When no agonist is present, a neutral antagonist will have no effect. An **inverse agonist**, first described by Tommaso Costa and Albert Herz for GPCRs in 1989, binds and results in a decrease in the response of a constitutively active receptor (a constituitively active receptor transduces a small amount of signal even in the absence of an activating ligand). In the presence of an agonist or the natural ligand, an inverse agonist will decrease the response, even below basal levels. The effect of each type of ligand is shown in **Figure 6.7**.

Typically, drugs bind either at **orthosteric sites** (same as natural ligand), where they bind competitively, or at **allosteric sites** (remote from where the natural ligand binds), where they bind noncompetitively. Drugs that bind at allosteric sites may act as either **positive allosteric modulators** (PAM) or **negative allosteric modulators** (NAM), depending on whether they increase or decrease activity of the natural ligand or agonist. For any type of drug, there are two important components to bioactivity: first, the drug must have binding affinity for the receptor, and second, upon binding, it must have efficacy, or an effect on signal transduction.

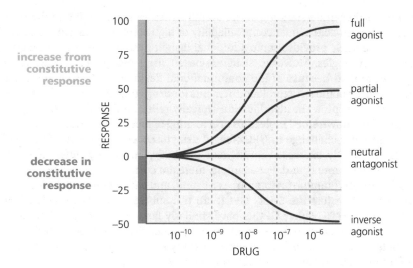

Figure 6.7 Effect of increasing concentrations of various types of ligands. The biological response of a receptor that has constitutive activity is set at zero in the graph. A full agonist, at some concentration, will afford a complete (100%) response; a partial agonist will give a less-than-full response, despite increasing concentrations; a neutral antagonist will cause no response and will prevent an agonist from activating the receptor; and an inverse agonist will decrease the constitutive or basal response. (Adapted from Boghog/Wikimedia Commons, CC BY-SA 4.0.)

The **affinity**, or binding strength, of a drug that acts at a receptor can be measured in a binding assay. This information reflects both strength of binding and mechanism (orthosteric versus allosteric). Strength of binding (affinity) depends on the dissociation of the drug–receptor complex as outlined in **Figure 6.8A**, where A = drug, R = receptor, and AR = drug–receptor complex (see Chapter 3). In practice, this can be determined by using a known radiolabeled ligand, allowing it to equilibrate with the receptor, and then washing to remove unbound ligand. While the concentrations

A: DETERMINATION OF K_d AND B_{max} (R_{tot})

$$A + R \underset{K_d \,(\text{off})}{\overset{K_b \,(\text{on})}{\rightleftharpoons}} AR$$

equilibrium of unbound/bound drug (A)

$$K_d = \frac{[A][R]}{[AR]} \text{ and } K_b = 1/K_d$$

dissociation constant of drug (K_d)

$$\frac{[AR]}{[A]} = \frac{B_{max} - [AR]}{K_d}$$

Scatchard equation

B: SCATCHARD PLOT TO DETERMINE K_d AND B_{max}

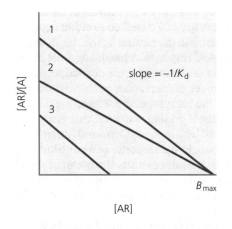

C: DETERMINATION OF IC_{50}

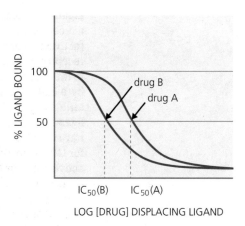

Figure 6.8 Binding affinity determinations. A: Equations used to determine K_d and B_{max} for a ligand, A binding to receptor R. The dissociation constant K_d can be derived from a series of experiments measuring the amount of bound drug in the presence of various concentrations of a known ligand. The binding constant K_b is the inverse of the dissociation constant ($1/K_d$). B: Scatchard plots of [AR]/[A] vs [AR] for (1) a known radiolabeled ligand, (2) a compound binding at an orthosteric site, and (3) a compound binding at an allosteric site (PAM or NAM). The slope of each line = $-1/K_d$, and the x-intercept = B_{max}. The line for the allosteric compound (3) will not intersect B_{max} (total number of binding sites) since it binds at a different site than in cases 1 and 2. C: Graph of concentration of known bound ligand vs concentration of two drugs tested. The concentration of drug that displaces 50% of the labeled ligand is known as IC_{50}. Drug B is more potent than drug A because it displaces 50% of the labeled ligand at a lower concentration than drug A.

of [A] (free ligand) and [AR] (bound ligand) can be measured because A is labeled, [R] (unoccupied receptor) cannot be measured and is equal to $[R]_{tot} - [AR]$ or the total number of receptors (R_{tot}) minus those bound to ligand (R_{tot} is also known as B_{max}). The dissociation constant (K_d) is determined by measuring [AR]/[A] at varying concentrations of the known ligand and plotting the ratio versus [AR] in a Scatchard plot. The binding constant (K_b) is the reciprocal of the K_d. Repeating the experiment in the presence of an unlabeled drug being tested indicates if the drug competes with the known ligand, as well as whether it works via an orthosteric or allosteric mechanism. In a Scatchard plot the slope of a line reflects affinity of the drug for the receptor, and the x-intercept is equal to B_{max}.

In the Scatchard plot in **Figure 6.8B**, line 1 is characteristic of an agonist and was generated from a known radiolabeled ligand. Line 2 is characteristic of a drug binding at an orthosteric site but with different affinity (K_d) compared to the compound evaluated in line 1. The slope of line 2 is different than that of line 1, but with enough radiolabeled ligand added, eventually all receptors will be displaced and the line will cross the x-axis at B_{max}. Line 3 is characteristic of a drug (a PAM or NAM) binding at an allosteric site. In this example, adding radiolabeled ligand will not displace the drug, but a conformational change makes fewer binding sites available for the radiolabeled ligand and B_{max} (x-intercept) decreases while the slope remains the same as the line 1.

An alternative plot compares the percent of bound known ligand versus the concentration of drug that decreases binding of that ligand (**Figure 6.8C**). The amount of drug required to decrease binding of a standard by 50% is known as IC_{50} (**Inhibitory Concentration**). A drug with higher binding affinity (drug B) will have a lower IC_{50} than a drug with lower binding affinity (drug A).

6.3 Drug activity is classified by examining biological response as compared to dose

The effect of a drug relies on efficacy as well as binding affinity, and in order to measure the biological effects of a drug, dose–response curves such as those in **Figure 6.9** are generated, where the physiological effect, such as changes in cAMP or Ca^{2+} levels, is measured as a function of compound concentration. The EC_{50} (**Effective Concentration**) of the drug is the concentration that produces 50% of maximal response and is derived from the graph. In practice, this value may be expressed as the pEC_{50} (known in earlier literature as pD_2), which is the negative logarithm of EC_{50} and expresses the potency of a drug. As in Figure 6.7, if the agonist generates the same maximal response (E_{obs}) as the natural ligand or a defined full agonist (E_{max}), it is considered 100% efficacious.

By use of these types of dose–response curves, the activity profile of a drug or small molecule probe can be determined, with different shapes of curves characteristic of agonists, partial agonists, neutral antagonists, and inverse agonists. A full agonist will reach a 100% response (considered 100% efficacious) as concentration increases. A partial agonist will increase response and plateau at a certain level of efficacy, never reaching 100% (**Figure 6.10A**).

Figure 6.9 Determination of EC_{50} of a full agonist. Concentration of the compound is plotted vs defined response (E_{obs}) as a fraction of maximal response (=1.0; E_{max}). EC_{50} is the dose producing 50% response. In this example, EC_{50} is 1×10^{-5} M. This may be expressed as $-\log EC_{50}$, which is pEC_{50} (also known as pD_2).

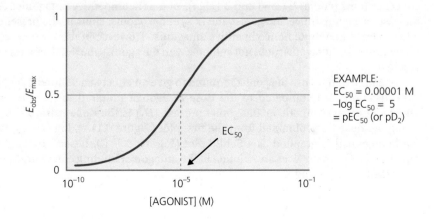

EXAMPLE:
$EC_{50} = 0.00001$ M
$-\log EC_{50} = 5$
$= pEC_{50}$ (or pD_2)

A: AGONIST AND PARTIAL AGONIST DOSE–RESPONSE CURVES

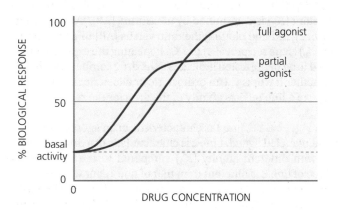

B: NEUTRAL ANTAGONIST AND INVERSE AGONIST DOSE–RESPONSE CURVES IN PRESENCE OF FULL AGONIST

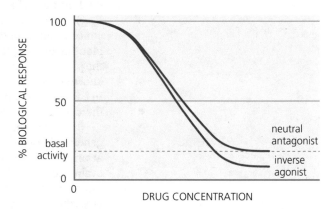

A neutral antagonist and an inverse agonist act in the presence of an agonist (such as the natural ligand); therefore, the response when no drug is present is, by definition, 100%. A neutral antagonist decreases the biological response to the baseline in a dose-dependent manner; an inverse agonist will further decrease the constitutive response, as seen in **Figure 6.10B**.

A drug discovery program, depending on the specific receptor target, may be aimed at modulating the activity of a GPCR in a variety of ways. For example, there are several GPCR targets that are involved in controlling serotonin levels, with different effects on the central nervous system. The anti-migraine drugs called triptans are agonists at the 5-HT$_{1B/1D}$ receptors and have the effect of constricting blood vessels in the brain, resulting in headache relief. Examples of antagonists at 5-HT receptors include some antipsychotic drugs, such as risperidone, that act on the 5-HT$_{2A}$ receptor and others, such as pimavanserin, are inverse agonists at the same (5-HT$_{2A}$) receptor. The serotonin receptor-binding drugs are just one example of the complexity of receptor subtypes and biological effects of agonists, partial agonists, antagonists, and inverse agonists.

The effect of a competitive antagonist can be measured by generating a dose–response curve for a known agonist (E_{obs}/E_{max} versus concentration of agonist) in the presence of different fixed concentrations of the antagonist (**Figure 6.11A**). Since a competitive antagonist directly prevents the natural or known ligand from binding and causing a response, increasing concentrations of the antagonist shift the EC$_{50}$ of the agonist to the right. In Figure 6.11A, the EC$_{50}$ of agonist alone is estimated to be 10^{-5}; at each higher concentration of antagonist (lines 2–4) it consistently shifts to larger (less potent) numbers.

A noncompetitive antagonist occupying an allosteric site may reduce or prevent the response caused by an agonist but may not prevent its binding. **Figure 6.11B** shows the dose–response curve for an agonist in the presence of different fixed concentrations (curves 2 (low) and 3 (high)) of a noncompetitive antagonist. As in the case of a competitive antagonist, the EC$_{50}$ of the agonist shifts in the presence of a fixed concentration of noncompetitive antagonist. However, in this case, since the noncompetitive antagonist does not compete with the agonist, maximal effect is never reached.

The ratio of the dose of agonist required to give an effect at a defined antagonist concentration (D_2) compared to the dose of agonist required to give the same effect without a competitive antagonist present (D_1) is the **dose ratio**, $r = D_2/D_1$. Using the dose ratio obtained from the first plot (Figure 6.11A), log ($r - 1$) versus log [antagonist] is graphed as a Schild plot (**Figure 6.11C**), based on the Schild equation (6.1), which gives an estimate of the antagonist binding constant K_b, often expressed as pA_2 = –log K_b.

Figure 6.10 Theoretical full agonist, partial agonist, neutral antagonist, and inverse agonist dose–response curves. A: Full agonists will achieve the maximal response at a given concentration; partial agonists never achieve 100% response regardless of increasing concentration. B: To measure a dose–response curve, neutral antagonists and inverse agonists are evaluated in the presence of an agonist-activated receptor; therefore, when no drug is present, there is 100% response. A neutral antagonist results in a reduction in response to the basal level with increasing concentration. An inverse agonist results in lower response than the system when no natural ligand is present and requires that the receptor have a level of constitutive activity.

A: DOSE–RESPONSE CURVES FOR AGONIST IN THE PRESENCE OF COMPETITIVE ANTAGONIST AT DIFFERENT CONCENTRATIONS

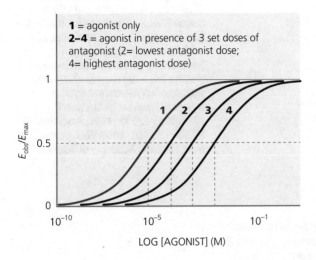

1 = agonist only
2–4 = agonist in presence of 3 set doses of antagonist (2= lowest antagonist dose; 4= highest antagonist dose)

E_{obs}/E_{max}

LOG [AGONIST] (M)

B: DOSE–RESPONSE CURVES FOR AGONIST IN THE PRESENCE OF NON-COMPETITIVE (ALLOSTERIC) ANTAGONIST AT DIFFERENT CONCENTRATIONS

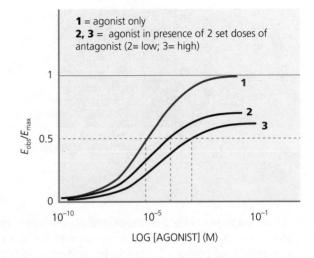

1 = agonist only
2, 3 = agonist in presence of 2 set doses of antagonist (2= low; 3= high)

E_{obs}/E_{max}

LOG [AGONIST] (M)

C: SCHILD PLOT OF LOG [ANTAGONIST] VERSUS LOG r–1

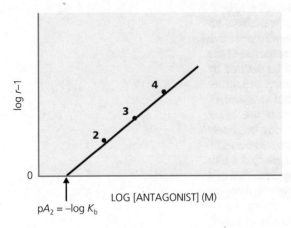

log r–1

LOG [ANTAGONIST] (M)

$pA_2 = -\log K_b$

D: COMPARISON OF COMPETITIVE ANTAGONISTS A AND B OF DIFFERENT POTENCIES

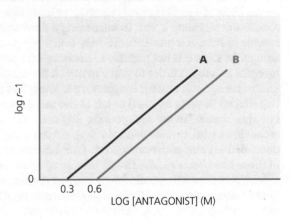

log r–1

0.3   0.6

LOG [ANTAGONIST] (M)

Figure 6.11 Characterization of antagonists based on dose–response curves.
A: Dose–response curves relating the biological effect E_{obs}/E_{max} to increasing concentrations of agonist in the presence of different fixed concentrations of a competitive antagonist. Curve 1 (red) shows the effect of agonist only; curves 2–4 show the effects of three different antagonist concentrations on the agonist dose–response curve. Dashed lines to the x-axis show agonist EC_{50} for each concentration of antagonist present. The right shift of the dose response curves as the concentration of antagonist increases is characteristic of a competitive antagonist. B: Dose–response curves for agonist in the presence of different fixed concentrations (curves 2 and 3) of noncompetitive antagonist; increasing agonist concentration will not achieve full biological effect. C: Schild plot of antagonist concentration vs log (dose ratio – 1), generated from agonist dose–response curves 2–4 in graph A. The x-intercept = pA_2, which is the concentration of antagonist where $r = 2$ (pA_2 may be used to estimate binding constant K_b, where $pA_2 = -\log K_b$). D: Comparison of Schild plots of two competitive antagonists of different potencies, where the higher pA_2 (x-intercept) corresponds to higher potency.

$$\log (r - 1) = \log [\text{antagonist}] - \log K_b \ (\text{or} + pA_2) \tag{6.1}$$

Solving the equation for when the dose of agonist must be doubled to reach full effect when $r = 2$ and $\log (r - 1) = 0$, then the x-intercept equals pA_2 for the antagonist. Because the value is on a log scale, a more potent antagonist will correspond to a higher pA_2 value. In **Figure 6.11D**, compound A has $pA_2 = 0.3$ M and compound B has $pA_2 = 0.6$ M. Comparing the pA_2 values, twice as much of compound A was required

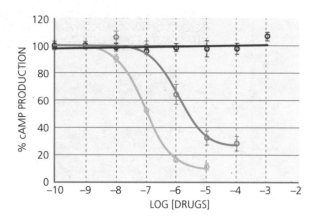

Figure 6.12 Dose–response curves showing effect of drugs acting at the H$_2$ receptor. Plots show percent of cAMP (the basal level set at 100%) vs log concentration of compound. Ranitidine (shown in green) and cimetidine (shown in blue) are both inverse agonists. Burimamide (shown in red) does not change the basal level of cAMP and therefore is a neutral antagonist. (Adapted from Smit MJ, Leurs R, Alewijnse AE et al. (1996) *Proc Natl Acad Sci USA* 93:6802–6807. With permission from National Academy of Sciences.)

to achieve a dose ratio of 2 as compound B; therefore compound B is the more potent antagonist. pA_2 may be used as an estimate of the binding constant, –log K_b, based on certain assumptions, which include competitive antagonism, reversible binding of agonist and antagonist, a system at equilibrium, and a biological response dependent upon occupancy and activation of the receptor.

It can be difficult to differentiate a competitive antagonist from an inverse agonist on the basis of a physiological response, as most often an agonist is present and both reduce the signaling event. In measuring a downstream pharmacological effect, an inverse agonist of a non-constitutively active receptor will behave like a competitive antagonist since it is not possible to measure a decrease if the resting response of the receptor is zero. In order to prove neutral antagonism, a system must be defined by an inverse agonist, since it is necessary to know that the constitutive level can either be reduced (inverse agonist) or left at the same response level (neutral antagonist). For this reason, many compounds originally classified as antagonists are being reclassified with further work. In fact, a 2004 study of 380 compounds originally described as competitive antagonists found that newly reported data showed that 85% of those have been reclassified as inverse agonists. For example, in a study done in 1996, it was shown that both cimetidine and ranitidine, drugs originally classified as a neutral antagonist of the H$_2$ receptor, are inverse agonists. In this case, the H$_2$ receptor exhibits basal activity, so a reduction in cAMP levels when no agonist is present can be observed (**Figure 6.12**). However, an early clinical candidate that also acts at the H$_2$ receptor, burimamide, is a neutral antagonist.

6.4   Theories have been developed to explain how drugs binding at the same receptor site may have different types of activity

Theories of how ligand–receptor and drug–receptor interactions affect bioactivity have evolved over the past century, with the goal of explaining how different drugs may bind to the same receptor but have different levels of activity and even different downsteam signaling effects. In 1937, A. J. Clark was the first to apply chemical laws to quantify drug–receptor activity, proposing that the fraction of receptors occupied was directly proportional to the biological response. Modification of this theory by Everhardus Ariens and R. P. Stephenson, and others, led to the current version of the **occupation theory**, which explains how partial agonists can occupy all receptors but not produce a full response. A key concept is that of **efficacy** or **intrinsic activity**: the degree to which a drug, by binding to a receptor, has the capacity to result in a biological response. In this theory the biological activity of a molecule is not only directly proportional to the fraction of occupied receptors but is also dependent on the molecule's intrinsic activity. The **rate theory**, developed by W. D. M. Paton and H. P. Rang, proposed that activity is a function of the rate of association and dissociation and not just the number of occupied receptors.

Figure 6.13 Extended ternary complex model for GPCRs. Three forms of free receptor (R_i, R_a, and R_a-G), shown at the bottom, are in equilibrium with each other, as well as three forms bound to ligand A (A-R_i, A-R_a, and A-R_a-G), shown at the top. Equilibrium constants K_a, αK_a, and $\alpha\gamma K_a$ characterize binding of ligand A to each form of the receptor. K_G and γK_G are characteristic of binding of the G protein to the free active form (R_a) and the bound active form (A-R_a), respectively. In this model, the terms α and γ are parameters characteristic of the specific ligand A and reflect affinity and efficacy.

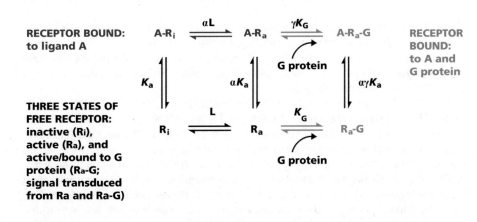

Multiple models of GPCR action have been developed and adopted, and each has been refined over time. One of the most commonly accepted models is the **extended ternary complex** (ETC) model first proposed in 1993 by Robert Lefkowitz (who was awarded the Nobel Prize in Chemistry 2012 "for studies of G protein-coupled receptors") and Philippe Samama. In this model, without a ligand (A) bound, three forms of the receptor exist: inactive (R_i), active (R_a), and active/bound to G protein (R_a-G), with the signal being transduced from the R_a or R_a-G state. In the absence of a ligand, the equilibrium between active and inactive receptors lies far towards the inactive state (R_i), and little, if any, signal is transduced. In the case of constitutively active receptors, a small percentage of receptors are in the active states, R_a or R_a-G, accounting for the modest amount of signal transduction. Binding of a ligand (A) to any one of the three forms changes the resting equilibrium (based on the equilibrium constants K_a and K_G) and leads to changes in signal transduction. This model is outlined in **Figure 6.13**.

This theory provides an explanation for how molecules that bind to the same putative site can exert vastly different effects. In the ETC model, an agonist has high affinity for the active R_a state and, upon binding, stabilizes the active form, shifts the equilibrium away from R_i to A-R_a and R_a-G, and increases the amount of signal transduced. In the case of a partial agonist, the equilibrium also shifts toward A-R_a and R_a-G but not to the same extent as a full agonist. An inverse agonist has high affinity for the R_i state and stabilizes the inactive form, shifting the equilibrium even further away from R_a and R_a-G, and thereby reducing any constitutive activity. A neutral antagonist binds, but does not change the equilibrium.

Differences in activity, as evidenced by dose–response curves, result from affinity for different forms of the receptor, and the parameters α and γ in the ETC are characteristic of the specific ligand and reflect activity and efficacy. Equilibrium constants K_a, αK_a, and $\alpha\gamma K_a$ characterize binding of ligand A to each form of the receptor.

The ETC model relies on three defined (unoccupied) receptor species as the resting population. A different way to explain ligand–receptor behavior is the use of a **probability model** or a model based on ensembles of conformations. In this model there is a large distribution (rather than just three) of resting receptor states or microconformations, and binding of a ligand shifts the overall distribution, increasing some states and decreasing others.

6.5 Drugs acting at GPCRs include drugs to treat allergy, cardiovascular disease, asthma, and ulcers

Many early drugs act at class A GPCRs and were discovered serendipitously or by using whole-animal models of diseases rather than by target-based drug design. Their mechanisms and specific targets were only determined well after the drugs were approved and widely used, and as described above, in many cases the characterization of these molecules as an agonist or antagonist has been revised. More recently, drug discovery for GPCRs has relied on design based on the natural ligand, when the natural ligand is a small molecule. With the availability of technology that allows efficient screening of GPCRs for functional activity, focused screening of specialty libraries is also common. The forefront of GPCR drug discovery takes advantages of the very recent advances in structural biology and the availability of high-resolution structures of small molecules bound to GPCRs.

The early antihistamine drugs such as diphenhydramine (**Figure 6.14**) act primarily on the H_1 subtype as antagonists of the natural ligand histamine, with activity in the periphery against the itching and inflammation associated with allergies. However they also act on H_1 receptors in the central nervous system (CNS), leading to sedation, and they have effects as an antagonist at another GPCR, the muscarinic receptor. Newer drugs such as cetirizine and loratidine do not penetrate the CNS and thus exert their activity only on peripheral receptors, so patients experience much lower levels of sedation. Although long categorized as antagonists, loratidine and diphenhydramine have recently been reclassified as inverse agonists. These compounds are also examples of drugs that were originally available only by prescription, and then, on the basis of their safety record, became available over the counter.

Drugs that are selective for the H_2 subtype act to prevent the effects of histamine on cells in the gut that secrete gastric acid, leading to their use as ulcer medications. One of the first drugs developed using the concept of modern drug design was cimetidine (Figure 6.14). Robin Ganellin and others at Smith, Kline & French designed a series of compounds based on the structure of the natural ligand, histamine (see Case Study 2 in Chapter 4).

Drugs acting at the adrenaline receptor are used to treat a variety of conditions, including asthma, heart failure, arrhythmia, and hypertension. These drugs are categorized by the receptor subtype that they act upon, as well as their agonist or antagonist activity. In 1948, two major subtypes of the adrenergic receptor, α and β, were recognized. These have been delineated further into $α_1$ and $α_2$ subtypes and $β_1$, $β_2$, and $β_3$ subtypes. Two of the most clinically useful categories of drugs are $β_2$ agonists and $β_1$ inverse agonists (originally classified as antagonists). Stimulation of $β_2$ receptors in the lung results in bronchodilation, and a number of agonists based on the phenylethanolamine structure of the natural ligand, adrenaline, have been developed to treat asthma (**Figure 6.15**). Increasing the size of the alkyl substituent on the nitrogen atom leads to efficacy at the $β_2$ receptors, with varying levels of selectivity over other adrenaline receptors. Isoproterenol (isoprenaline), containing an isopropyl group in place of the methyl group in adrenaline, is an early example of an agonist at the $β_2$ receptor, and use of it results in bronchodilation in patients. However, the catechol is rapidly metabolized to an inactive metabolite. Homologation of one of the catechol hydroxyl groups to a benzylic alcohol increased the duration of action, and this modification combined with further incorporation of steric bulk led to *rac*-albuterol (salbutamol), a drug commonly used to treat asthma. Treatment with the optically pure *R*-isomer, levosalbutamol, avoids the inflammatory side effects of the *S*-isomer.

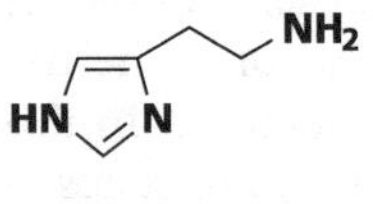

Figure 6.14 Examples of drugs acting at histamine receptors and natural ligand histamine. Diphenhydramine, cetirizine, and loratidine are all antagonists or inverse agonists at the H_1 receptor. Diphenhydramine, certirizine, and loratidine act at the H_1 subtype and are used to treat allergies, while cimetidine acts at the H_2 subtype and is used to treat gastric ulcers.

histamine
(natural ligand)

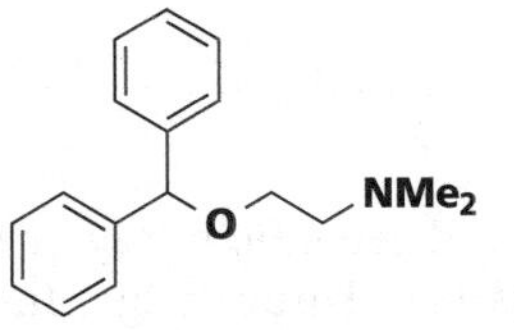

diphenhydramine
Benadryl
1946
H_1 antagonist/inverse agonist

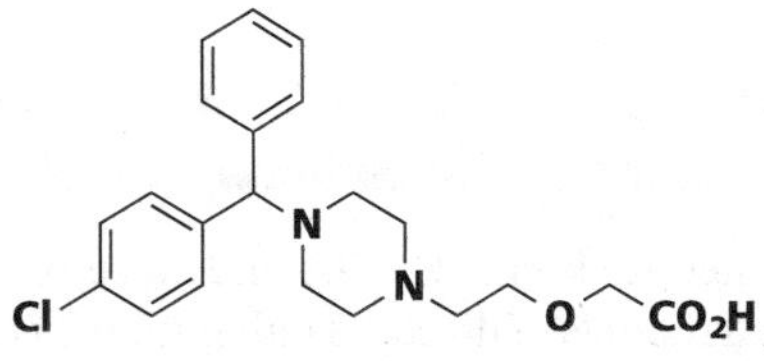

cetirizine
Zyrtec
1996
H_1 inverse agonist

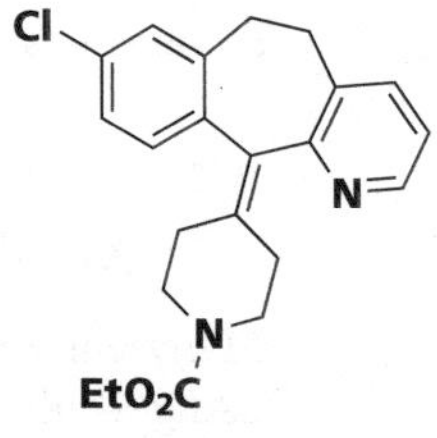

loratidine
Claritin
1993
H_1 inverse agonist

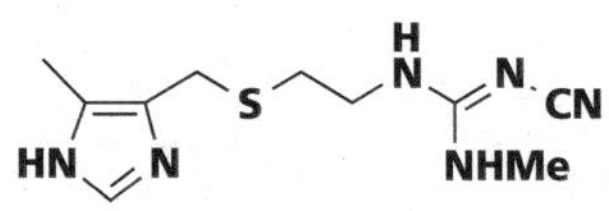

cimetidine
Tagamet
1979
H_2 inverse agonist

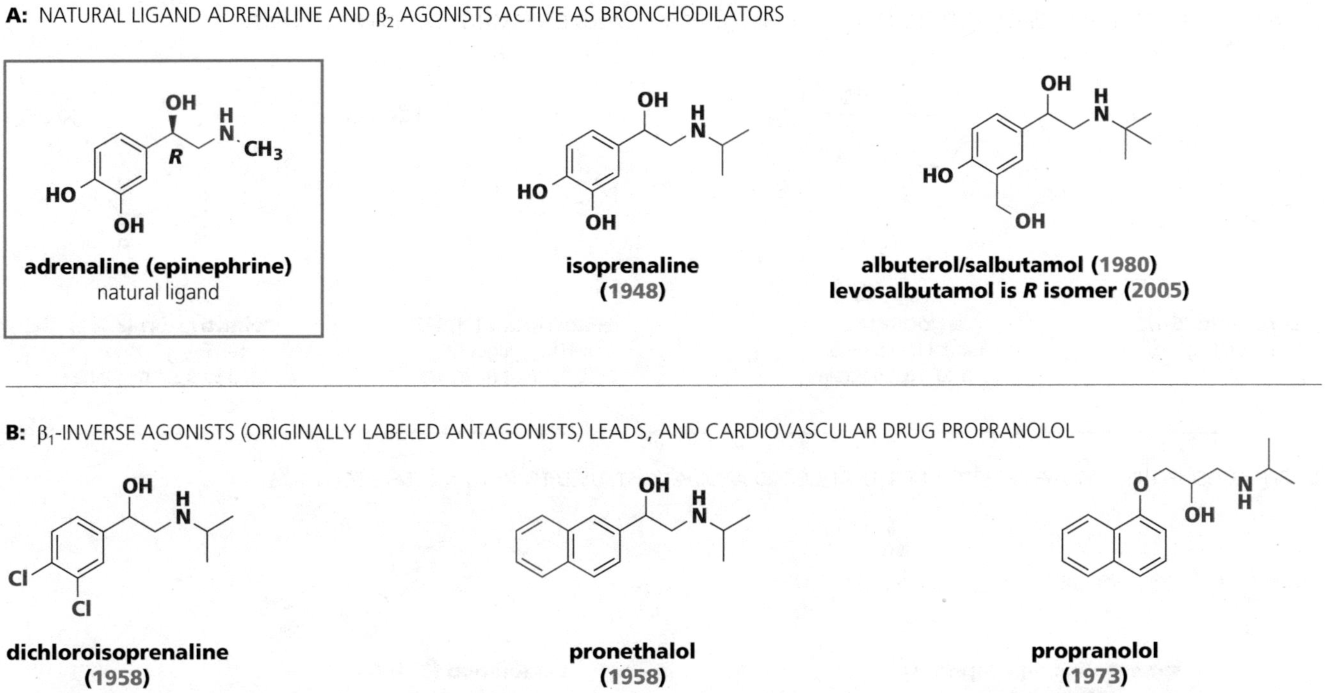

A: NATURAL LIGAND ADRENALINE AND β_2 AGONISTS ACTIVE AS BRONCHODILATORS

adrenaline (epinephrine)
natural ligand

isoprenaline
(1948)

albuterol/salbutamol (1980)
levosalbutamol is *R* isomer (2005)

B: β_1-INVERSE AGONISTS (ORIGINALLY LABELED ANTAGONISTS) LEADS, AND CARDIOVASCULAR DRUG PROPRANOLOL

dichloroisoprenaline
(1958)

pronethalol
(1958)

propranolol
(1973)

Figure 6.15 Examples of drugs acting at adrenergic receptors and the natural ligand adrenaline. A: β_2 Receptor agonists isoprenaline and albuterol, both containing the phenylethanolamine moiety found in adrenaline, are effective as bronchodilators (modifications are shown in red). Increasing steric bulk at the nitrogen atom increases potency; extension of alcohol by a carbon atom improves duration of action. Levosalbutamol is the R-enantiomer of albuterol B: β_1 Receptor inverse agonist lead dichloroisoprenaline, along with pronethalol and propranolol, which is used as a cardiovascular drug (modifications are shown in red). Propranolol, containing an aryloxypropanolamine scaffold, is the prototypical β-blocker.

Removing the hydroxyl groups of the aromatic ring in adrenaline leads to activity as an inverse agonist rather than agonist activity. Dichloroisoprenaline, which blocked the effects of adrenaline on bronchodilation and cardiac stimulation, as well as on uterine relaxation in animal models, is a representative compound. Replacing the di-chloro phenyl scaffold with a naphthalene led to pronethalol, the first β_1 inverse agonist marketed. However, it was found to cause thymic tumors and was withdrawn from the market. Further modification, by reorientation and homologation of the side chain through insertion of an $-OCH_2$ group, led to the first example of an important class of drugs characterized by the aryloxypropanolamine scaffold, commonly known as β-blockers. Propranolol is a prototypical β-blocker that is widely used to treat both cardiac arrhythmia and hypertension. Sir James Black was awarded the Nobel Prize in Physiology or Medicine 1988 for his discovery of this drug as well as cimetidine.

Drugs acting at GPCRs found in the CNS are numerous and are important analgesics and antipsychotic medications. These include opiates such as morphine, codeine, and fentanyl to treat pain and antipsychotic drugs acting at dopamine receptors, such as Thorazine, haloperidol, and clozapine. All of these drugs act at GPCRs and are discussed in detail in Chapter 13.

A relatively recent class of drugs is the anti-migraine serotonin receptor agonists such as sumatriptan and zolmitriptan (**Figure 6.16A**). The triptans were first developed at Glaxo in the 1970s and were based on the vasoconstriction effects of the natural ligand serotonin and of the natural product ergotamine, which was approved to treat migraine. The triptans, the natural ligand, and ergotamine all contain an indole ring and a pendant amine function. Sumatriptan, approved in 1991 and zolmitriptan (2001), are selective for the 5-HT$_{1B/1D}$ subtypes of the serotonin receptors and constrict blood vessels in the brain.

Fingolimod, (**Figure 6.16B**) the first disease-modifying drug approved to treat multiple sclerosis, also acts at a GPCR. It is phosphorylated and that product, a monophosphate, is an agonist at the sphingosine 1-phosphate receptor (S1PR1), a lipid-activated GPCR involved in the immune response.

One active area of research is the development of compounds that act at cannabinoid receptors. The natural ligands, anandamide (**Figure 6.16C**) and other metabolites of arachidonic acid, indiscriminately activate the receptors, which results in numerous effects including psychoactive effects, analgesia, and increased appetite. Tetrahydrocannabinol (THC), the active constituent of marijuana, is a nonselective

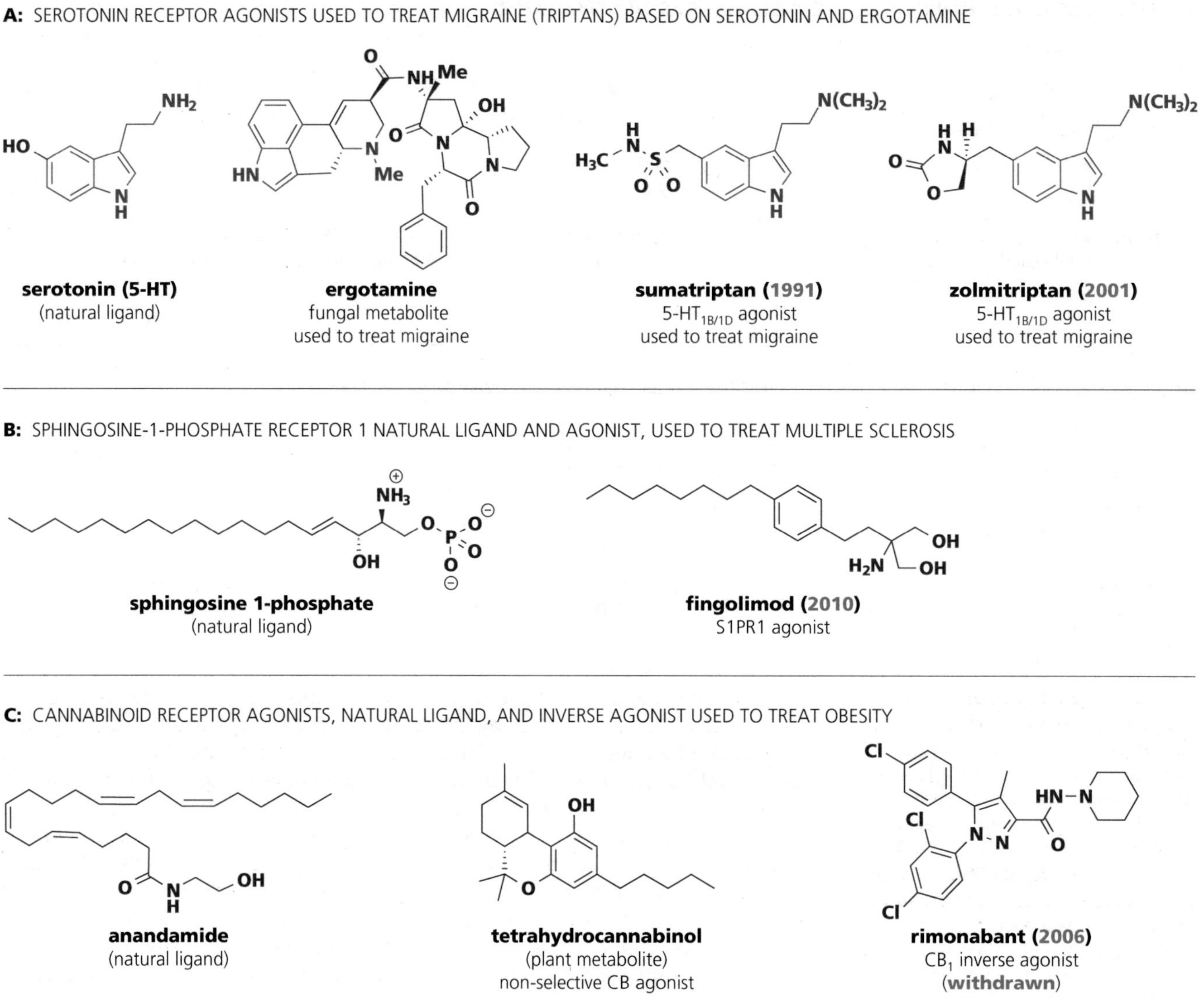

A: SEROTONIN RECEPTOR AGONISTS USED TO TREAT MIGRAINE (TRIPTANS) BASED ON SEROTONIN AND ERGOTAMINE

serotonin (5-HT)
(natural ligand)

ergotamine
fungal metabolite
used to treat migraine

sumatriptan (1991)
5-HT$_{1B/1D}$ agonist
used to treat migraine

zolmitriptan (2001)
5-HT$_{1B/1D}$ agonist
used to treat migraine

B: SPHINGOSINE-1-PHOSPHATE RECEPTOR 1 NATURAL LIGAND AND AGONIST, USED TO TREAT MULTIPLE SCLEROSIS

sphingosine 1-phosphate
(natural ligand)

fingolimod (2010)
S1PR1 agonist

C: CANNABINOID RECEPTOR AGONISTS, NATURAL LIGAND, AND INVERSE AGONIST USED TO TREAT OBESITY

anandamide
(natural ligand)

tetrahydrocannabinol
(plant metabolite)
non-selective CB agonist

rimonabant (2006)
CB$_1$ inverse agonist
(**withdrawn**)

---

agonist and is approved to treat anorexia in AIDS patients and as a second-line therapy to treat nausea and vomiting in chemotherapy patients. Recent efforts have focused on identifying subtype-selective agonists and antagonists in the hope of separating some of the beneficial effects of marijuana and THC from the psychoactive effects. For example, inverse agonists or antagonists of the CB$_1$ receptor were expected to reduce the activity of the receptor and therefore suppress appetite, with potential as effective anti-obesity agents. Initially, CB$_1$-selective inverse antagonists such as rimonabant showed great promise as a treatment for obesity; however, rimonabant was withdrawn from the market due to side effects including depression and anxiety, perhaps due to excessive reduction of receptor activity. There are also a number of cannabinoid agonists in development to treat a variety of conditions including pain, nausea, and anxiety.

ION CHANNELS (IONOTROPIC RECEPTORS) AS DRUG TARGETS

Ion channels are proteins that span the cell membrane and regulate the highly selective transport of ions from the outside of the cell to the inside. Their function is critical to physiological processes such as muscle contraction and neurotransmission. There are hundreds of genes that code for ion channels, and many conditions are related

Figure 6.16 Examples of drugs acting at GPCRs with diverse bioactivities. A: 5-HT receptor natural ligand, serotonin (5-HT); natural product, ergotamine which causes vasoconstriction and is used to treat migraine; and two triptans, sumatriptan and zolmitriptan, which are serotonin 5-HT$_{1B/1D}$ agonists (common structural features are shown in red). B: S1PR1 receptor natural ligand, sphingosine-1-phosphate, and fingolimod, used to treat multiple sclerosis. Phosphorylation of fingolimod generates the phosphate, which is an agonist at the S1P1 receptor. C: CB receptor natural ligand, anandamide; natural product tetrahydrocannabinol (THC), an agonist; and rimonabant, a CB$_1$ inverse agonist. CB$_1$ inverse agonists or antagonists have potential as anti-obesity drugs.

to malfunction of those channels. Examples include cardiovascular diseases related to malfunction of calcium channels; depression and anxiety, which can be caused by dysfunction of γ-aminobutyric acid (GABA) chloride ion channels; and pain, which can be affected by sodium channels. Ion channels are made up of multiple subunits that combine to form a cylindrical structure with a central pore. The pore is lined with hydrophilic residues that are arranged in a specific geometry (**Figure 6.17A**). This geometry serves to select, usually by size, which specific ions are transported and which are excluded. Ion selectivity is regulated by an ion filter (for charge and/ or size) and a gate that allows the selected ions to pass into the cell. Ion channels are classified as either voltage-gated ion channels (VGIC) or ligand-gated ion channels (LGIC), depending on whether a change in membrane potential or binding of a ligand initiates their opening or closing. LGICs are also referred to as ionotropic receptors. In addition, ion channels can be classified according to the ions they transport.

Under normal physiological conditions, an ion channel exhibits a range of resting (open), activated (open), and inactivated (closed) states over a given period of time (**Figure 6.17B**). The equilibrium between these states is affected by ligands in the case of LGICs and by changes in membrane potential in the case of VGICs.

Natural products have been an excellent source of small molecules that act at ion channels. These structures, sometimes themselves drugs, are often used as starting points for drug discovery and medicinal chemistry activities. In addition, high-throughput screening and ligand-based screening are also common starting points. The first X-ray structure of an ion channel (a bacterial K^+ channel) was solved in 1998, and like the GPCRs, this field is evolving as new structural information becomes available. Recent successful solution of X-ray and cryo-EM structures illustrating ion channels in various points of opening has further supported the use of structure-based design.

Assaying for activity at ion channels is simpler than for GPCRs, since the downstream event is an immediate change in membrane potential due to release of ions. A widely used assay is the patch clamp assay, developed in the late 1970s by

A: ION CHANNEL EMBEDDED IN CELL MEMBRANE

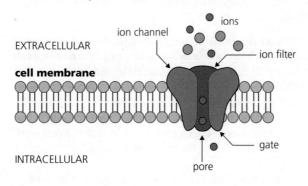

Figure 6.17 Ion channels. A: General structure of ion channel (shown in blue) embedded in cell membrane. Ions of various sizes (shown in green and pink) on the outside of a cell pass through an ion selectivity filter into the hydrophilic pore. Only those with the appropriate size and charge (here shown in pink) proceed through a gate into the cell. B: Different activation states of ion channels. At resting state, there is some basal level of ion flow; in the activated state, there is increased ion flow; and in the inactivated state, ion flow is blocked or decreased from basal level.

B: DIFFERENT STATES OF ION CHANNELS IN EQUILIBRIUM

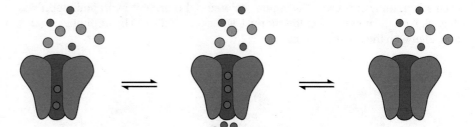

RESTING STATE: some intermittent ion flow

ACTIVATED STATE: increased ion flow

INACTIVATED STATE: blocked ion flow

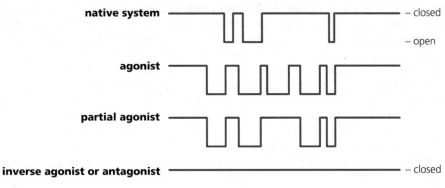

y-axis = amperes; x-axis = time

Figure 6.18 Patch clamp assays. Time is plotted vs conductance (measured in amperes) reflecting open or closed channel. Top trace shows the native system and changes in conductance at resting state. The effect of an agonist is increased ion flow through the open channel, which may open more often and/or for longer periods of time. The effect of a partial agonist is increased flow but less than for a full agonist. The effect of an inverse agonist or antagonist (blockers) is decreased or no opening of the channel.

Erwin Neher and Bert Sakmann, for which they won the Nobel Prize in Physiology or Medicine 1991. In this assay, a patch of membrane containing as few as one ion channel is used, and the voltage change can be measured with a microelectrode over millisecond time periods, indicating whether the ion channel is open or closed. As shown in **Figure 6.18**, an agonist or opener will cause the channel to open for a given period of time or cause it to stay open longer or to open more frequently than the native system. A partial agonist will open the channel but for a shorter time period and/or less frequently than a full agonist. Antagonists and inverse agonists (also called channel blockers) prevent the channel from opening.

Patch clamp assays have been modified and automated for use in HTS, as have other assay techniques. These include the use of flash luminescence assays for calcium channels, which rely on Ca^{2+}-sensitive photoproteins that emit a burst of light upon calcium binding, as well as fluorescence-based assays that respond to changes in ion concentration.

6.6   Ligand-gated ion channels open or close in response to binding of a drug or natural ligand

Ligand-gated ion channels all have a cylindrical shape made of protein subunits with a hydrophilic internal surface that, when open, allows the passage of ions through the pore. When closed, the pore is locked until an agonist or natural ligand binds. Binding causes a conformation change that opens the gate and allows the ions to pass through. In addition to being classified according to the type of ion allowed to pass through, LGICs are also characterized by the ligand or agonist that binds and according to the arrangement of their transmembrane regions. LGICs may open or close in response to neurotransmitters or other small molecules or to the presence of calcium ions or cAMP as second messengers.

The superfamilies of LGICs include the pentameric Cys-loop family, the tetrameric ionotropic glutamate receptors (iGluR), and the trimeric purinergic ATP-gated channels (P2X). **Figure 6.19** highlights the general structural differences between the families of LGICs, based on the number and arrangement of subunits. A top view of each superfamily is shown. The regions colored red represent hydrophilic portions that align on the inner core of the channel, while blue indicates hydrophobic regions that align with the cell membrane.

Figure 6.19 General schematic of families of ligand-gated ion channels. Top views are shown. Blue (hydrophobic) and red (hydrophilic) portions are grouped in the transmembrane-spanning regions that make up each subunit (yellow circles). Although not designated in this general view, each subunit may consist of separate units called α, β, γ, or δ. Cys-loop channel consists of five subunits, the ionotropic glutamate ion channel has four subunits, and the P2X ion channel consists of three subunits.

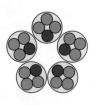

Cys-loop

ionotropic glutamate   **P2X**

The Cys-loop receptors are characterized by five subunits, usually two α and three among β, γ, and δ, which have different sequence homology. Near the N-terminal extracellular region, there is a disulfide linkage between two cysteine residues that forms a loop. The ionotropic glutamate receptors have four subunits, and the P2X receptors have three. **Table 6.2** illustrates examples of LGICs and the ions they transport, their natural ligands, drugs that target each and the approved indication.

One of the most well-studied LGICs is the nicotinic acetylcholine receptor (nAChR). In 1903, John Langley proposed the existence of specific receptive substances for nicotine and curare, which we know today as the nAChR. He noted that curare, a muscle relaxant that is the ingredient in a South American blow dart poison, antagonized the action of nicotine, a muscle contractant. The N2 subtype of the nAChR is a pentameric Cys-loop channel composed of two α_2 and one each β, γ, and δ subunits that allows passage of Na^+ ions as well as K^+ and Ca^{2+} ions. The N2 subtype receptors are located on the surface of muscle cells, near the synapse between neurons and muscle cells. In the normal course of action, two molecules of the natural ligand, acetylcholine, bind to each of the α subunits, resulting in channel opening and the passage of Na^+ ions. This opening causes depolarization of the postsynaptic membrane. As the potential spreads along the muscle, the muscle contracts. **Figure 6.20** shows a diagram of the N2 nAChR based on an X-ray structure.

Table 6.2   Examples of ligand-gated ion channel receptors, their ligands, ions transported, drugs targeting it, and the approved indication.

Natural ligand	Receptor	Ion(s) transported	Drug or ligand examples	Indication
Cys-loop Receptors				
acetylcholine	nicotinic AChR (neuromuscular)	Na^+, K^+	vecuronium, pancuronium	paralytics
	nicotinic AChR (neuronal)	Na^+, K^+	nicotine, varenicline	partial agonist, smoking cessation
glycine	GlyR	Cl^-	strychnine[a], brucine[a]	
γ-aminobutyric acid	GABA_A	Cl^-	benzodiazepines	sedative
			barbiturates, ethanol, inhaled anesthetics	muscle relaxants, sedatives
serotonin (5-HT)	5-HT_3	Na^+, K^+	ondansetron	nausea
Ionotropic Glutamate Receptors				
α-amino-3-hydroxy-5-methyl-4-isoxazole-propionic acid	AMPA	Na^+, K^+, Ca^{2+}	quisqualate[a], 5-methyl-4-aniracetam[a]	
N-methyl-D-aspartate	NMDA	Na^+, K^+	ketamine	anesthetic
			phencyclidine (PCP)[a]	
kainate, glutamate	KAR, GluR_{5-7}	Na^+, K^+	tezampanel[a]	
P2X Receptors				
ATP	P2X_{1-7}	Na^+, Ca^{2+}	suramin[a]	

[a]Ligand is not used clinically and either is a probe molecule, is in development, or has been removed from the market.

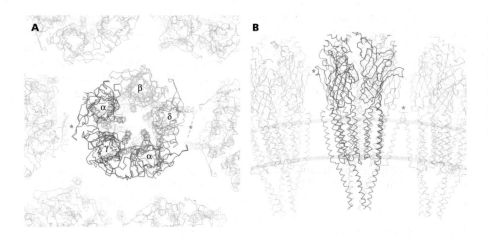

Figure 6.20 Structure of the N$_2$ nicotinic acetylcholine receptor based on X-ray. Views from the top (left image) and the side (right image) relative to the membrane are shown. Subunits α, β, γ, and δ are colored and labeled in the left image. (From Unwin N [2005] *J Mol Biol* 346:967–989. With permission from Elsevier.)

6.7   Neuromuscular blockers, sedatives, and anti-nausea agents are examples of drugs acting at LGICs

Drugs that act as antagonists at the N2 nAChR are used as neuromuscular blocking agents in anesthesia. One of the simplest examples is succinylcholine, which can be thought of as two units of the natural ligand (acetylcholine) linked together. Pancuronium and vecuronium are steroids based on the natural product malouetine (**Figure 6.21**). One of the earliest natural products acting on the nAChR used was tubocurarine, described in Chapter 1. The effects of these compounds can be profound, with pancuronium being one of several drugs used for lethal injections. The common structural feature of these compounds is the presence of two quaternary amines positioned to interact with two separate α subunits of the ion channel.

The partial agonist varenicline was developed at Pfizer and is used to treat nicotine addiction. Dependence on nicotine is related to its activation of an α$_4$β$_2$ subtype of the ion channel, which results in increased dopamine levels. Varenicline is selective for neuronal α$_4$β$_2$ ion channels. Its structure is based on cytisine, a natural product found in a number of plants, including *Cytisus laburnum*, the leaves of which have been used as a tobacco substitute and as a natural smoking cessation aid.

Benzodiazepines such as diazepam act at the Cys-loop GABA$_A$ chloride ion channel and bind to an allosteric binding site, now termed the benzodiazepine (BZ) site, located between the α and γ subunits. The natural ligand, GABA, binds between the α and β subunits and is an inhibitory neurotransmitter, meaning it decreases the likelihood that the postsynaptic neuron will generate an action potential. Other allosteric agonists include barbiturate sedatives, ethanol, and inhaled anesthetics such as isoflurane.

Figure 6.21 Examples of drugs acting at various nicotinic acetylcholine receptors. Antagonists such as succinylcholine, vecuronium and malouetine are used as neuromuscular blockers (common quaternary amines are shown in red). The partial agonist varenicline is used for smoking cessation and was based on the natural product cytisine.

ANTAGONISTS AT N2 nAChR

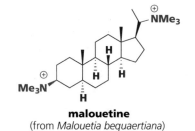

succinylcholine

vecuronium bromide
(pancuronium = A-ring *N*-methyl piperidine analog)

malouetine
(from *Malouetia bequaertiana*)

AGONISTS AT NEURONAL nAChR

varenicline
(partial agonist)

cytisine
(partial agonist)

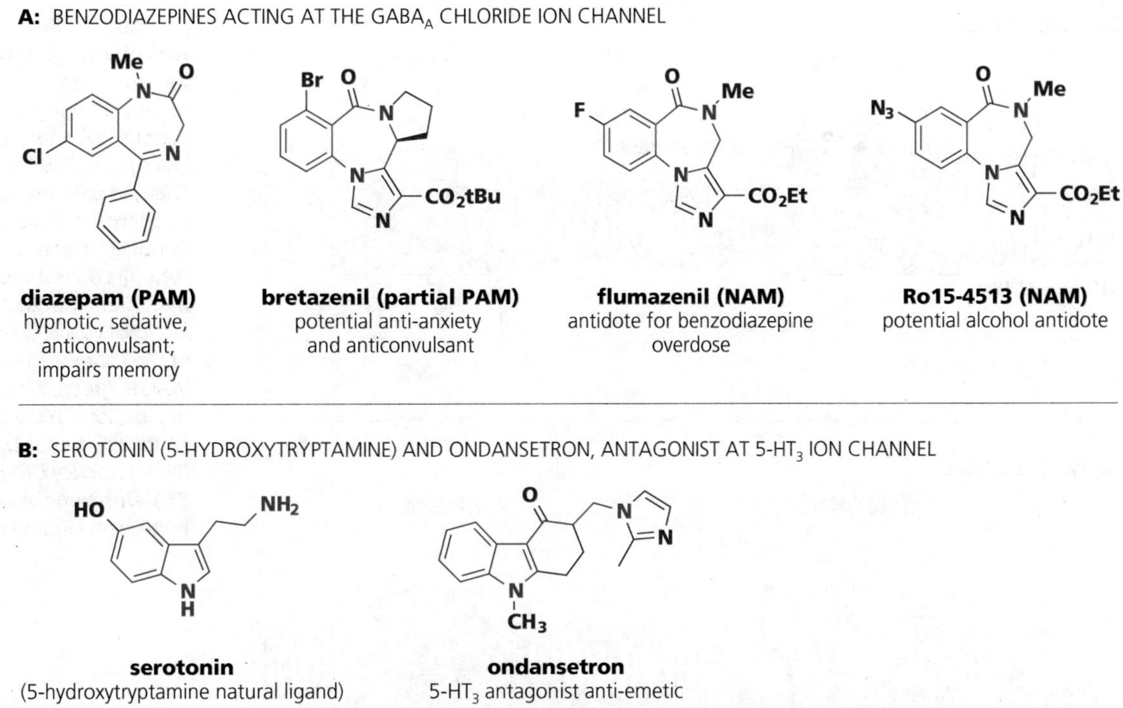

A: BENZODIAZEPINES ACTING AT THE GABA$_A$ CHLORIDE ION CHANNEL

diazepam (PAM)
hypnotic, sedative,
anticonvulsant;
impairs memory

bretazenil (partial PAM)
potential anti-anxiety
and anticonvulsant

flumazenil (NAM)
antidote for benzodiazepine
overdose

Ro15-4513 (NAM)
potential alcohol antidote

B: SEROTONIN (5-HYDROXYTRYPTAMINE) AND ONDANSETRON, ANTAGONIST AT 5-HT$_3$ ION CHANNEL

serotonin
(5-hydroxytryptamine natural ligand)

ondansetron
5-HT$_3$ antagonist anti-emetic

Figure 6.22 Examples of drugs acting at GABA$_A$ and 5-HT$_3$ ion channels.
A: Benzodiazepines acting at the GABA$_A$ chloride ion channel, with common benzodiazepine structure shown in red. PAMs such as diazepam and bretazenil are anti-anxiety drugs and can be anti-convulsants. The NAM flumazenil is an antidote for benzodiazepine overdose and the experimental NAM Ro15-4513 was a potential alcohol antidote. B: Structures of serotonin (natural ligand) and ondansetron, an antagonist at the 5-HT$_3$ ion channel, use to treat nausea (common features in red).

The benzodiazepines are an example of a family of drugs where small structural modifications lead to differences in intrinsic activity. Early benzodiazepines, such as diazepam, act as positive allosteric modulators and amplify the effects of GABA, resulting in opening of the channel. The benzodiazepines are widely used as anti-anxiety drugs and as anticonvulsants, but they also impair memory. Minor changes in the structure lead to differences in efficacy, although they all bind at the benzodiazepine site. For example, while diazepam is a full PAM, the analog bretazenil is a partial PAM (**Figure 6.22A**) that maintains anti-anxiety activity, although it is not marketed. The structurally similar flumazenil is a negative allosteric modulator (NAM) and is used to treat benzodiazepine overdose. The NAM Ro15-4513, an experimental agent, is identical to flumazenil except for the replacement of the fluorine atom with an azide. While not as effective as flumazenil against benzodiazepine overdose, Ro15-4513 was effective as an antidote to alcohol poisoning in animal models, although it also caused seizures. One physiological effect of NAMs is an enhancement in memory; however, this is offset by anxiogenic and convulsant properties.

Although the other subtypes of serotonin receptors are GPCRs, the 5-HT$_3$ receptor is a sodium/potassium ion channel found in several regions of the nervous system that responds to 5-hydroxytryptamine (serotonin). Antagonists such as ondansetron, structurally similar to the natural ligand serotonin, are used primarily to treat nausea associated with chemotherapy in cancer patients (**Figure 6.22B**).

6.8 Voltage-gated ion channels open or close in response to changes in membrane potential

Voltage-gated ion channels (VGICs) open or close in response to a change in membrane potential and may be selective for Na$^+$, K$^+$, Ca^{2+}, or Cl$^-$ ions. Like LGICs, they exist in equilibrium between three states: resting, open, and inactivated. While the states vary depending on membrane potential, drugs that act at these ion channels have affinity for one form over another and hence affect their equilibrium. Voltage-gated channels typically contain four transmembrane domains with a selectivity filter at the top surrounded by four voltage sensors. The voltage-sensing domain responds to membrane depolarization, causing opening of the channel. Several models for the function of VGICs have been proposed, including a piston-type model, a flap model, and a transporter-type model (**Figure 6.23**).

A: PISTON MODEL

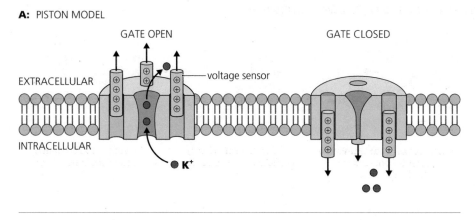

B: PADDLE MODEL

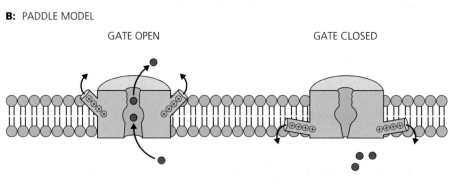

C: TRANSPORTER MODEL

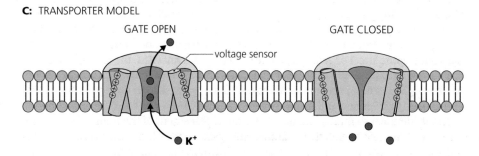

Figure 6.23 Several models proposed for voltage-gated ion channel opening and closing. A: Piston model, showing movement of charged pistons (cylinders) as ion concentration changes. B: Paddle model, showing charged paddles that move as levers to open and close the ion channel. C: Transporter model, where charged subunits do not move through the membrane but translocate within the receptor to affect opening and closing of the channel (membrane in pink; VGIC in green, with charges on pistons in pink, ions in blue). (Adapted from Ashcroft F, Benos D, Bezanilla F et al. [2004] *Nat Rev Drug Discovery* 3:239–278. With permission from Macmillan Publishers Limited.)

In the piston model, the voltage-sensing domains move up or down, as would a piston, resulting in a conformational change that allows ions through the pore. On the basis of an X-ray structure of a bacterial K^+ voltage-gated channel, this model has been disfavored, and ones where the voltage-sensing domains are more like paddles that either move through the membrane, as in the paddle model, or simply pivot along an axis, as in the transporter model, are now preferred.

Unlike GPCRs and LGICs, VGICs do not respond to binding by a natural ligand for their activation (or opening and closing); therefore, hit identification cannot rely on knowledge of the structure of a natural ligand. As such, drug discovery targeting VGICs has not been as active an area as it has been for GPCRs and LGICs. Most drugs in this category were discovered serendipitously, without knowledge of their mechanism of action. Many plant and animal toxins have activity at VGICs, including tetrodotoxin from pufferfish and saxitoxin from shellfish, as well as batrachotoxin, found in frogs. More recent examples of drugs have been based on pharmacophore models developed from such discovered ligands. Compounds that act to open the channel are known as **channel activators**, and those that keep the channel closed are termed **channel blockers**. Significant advances in miniaturization and standardization of techniques to measure ion flux have been developed, and these techniques now allow high-throughput screening as a viable approach to hit identification and optimization. Like other receptors, selectivity for one LGIC in the presence of many others that transport the same ion is often a significant hurdle. Some therapeutically important VGICs are listed in **Table 6.3**.

Table 6.3 Examples of voltage-gated ion channel receptors, ions transported, ligands or drugs targeting it, their mechanism of action and approved indication.

Channel	Ion(s) transported	Drug or ligand examples	Mechanism	Indication
L-type Ca$_v$	Ca^{2+}	verapamil, diltiazem, nifedipine	blocker	cardiovascular disease
Na$_v$	Na$^+$, K$^+$	lidocaine	blocker	anesthetic
		carbamazepine, phenytoin	blocker	anticonvulsants
Ca$_v$ ($\alpha_2\delta$)	Ca^{2+}	gabapentin, pregabalin	activator	anticonvulsant, analgesic
Ca$_v$2.2	Ca^{2+}	ziconotide	blocker	analgesic
influenza M2	H$^+$	amantadine	blocker	influenza

6.9 Blockers of sodium, calcium and potassium VGICs include local anesthetics, anticonvulsants, and anti-arrhythmia drugs

Drugs typically have affinity for either the activated (open) or inactivated (closed) state of the VGIC, binding either directly to the ion channel subunits or to auxiliary subunits. Historically, important drugs that act through voltage-gated sodium channels include the "caine" anesthetics. Although illegal today, the natural product cocaine was used as a local anesthetic in the late 1880s, and that bioactivity was later attributed to action at a voltage-gated sodium channel. However, cocaine has multiple effects, and today a number of much more selective caine anesthetics are available and are used as local anesthetics. The sodium channel involved initiates and propagates the action potentials in neurons. These molecules bind to the open and inactivated states with high affinity. Early ester analogs of cocaine included amylocaine (Stovaine) and the more commonly used procaine (Novocaine), which was introduced in 1905. Problems with procaine include its short duration of action and instability. The search for a more stable analog led to the amide analogs lidocaine (Xylocaine) and prilocaine (**Figure 6.24**). Lidocaine was originally derived from a synthetic intermediate prepared during a synthesis of isogramine, a natural product found in a barley plant that, like cocaine, has activity as a local anesthetic. Isogramine itself is too irritating to be a useful anesthetic, and the chemists Nils Löfgren and Holger Erdtman prepared many analogs of isogramine, as well as its synthetic precursor, before identifying lidocaine.

A number of drugs that are used to treat convulsions act at the Na$_v$ or sodium VGICs. Convulsions can occur when neurons are depolarized and active for long periods of

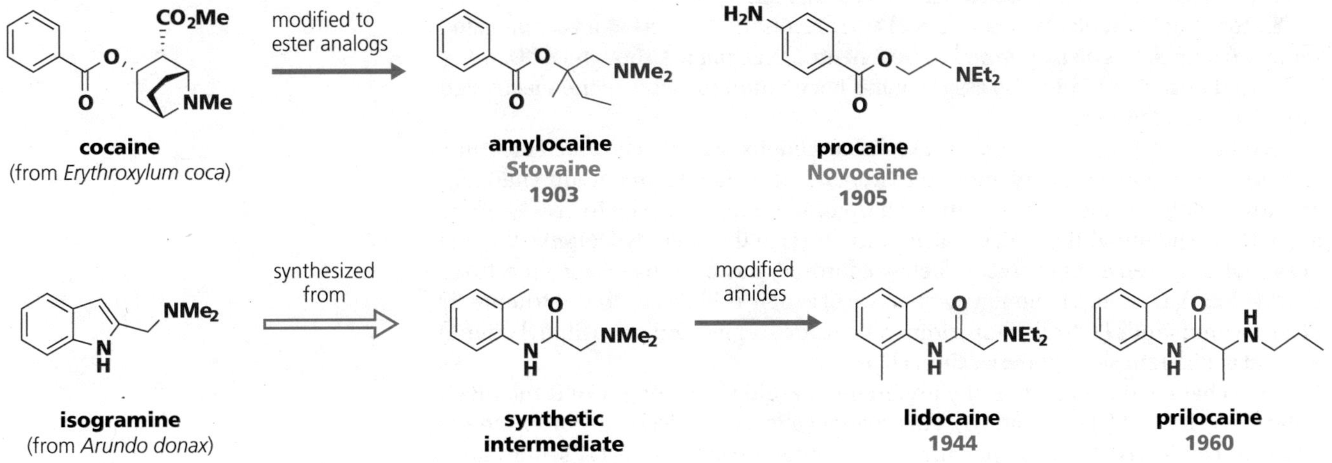

Figure 6.24 Examples of caine anesthetics. (Top) Cocaine was modified to give ester analogs amylocaine and procaine, commonly used anesthetics (modifications shown in red). (Bottom) Lidocaine and procaine (amide groups shown in red) were derived from a synthetic intermediate used to make the natural product isogramine. Both are frequently used as local anesthetics.

cocaine
(from *Erythroxylum coca*)

modified to ester analogs

amylocaine
Stovaine
1903

procaine
Novocaine
1905

isogramine
(from *Arundo donax*)

synthesized from

synthetic intermediate

modified amides

lidocaine
1944

prilocaine
1960

A: ANTICONVULSANTS THAT BLOCK SODIUM VGICs (Na$_v$)

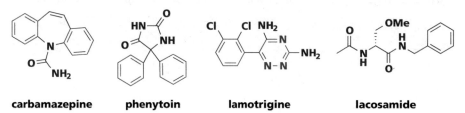

carbamazepine   phenytoin   lamotrigine   lacosamide

B: MODEL OF LAMOTRIGINE BOUND IN INACTIVATED STATE OF Na$_v$

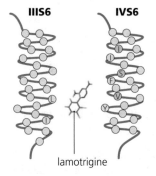

mutation of green and blue residues to
alanine decreases binding of lamotrigine

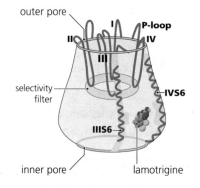

Figure 6.25 Anticonvulsant drugs acting at voltage-gated ion channels. A: Carbamazepine, phenytoin, lamotrigine, and lacosamide all block sodium VGICs. Common structural features of the first three are shown in red. B: Model of lamotrigine localized at its binding site in the brain Na$_v$. (Left) Close-up view of binding site: IIIS6 and IVS6 are subunits in the pore region, and lamotrigine binds between them. Amino acids mutated (green and blue) to identify binding site. (Right) Model of the Na$_v$ pore: I–IV (red lines) each represent an α subunit, each of which has six segments (S1-S6); the wall of the ion channel is formed by S5 and S6 α helices, with the IIIS6 and IVS6 that contain the binding site highlighted. The outer pore and selectivity filter are formed by P loops that connect the subunits. (Adapted from Rogawski MA & Löscher W [2004] *Nat Rev Neurosci* 5:553–564. With permission from Macmillan Publishers Limited.)

time. Most anticonvulsant drugs were discovered through phenotypic assays rather than by design, and those that act at sodium VGICs include diverse structures such as carbamazepine, phenytoin, lamotrigine, and most recently lacosamide (**Figure 6.25A**). Their overall mechanism is stabilization of the inactivated state of the receptor, preventing channel opening and ending the action potential that leads to convulsions. Carbamazepine was discovered in the 1950s and first marketed in the 1960s as an anticonvulsant. While it stabilizes the inactivated state of the ion channel, it is not selective and also acts as a GABA agonist. Phenytoin, approved in 1953, was discovered in the early 1900s as a non-sedating analog of the barbiturates. It also binds to the inactivated state of the ion channel. Lamotrigine, approved in 1994 as an anticonvulsant, acts by blocking the inactivated form of Na$_v$. While these three compounds are from distinct scaffolds, they bind at a common site and contain two pendant aryl rings as a common structural feature. On the basis of site-directed mutagenesis studies of the brain type II Na$_v$ ion channel, lamotrigine does not physically block the pore but is proposed to bind to hydrophobic amino acids, in two particular α-helices in the pore region of the ion channel (**Figure 6.25B**). Structurally, this channel is composed of four homologous α-subunits (I-IV), each composed of six α-helical segments (S1-S6).

Lacosamide is a relatively new (2007) anticonvulsant that acts at a voltage-gated sodium channel. It is also approved to treat neuropathic pain. Although its discovery was based on activity in *in vivo* assays, it has been found to stabilize the inactivated form of the ion channel.

A number of drugs to treat cardiovascular conditions, such as high blood pressure, arrhythmia, angina, coronary artery disease, and heart failure, act at ion channels. These include drugs such as nifedipine, diltiazem, and verapamil, which act as blockers at the L-type potential-dependent calcium channels in the heart. Nifedipine, the first of the 1,4-dihydropyridine structural class approved, has been used since the 1970s (**Figure 6.26**). Despite a common mechanism of action as blockers, these structurally diverse compounds (1,4-dihydropyridines, benzothiazepine and phenylbutyl amine) all bind at different sites on the calcium channel.

One channel that is particularly important to avoid interacting with is the hERG potassium channel (see Chapter 5). This channel affects the electrical current in the heart, and inhibition leads to a potentially fatal condition called long QT syndrome.

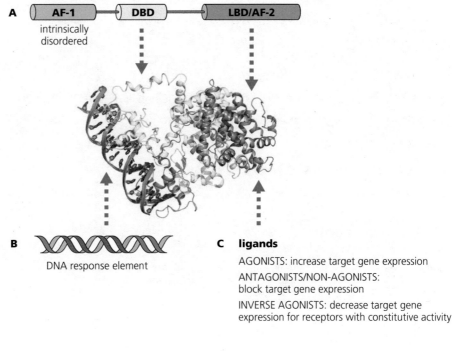

nifedipine   **diltiazem**   **verapamil**

Figure 6.26 Cardiovascular drugs that target L-type Ca^{2+} channels. Examples are structurally diverse and include nifedipine, diltiazem, and verapamil. Each is a channel blocker, but they bind at distinct sites.

NUCLEAR RECEPTORS AS DRUG TARGETS

Nuclear receptors, like GPCRs, are proteins that transduce a signal based on binding of a ligand. Unlike GPCRs and ion channels, however, they do not span the cell membrane but instead are intracellular receptors. After binding of a ligand, they function as transcription factors that regulate gene expression. The processes affected include reproduction, energy homeostasis, immunity, circadian rhythm, and metabolic processes, among many others. The natural ligands of nuclear receptors are often lipophilic small molecules such as estradiol, androgens, calcitriol (metabolite of vitamin D), and retinoic acid (vitamin A). However, there are also a number of orphan nuclear receptors, for which the natural ligand is unknown. Nuclear receptors and their signaling mechanisms are highly complex. The same receptors may be located in multiple tissues, but may have very distinct responses to the same ligand binding. Their role in a variety of physiological and pathophysiological processes, as well as the small-molecule nature of their ligands makes them a popular target for drug discovery. In fact, approximately 16% of drugs target nuclear receptors.

Structurally, the nuclear receptors share a common N-terminus, which is composed of the activation function (AF-1), a highly conserved DNA-binding domain (DBD), a linking domain, and the ligand-binding domain (LBD), which is part of the second activation function (AF-2). **Figure 6.27** illustrates some of the general features of a nuclear receptor, as seen in an X-ray structure of a truncated form of peroxisome proliferator-activated receptor (PPARγ) receptor bound to DNA and the retinoid X receptor (RXR). The DNA-binding domain is a zinc finger, characterized in this case by a pattern of eight cysteine residues that coordinate with two zinc atoms. This coordination results in formation of two peptide loops: one is involved in binding to

Figure 6.27 Structure of nuclear receptors and actions of ligands. Shown is the complex of truncated PPARγ (yellow) and RXRα (purple) bound to DNA (orange/blue) and sites for ligands and regulator peptides (green). The AF-1 region is intrinsically disordered, and therefore not visible in X-ray. A: Schematic of nuclear receptor: N-terminal domain with activation function 1 (AF-1) linked to the DNA binding domain (DBD) and the ligand binding domain (LBD) and activation function 2 (AF-2). B: DNA response element, a fragment of DNA (orange) in the context of a larger DNA molecule (blue). C: Ligand types and results: agonists increase target gene expression; antagonists block gene expression, and inverse agonists decrease gene expression. (Adapted from Kojetin DJ & Burris TP (2013) *Mol Pharmacol* 83:1–8. With permission from The American Society for Pharmacology and Experimental Therapeutics.)

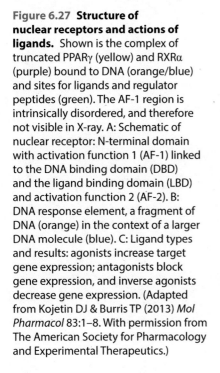

A AF-1 — DBD — LBD/AF-2

intrinsically disordered

B DNA response element

C ligands

AGONISTS: increase target gene expression

ANTAGONISTS/NON-AGONISTS: block target gene expression

INVERSE AGONISTS: decrease target gene expression for receptors with constitutive activity

DNA response elements, which are short DNA sequences that recognize the receptors, and the other is involved in receptor dimerization. After binding of the ligand at the LBD, the receptor undergoes a conformational change, which allows other proteins (termed co-regulator proteins) to bind to AF-2, and the receptor to bind to the DNA response element, leading to eventual changes in gene expression.

Nuclear receptors are characterized as class 1 (steroid receptors), class 2, or class 3. **Table 6.4** gives examples of common class 1 and 2 nuclear receptors that are drug targets, their ligands, drugs that target each, and the therapeutic indication. **Steroid receptors** include the estrogen receptor (ER), androgen receptor (AR), progesterone receptor (PR), glucocorticoid receptor (GR), and mineralocorticoid receptor (MR), all of which are targets of important drugs. Class 2 receptors include thyroid, vitamin D, retinoic acid, and peroxisome proliferator-activated receptors, also targets of a number of drugs. Class 3 comprises orphan receptors, which have been identified by sequence similarity to known nuclear receptors but, as yet, have no identified endogenous ligands.

Although the nuclear receptors are structurally related, the mechanisms of each class differ. Steroid receptors (class 1) are bound in the cytoplasm to heat-shock proteins (HSPs). When their ligand diffuses into the cell, it binds to the receptor, which then releases the HSP, translocates into the nucleus, and binds to DNA hormone response elements (HREs) near the target genes. DNA binding results in transcriptional activation. Class 2 receptors are located in the nucleus, bound to DNA as heterodimers with the retinoic X receptor (RXR). The ligand migrates, binds to the LBD, and typically recruits additional co-regulatory proteins prior to gene transcription. Orphan receptors (class 3) are least understood and primarily function as monomers (**Figure 6.28**). This class may cause gene transcription as a result of phosphorylation by kinases such as MAPK or PKA.

As with GPCRs and LGICs, the activity of nuclear receptors can be modulated by small-molecule agonists, partial agonists, antagonists, and inverse agonists. Methods for measuring drug–nuclear receptor affinity and efficacy include detection of direct

Table 6.4   Examples of nuclear receptors, their ligands, drugs targeting it, and the approved indication.

Natural ligand	Receptor	Drug or ligand[a] examples	Indication
Steroid Receptors (Class 1)			
estrogen	estrogen (ER)	tamoxifen, raloxifene	breast cancer, osteoporosis
testosterone, dihydrotestosterone	androgen (AR)	flutamide, bicalutamide	anti-androgens, prostate cancer, hirsutism
progesterone	progesterone (PR)	mifepristone	abortifacient
cortisol	glucocorticoid (GR)	dexamethasone	anti-inflammatory
aldosterone	mineralocorticoid (MR)	fludrocortisone	salt imbalance
Class 2			
thyroxine	thyroid	thyroxine[a]	hypothyroidism
vitamin D	calcitriol or vitamin D (VDR)	calcitriol	osteoporosis
retinoic acid	retinoic acid	isotretinoin, tretinoin	acne
fatty acids	peroxisome proliferator-activated receptors (PPAR)	rosiglitazone, pioglitazone	diabetes

[a]Natural ligand, also used as a drug.

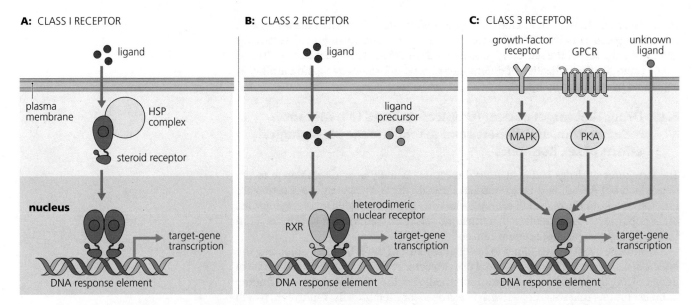

A: CLASS I RECEPTOR

B: CLASS 2 RECEPTOR

C: CLASS 3 RECEPTOR

Figure 6.28 Mechanisms of nuclear receptors. A: Steroid receptor (class 1) mechanism: ligand binding causes release of HSP from the receptor–HSP complex and is followed by translocation of the nuclear receptor into nucleus and binding as a homodimer to DNA response element, resulting in gene transcription. B: Class 2 receptor mechanism: Diffusion of the ligand into the nucleus and binding to pre-associated receptor–RXR heterodimer causes the complex to bind to DNA response element and results in gene transcription. The ligand may be extracellular, or may be produced from a precursor in the cell. C: Orphan receptor mechanism: receptors mainly act as monomers (shown), where ligand binding causes binding to DNA response element, resulting in gene transcription, which may be the result of phosphorylation by kinases such as mitogen-activated protein kinase (MAPK) or protein kinase A (PKA). (Adapted from Glass CK & Ogawa S [2006] *Nat Rev Immunol* 6:44–55. With permission from Macmillan Publishers Limited.)

binding to the nuclear receptor by use of biophysical methods and reporter assays that measure levels of gene transcription, respectively. Hit identification methods include those based on the structure of the natural ligand, high-throughput screening, and structure-based drug design. The observation that some modulators of nuclear receptors have distinct effects depending on where the receptor is located complicates certain aspects of drug discovery programs aimed at these targets. The existence of multiple subtypes of specific receptors that respond to the same natural ligand opens up the possibility of designing selective drugs that modulate some of the effects of the natural ligand but not all. The X-ray crystal structures of domains of multiple steroid receptors have been solved. One of the earliest examples (1997) of the structure of the ligand-binding domain (LBD) of the estrogen receptor illustrated the drastically different conformer of the receptor when an agonist versus an antagonist is bound. As seen in **Figure 6.29**, when estradiol, an agonist (shown in yellow) is bound (left

Figure 6.29 X-ray structures of ligands bound to ligand-binding domain of the estrogen receptor in two conformations. The receptor is shown in red with helix 12 highlighted. (Left) X-ray structure of ER LBD bound to estradiol, an agonist (shown in yellow); helix 12 is shown in blue. (Right) X-ray structure of ER LBD bound to raloxifene, an antagonist (shown in yellow); helix 12, shown in green, rotates by 130° compared to agonist bound structure. Residue K362 (shown in pink) is a lysine required for receptor activation, which is partially buried by the proximity of helix 12 when an antagonist binds. (From Brzozowski AM, Pike ACW, Dauter Z et al. [1997] *Nature* 389:753–758. With permission from Macmillan Publishers Limited.)

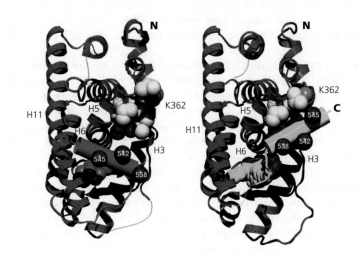

structure), helix 12 (shown in blue) is in one conformation, but when the antagonist raloxifene (yellow) is bound (right structure), helix 12 (shown in green) rotates by 130°, while the rest of the receptor (shown in red) undergoes minimal change. This is a nice example of stabilization of different receptor conformers by ligand binding, as explained by receptor theory.

6.10 Drugs that target nuclear receptors are used to treat cancer, inflammation, and diabetes and to regulate the physiological effects of sex hormones

The structures of drugs acting at steroid receptors usually bear resemblance to the natural steroid ligand, and they often have broad effects since steroid receptors are found throughout the body. For example, the wide use of estrogens to treat symptoms of menopause (estrogen replacement therapy) was restricted when it was understood that they may also promote certain cancers.

A stilbene scaffold was found to be an antagonist of the ER, thereby blocking the effects of estrogen and having potential use as a contraceptive. In addition, the idea of antagonizing the ER to treat breast tumors emerged in the 1970s, based on the finding of breast tumors that were dependent on estrogen for their growth. Tamoxifen, which contains the stilbene scaffold (red), was unsuccessful as a contraceptive but found wide use to treat breast tumors that are dependent on estrogen. The chroman ormeloxifene (centchroman), which can be considered a constrained stilbene structure, is used as a contraceptive in some countries. Raloxifene, which bears some structural similarity to ormeloxifene and tamoxifen, was ineffective as an anti-cancer agent but is effective in preventing and treating osteoporosis. The effects of tamoxifen and raloxifene are complex. They are termed **selective estrogen receptor modulators** (SERMs) because their activity on the ER varies depending on the location of the receptor. For example, tamoxifen and toremifine block breast tissue ER but not uterine or endometrial tissue ER, and are used to treat certain breast cancers. Raloxifene mimics estrogen's effects (acts as an agonist) in skeletal tissues (strengthening bones) but blocks estrogen effects (antagonist) in breast and endometrial tissue (proliferation).

In addition to being selective for specific locations of the estrogen receptor (ER), compounds may be selective for specific forms of it. There are two forms of the ER, α and β, and the activated receptor dimers can be either homodimeric or heterodimeric. Selective ERβ agonists have the potential to be used as anti-inflammatory drugs and as neuroprotectants, while selective ERα agonists may be useful to promote cardiovascular health. Although no drugs in this category have yet been approved, ERB 041 advanced to phase II clinical trials as a treatment for rheumatoid arthritis. Designing drugs to target the ER is further complicated by the involvement of co-activators or co-repressors, proteins that interact with the ER and either increase or decrease gene expression. For example, tamoxifen's differential activity (antagonist in breast tissue, agonist in bone) is believed to be due to different levels of specific co-activator proteins in breast and bone tissue. Further complicating the understanding of this system is the discovery of other receptors, such as the G protein-coupled receptor GPR30, which was recently found to be activated by estrogen. Structures of the natural ligand estradiol, as well as synthetic ER modulators, are shown in **Figure 6.30**.

Drugs acting at androgen receptors (**Figure 6.31**), known as selective androgen receptor modulators (SARMs), are useful to treat prostate cancer (antagonists) as well as for their anabolic effects on bone and muscle. The natural ligands for the androgen receptors are testosterone and its reduction product, 5α-dihydrotestosterone (see Figure 6.31A). Testosterone is also converted to estrogen via an aromatase enzyme. Examples of SARMs include the agonist stanozolol, used for its anabolic effects in building muscle mass, and the antagonists flutamide and bicalutamide, used to treat prostate cancer and other disorders caused by overactive androgen receptors. Other uses for SARMs include treatment of alopecia (hair loss) and acne. Some side effects that arise with drugs that are analogs of endogenous steroids are due to their activity at other steroid receptors, as well as the fact that they may be substrates for enzymes that act on steroid-like substrates. These may include virilism due to 5α-reductase activity and feminization due to aromatase substrate activity.

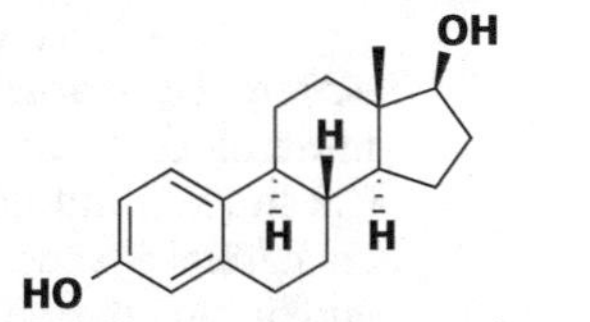

estradiol
(natural ligand)

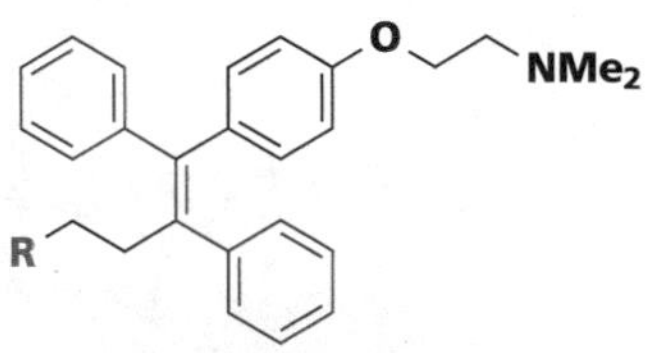

tamoxifen (R = H)
toremifene (R = Cl)
(breast cancer)

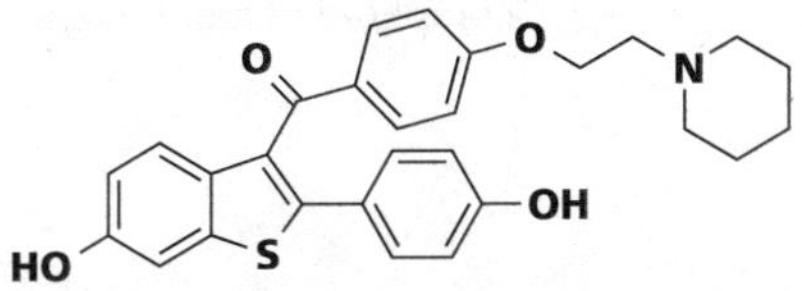

raloxifene
(breast cancer and osteoporosis)

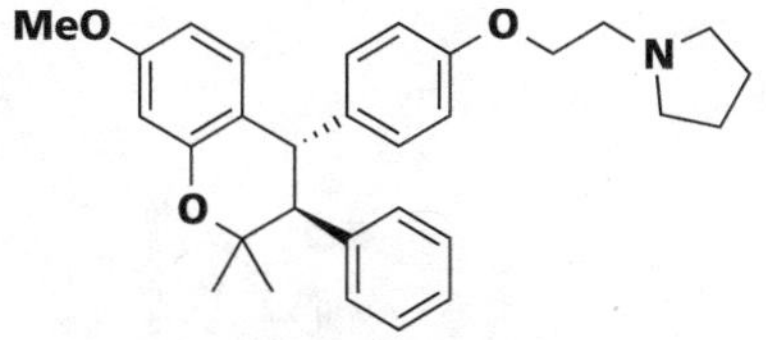

ormeloxifene
(oral contraceptive)

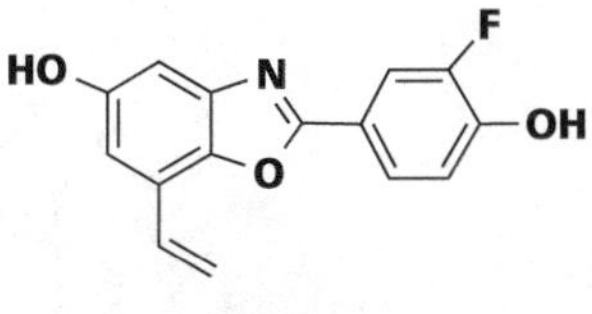

ERB 041
(selective ERβ agonist)

Figure 6.30 **Examples of compounds acting at estrogen receptors.** The natural ligand, estradiol, styrenes tamoxifen and toremifene (styrene in red); and related analogs raloxifene and ormeloxifene. The last four are considered SERMs and are approved for various uses including breast cancer, contraception, and osteoporosis. ERB 041 is an experimental compound that only interacts with one form of the ER.

Other steroid receptors include the glucocorticoid (GR) and mineralocorticoid (MR) receptors. The glucocorticoid receptor has a role in inflammation as well as in fat metabolism, glucose regulation, and bone formation. The natural ligand, cortisol, is used as an anti-inflammatory drug, as is the synthetic analog dexamethasone (Figure 6.32). Cortisol binds at both GR and MR; however, the natural ligand for MR is aldosterone. This steroid is involved in regulation of plasma Na^+ and K^+ levels and affects blood pressure. The synthetic agonist fludrocortisone is used in conditions such as Addison's disease, where there is a deficiency of aldosterone.

The three **peroxisome proliferator-activated receptors** (PPARs) α, γ, and δ, which are involved in carbohydrate and lipid metabolism and adipose tissue differentiation, are another important nuclear receptor drug target. Their natural ligands are fatty acids and eicosanoids, and binding of those ligands results in the formation of heterodimers with the retinoid X receptor (RXR). The heterodimers then bind to peroxisome proliferator response elements (PPRE), resulting in transcription of target genes. These receptors are affected by the drug class called

A: ANDROGEN RECEPTOR NATURAL LIGANDS TESTOSTERONE AND 5α-DIHYDROTESTOSTERONE

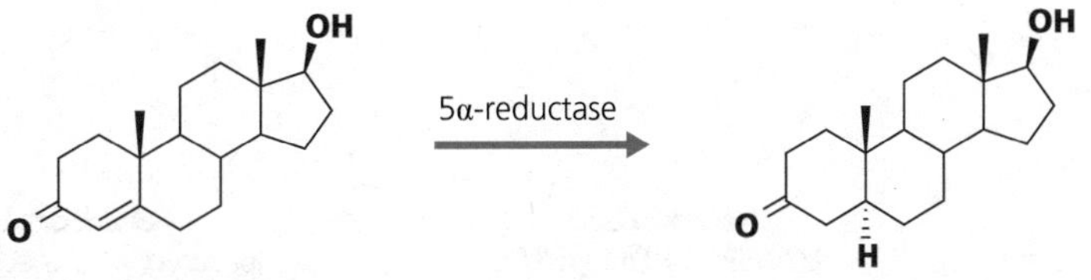

testosterone
(natural ligand)

5α-dihydrotestosterone

B: SYNTHETIC ANALOGS

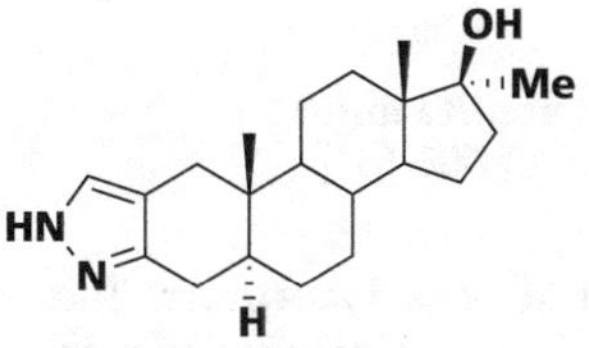

stanozolol: AGONIST
(anabolic steroid)

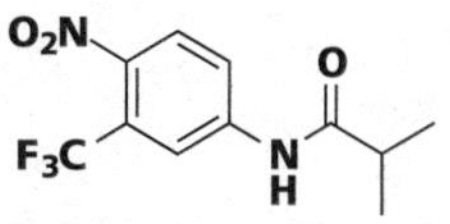

flutamide: ANTAGONIST
(prostate cancer)

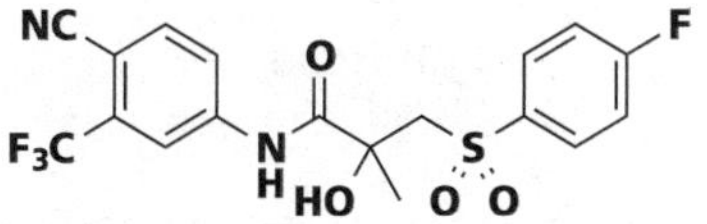

bicalutamide: ANTAGONIST
(prostate cancer)

Figure 6.31 **Examples of compounds acting at androgen receptors.** A: Testosterone, and its reduction product, 5α-dihydrotestosterone, natural ligands of the AR. B: Structures of selective androgen receptor agonist stanozolol and antagonists flutamide and bicalutamide. Antagonists are approved for indications such as prostate cancer and others that result from overactive AR.

cortisol
(natural ligand)

dexamethasone

aldosterone
(natural ligand)

fludrocortisone

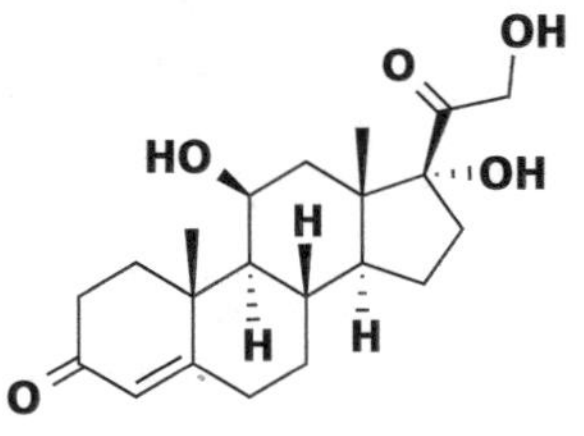

Figure 6.32 **Examples of compounds acting at glucocorticoid and mineralocorticoid receptors.** Cortisol (GR and MR) and aldosterone (MR) are natural ligands. Both cortisol and dexamethasone, an agonist, are used as anti-inflammatory drugs, and fludrocortisone (MR agonist) is used in diseases where there is a deficiency of aldosterone. Changes in dexamethasone and fludrocortisone, compared ot natural ligand are in red.

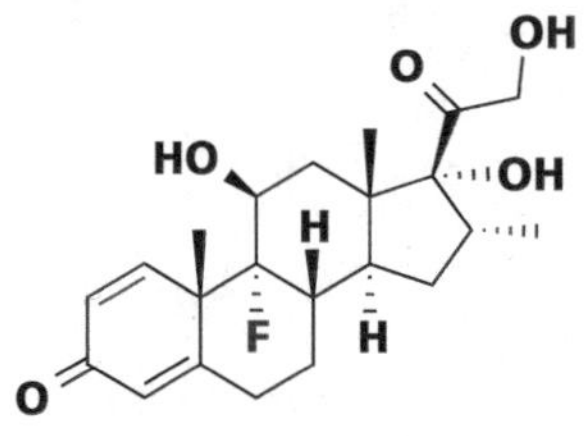

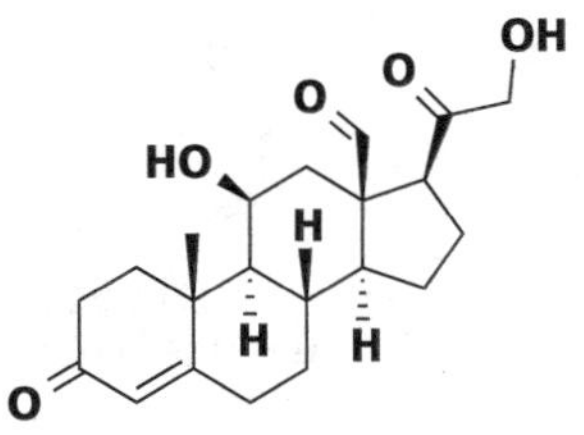

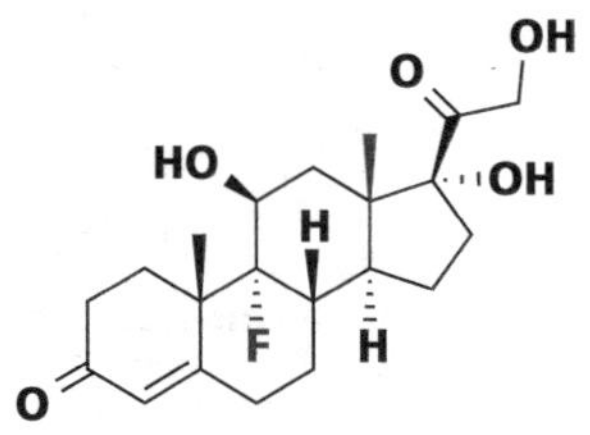

fibrates. Clofibrate was reported in the 1960s by ICI Pharmaceuticals and approved as a lipid- and cholesterol-lowering agent. It is a prodrug that generates the active carboxylic acid *in vivo*. It has since been replaced by safer analogs such as the agonists gemfibrozil and fenofibrate, which are used to treat hypercholesteremia and hyperlipidemia (**Figure 6.33**). The mechanism of the fibrates, not determined until 1990, involves activation of the PPARs, with approximately 10-fold selectivity for PPARα as compared to PPARγ.

Thiazolidinediones, exemplified by rosiglitazone and pioglitazone in Figure 6.33, are used to treat diabetes, and are agonists at PPARγ. Like the fibrates, this class of drugs was identified on the basis of their anti-diabetic activity, and the mechanism of action was not discovered until later. The discovery of rosiglitazone is described in Case Study 2 at the end of this chapter.

DRUGS ACTING AT PPARS

clofibrate
(prodrug: acid is active form)
LOWERS CHOLESTEROL

gemfibrozil
LOWERS CHOLESTEROL

fenofibrate
(prodrug: acid is active form)
LOWERS CHOLESTEROL

rosiglitazone
DIABETES

pioglitazone
DIABETES

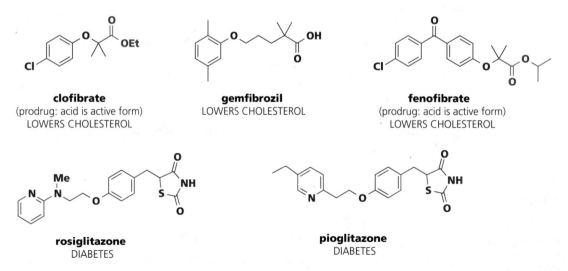

Figure 6.33 **Drugs acting at peroxisome-proliferator-activated receptors.** The fibrates clofibrate, gemfibrozil and fenofibrate activate PPARα, and are used to lower cholesterol levels (esters of prodrugs in red). The thiazolidinediones rosiglitazone and pioglitazone activate PPARγ, and are used to treat diabetes.

TRANSPORTERS AS DRUG TARGETS

Transporters are membrane-bound proteins that, like receptors, respond to a signal outside the cell. They are related to ion channels in that they are active or inactive based on the concentration of the ligand they transport. Unlike ion channels, they bind and transport far fewer ligands per cycle. These ligands include amino acids, carbohydrates, and neurotransmitters. Transporters are classified as uniporters, symporters, and antiporters (**Figure 6.34**). Whereas uniporters transport one molecule or ion at a time along a concentration gradient, symporters and antiporters couple the transport of two molecules or ions. A symporter couples movement of one molecule against its concentration gradient with movement of a different molecule along its concentration gradient. An antiporter transports two different molecules or ions in opposite directions, one with and one against its gradient. Transporters play an important role in maintaining the appropriate concentrations of nutrients, ions, and neurotransmitters.

Structural details of transporters have been clarified with the solution of several X-ray structures, such as bacterial LeuT, a sodium-coupled leucine symporter. All transporters have in common a series of structural repeats, each of which has several contiguous transmembrane segments (TM), which form folds. These folds result in a membrane-spanning complex with an outward side and an inward side, as shown in **Figure 6.35**. In a simplified model for neurotransmitter sodium symporters, binding of Na^+ in the outward open state facilitates binding of the ligand. The outward side closes, followed by opening of the inward side and release of Na^+ and ligand.

Assays for transporter activity rely on making synaptosome preparations from homogenization of tissue rich in these receptors or use of engineered cells that overexpress the transporter of interest. By tagging the natural ligand (with radioactivity, fluorescence, etc.), the rate of uptake can be measured by adding tagged ligand to the suspension for a specified period of time and detecting and measuring the movement of the tag. Drugs that inhibit transporters will slow or inhibit the protein's ability to take up the tagged ligand as a function of concentration of the drug. To date, only a handful of drug targets are transporters, although the most widely used antidepressants inhibit the serotonin transporter. Most drugs that act on transporters are structurally related to the ligand they transport, and identification often relies on design based on the natural ligand or a known active compound. An important area that has exploited transporters is the development of imaging agents. In these cases, the localization of specific transporters in certain cell types (for example, tumors) can be exploited to transport labeled molecules, for example, those containing a positron-emitting atom, as an imaging agent. Another emerging area is the use of transporters to selectively deliver drugs to certain organs. **Table 6.5** lists examples of transporters and the drugs or tools that bind to them.

Figure 6.34 General structural features of transporters. Uniporters transport one ion or small molecule (black) along a concentration or electrochemical gradient. A symporter transports two different molecules or ions in the same direction, one with the gradient (A, red) and one (B, blue) against it. An antiporter transports two different molecules or ions (A, red; B, blue) in opposite directions, one with the gradient and one against (transporters in green, membrane in pink, gradient in gray triangles).

ion or small molecule

EXTRACELLULAR

INTRACELLULAR

UNIPORTER

transports ion or small molecule along gradient

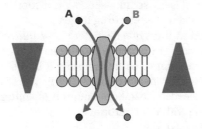

ion or small molecules A and B

A   B

SYMPORTER

transports ion/small molecule A into cell along gradient and ion/small molecule B into cell against gradient

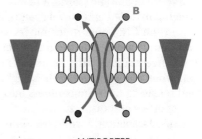

ion or small molecules A and B

B

ANTIPORTER

transports ion/small molecule A out of cell against gradient and B into cell along gradient

A

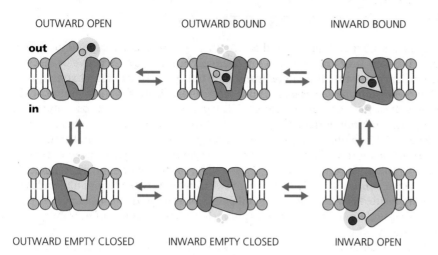

OUTWARD OPEN   OUTWARD BOUND   INWARD BOUND

out

in

OUTWARD EMPTY CLOSED   INWARD EMPTY CLOSED   INWARD OPEN

Figure 6.35 Representation of neurotransmitter symporter. The protein equilibrates between states by movement of flaps. In the scheme, the symporter (blue) starts with extracellular flaps open. As molecules or ions bind (red or green circles), the outward flaps close; as molecules or ions move toward the intracellular side, the inward flaps open releasing the two substrates inside the cell. When the symporter is empty, the inward flaps then close to give the state where both inward and outward flaps are closed. (Adapted from Boudker O & Verdon G [2010] *Trends Pharmacol Sci* 31:418–426. With permission from Elsevier.)

Table 6.5   Examples of transporters, their ligands and drugs, and approved indication.

Natural ligand	Transporter	Drug or ligand examples	Indication
serotonin	serotonin transporter (SERT)	fluoxetine, paroxetine	depression
norepinephrine	norepinephrine transporter	methylphenidate	attention deficit hyperactivity disorder (ADHD)
Na^+/Cl^-	sodium-chloride cotransporter (NCC)	hydrochlorothiazide	diuretics, hypertension
$Na^+/K^+/2Cl^-$	sodium-potassium-chloride cotransporter (NKCC)	furosemide	diuretics, hypertension
glucose	sodium-glucose transporter (SGLT)	canagliflozin	diabetes
		^{18}F-fluorodeoxyglucose	tumor imaging agent

6.11   Drugs acting at transporters treat a wide array of neuropsychiatric disorders, hypertension, and diabetes

Transporters are important drug targets in CNS diseases such as depression, where neurotransmitter transporters are involved in regulation of levels of serotonin, noradrenaline, and dopamine. They are also an important target for the treatment of hypertension, where modulating Na^+/Cl^- and $Na^+/K^+/Cl^-$ symporters in the kidney can result in diuretic effects. A relatively new target is the sodium-glucose transporter, which is involved in removal of glucose and is an anti-diabetic drug target.

In the CNS, neurotransmitters are released at the synapse, where they diffuse across and bind to receptors on the post-synaptic cell. Transporters in neurons regulate the concentration of the neurotransmitter at the synapse by transporting it into the cell when the concentration is high. Examples of transporters working in reverse and releasing neurotransmitters into the synapse also exist. Some neurotransmitter transporters cotransport ions, usually Na^+, along with the neurotransmitters and are classified as neurotransmitter sodium symporters (NSS).

Drugs that act at NSS sites include neurotransmitter reuptake inhibitors (**Figure 6.36**), which are widely used to treat anxiety and depression. Selective serotonin reuptake inhibitors (SSRIs) such as fluoxetine, sertraline, paroxetine, and citalopram block the serotonin transporter, resulting in higher concentrations of serotonin in the synapse. These compounds have revolutionized the treatment of depression. Norepinephrine

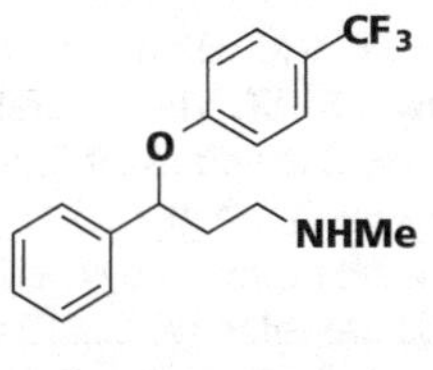

fluoxetine
Prozac
serotonin reuptake inhibitor

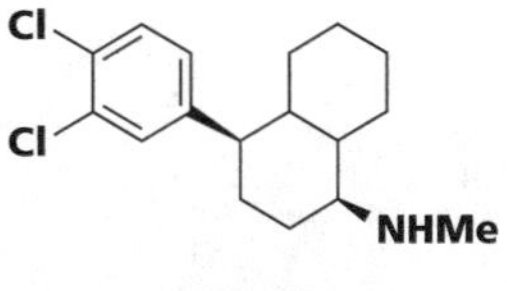

sertraline
Zoloft
serotonin reuptake inhibitor

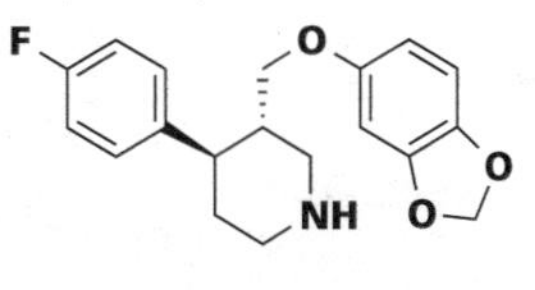

paroxetine
Paxil
serotonin reuptake inhibitor

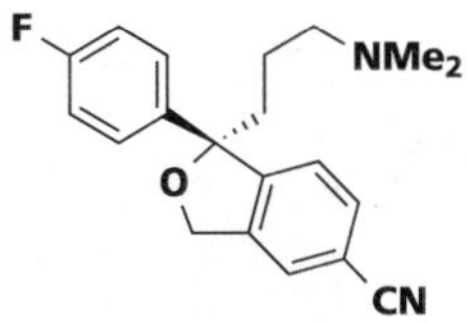

citalopram
Celexa
serotonin reuptake inhibitor

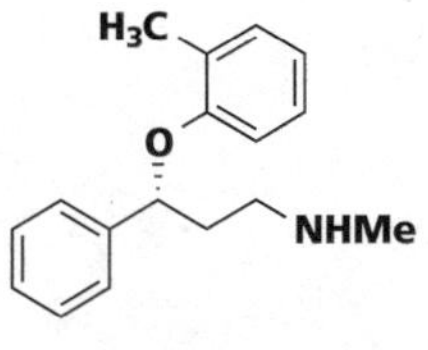

atomoxetine
Strattera
norepinephrine reuptake inhibitor

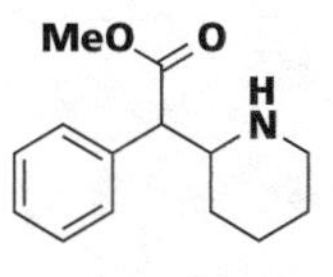

methylphenidate
Ritalin
dopamine and norepinephrine
reuptake inhibitor

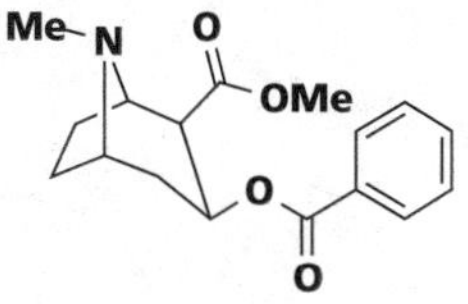

cocaine
dopamine, serotonin,
and norepinephrine
reuptake inhibitor

Figure 6.36 Drugs acting at neurotransmitter transporters. The serotonin reuptake inhibitors fluoxetine, sertraline, paroxetine, and citalopram are used as anti-depressants. Norepinephrine reuptake inhibitors atomoxetine and methylphenidate are used to treat ADHD. Cocaine, a drug of abuse, has activity at several neurotransmitter transporters.

reuptake inhibitors (NRIs), such as atomoxetine and methylphenidate, are often used to treat attention deficit hyperactivity disorder (ADHD). The success of the SSRIs has led to the development of combined serotonin–norepinephrine reuptake inhibitors (SNRIs) to treat depression and anxiety. Drugs of abuse, including cocaine and amphetamines, also affect dopamine and norepinephrine reuptake as part of their mechanism of action. Many drugs in this category will be discussed in more detail in Chapter 13.

There are two classes of diuretics that act on cotransporters and are widely used to treat hypertension and cardiovascular disease. One class includes thiazides such as chlorothiazide, hydrochlorothiazide, and chlorthalidone, which were initially discovered in the 1950s during investigations of sulfonamide antibacterial agents. The sulfonamides in this class are not antibacterial and instead act as diuretics. Long after they were introduced, the mechanism of action was identified as inhibition of cotransporters in the kidney. Chlorothiazide and hydrochlorothiazide block the Na^+/Cl^- cotransporter in the distal convoluted tubule of the kidney. Prevention of Na^+ and Cl^- absorption leads to increased elimination of fluid. The other class of diuretics target the $Na^+/K^+/2Cl^-$ cotransporter (NKCC) in the loop of Henle in the kidney. Diuretics blocking this target include furosemide, bumetanide, and torasemide, with some evidence that they compete for the chloride ion site on the transporter (**Figure 6.37**).

A: DIURETICS ACTING ON THE Na^+/Cl^- SYMPORTER

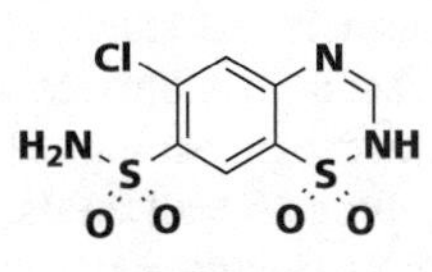

chlorothiazide

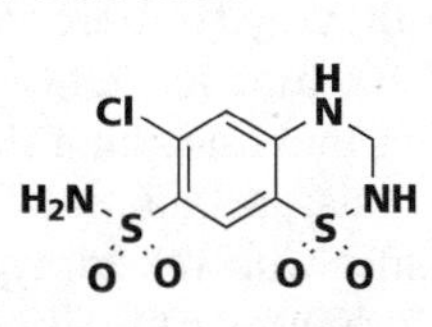

hydrochlorothiazide

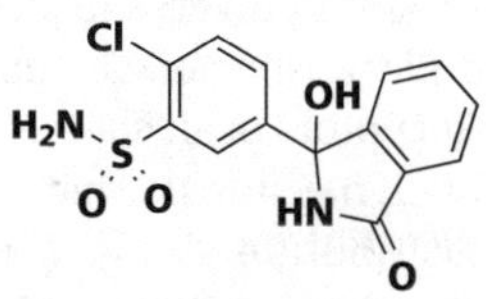

chlorthalidone

B: DIURETICS ACTING ON THE $Na^+/K^+/2Cl^-$ SYMPORTER

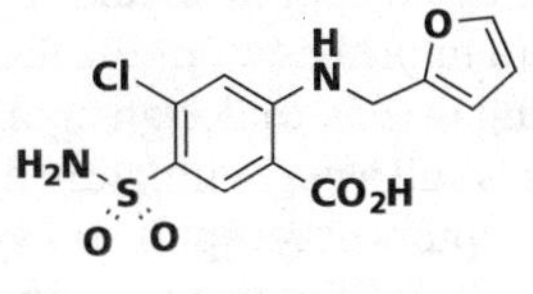

Figure 6.37 Diuretics acting on symporters. A: The thiazide class (chlorothiazide, hydrochlorothiazide, and chlorthalidone) act on the Na^+/Cl^- cotransporter in the distal convoluted tubule and are used as diuretics. B: Drugs acting on the $Na^+/K^+/2Cl^-$ cotransporter in the loop of Henle, furosemide, bumetanide and torasemide, are also used as diuretics.

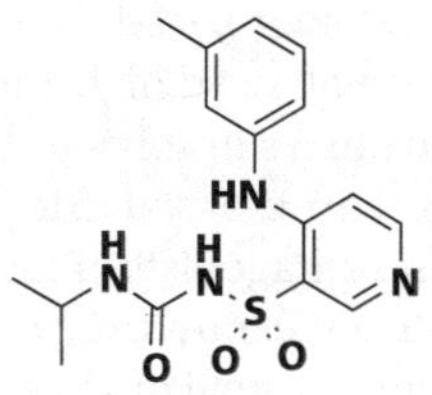

furosemide

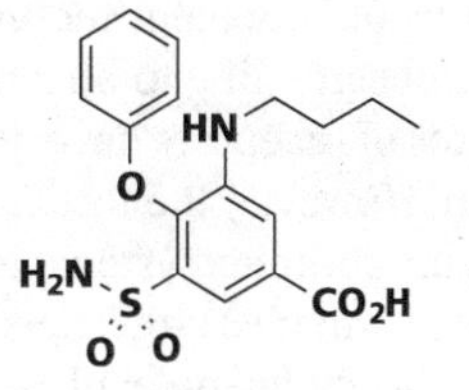

bumetanide

torasemide

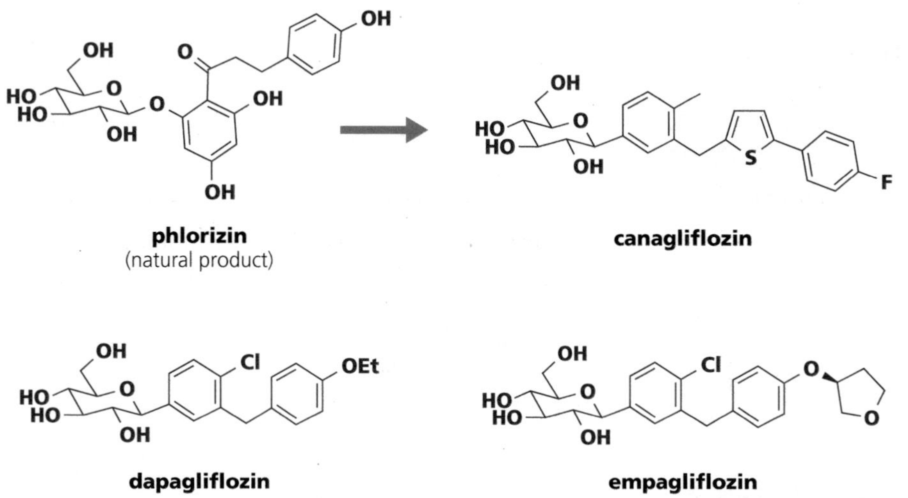

Figure 6.38 Phlorizin and analogs that target SGLT. The natural product phlorizin was found to inhibit SGLT. Analogs where the glycosidic phenol groups were replaced by C-aryl glycoside are selective SGLT2 and are approved to treat diabetes. This class, called glifozins, includes canaglifozin, dapagliflozin, and empagliflozin.

Several of these diuretics have been banned from use by athletic organizations, due to their ability to mask illicit drugs by increasing their elimination in urine.

Recent interest in sodium-glucose transport proteins (SGLT) has stemmed from efforts to identify new targets to treat diabetes, as these proteins are involved in reabsorption of glucose. Specifically, subtype 2 (SGLT2), is responsible for glucose reabsorption in the kidney, as opposed to subtype 1 (SGLT1), which operates in the intestine. Blocking reabsorption of glucose in the kidney leads to elimination of glucose through urine and lower levels of blood glucose, so selective SGLT2 blockers would be effective anti-diabetic drugs. In the early 2000s phlorizin was identified as a nonselective SGLT inhibitor. This is a compound found in apple trees that had shown to induce excretion of glucose through the urine (glucosuria) in the 1880s. Analogs of phlorizin with lipophilic groups replacing the phenols exhibited selectivity for SGLT2, and both O- and C-glycosides were investigated by several research groups. Stability to glucosidases as well as selectivity and potency were achieved with the C-aryl analogs. Drugs in the SGLT2 inhibitor class include canagliflozin, dapagliflozin, and empagliflozin, and these have been recently approved to treat type 2 diabetes (**Figure 6.38**).

Canagliflozin was approved in 2013 in the U.S., with dapagliflozin and empagliflozin approved the following year.

SUMMARY

Receptors, as a broad class, are the target of more than two-thirds of all marketed drugs. Although diverse in structure and function, GPCRs, ion channels, nuclear receptors, and transporters are all proteins that transmit a signal to effect a physiological result. Receptors of all classes usually exist as multiple subtypes, and the physiological result of signal transmission may differ with the subtype of receptor as well as its tissue distribution. Drugs acting at receptors can either increase or decrease the level of signal transmission. Many older drugs act at receptors, but their mechanism of action was discovered well after they were in clinical use. Natural ligands for receptors, as well as natural products, have been a valuable source of starting points for drug discovery projects that target receptors. As such, medicinal chemistry optimization approaches often rely on knowledge of the structure of the natural ligand or on pharmacophore modeling based on known ligands. Recent technical advances in assay techniques have allowed high-throughput screening to be a more feasible approach, and recent advances in solving structures of receptors have started to inform new approaches in structure-based drug design. However, the understanding of how to design agonists and antagonists of these highly complex systems *a priori* is still a very immature field. Most recently, drug discovery strategies target specific receptors or receptor subtypes, with the goal of generating efficacious molecules that do not exhibit many of the side effects that plague older compounds.

CASE STUDY 1 DISCOVERY OF RAMELTEON

Insomnia, characterized by an inability to go to sleep or to stay asleep, is estimated to affect about one-third of all Americans. Standard treatment includes benzodiazepines, zolpidem (Ambien), and eszopiclone (Lunesta), all of which act at the $GABA_A$ receptor. However, their long-term use is discouraged due to abuse potential. Sleep patterns are affected by melatonin, a hormone that has a role in regulating circadian rhythms. The hormone itself has a short half-life and there are few data on its long-term safety, although it is sold over the counter and used as a dietary supplement to promote sleep. It binds to the melatonin receptor (MT), a GPCR that exists as three subtypes. Both the MT_1 and MT_2, subtypes are involved in regulating circadian rhythm patterns. The MT_1 subtype is expressed throughout the brain, while MT_2 is found primarily in the retina. A third subtype, MT_3, has been identified as a form of the enzyme quinone reductase, but its function is unknown. Osamu Uchikawa and others at Takeda Pharmaceuticals began a program to find melatonin receptors agonists that would have selectivity for the MT_1 receptor, based on the assumption that its localization in the brain made it the more important target for regulating sleep patterns. Their initial study, based on a CoMFA analysis of 133 compounds that bound to the melatonin receptor, indicated that the pyrrole of melatonin (**Figure 6.39**) was not necessary for binding but the methoxy and amide groups (shown in red) were needed. To this end, a series of benzocycloalkenes were synthesized, with variations in ring size (n), olefin position, aryl substitution (R^2, OR^1), and amide substituent (R^4).

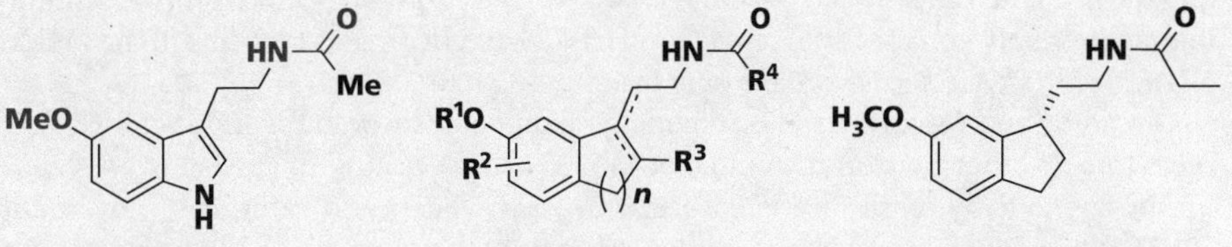

Figure 6.39 Structures of early analogs leading to development of ramelteon. The natural ligand melatonin, along with 132 other compounds, were used in a CoMFA analysis. The analysis indicated that the methoxy and amide of melatonin were required (in red), but the pyrrole was not. This led to synthesis of a series of benzocycloalkenes. The optimal structure in this series was compound **1** based on potency and selectivity.

melatonin   benzocycloalkenes   compound 1

The five-membered ring analogs ($n = 1$) were twice as active as those containing a six-membered ring ($n = 2$), and S-enantiomers of the saturated compounds exhibited the highest selectivity for MT_1 over MT_3. The optimal structure in this series was found to be **1**, with the S-configuration. Compounds were assayed for inhibition of binding of 2-[^{125}I]iodomelatonin to both MT_1 and MT_3 receptors, and **1** showed excellent selectivity (for MT_1, $K_i = 0.041$ nM; for MT_3, $K_i = 3570$ nM).

Based on a homology model of the MT_1 receptor derived from bovine rhodopsin, the oxygen of the methoxy group is proposed to bind to a histidine residue (His195) via a H-bond, the amide NH is thought to bind to a serine OH side chain (Ser144), and the amide carbonyl participates in a H-bond with the OH of another serine (Ser110), as seen in **Figure 6.40**.

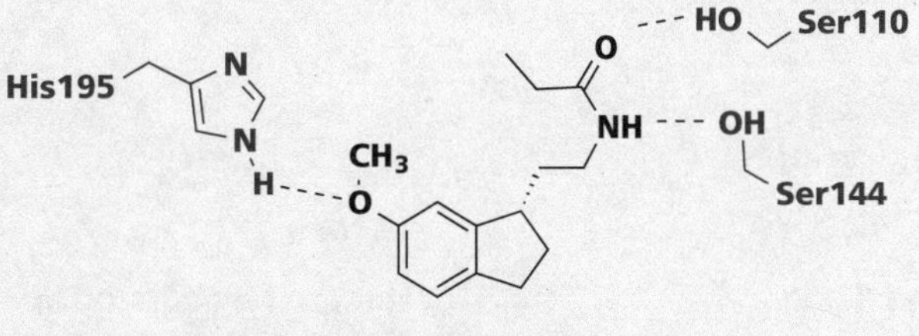

Figure 6.40 Proposed binding interactions between compound 1 and MT$_1$ receptor. Based on a homology model of the MT$_1$ receptor, the methoxy oxygen is proposed to hydrogen-bond to His195, with other H-bonds from the amide NH to Ser144 and the amide carbonyl to Ser110.

To optimize the orientation of the methoxy oxygen lone pair for hydrogen bonding, the next series added a ring constraint by synthesizing tricyclic analogs. The angular fused system was more potent than the linear fused system and had similar or slightly reduced potency compared to **1**. For example the linear compound **2** had >300× less

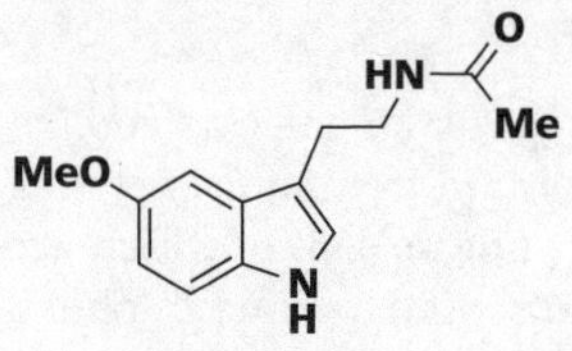

melatonin
MT$_1$ K_i = 0.0823 nM
MT$_3$ K_i = 27.6 nM

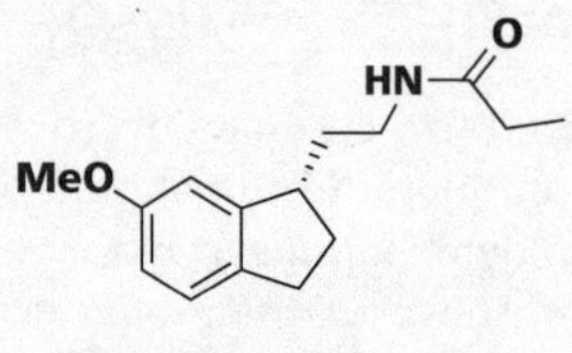

compound 1
MT$_1$ K_i = 0.041 nM
MT$_3$ K_i = 3570 nM

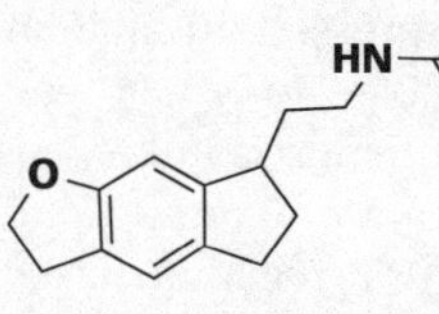

compound 2 (linear)
MT$_1$ K_i = 483 nM
MT$_3$ K_i = 287 nM

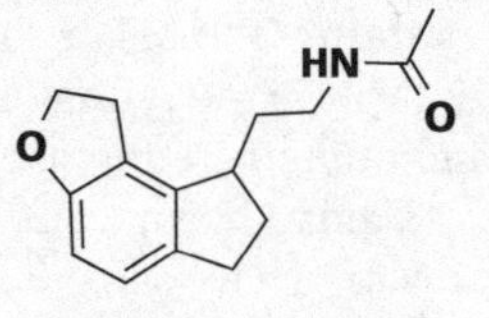

compound 3 (angular)
MT$_1$ K_i = 0.126 nM
MT$_3$ K_i = 5960 nM

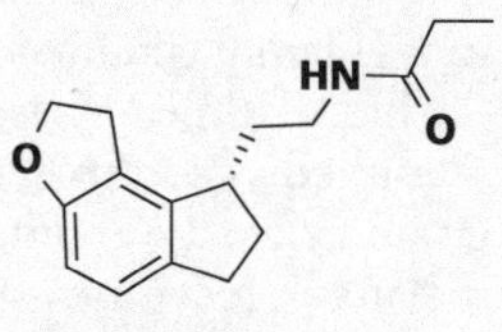

ramelteon
MT$_1$ K_i = 0.0138 nM
MT$_3$ K_i = 2600 nM

Figure 6.41 Structure and potencies of melatonin and synthetic analogs. Compound 1 is more potent and selective for MT$_1$ vs. MT$_3$ as compared to melatonin. A series of tricyclic analogs use ring constraint to optimize the orientation of the ether oxygen. The linear tricyclic analog **2** is less potent and less selective than the angular tricyclic analog **3**. Ramelteon, containing the propanamide with the S-configuration, was approved in 2005 for insomnia.

affinity for MT$_1$ than the angular compound **3**, as well as much less selectivity versus MT$_3$ (**Figure 6.41**).

Increasing the size of the tetrahydrofuran ring to a six-membered ring or substituting a nitrogen into that ring did not further improve activity. Overall, the optimized candidate based on potency and selectivity was ramelteon, which contained the S-configuration and the propanamide. Docking ramelteon into an MT$_1$ homology model shows binding interactions between the furan oxygen and His195 and hydrogen-bonding of the amide NH and carbonyl to serine and tyrosine residues (**Figure 6.42**).

In addition to M$_1$ versus MT$_3$ selectivity, ramelteon showed no affinity for GABA$_A$ receptors or other neurotransmitter receptors. *In vivo* testing in cats showed sleep-promoting activity, with an increase in slow-wave sleep and rapid eye movement (REM) sleep. Ramelteon entered clinical trials in both younger and older adults with chronic insomnia. Both studies showed a decrease in the amount of time to enter sleep as compared to placebo. No evidence for abuse, withdrawal, or residual effects was found, and ramelteon was approved by the FDA in 2005.

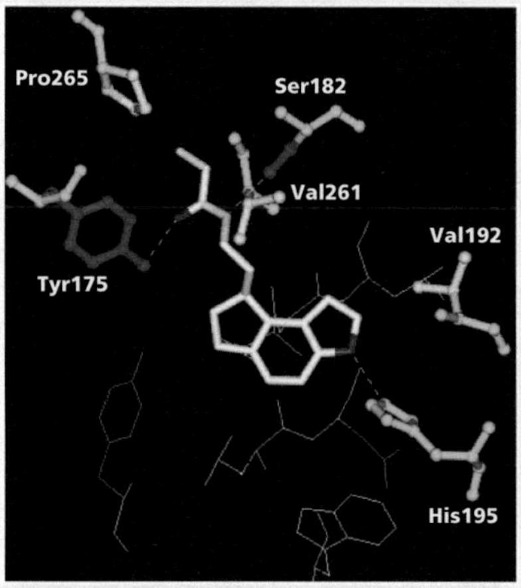

CASE STUDY 2   DISCOVERY OF ROSIGLITAZONE

In the early 1990s, the most widely used drugs for treating non-insulin-dependent diabetes mellitus (NIDDM) were the sulfonylureas, which act by increasing insulin secretion. Undesirable side effects include hypoglycemia and weight gain. At Glaxo, the glitazone compound, ciglitazone, was found by screening compounds for their effects in rodent models of insulin resistance. Interestingly, the same compound (ADD-3878) had been reported much earlier, in 1982, by a different pharmaceutical company, Takeda, as having anti-diabetic activity in animal models (**Figure 6.43**).

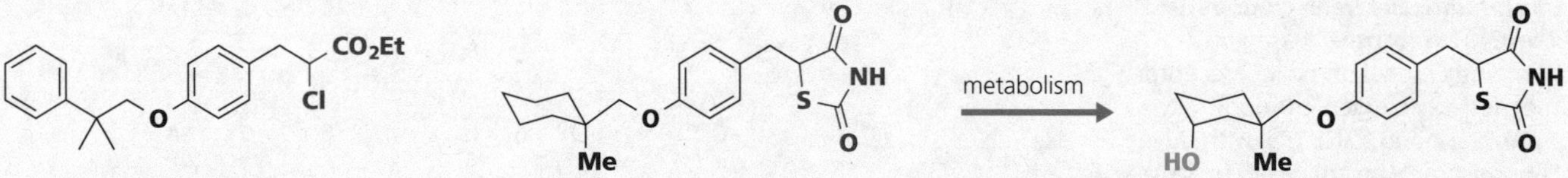

Figure 6.42 Model of ramelteon in binding site of MT$_1$ receptor. Using a homology model, key interactions include the furan oxygen to His195, and H-bonds of the amide NH and carbonyl to Ser185 and Tyr175, respectively. (From Uchikawa O, Fukatsu K, Tokunoh R et al. [2002] Synthesis of a novel series of tricyclic indan derivatives as melatonin receptor agonists. *J Med Chem* 45:4222–4239. With permission from American Chemical Society.)

AL-294 (lead)
1982

ciglitazone (ADD-3878)
1982
(clog*P* = 3.5)

metabolism

(AD-4743)
(clog*P* = 1.48)

Figure 6.43 Early leads in the development of rosiglitazone. The initial lead, compound AL-294, was modified at Takeda by substitution of a thiazolidinedione (red) for the chloroester to give ciglitazone (ADD-3878), the same compound was identified as a lead in a screening program at Glaxo. The less lipophilic metabolite AD-4743 was more potent in mice.

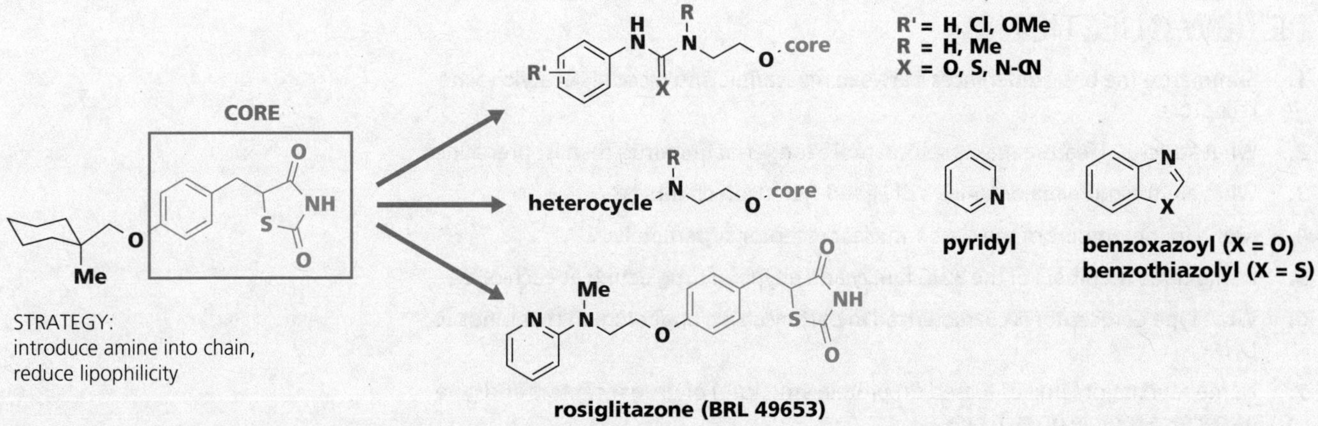

Figure 6.44 Amine analogs of ciglitazone lead. A library of amine analogs of ciglitazone were prepared in order to reduce lipophilicity by replacing the cyclohexyl while retaining the thiazolidinedione core (blue). Substitutions included phenylureas (top) and heterocyclic amines (middle). The heterocycles were the most potent and the pyridyl compound, rosiglitazone, was approved to treat diabetes.

At that time, scientists at Takeda had synthesized ADD-3878 as a derivative of their lead compound, AL-294, and reported that substitution of the thiazolidinedione for the α-chloro ester improved hypoglycemic activity and decreased toxicity. The overall mechanism in insulin-resistant animal models was an increase in sensitivity to endogenous insulin rather than an increase in secretion.

Scientists at Glaxo took advantage of the observation that the less lipophilic (clogP = 1.48 vs. 3.5) hydroxyl metabolite AD-4743 was a more potent anti-hyperglycemic agent in genetically obese or glucose-intolerant mice than ciglitazone. Replacement of the cyclohexylmethyl with various amine groups lowered lipophilicity and in some cases increased activity. They prepared a library of analogs with amines incorporated into the side chain (**Figure 6.44**). Aryl urea and thiourea analogs in some cases improved activity over ciglitazone, and heterocyclic analogs were up to 300 times more active than the parent compound.

One of the most potent compounds, BRL 49653 (rosiglitazone), had a minimum effective dose of 3 μmol/kg of diet. Although the clogP of rosiglitazone is 1.53, it was found that other analogs with similar lipophilicity were 100 times less active, indicating that lipophilicity is not the sole determining factor for activity. Screening of several of the more potent analogs for toxicity was based on their ability to lower blood hemoglobin levels; rosiglitazone had the best profile, with no effect on hemoglobin at doses 100-fold greater than the anti-hyperglycemic dose level.

Although screening and drug development were based on animal models of anti-hyperglycemia, rosiglitazone was later found to act as a selective PPARγ agonist. This receptor is primarily expressed in adipose tissue, and activation leads to adipocyte differentiation and improved insulin signaling in mature adipocytes.

Rosiglitazone is one of several thiazolidinediones that received FDA approval to treat type II diabetes, with other examples including pioglitazone and troglitazone (**Figure 6.45**). Since their introduction, all have had some issues with side effects: troglitazone was withdrawn due to liver toxicity, pioglitazone conferred an increased risk for bladder cancer, and rosiglitazone increased the risk of heart attack.

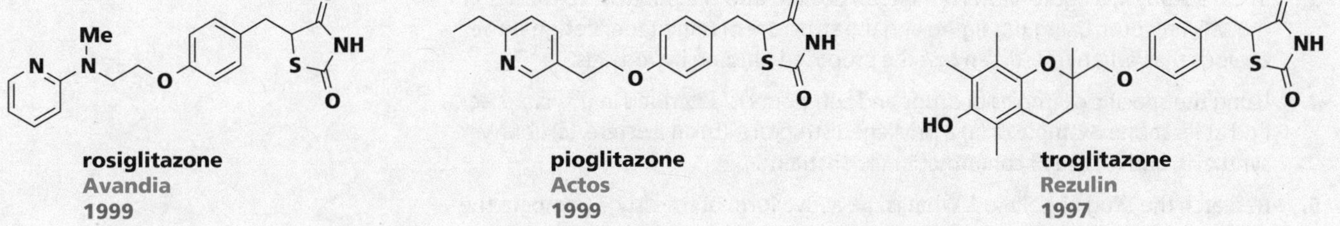

Figure 6.45 Structures of anti-diabetic thiazolidinediones. Rosiglitazone, pioglitazone and troglitazone all received FDA approval to treat diabetes although the latter two have been withdrawn due to toxicity issues.

REVIEW QUESTIONS

1. Summarize the basic differences between muscarinic and nicotinic acetylcholine receptors.

2. What structural feature makes salbutamol a longer-acting drug than isoprenaline?

3. What are the three major families of ligand-gated ion channels?

4. Name four members of the class 1 nuclear receptor superfamily.

5. Name three members of the VGIC family and a type of drug acting at each one.

6. What type of receptor is characterized in part by a zinc finger region that binds to DNA?

7. Name four major families (based on protein structure) of drug receptors and give a specific example of each one.

8. Explain the difference between an agonist and an antagonist.

9. LGICs, VGICs, and neurotransmitter transporters all allow ions to pass through. Explain how they differ.

10. What hit identification strategies are typically used to start drug discovery programs with GPCR targets, ion channel targets, nuclear receptor targets, and transporter targets? For each specific target class, explain why that strategy is used more than others and why some strategies are not often used.

APPLICATION QUESTIONS

1. A Schild plot is shown for two antagonists, **1** and **2**. Which compound is more active? What is the pA_2 of each compound? Explain what r is.

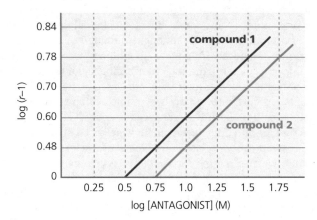

2. Research the drug lorcaserin. What is its structure? What GPCR does it affect? What is its selectivity profile against related GPCRs? Is it an agonist or an antagonist? Compare its structure to that of the natural ligand of its GPCR target. Draw a pharmacophore that is consistent with the two structures.

3. In Case Study 1, a figure shows ramelteon docked into the putative active site of the MT_1 receptor. Using this figure and the structure of ramelteon, design three analogs that, when tested, can test the proposed binding hypothesis.

4. Using the specific examples of drugs and compounds described in this chapter, find at least one example of (a) a privileged structure, (b) an isostere, (c) library synthesis, and (d) use of conformational constraint.

5. Research the drug fingolimod. What is the active form of the drug? Compare the structure of the active form to the natural substrate of the S1PR1. Research how the compound myriocin was important to the discovery and development of fingolimod.

6. Figure 6.36 shows the structures of four well-known selective serotonin reuptake inhibitors. Of the four structures, choose two of them and draw pharmacophore models based on their structures. Explain your rationale for the model and which features of the two chosen compounds fit this model. For the two compounds you did not choose: do they fit your pharmacophore model? Explain why or why not.

7. Natural products have been an abundant source of modulators of receptors. Research the structure of two different natural products (not described in this chapter) that exert their effects on receptors. What is their structure, what class of receptor do they target, and what is their physiological effect?

8. Design three new analogs of the PPAR agonist gemfibrozil in Figure 6.33 by incorporating different acid isosteres.

9. Research the Nobel Prize in Chemistry 2003. Who received the award and for what work?

10. Do the structures of estradiol and raloxifene (shown in Figure 6.30) adhere to Lipinski's rules? Use an online program or ChemDraw to find the log$P$.

FURTHER READING

General

Santos R, Ursu O, Gaulton A et al. (2016) A comprehensive map of molecular drug targets. *Nat Rev Drug Discovery* 16:19–34.

Overington JP, Al-Lazikani B & Hopkins AL (2006) How many drug targets are there? *Nat Rev Drug Discovery* 5:993–996.

Hopkins AL & Groom CR (2002) The druggable genome. *Nat Rev Drug Discovery* 1:727–730.

Maehle A-H (2004) Receptive substances: John Newport Langley (1852–1925) and his path to a receptor theory of drug action. *Med Hist* 48:53–174.

Leff P (1995) The two-state model of receptor activation. *Trends Pharmacol Sci* 16:89–97.

Kenakin T (2004) Principles: receptor theory in pharmacology. *Trends Pharmacol Sci* 25:186–192.

Neubig RR, Spedding M, Kenakin T & Christopoulos A (2003) International union of pharmacology committee on receptor nomenclature and drug classification. XXXVII. Update on terms and symbols in quantitative pharmacology. *Pharmacol Rev* 55:597–606.

Alexander SPH, Kelly E, Marrion N et al. (2015) The concise guide to pharmacology 2015/16: Overview. *Brit J Pharmacol* 172: 5729-5743.

G protein-coupled receptors

Bjarnadottir TK, Gloriam DE, Hellstrand SH et al. (2006) Comprehensive repertoire and phylogenetic analysis of the G protein-coupled receptors in human and mouse. *Genomics* 88:263–273.

Fredriksson R, Lagerstrom MC, Lundin L-G & Schioth HB (2003) The G-protein-coupled receptors in the human genome form five main families. Phylogenetic analysis, paralogon groups, and fingerprints. *Mol Pharmacol* 63:1256–1272.

Marinissen MJ & Gutkind JS (2001) G-protein-coupled receptors and signaling networks: emerging paradigms. *Trends Pharmacol Sci* 22:368–376.

Congreve M, Langmead CJ, Mason JS & Marshall FH (2011) Progress in structure based drug design for G protein-coupled receptors. *J Med Chem* 54:4283–4311.

GPCR structure review: Topiol S & Sabio M (2009) X-ray structure breakthroughs in the GPCR transmembrane region. *Biochem Pharmacol* 78:11–20.

Costanzi S (2008) On the applicability of GPCR homology models to computer-aided drug discovery: a comparison between *in silico* and crystal structures of the β_2-adrenergic receptor. *J Med Chem* 51:2907–2914.

Smit MJ, Leurs R, Alewijnse AE et al. (1996) Inverse agonism of histamine H2 antagonists accounts for upregulation of spontaneously active histamine H2 receptors. *Proc Natl Acad Sci USA* 93:6802–6807.

Ion channels

Bagal SK, Brown AD, Cox P et al. (2013) Ion channels as therapeutic targets: a drug discovery perspective. *J Med Chem* 56:593–624.

Anger T, Madge DJ, Mulla M & Riddall D (2001) Medicinal chemistry of neuronal voltage-gated sodium channel blockers. *J Med Chem* 44:115–137.

Pallotta B (1991) Single ion channel's view of classical receptor theory. *FASEB J* 5:2035–2043.

Unwin N (2005) Refined structure of the nicotinic acetylcholine receptor at 4 Å resolution. *J Mol Biol* 346:967–989.

Ashcroft F, Benos D, Bezanilla F et al. (2004) Twenty questions. *Nat Rev Drug Discovery* 3:239–278.

Nuclear receptors

Kojetin DJ & Burris TP (2013) Small molecule modulation of nuclear receptor conformational dynamics: implications for function and drug discovery. *Mol Pharmacol* 83:1–8.

Glass CK & Ogawa S (2006) Combinatorial roles of nuclear receptors in inflammation and immunity. *Nat Rev Immunol* 6:44–55.

Brzozowski AM, Pike ACW, Dauter Z et al. (1997) Molecular basis of agonism and antagonism in the oestrogen receptor. *Nature* 389: 753–758.

Transporters

Boudker O & Verdon G (2010) Structural perspectives on secondary active transporters. *Trends Pharmacol Sci* 31:418–426.

Focke PJ, Wang X & Larsson HP (2013) Neurotransmitter transporters: structure meets function. *Structure* 21:694–705.

Levine M, Cuendet MA, Khelashvili G & Weinstein H (2016) Allosteric mechanisms of molecular machines at the membrane: transport by sodium-coupled symporters. *Chem Rev* 116:6552–6587.

Ramelteon

Fukatsu K, Uchikawa O, Kawada M et al. (2002) Synthesis of a novel series of benzocycloalkene derivatives as melatonin receptor agonists. *J Med Chem* 45:4212–4221.

Uchikawa O, Fukatsu K, Tokunoh R et al. (2002) Synthesis of a novel series of tricyclic indan derivatives as melatonin receptor agonists. *J Med Chem* 45:4222–4239.

Buysse D, Bate G & Kirkpatrick P (2005) Ramelteon. *Nat Rev Drug Discovery* 4:881–882.

Rosiglitazone

Willson TM, Brown PJ, Sternbach DD & Henke BR (2000) The PPARs: from orphan receptor to drug discovery. *J Med Chem* 43:527–550.

Cantello BCC, Cawthorne MA, Cottam GP et al. (1994) [[ω-(Heterocyclylamino)-alkoxy]benzyl]-2,4-thiazolidinediones as potent antihyperglycemic agents. *J Med Chem* 37:3977–3985.

Sohda T, Mizuno K, Imamiya E et al. (1982) Studies on antidiabetic agents. II. Synthesis of 5-[4-(1-methylcyclohexylmethoxy)-benzyl] thiazolidine-2,4-dione (ADD-3878) and its derivatives. *Chem Pharm Bull* 30:3580–3600.

Edvardsson U, Bergstrom M, Alexandersson M et al. (1999) Rosiglitazone (BRL49653), a PPARγ-selective agonist, causes peroxisome proliferator-like liver effects in obese mice. *J Lipid Res* 40:1177–1184.

Web sites

GPCR action: (a) Signal transduction pathways, Bozeman Science, 2011, http://www.youtube.com/watch?v=qOVkedxDqQo; (b) G protein signaling, Garland Science, 2009, http://www.youtube.com/watch?v=V_0EcUr_txk&feature=related; (c) GPCR Claymation, 2011, http://www.youtube.com/watch?v=pRBg8Q2pR1s

Cimetidine discovery: https://www.acs.org/content/acs/en/education/whatischemistry/landmarks/cimetidinetagamet.html

Nobel lecture by Sir James W. Black (1988): http://www.nobelprize.org/mediaplayer/index.php?id=1669

Nobel lecture by Roderick MacKinnon (2003): http://www.nobelprize.org/mediaplayer/index.php?id=550

Pharmacological targets and ligands guide: http://www.guidetopharmacology.org/

Modeling of molecular machines: http://www.scidacreview.org/0803/html/molecular.html

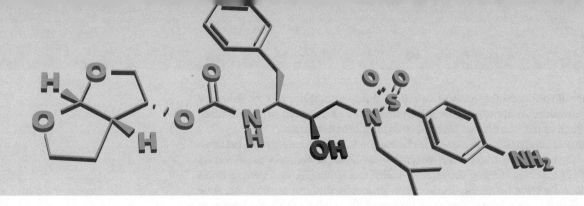

Enzymes as drug targets

7

LEARNING OBJECTIVES

- Learn general mechanisms of several classes of enzymes including proteases, kinases, polymerases, and phosphodiesterases.
- Understand the use of enzyme kinetics to characterize modes of enzyme inhibition.
- Recognize when to apply specific medicinal chemistry strategies according to the class of enzyme being targeted.
- Learn examples of drugs that target various enzyme classes.

Enzymes are a broad class of proteins that catalyze chemical reactions involving conversion of an enzyme substrate to a product. They are ubiquitous and are involved in numerous physiological processes such as digestion, blood coagulation, energy production, neurotransmission, and DNA replication. Several of their specific functions include the following:

- Synthesis of amino acids, nucleic acids, fatty acids, coenzymes, vitamins, and proteins

- Degradation of proteins, lipids, carbohydrates, nucleic acids, and small-molecule xenobiotics

- Replication of DNA and RNA

- Activation or inactivation of proteins

- Processing of proteins and nucleic acids by adding or removing specific functional groups such as carbohydrates, methyl groups, acetate groups, or prenyl groups

Enzymatic reactions range from very simple reactions, such as the hydrolysis of an ester substrate to generate an acid and alcohol, catalyzed by an esterase, to complex multicomponent reactions like those involved in cellular respiration. An example of a multicomponent enzyme is pyruvate dehydrogenase, a complex that consists of multiple copies of three different enzymes along with associated coenzymes, that converts pyruvate to acetyl-CoA, which is then used in the citric acid cycle for cellular respiration. Some enzymes are highly specific, acting only on certain molecular substrates, while others are much less selective and will catalyze reactions at a certain position on the substrate, regardless of the specific structure. Enzymes that exhibit high specificity rely on recognition of the substrate and can often discriminate between very similar substrates on the basis of structural differences quite remote from the active site. Localization of the enzyme in certain organs and tissues, or surrounding conditions such as pH, can also impact selectivity in a broader sense.

All chemical catalysis is centered on reducing the activation energy of a reaction in order for it to proceed faster. With enzymatic catalysis, a reaction catalyzed by an enzyme (E) involves starting material(s), called substrate (S), and generates an enzyme·substrate complex (E·S). The reaction proceeds through a transition state and eventually forms an enzyme·product complex (E·P), finally releasing the product (P) and the regenerated enzyme (E) (Equation 7.1). The location in the enzyme where this process occurs is called the **active site**.

$$E+S \underset{k_d}{\overset{k_a}{\rightleftharpoons}} E \cdot S \overset{k_{cat}}{\rightleftharpoons} E \cdot P \rightleftharpoons E+P \tag{7.1}$$

Scientists can describe an enzyme's activity mathematically, using equations that describe kinetics. In Equation 7.1, K_d represents the dissociation constant (see Chapter 3), which is a measure of the affinity between the enzyme and substrate. The term k_{cat} is the rate constant for the catalytic step, measured in units of seconds^{-1}. This number reflects how many molecules of substrate one molecule of enzyme can turn over in one second when the enzyme is fully saturated with substrate. Other values used in describing the activity of an enzyme are V_{max}, the maximum rate of the reaction, and K_m (Michaelis–Menten constant), which reflects not only the affinity between the enzyme and substrate but the rate of the reaction as well.

The role of the enzyme in most cases is to stabilize the transition state, effectively lowering the energy barrier for the reaction to occur (**Figure 7.1**). In some cases, enzymes increase the strain energy of the substrate, with the same overall result of reducing the activation energy.

There are several common features of enzyme-catalyzed reactions that are relevant to understanding how drugs work when they act as enzyme inhibitors. Enzymes enhance the rate of chemical reactions via **proximity and orientation effects**. Just bringing the reactants together (proximity) and in optimal alignment for reaction (orientation) in the active site provides a considerable rate enhancement compared to the uncatalyzed or nonenzymatic reaction. **Stabilization of the transition state** is a another fundamental means by which enzymes accelerate reaction rates.

Different enzymes catalyze distinct chemical reactions, but many individual enzymes and general classes of enzymes (several described in later sections) rely on some common mechanisms:

- Covalent bonds can be formed between a nucleophilic side chain of an amino acid such as serine, threonine, cysteine, or lysine and an electrophilic site in the substrate. Certain proteases utilize this **covalent catalysis** mechanism.

- Enzymes that utilize **metal ion catalysis** require a metal ion as a cofactor (commonly Zn^{2+}, Mg^{2+}, Fe^{2+}, Fe^{3+}, Cu^{2+}, Co^{2+}, or Mn^{2+}) for reaction acceleration. The metal ion can play a variety of roles, including binding to substrate and appropriately orienting it for reaction, acting as a reversible oxidant or reductant, and stabilizing electrostatic charges, possibly by shielding negative charges on either substrates or developing transition states.

- **Acid–base catalysis** is a common mechanism used by enzymes to lower the activation barriers of certain reactions. Proton transfer and relay between amino acid side chains in the active site, substrates, and products is an efficient mechanism. Enzymes that rely on acid–base catalysis will be sensitive to pH.

Examples of some of these features and mechanisms are illustrated in hydrolysis of the neurotransmitter acetylcholine, catalyzed by the enzyme acetylcholinesterase (**Figure 7.2**). The substrate, acetylcholine, is localized in a deep gorge within the active site of the enzyme, and the carbonyl of the acetate group is attacked by Ser203 of the enzyme. This step is initiated by acid–base catalysis, where Glu334 deprotonates the nearby His447, which then removes a proton from Ser203 to allow the serine oxygen to form a covalent bond to the carbonyl. The anionic transition-state intermediate

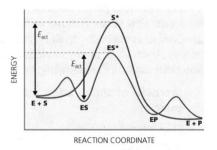

REACTION COORDINATE

Figure 7.1 General energy diagram of an enzyme-catalyzed reaction versus an uncatalyzed reaction. In an uncatalyzed reaction (red line), substrate (S) is converted to product (P) via transition state S*, requiring a specific energy of activation (E_{act}). In an enzyme-catalyzed reaction (purple line), enzyme (E) forms an E·S complex and the transition state (E·S*) has a lower E_{act} than the uncatalyzed reaction. The E·S complex proceeds to an E·P complex, which is converted to E + P. (Adapted from Gluza K & Kafarski P [2013] Transition state analogues of enzymatic reaction as potential drugs. In Drug Discovery [El-Shemy H ed]. InTech. DOI: 10.5772/52504.)

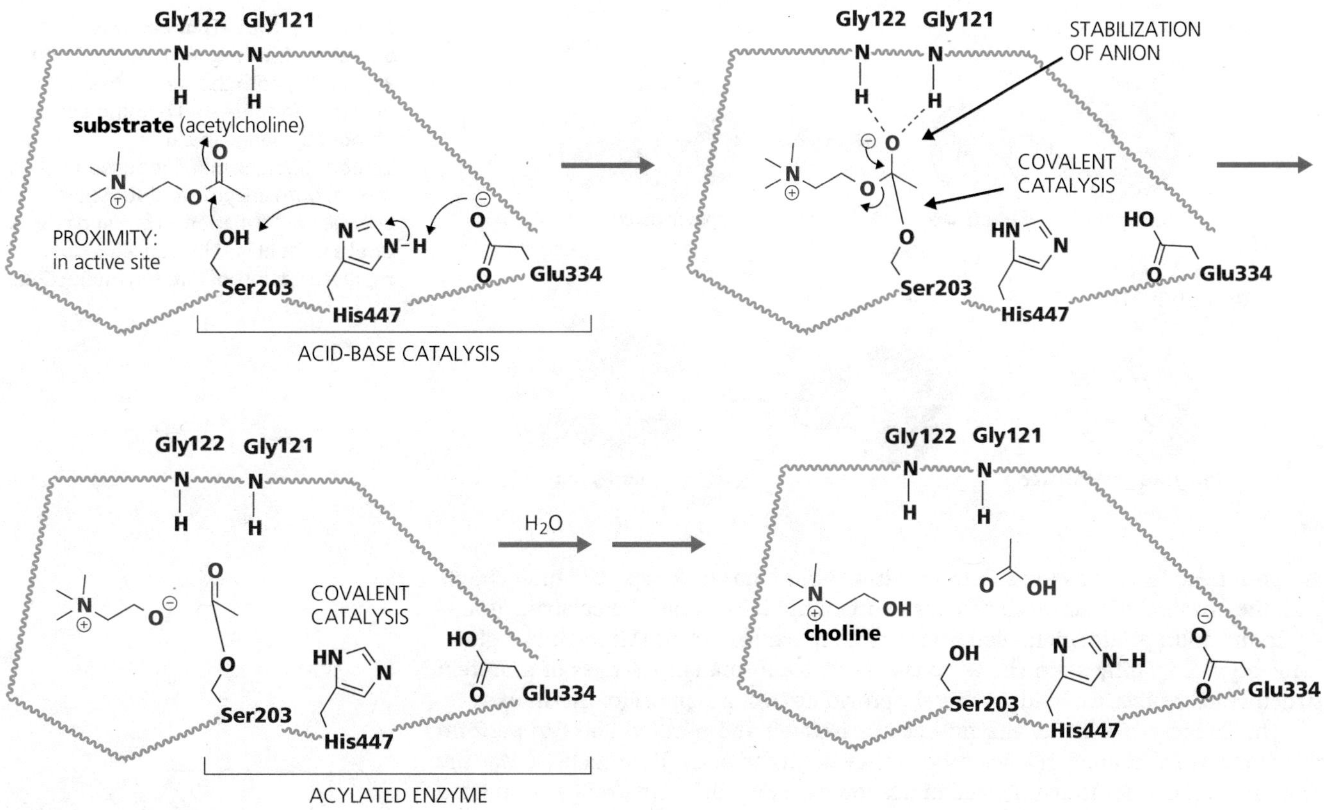

catalysis mechanisms:

PROXIMITY:
substrate localized in active site

ACID–BASE:
proton transfer from His447 to Glu334, His447 removes H from Ser203

COVALENT:
Ser203 adds to carbonyl

TRANSITION-STATE STABILIZATION
in oxyanion hole by backbone NH groups of Gly121 and Gly122

Figure 7.2 Mechanism for hydrolysis of acetylcholine catalyzed by acetylcholinesterase. The substrate (acetylcholine, shown in red) is localized in the active site; acid–base catalysis by Glu334 and His447 activates Ser203, which then forms a covalent bond to the carbonyl of the substrate. The resulting transition-state anion is stabilized in the oxyanion hole by backbone NH groups of Gly121 and Gly122. Completion of the reaction occurs with release of choline, as the oxyanion, and the acetylated enzyme. Further acid-base catalyzed hydrolysis (not shown) generates the protonated choline and activates a water molecule to hydrolyze the acylated enzyme and regenerate it.

is stabilized by interaction with backbone amide N-Hs of glycine residues (121 and 122) in what is termed the oxyanion hole. Collapse of the tetrahedral intermediate releases the choline product as the oxyanion and acetylated Ser203. Further acid–base catalysis is involved in donating a proton to the choline product, as well as activating a water molecule in a hydrolysis reaction of the acetylated enzyme, which then releases acetate and the enzyme.

Models to describe the interaction of an enzyme with a substrate have been developed, and since a number of drugs mimic the enzyme substrate, these models have implications for drug design and medicinal chemistry. One of the earliest, the **lock and key model** (Figure 7.3A), was proposed by Emil Fischer in 1894 to explain the high specificity exhibited by enzymes. This model suggests that the enzyme and its substrate are of rigid, precise complementary shapes. Only a substrate (key) of a precise shape and size will fit into the active site (lock) to allow the enzymatic reaction to occur. This model does not account for the dynamic nature of proteins, nor the concept that enzymes stabilize transition states. In the late 1950s, Daniel Koshland proposed the **induced-fit model** (Figure 7.3B), which addresses some of the shortcomings of the lock and key model. In this model, the enzyme and substrate

A: LOCK AND KEY

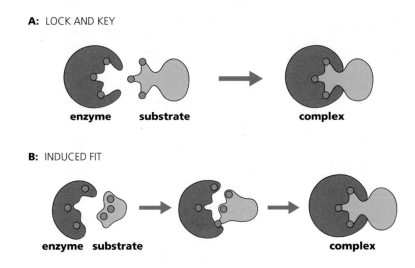

Figure 7.3 Models of enzyme–substrate binding. A: In the lock and key model, both the substrate and the enzyme are static, and binding occurs without a change in either's conformation. B: In the induced-fit model, both enzyme and substrate change conformation as binding occurs until a tight fit is achieved. Blue dots represent points of binding interactions.

B: INDUCED FIT

are both flexible, and as the substrate starts to bind and make specific interactions with the enzyme, the active site moves to accommodate it until the catalytic groups are in the appropriate orientation for reaction, much like a hand fitting into a glove. X-ray crystallography often shows considerable conformation changes of a protein structure after substrate binding, thereby providing strong support for this model.

Unlike receptors, many enzymes can be isolated and purified and can perform their function as readily in a test tube as they do in the body. Ribonuclease was the first functional enzyme synthesized in a laboratory. Two different groups completed this feat: Bruce Merrifield and Bernd Gutte from Rockefeller University used solid-phase synthesis methods, and a separate research group from Merck Sharpe and Dohme, led by Ralph Hirschmann and Robert Denkewalter used solution methods. This scientific breakthrough was reported on the front page of *The New York Times* on January 17, 1969. The ability to prepare and purify large quantities of enzymes allows them to succumb to structure elucidation via spectroscopic methods such as NMR or X-ray crystallography. These types of studies have provided significant advances in understanding how specific enzymes function. In addition, access to large quantities of proteins enables a number of drug discovery and medicinal chemistry strategies such as high-throughput screening and structure-based drug design.

EFFECT OF SMALL-MOLECULE MODULATORS ON ENZYMES

While the previous section described the function and effects of enzymes on their natural substrates, the focus in this section is on how small-molecule drugs change the course of the natural, enzyme-catalyzed conversion of substrate to product. As with receptor modulators, enzyme modulators may resemble the natural substrate or may have a significantly different structure. Regardless of the structure, however, most drugs that act on enzymes work through inhibition of the enzyme and are termed **inhibitors**. Drugs that activate an enzyme (**activators**) are less common than inhibitors.

7.1 Modulators are classified by how they interact with an enzyme

Small-molecule enzyme modulators are classified by two primary characteristics: the location of their binding to the enzyme and the extent of their binding. The extent of binding is related to the reversibility of binding, and enzyme inhibitors (I) can be classified as either reversible or irreversible. **Reversible inhibitors** form a complex (often noncovalent, but not always) with the enzyme, [E·I], and both the enzyme and the inhibitor can be recovered intact (**Figure 7.4**). Reversible inhibitors may also be **slow tight-binding inhibitors**, which have such a slow off rate that they are nearly

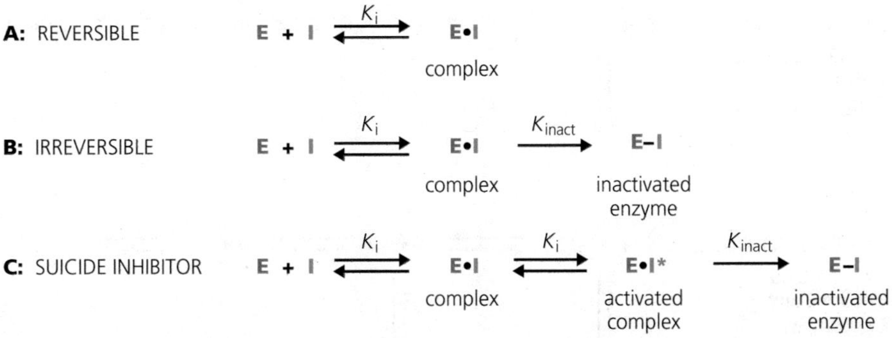

Figure 7.4 Three types of interaction of an enzyme with an inhibitor.
A: Reversible interaction of an enzyme (E) with an inhibitor (I) gives an enzyme/inhibitor complex E · I in equilibrium with E and I. B: Irreversible inhibition leads to the complex E · I and then formation of a permanent, covalent bond to generate covalently modified enzyme E–I. C: A suicide inhibitor leads to the complex E · I and then formation of an activated complex E · I*, which proceeds to inactivated enzyme E–I.

A: REVERSIBLE $E + I \underset{}{\overset{K_i}{\rightleftharpoons}} E{\bullet}I$
   complex

B: IRREVERSIBLE $E + I \underset{}{\overset{K_i}{\rightleftharpoons}} E{\bullet}I \xrightarrow{K_{inact}} E{-}I$
   complex   inactivated enzyme

C: SUICIDE INHIBITOR $E + I \underset{}{\overset{K_i}{\rightleftharpoons}} E{\bullet}I \underset{}{\overset{K_i}{\rightleftharpoons}} E{\bullet}I^* \xrightarrow{K_{inact}} E{-}I$
   complex   activated complex   inactivated enzyme

irreversible. The inhibitor constant (K_i) is a measure of the affinity of the inhibitor for the enzyme. As described in Chapter 3, K_i can be directly related to the Gibbs free energy of binding. Another value frequently used to quantify enzyme inhibition, IC_{50}, is the concentration of inhibitor at which 50% of the enzyme activity is inhibited. This value will vary according to the conditions of the assay, such as substrate concentration. In contrast, the K_i is constant, regardless of conditions.

Classical irreversible inhibitors bind through covalent interactions and do not dissociate from the enzyme. In these cases, K_{inact} is an indication of the rate of formation of the inactivated enzyme. A specific type of irreversible inhibitor is a **suicide inhibitor** or **mechanism-based inactivator**. This is usually a modified version of the substrate, and the initial complex is acted upon by the enzyme to generate an activated complex E · I*, which then covalently modifies the enzyme, resulting in its irreversible inhibition.

The location of binding is another way in which enzyme modulators are characterized (**Figure 7.5**). **Active-site inhibitors** bind at the reaction site and prevent substrate from binding (see Figure 7.5B). **Allosteric modulators** are small molecules that bind to a site remote from the active site and affect enzymatic activity through either inhibition or activation. Allosteric modulators can function through multiple mechanisms; Figure 7.5C illustrates one way in which binding at a remote site can inhibit enzymatic activity.

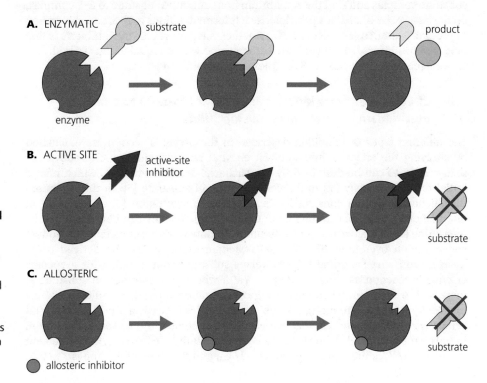

A. ENZYMATIC   substrate   product
enzyme

B. ACTIVE SITE   active-site inhibitor   substrate

C. ALLOSTERIC   substrate

● allosteric inhibitor

Figure 7.5 Modes of inhibition based on location of binding. A: With no inhibition, enzyme and substrate bind, and product is formed. B: An active-site inhibitor binds at the same site as the substrate, so that substrate cannot bind and no product is formed. C: One type of allosteric inhibitor binds at a site remote from the active site and changes the conformation of the active site such that substrate can no longer bind efficiently; no product is formed.

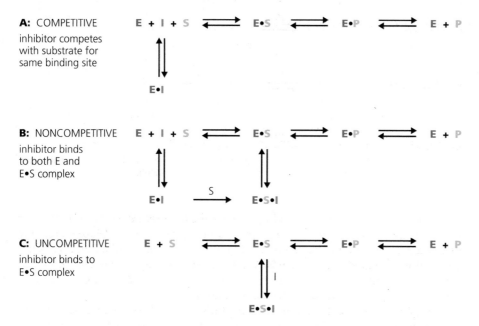

A: COMPETITIVE
inhibitor competes
with substrate for
same binding site

B: NONCOMPETITIVE
inhibitor binds
to both E and
E•S complex

C: UNCOMPETITIVE
inhibitor binds to
E•S complex

Figure 7.6 Effect of types of inhibition on reaction of an enzyme with a substrate in the presence of an inhibitor. A: Competitive inhibitors compete directly with substrate to give an E·I complex. B: Noncompetitive inhibitors can bind to both the E and the E·S complex, producing an E·I and E·S·I complex. C: An uncompetitive inhibitor binds to the E·S complex, giving an E·S·I complex.

In addition to location and extent of binding, enzyme inhibitors are also classified with respect to how they influence binding of the natural substrate(s), as shown in **Figure 7.6**. **Competitive inhibitors** are active-site inhibitors; they bind to the enzyme at the same site as the substrate and compete with it for binding (see Figure 7.6A). When the enzyme has multiple substrates, the substrate with which the inhibitor is competitive is noted. In these cases, increasing the amount of substrate will decrease the degree of inhibition by the inhibitor.

Noncompetitive inhibitors are usually allosteric inhibitors, but can also bind near the active site without competing with the substrate for binding. They bind to the enzyme and the enzyme·substrate complex with equal affinity, resulting in a situation where the activity of the enzyme is reduced but substrate binding is not affected (see Figure 7.6B).

Uncompetitive inhibitors are allosteric inhibitors that bind to the enzyme· substrate complex and shift the equilibrium from unbound substrate to E·S complex, on the basis of Le Chatelier's principle. As it is formed, I binds to E·S, and conversion to product is limited (see Figure 7.6C). Another category of enzyme inhibitors is that of **mixed inhibitors**, where the inhibitor may bind with unequal affinity to both free enzyme (competitively) and E·S complex (uncompetitively).

7.2   Effects on enzyme kinetics are used to characterize the mechanism of small-molecule modulators

The different types of inhibition described in the previous section are elucidated by studying the effect of inhibitors on enzyme reaction kinetics. The activity of many enzymes can be described by the Michaelis–Menten equation, which relates initial reaction velocity (V) to the concentration of substrate [S]. In this equation, the Michaelis–Menten constant K_m is substrate concentration [S] at the point of one-half of V_{max} (the maximum rate of the reaction). Velocity can be determined by measuring either decrease in substrate concentration over time or increase in product concentration over time. The Michaelis–Menten constant may be derived using a **saturation curve** plotting velocity versus substrate concentration for a specific enzymatic reaction as shown in **Figure 7.7B**, where concentration of substrate is increased to the point where increasing concentration no longer results in change in velocity (that is, saturation). A double-reciprocal (Lineweaver–Burk) plot of 1/[S] versus $1/v$ gives a linear plot that can also be used to obtain the same information, based on the reciprocal of the Michaelis–Menten equation. In this case, the y-intercept is equal to $1/V_{max}$, the x-intercept equals $-1/K_m$, and the slope of the line is K_m/V_{max} (**Figure 7.7C**).

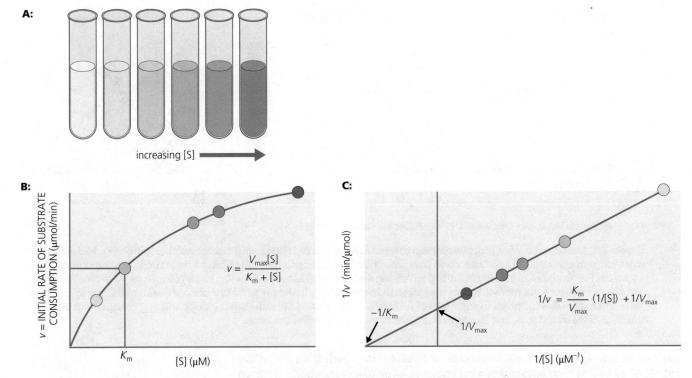

Figure 7.7 Equations and graphs used to characterize enzyme kinetics. A: Representation of increasing substrate concentration [S]. B: Michaelis–Menten equation and representation of a saturation curve for an enzymatic reaction, plotting substrate concentration [S] versus velocity. The Michaelis constant, K_m is the substrate concentration at half of the maximal reaction velocity. C: Reciprocal Michaelis–Menten equation and linear (Lineweaver–Burk) plot for an enzymatic reaction. In this plot, the slope = K_m/V_{max}, the x-intercept = $-1/K_m$, and the y-intercept = $1/V_{max}$. (From Alberts B, Bray D, Hopkin K et al. [2013] Essential Cell Biology, 4th ed. Garland Science.)

When the Michaelis–Menten equation is used to distinguish between competitive and noncompetitive inhibitors, the control curve or plot when no inhibitor is present is compared to the curve or plot in the presence of a fixed amount of inhibitor. If the inhibitor is competitive, then K_m will increase since more substrate is required to reach a given velocity of $1/2$ V_{max}, but V_{max} will not change, since at a high enough [S], the substrate will displace all of the inhibitor and the reaction will proceed as it does without inhibitor present. When graphed, the x-intercept ($-1/K_m$) will change, as will the slope (K_m/V_{max}) of the line compared to the graph of substrate alone. In contrast, if the inhibitor is noncompetitive, $-1/K_m$ will remain the same but V_{max} can never be reached, so in a Lineweaver–Burk plot, the slope of the line will change, due to the change in V_{max}, with the reciprocal $1/V_{max}$ being a larger number with inhibitor present, but the x-intercept ($-1/K_m$) remaining the same. If the inhibitor is uncompetitive, K_m and V_{max} will both decrease, changing both the x- and y- intercepts, but the slope of the line will remain the same. These examples are illustrated in **Figure 7.8**.

Molecules that activate an enzyme (activators) could do so by increasing the affinity of the enzyme for the substrate (K_d) or affecting the maximum rate of the enzymatic reaction (V_{max}). A more detailed discussion of enzyme biochemistry is beyond the scope of this chapter; however, characterization of enzyme inhibitors is an essential component of medicinal chemistry and drug discovery programs.

In the context of drug discovery, human diseases can be caused by or exacerbated by enzymes that are overactive, underactive, or misactive. The goal then is to find a drug that will target only the particular human enzyme that contributes to or causes the disease targeted. Given the similarity in function and structure of various enzyme classes, this is a challenging prospect. In addition to targeting human enzymes, infectious agents such as bacteria and viruses may rely on their unique enzymes in order to replicate. Therefore, bacterial and viral enzymes are frequently

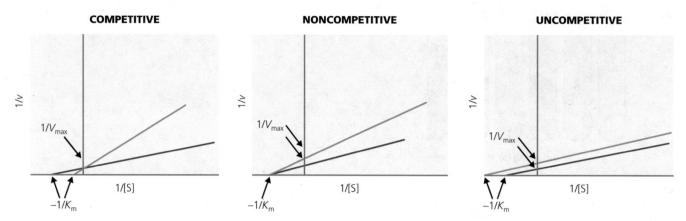

*Red lines = substrate alone; blue lines = inhibitor (fixed concentration) + substrate

Figure 7.8 Lineweaver–Burk plots describing competitive, noncompetitive, and uncompetitive inhibition. Red lines show increasing concentration of substrate alone; blue lines show fixed concentration of inhibitor + increasing concentration of substrate. For a competitive inhibitor, adding increasing amounts of substrate allows V_{max} to be reached, so it remains the same, but K_m will increase since more substrate is required to reach 1/2 V_{max}. In the presence of a noncompetitive inhibitor V_{max} cannot be reached regardless of increasing amounts of substrate, so K_m remains the same but the slope and V_{max} change. With an uncompetitive inhibitor, K_m and V_{max} both change, and the slope remains the same.

targeted as a treatment for these infections. In diseases that result from overactive enzymes, as well as with bacterial or viral enzymes, drug discovery efforts focus on inhibitors. Underactive enzymes require activators, and depending on the specific circumstances, diseases caused by misactive enzymes can be treated by either inhibitors or activators.

7.3   Enzymes are frequent targets of drug action

As described previously, because of their roles in numerous physiological and pathophysiological processes, enzymes are an important class of drug targets and are considered readily druggable (particularly inhibitors) for the following reasons:

- Enzymes are often isolable, well-characterized, and available in significant quantity; therefore, development of assays for hit identification and optimization is usually straightforward.

- Characterization of inhibitors and activators can rely on established biochemistry and enzyme kinetics principles.

- Enzyme substrate mimics and transition-state analogs, as described in Chapter 4, are often excellent starting points for hit and lead generation.

- Enzymes and enzyme–inhibitor complexes are amenable to structure elucidation via methods such as X-ray crystallography and NMR, which affords opportunities for virtual screening, fragment-based screening and structure-based drug design approaches.

However, there are also challenges in targeting enzymes that are distinct from other target classes, which include the following:

- Specificity for one enzyme over many related enzymes may be difficult to achieve.

- Certain enzyme substrates occur in very high concentrations in the body, thereby requiring extremely potent modulators to compete with the natural substrate.

- Physical properties of enzyme inhibitors are often at odds with druglike properties, such as permeability and metabolic stability.

Some common classes of enzymes that are frequent medicinal chemistry targets, as well as specific examples of drugs that affect a specific enzyme in that class, are listed in **Table 7.1**.

Table 7.1   Common enzyme drug targets, the reaction catalyzed and substrates, and select drug examples.

Class of enzyme	Reaction catalyzed	Substrate	Select drug examples		
			Drug	Mechanism	Indication
kinase	phosphorylation	protein, lipid, or small molecule	imatinib	Bcr-Abl kinase inhibitor	cancer
			tofacitinib	JAK inhibitor	autoimmune diseases
protease	hydrolysis of peptide bond	peptide or protein	captopril	ACE inhibitor	cardiovascular disease
			indinavir	HIV protease inhibitor	HIV infection
			penicillin	penicillin-binding protein inhibitor	bacterial infection
polymerase or reverse transcriptase	formation of phosphodiester bond	DNA or RNA	AZT	HIV reverse transcriptase inhibitor	HIV infection
			sofosbuvir	HCV RNA polymerase inhibitor	hepatitis C infection
esterase and phosphodiesterase	hydrolysis of carboxylic acid and phosphate esters	small-molecule second messengers, lipids, proteins, nucleic acids	orlistat	lipase inhibitor	obesity
			donepezil	acetylcholinesterase inhibitor	Alzheimer's disease
			sildenafil	phosphodiesterase inhibitor	erectile dysfunction
oxidoreductase	oxidation and reduction	small-molecule building blocks for endogenous molecules, proteins, lipids	statins	HMG-CoA reductase inhibitor	cardiovascular risk, cholesterol lowering
			methotrexate	dihydrofolate reductase inhibitor	cancer; autoimmune diseases
topoisomerase	cleavage and formation of nucleotide bond	DNA and RNA	quinolone antibacterial compounds	DNA gyrase inhibitors	bacterial infection
			camptothecins, etoposide	topoisomerase II inhibitors	cancer
glucokinase	phosphorylation of glucose at C6	glucose	piragliatin*	glucokinase activator	diabetes

*Indicates a compound not approved as a drug.

In the following sections, some specific enzyme classes are described along with representative examples of enzyme inhibitor drugs. To date, no drugs that work by enzyme activation have been approved, although numerous probe molecules exist, and several glucokinase activators have advanced to clinical trials as potential anti-diabetic drugs, although most were terminated after phase II trials.

KINASES AND KINASE INHIBITOR DRUGS

Kinases are enzymes that catalyze phosphorylation of a substrate. The number of distinct human kinases is estimated to be >500, and these play essential roles in numerous physiological events. Many are receptor kinases; that is, they span the

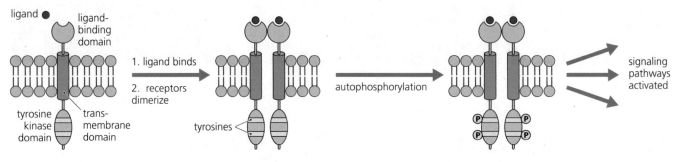

EXTRACELLULAR

INTRACELLULAR

Figure 7.9 Structure and function of a receptor tyrosine kinase. A receptor tyrosine kinase has an extracellular ligand-binding domain, a transmembrane region, and an intracellular tyrosine kinase domain. Upon ligand binding, two receptors dimerize, resulting in activation by self-phosphorylation. The active phosphorylated form then acts as a kinase, phosphorylating substrates and resulting in downstream effects by activating signaling pathways.

plasma membrane and contain an extracellular binding site and an intracellular catalytic site. There is also a smaller family of non-receptor intracellular kinases. Many receptor kinases are an integral part of a signaling cascade and regulate cell growth, proliferation, and differentiation, making them frequent targets for cancer drugs. **Figure 7.9** illustrates a receptor tyrosine kinase. Typically, receptor kinases are composed of an extracellular ligand-binding domain, a membrane-spanning region, and an intracellular domain containing the phosphorylating enzymatic activity. Upon binding of a ligand, two receptors dimerize, resulting in activation by autophosphorylation (tyrosine in figure, but can also be serine or threonine) using ATP as the phosphate source. The active, phosphorylated form then phosphorylates substrates, activating signaling pathways and leading to a downstream effect such as cell proliferation.

In addition to cancer, other disorders that are marked by uncontrolled cell proliferation, such as inflammatory diseases and autoimmune disorders, may also be treated by kinase inhibitors.

The kinase substrate may be a protein or a bioactive small molecule, such as a nucleic acid, a carbohydrate, or a lipid that contains a free hydroxyl group. When the substrate is a protein, phosphorylation usually occurs on a serine, threonine, or tyrosine hydroxyl group; these kinases are termed serine/threonine kinases or tyrosine kinases, respectively. The reaction involves transfer of a phosphate group from a nucleoside triphosphate, usually adenosine triphosphate (ATP) but sometimes guanosine triphosphate (GTP), to a substrate containing a hydroxyl group. The products of the reaction are the phosphorylated substrate and the nucleoside diphosphate, ADP (or GDP), as shown in **Figure 7.10**.

Kinase-mediated phosphorylations proceed through a complex mechanism. A condensed version is illustrated in **Figure 7.11,** using an ATP-dependent kinase as an example. It involves complexation of the triphosphate of ATP by two magnesium

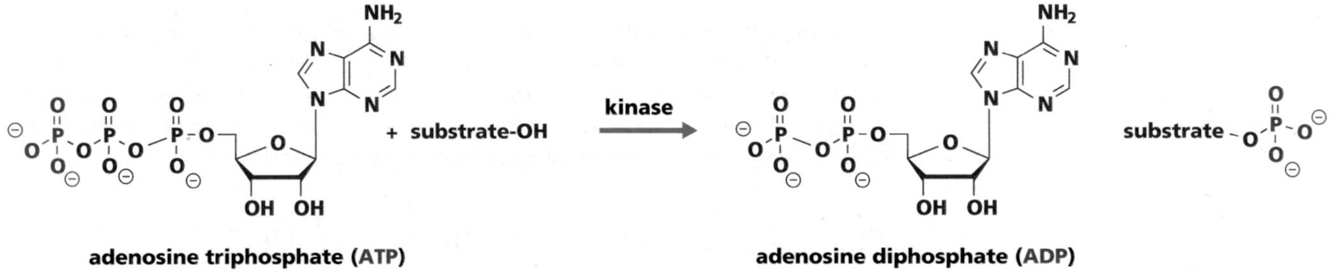

adenosine triphosphate (ATP)

adenosine diphosphate (ADP)

Figure 7.10 Phosphorylation of the hydroxyl of a substrate catalyzed by a kinase. A substrate (either a small molecule containing a hydroxyl group or a protein containing a serine, threonine, or tyrosine) is phosphorylated. In this example, ATP is a second substrate and donates the phosphate group (shown in red), producing ADP and phosphorylated substrate.

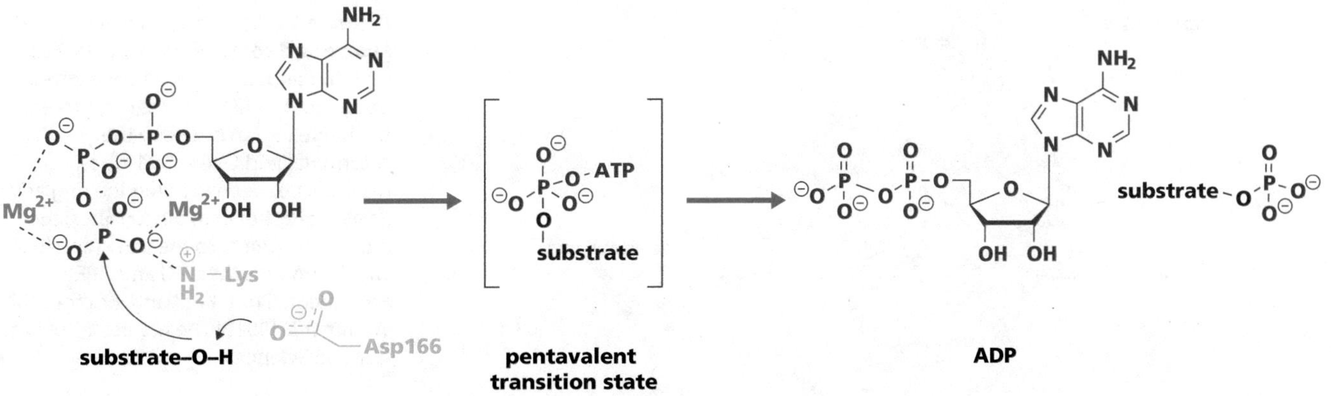

Figure 7.11 Condensed reaction mechanism of ATP-dependent kinase phosphorylation of a substrate. Metal and amino acid coordination to the phosphate groups in the active site and acid–base catalysis, enable reaction between the substrate and ATP to generate a pentavalent transition state. Completion of the reaction generates phosphorylated substrate and ADP. Key: red = ATP, ADP, transferred phosphate; blue = Mg^{2+}; green = protein kinase residues; black = substrate.

ions and also to amino acids in the protein. This coordination (metal ion catalysis) appropriately orients and activates the terminal phosphate toward nucleophilic attack. The substrate hydroxyl group is deprotonated by an amino acid (Asp in figure) of the kinase via acid–base catalysis. Phosphate transfer from ATP to the substrate generates a pentavalent transition state, which leads to the newly formed ADP molecule and phosphorylated substrate. When the substrate is a protein or peptide, kinases often recognize up to four amino acid residues to either side of the phosphorylation site, meaning that phosphorylation will not occur unless this specific consensus sequence is present. However, while the kinase may accept a smaller peptide substrate containing the consensus sequence, the entire protein substrate contributes to binding and recognition, and enzymatic reactions are most efficient on the natural substrate.

The structure of the active site of kinases is highly conserved and is located in the kinase domain (also called the catalytic domain) of the much larger protein. The ATP-binding site is buried deep inside the protein, in a cleft between two lobes of the protein. One lobe consists of the N-terminal region, composed of β-sheets and a glycine-rich region, and the other is the α-helix-rich C-terminal region; the area between the two lobes is termed the hinge region, with the first amino acid here designated the gatekeeper residue. The adenine base of ATP makes a series of H-bonds to this hinge region of the kinase, while the furanose and triphosphate of ATP sit in a hydrophilic pocket that extends towards the substrate-binding site. An activation loop, marked by the conserved amino acid triads DFG (Asp-Phe-Gly) and APE (Ala-Pro-Glu), sits near the substrate-binding site and acts as a door for the substrate. This loop is often phosphorylated as part of a regulation mechanism, and this modification often substantially increases enzymatic efficiency. **Figure 7.12** shows the structure of the Abl tyrosine kinase bound to ATP and some of its key features.

In addition to phosphorylation, kinases are regulated by other mechanisms. In many cases, an effector protein is required to bind (often at a site remote from the active site) to the kinase to render it capable of phosphorylation. Mechanisms that control kinase activity include other modifications of the protein (such as acylation or isoprenylation) and localization. These regulatory elements can also be targeted by small molecules to modify the activity of the kinase.

Recent advances in solving X-ray structures of kinases bound to inhibitors and substrates, as well as the continued interest in kinase inhibitors as drug targets and their therapeutic success, has led to an explosion in the medicinal chemistry of small-molecule inhibitors. Traditional high-throughput screening can be used for hit identification. However, focused screening approaches, which test a small library of hundreds to thousands of molecules that are either designed to or known to target the kinase ATP-binding domain, are more common. The similarity across kinase binding domains virtually assures that hits will be identified; however, optimizing selectivity for the desired kinase is often a significant effort. Due to the availability of X-ray structures and/or homology models of kinases, fragment-based screening and virtual

Abl kinase

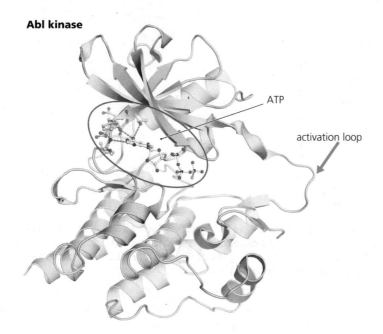

ATP

activation loop

Figure 7.12 Structure of Abl tyrosine kinase and some of its key features. Ribbon diagram of Abl tyrosine kinase bound to ATP. ATP (gray sticks) binds in the hinge region between the N-terminal and C-terminal lobes. H-bonds between the adenine ring and protein are shown in dotted lines; the blue arrow points to the activation loop, which contains the DFG and APE sequences. (From Kuriyan J, Konforti B & Wemmer D [2012] The Molecules of Life. Garland Science.)

screening strategies are often also successful. Application of transition-state mimic strategies for kinase inhibition has not been particularly useful due to the fact that mimicking a highly charged, pentavalent phosphate transition state (see Figure 7.11) is not readily achieved with standard organic small molecules.

7.4   Kinase inhibitors work through multiple binding modes and are effective anti-cancer drugs and anti-inflammatory agents

Many approved drugs that act on kinases are inhibitors of tyrosine kinases and bind at or near the active site. They are primarily used to treat cancers that either overexpress certain growth factor receptor kinases or have mutant forms of those kinases. Allosteric modulators and activators are much less common, as are inhibitors of kinases that act on small-molecule substrates. However, significant advances in the field have led to approval of the first small-molecule allosteric modulators, and some activators have advanced to clinical trials. Inhibitors of kinases that phosphorylate lipids (such as sphingosine) or nucleosides have also been reported.

A number of clinically used kinase inhibitors bind at the hinge region in the active kinase conformation, called the DFG-in conformation, and make similar H-bonding contacts as the adenine moiety of ATP. By definition these are active-site competitive inhibitors, and they mimic one of the substrates (ATP). These are classified as type I inhibitors. By taking advantage of cysteine residues in the vicinity of the ATP site, covalent active-site inhibitors have also been designed.

Representative noncovalent type I inhibitor structures, which will be discussed further in Chapter 10, are shown in **Figure 7.13**. Gefitinib and erlotinib inhibit epidermal growth factor receptor (EGFR) kinase activity and therefore prevent receptor signaling in cells. They are approved to treat certain cancers that overexpress EGFR. Activities against other kinases have also been reported. Vandetanib, sunitinib, and dasatanib inhibit a number of receptor tyrosine kinases including platelet-derived growth factor (PDGF) and vascular endothelial growth factor (VEGF).

The activity of these compounds against multiple kinases can be attributed to their binding to the ATP site, which is highly conserved across most kinases. **Figure 7.14** illustrates binding of a kinase inhibitor (structurally related to gefitinib and other aminoquinazolines) to the ATP-binding site of Abl1 when the kinase is in an active conformation, required for phosphorylation. Highlighted are the H-bonds made to the hinge region and hydrophobic pockets found where the ATP substrate binds. Also indicated is the gatekeeper residue, in this case a threonine, which is frequently mutated when resistance develops.

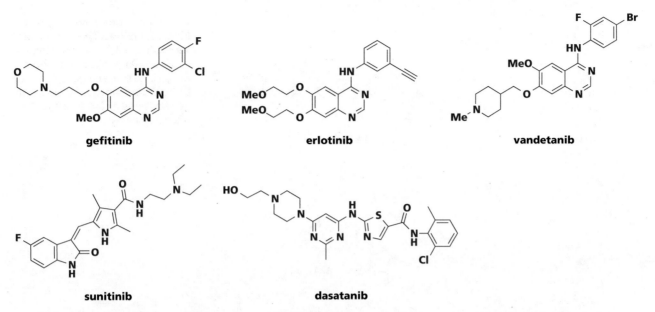

gefitinib
erlotinib
vandetanib

sunitinib
dasatanib

Figure 7.13 Structures of active-site kinase inhibitors that bind to the DFG-in conformation. Gefitinib and erlotinib inhibit epidermal growth factor receptor (EGFR) kinase activity and are approved to treat certain cancers that overexpress EGFR. Vandetanib, sunitinib, and dasatanib inhibit a number of receptor tyrosine kinases including platelet-derived growth factor (PDGF) and vascular endothelial growth factor (VEGF).

A second class of noncovalent inhibitors has been developed that bind to an inactive kinase conformation, called the DFG-out conformation. This conformation exposes hydrophobic binding sites near the ATP site. These inhibitors prevent binding of substrates because the active site is occluded by the activation loop of the protein. In these examples, the compounds bind to the ATP site but also occupy a newly revealed hydrophobic pocket that is not present in the active form of the kinase. Examples of these type II inhibitors (also described in Chapter 10) include imatinib, sorafenib, nilotinib, and lapatinib, shown in **Figure 7.15**.

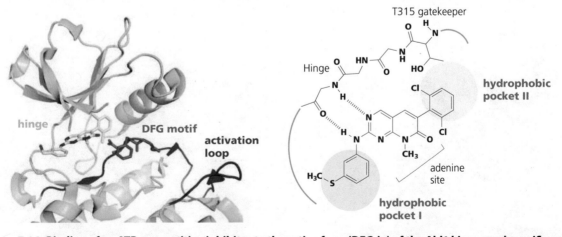

Figure 7.14 Binding of an ATP-competitive inhibitor to the active form (DFG-in) of the Abl1 kinase and specific molecular interactions. Left: The inhibitor (light blue) binds to the ATP binding site in the hinge region, with the conserved activation loop shown in dark blue and individual side chains of DFG shown in pink. B: The inhibitor is shown engaged in key H-bonds to the hinge region and occupying hydrophobic pockets I and II. The gatekeeper residue, in the case of Abl1, Thr315, is also indicated. (From Zhang J, Yang PL & Gray NS [2009] *Nat Rev Cancer* 9:28–39. With permission from Macmillan Publishers Limited.)

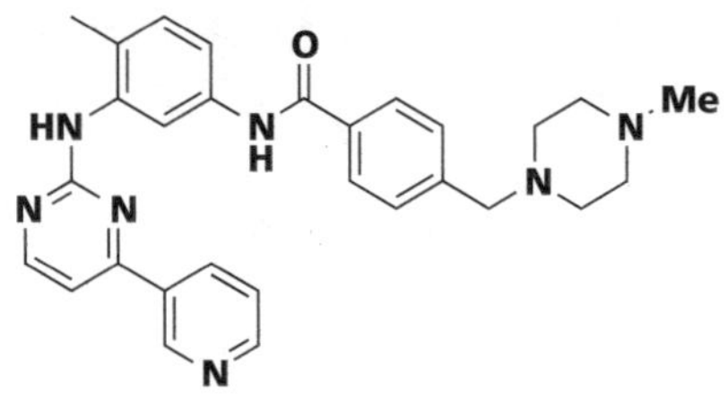

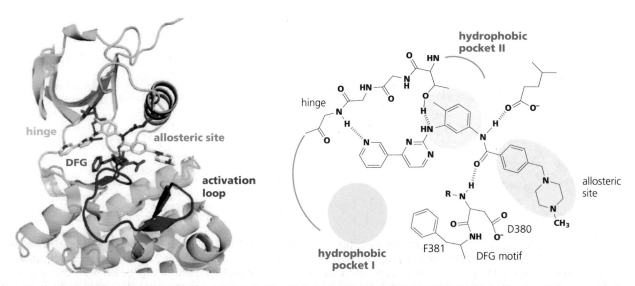

imatinib

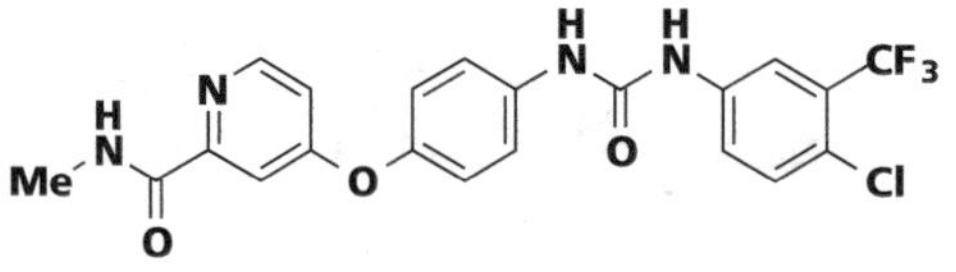

sorafenib

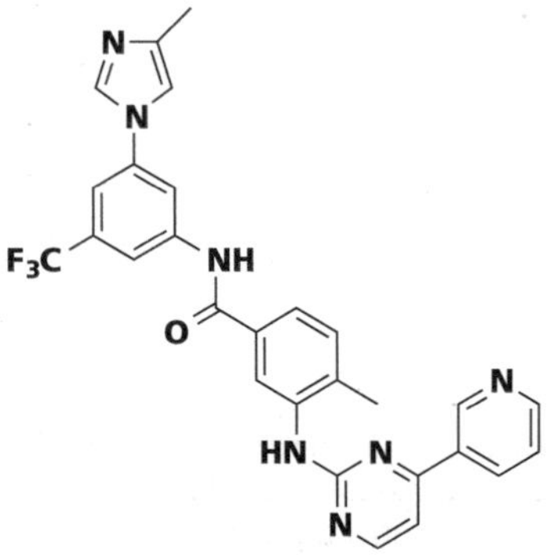

nilotinib

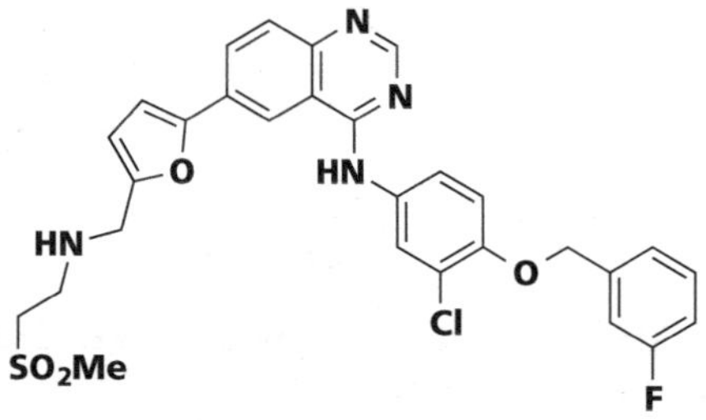

lapatinib

Figure 7.15 Structures of type II kinase inhibitors. Type II inhibitors, such as imatinib, sorafenib, nilotinib, and lapatinib (all approved cancer drugs) bind in the hinge region of the DFG-out conformation of kinases. In general, these molecules target multiple kinases.

Figure 7.16 shows a representative example of the type II inhibitor imatinib bound to an inactive form of Abl kinase. In this figure, the molecule occupies part of the ATP binding site (hydrophobic pocket II) but does not occupy the entire site (hydrophobic pocket I), as do the DFG-in binders. In addition, a new site (allosteric site), not present in the DFG-in conformation, is occupied. A number of hydrogen-bonds are also made to the protein, including one to the gatekeeper residue.

The therapeutic success of targeting kinases mutated in cancers has been tempered by the development of resistance to the drugs. This is due to secondary mutations that form after months of treatment. In an effort to combat these secondary mutations, there has been interest in developing covalent inhibitors. These molecules were

Figure 7.16 Ribbon diagram of DFG-out inhibitor imatinib bound to Abl1. Left: The inhibitor (light blue) partially occupies the ATP binding site in the hinge region. The activation loop is shown in dark blue, with side chains of the DFG motif shown in pink. Right: Inhibitor makes multiple H-bonds to the protein, including in the hinge region (not all shown) and occupies one of the hydophobic pockets. Additional interactions are made, including occupation of a newly revealed allosteric site observed only in the DFG-out conformation. (From Zhang J, Yang PL & Gray NS [2009] *Nat Rev Cancer* 9:28–39. With permission from Macmillan Publishers Limited.)

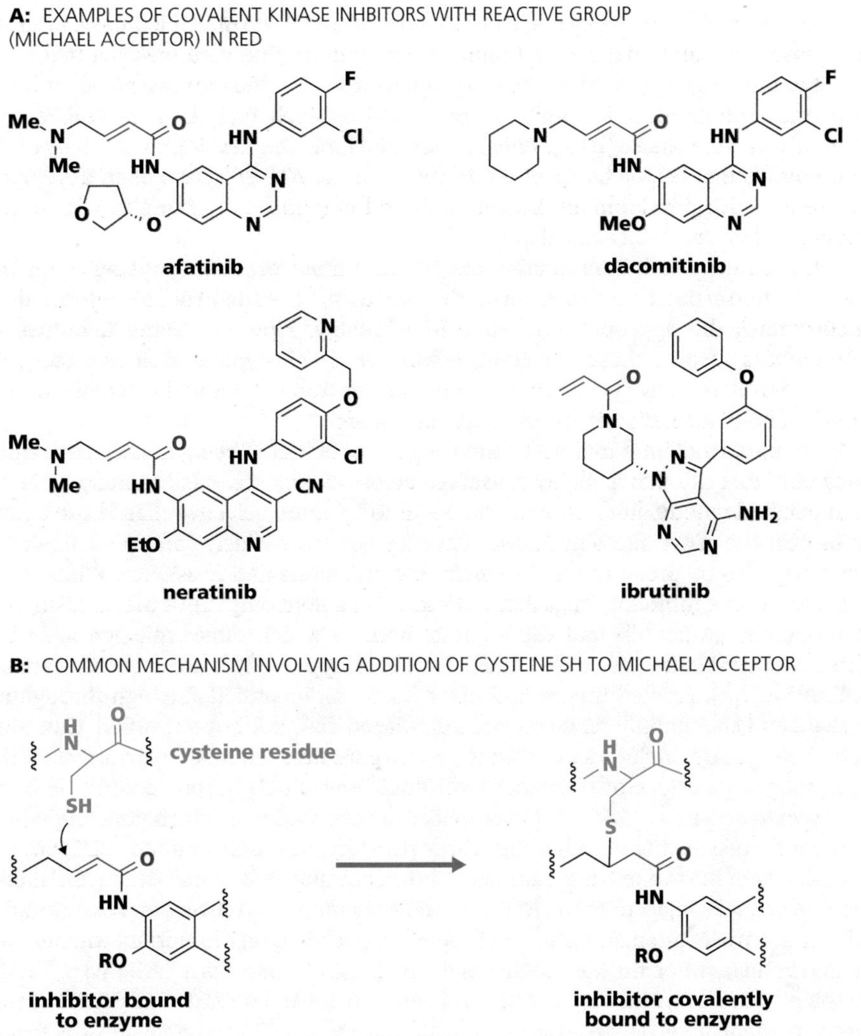

Figure 7.17 Covalent kinase inhibitors. A: Structures of afatinib, dacomitinib, neratinib, and ibrutinib; afatinib and ibrutinib have been approved to treat specific cancers. B: Common mechanism of inhibition involving addition of a cysteine thiol (blue) near the inhibitor binding site to a Michael acceptor (red) to give a covalent adduct.

A: EXAMPLES OF COVALENT KINASE INHBITORS WITH REACTIVE GROUP (MICHAEL ACCEPTOR) IN RED

afatinib

dacomitinib

neratinib

ibrutinib

B: COMMON MECHANISM INVOLVING ADDITION OF CYSTEINE SH TO MICHAEL ACCEPTOR

cysteine residue

inhibitor bound
to enzyme

inhibitor covalently
bound to enzyme

designed to bind in the ATP site and react with a noncatalytic cysteine via a Michael acceptor, such as an acrylamide. Several examples of covalent kinase inhibitors are shown in **Figure 7.17**, along with a common mechanism of covalent bond formation.

This type of inhibition results in a longer residence time of the inhibitor, which usually results in improved efficacy and can also limit the emergence of certain resistant mutations. **Figure 7.18** shows an X-ray structure of afatinib, the first covalent

Figure 7.18 X-ray structure of afatinib bound to epidermal growth factor receptor. Close-up of afatinib bound to EGFR (left), with complete structure of kinase domain/afatinib complex in the center, and afatinib structure on the right. Left: Red dotted line shows a hydrogen bond between the quinazoline nitrogen and Met793 in the hinge region. A covalent bond (shown in yellow) forms between Cys797 and the crotonamide Michael acceptor (red). (From Solca F, Dahl G, Zoephel A et al. [2012] *J Pharmacol Exp Ther* 343:342–350. With permission from American Society for Pharmacology and Experimental Therapeutics.)

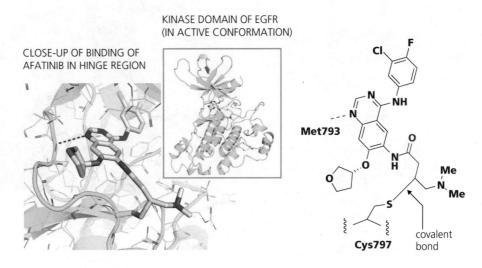

CLOSE-UP OF BINDING OF
AFATINIB IN HINGE REGION

KINASE DOMAIN OF EGFR
(IN ACTIVE CONFORMATION)

Met793

Cys797

covalent
bond

kinase inhibitor approved by the FDA, bound to the ATP site of EGFR kinase. Afatinib is a close structural analog of gefitinib, and its quinazoline core makes a hydrogen bond to the hinge region of the protein. The nearby cysteine makes a covalent bond with the crotonamide. Ibrutinib is approved for B-cell malignancies and targets Bruton's tyrosine kinase (BTK), which is essential for B-cell development. Many other compounds that act via covalent modification of the ATP site have been developed or are in active development. Dacomitinib and neratinib are examples of two that progressed to advanced clinical trials.

This strategy to inhibit kinases has become more prevalent and relies on the identification of potent noncovalent binders and then, based on structural information, incorporates the appropriate reactive functionality. However, some liabilities of compounds such as these, including inhibition of wild-type as well as oncogenic mutated proteins, have been reported, and further study of optimal reactivity toward covalent bond formation is an active area of research.

Inhibitors that bind to the ATP site have the potential of being nonselective since they bind to a site that is highly conserved across all kinases. It is generally believed that allosteric modulators have the potential to be more selective than those acting at or near the active site, since these sites may not be as widely conserved; however, they may also be prone to rapidly generating mutations and resistance. While there are few enzyme inhibitor drugs that work through a noncompetitive mechanism, two compounds, trametinib and cobimetinib, both of which target mitogen-activated protein kinase kinase (also called MEK), have been approved for use in certain cancers (**Figure 7.19A**). Trametinib was optimized from a hit identified in a high-throughput screen, and cobimetinib relied on structure-based design for optimization. Common structural features include a diaryl amine with a para-halogen substituent on one of the aryl groups, a polar group that interacts with the ATP terminal phosphate, and an H-bond acceptor to Ser212. **Figure 7.19B** exemplifies the orientation in which noncompetitive inhibitors such as these bind. In this X-ray structure, the MEK inhibitor PD318088, a para-halogen substituted diaryl amine, is shown binding to the kinase when ATP is also bound, at a site adjacent to the ATP site. The substituted aryl B-ring makes a number of van der Waals interactions in a hydrophobic pocket. Other important interactions include one between the para-iodine of the B-ring and a backbone carbonyl of Val127 in the hinge region, and a hydrogen bond between the aryl fluoride and Ser212. There are also interactions between the polar hydroxyls and the ATP terminal phosphate and Lys97. It is suggested that binding of these types of molecules stabilizes an inactive conformation of the kinase. As predicted on the basis of their binding to an allosteric site, these compounds are highly selective for MEK1 and MEK2, and they do not inhibit other kinases or members of the same kinase family. This selectivity is likely because the inhibitors bind to a site that has little sequence homology to other kinases.

Figure 7.19 Structures of allosteric inhibitors of MEK and X-ray structure of inhibitor bound near active site. A: Structures of approved drugs trametinib and cobimetinib. B: X-ray crystal structure of MEK inhibitor PD318088 (orange) bound in allosteric site of MEK1 along with ATP (green). Key interactions include van der Waals interactions of the B-ring in a hydrophobic pocket, an interaction between the iodine of the B-ring and a backbone carbonyl of Val127 in the hinge region, a hydrogen bond between the aryl fluoride and Ser212, and interactions between the polar hydroxyls and the ATP terminal phosphate and Lys97 (Adapted from Heald RA, Jackson P, Savy P et al. [2012] *J Med Chem* 55:4594–4604. With permission from American Chemical Society.)

A: STRUCTURES OF NON-COMPETITIVE KINASE INHIBITORS

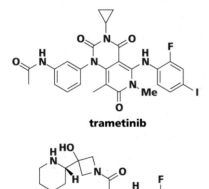

trametinib

cobimetinib

B: X-RAY CRYSTAL STRUCTURE OF MEK INHIBITOR BOUND NEAR ACTIVE SITE

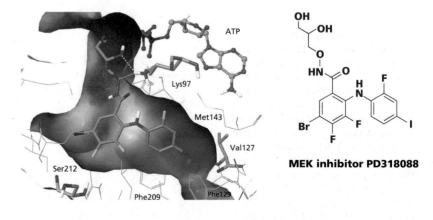

MEK inhibitor PD318088

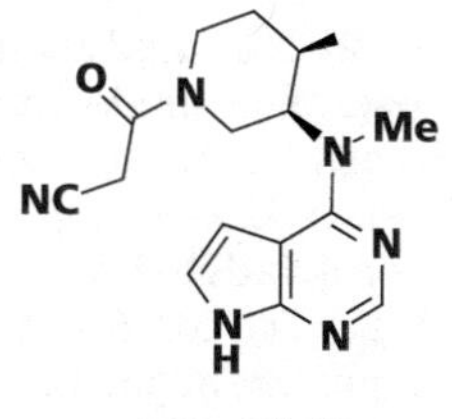

tofacitinib

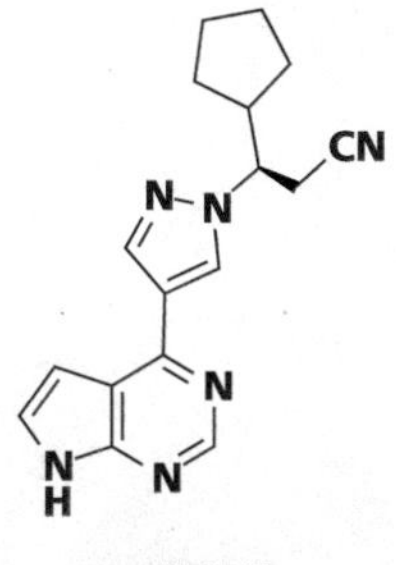

ruxolitinib

Figure 7.20 Structures of JAK inhibitors. The active site inhibitor tofacitinib is approved by the FDA for treatment of rheumatoid arthritis. Ruloxitinib, also an active site inhibitor (Class I), is approved for certain types of cancer and under investigation to treat psoriasis.

While the first kinase inhibitors found success as anti-tumor drugs, more recently several kinase inhibitors have also been approved to treat immunological disorders such as rheumatoid arthritis (RA). These target intracellular kinases such as the Janus kinases (JAK) and spleen tyrosine kinases (SYK). The Janus kinases are part of the JAK-STAT signaling pathway, which is involved in regulation of the immune system, with some mutant forms involved in certain types of cancer. JAKs are tyrosine kinases that bind to and phosphorylate interleukin cytokine receptors, resulting in production of cytokines. Tofacitinib was the first JAK inhibitor to be approved by the FDA for treatment of RA. It was based on a lead that was discovered at Pfizer by high-throughput screening of a 400,000 compound library against JAK-3 kinase. Modifications led to the development of tofacitinib, an active site inhibitor. A second JAK inhibitor, ruxolitinib, which is a Class I inhibitor, was developed by Incyte and Novartis and received approval in 2011 to treat myelofibrosis, a bone marrow cancer (**Figure 7.20**). It is also under investigation for the treatment of psoriasis.

The kinase inhibitors are excellent examples of combining screening, particularly focused screening, with structure-based design in order to optimize drug candidates. The availability of numerous X-ray structures of various kinases bound to inhibitors, as well as the ability to characterize their modes of inhibition, allows rapid progress in improving their biological, pharmaceutical, and physical properties. Kinase inhibitors, active-site as well as allosteric inhibitors, will continue to be an active area of research. While no drugs yet work via activating a kinase, several have reached clinical trials, and that area is also likely to see more progress in the future.

PROTEASES AND PROTEASE INHIBITORS

Proteases catalyze the hydrolysis of an amide bond in a highly controlled and regulated manner. Like kinases, they are ubiquitous in the body and are involved in numerous physiological processes such as digestion, blood coagulation, catabolism, apoptosis, and regulation of signaling. Their overactivity or misactivity is associated with disease states, making them frequent drug discovery targets. In addition, infectious agents such as bacteria, viruses, and parasites also rely on proteases for their replication. Drugs that target these proteases, such as antibacterial β-lactam compounds and antiviral HIV protease inhibitors, have found widespread use.

At neutral pH, the amide bond is highly stable, with a half-life in water estimated at up to 1000 years. This stability ensures the fidelity of peptides and proteins essential for normal physiological processes. However, when essential for a particular physiological process, proteases catalyze the cleavage of specific amide bonds in a peptide or protein. By convention, the bond that a protease cleaves is termed the **scissile bond**. Amino acid residues at the N-terminal side are numbered P1, P2, P3, etc., moving away from the site of reaction, and amino acid residues at the C-terminal side are numbered P1′, P2′, P3′, etc. (**Figure 7.21**). These correspond to binding sites S1–S3, etc. and S1′–S3′ etc. on the enzyme. Proteases can be highly specific or very general. For example, exopeptidases cleave a terminal amino acid, regardless of its identity; the serine protease chymotrypsin is selective for cleavage of any peptide bond that contains an aromatic amino acid (phenylalanine, tyrosine, or tryptophan) or large hydrophobic amino acid (such as methionine) at the P1 site. In contrast, the highly specific HIV protease recognizes eight specific amino acids in its substrate.

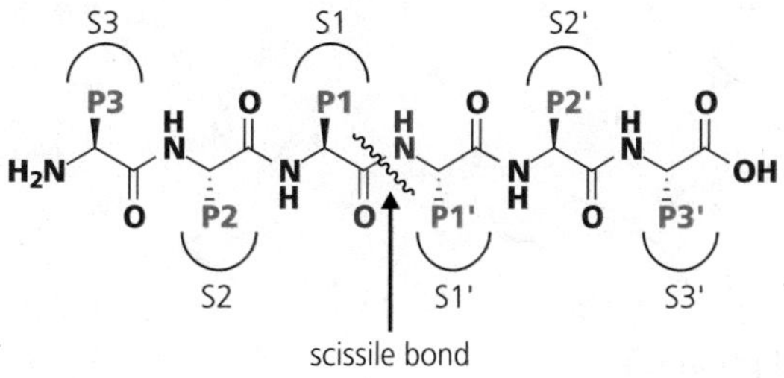

Figure 7.21 Protease substrate nomenclature and conventions. The amide bond that is cleaved by a protease is termed the scissile bond (red). For a six amino acid peptide cleaved by a protease, the three amino acids at the N-terminal are named P1–P3; and P1′–P3′ at the C-terminal. These correspond to S1–S3 and S1′–S3′ sites on the enzyme, respectively.

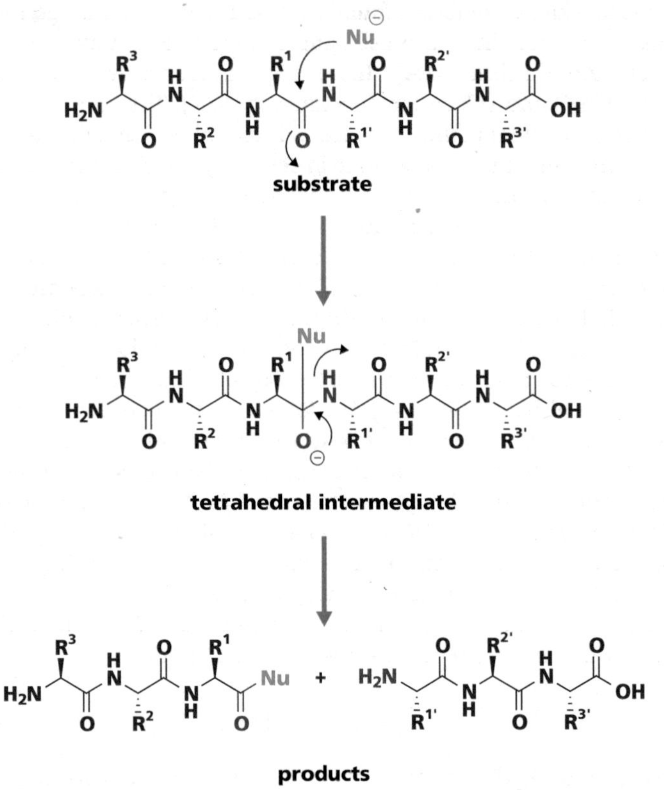

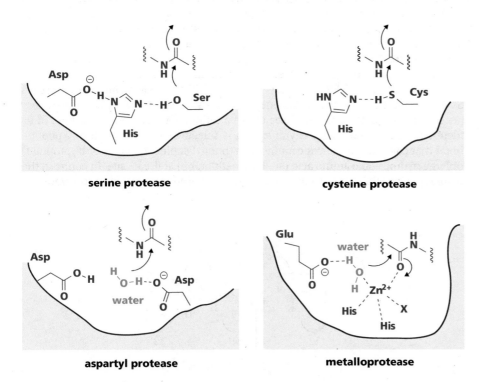

Figure 7.22 Abbreviated mechanism for hydrolysis of an amide bond in a peptide by a protease. Addition of the nucleophile (Nu⁻, blue) to a specific amide carbonyl leads to a tetrahedral intermediate, which collapses to give two smaller peptide fragments, the nucleophile being incorporated into the N-terminal fragment. The scissile bond is shown in red.

A very general mechanism for the protease reaction is shown in **Figure 7.22**. A nucleophile (Nu⁻) attacks the carbonyl group of the amide and generates a tetrahedral intermediate. Collapse of the intermediate generates two peptide fragments, one containing the newly formed acyl-nucleophile.

Proteases are classified according to their reaction mechanism, and their active sites are highly conserved. Serine and cysteine proteases (**Figure 7.23**) are similar in that the nucleophile is a serine or cysteine residue found at the protease's active site.

Figure 7.23 Active sites of serine, cysteine, aspartyl, and zinc metalloproteases (substrate in red). In a serine protease active site, acid–base catalysis, mediated by Asp and His residues activates a serine side chain, which acts as a nucleophile and reacts with the peptide carbonyl (shown in red). Cysteine proteases act by a related mechanism and rely on a histidine residue to activate a cysteine residue to accelerate reaction with the substrate carbonyl. Aspartyl proteases use two aspartates to deprotonate a water molecule in the active site, which then adds to the substrate. Metalloproteases use a metal to coordinate to the carbonyl of the substrate as well as to an activated water molecule in the active site; this nucleophile then reacts with the peptide carbonyl.

In these cases, as seen in the mechanism shown in Figure 7.22, the first products are the newly formed amine and an acyl-enzyme product, which is rapidly hydrolyzed in a second step to generate the carboxylic acid fragment and regenerate the enzyme. Key residues at the active site (Asp and His in the case of serine proteases, His in the case of cysteine proteases) are involved in acid–base catalysis to activate the nucleophile (serine and cysteine residue, respectively) by deprotonation. Aspartyl proteases and metalloproteases use water as the nucleophile (Nu = OH in Figure 7.22) and generate the amino and carboxyl fragments directly. Aspartyl proteases are characterized by the presence of two aspartic acid residues at the active site that act as general acid–base catalysts to deprotonate a water molecule. Metalloproteases contain a conserved metal cation (usually Zn^{2+}) that can serve as a Lewis acid to activate the water nucleophile and/or amide carbonyl as well as stabilize various intermediates via metal ion catalysis.

7.5   Protease inhibitors are designed on the basis of the enzyme's mechanism of action and are useful for treating HIV and bacterial infections as well as cardiovascular disease

Drug design targeting proteases relies on understanding the mechanism of action of the specific protease of interest. For example, drugs that inhibit **aspartyl proteases** often mimic the tetrahedral intermediate of the enzyme substrate, as described in Chapter 5. These include a series of HIV protease inhibitors such as darunavir, lopinavir, saquinavir, and indinavir (**Figure 7.24**). The HIV protease is an essential enzyme that is required for maturation of the human immunodeficiency virus and its replication. It cleaves at very specific sites that are unique to HIV, including one that contains Phe-Pro at the scissile site. In these examples, a substrate-like peptidic molecule was used as a starting point, and the scissile bond was replaced with various transition-state mimetics, such as hydroxyethylene. Further optimization, remote from the transition-state mimetic, led to the final drugs. Some of the structures in Figure 7.24, particularly saquinavir and indinavir, still bear some resemblance to the original Phe-Pro peptide starting point. Chapter 11, on antiviral agents, will describe these compounds in more detail.

Drugs targeting **serine/threonine proteases** include the penicillins and other β-lactam antibacterial compounds, which will be discussed further in Chapter 12, as well as the proteasome inhibitors described in Chapter 10. Like other protease inhibitors, the molecules mimic the natural substrate; however, they contain a **warhead**, an electrophilic moiety that reacts with the active-site nucleophile (serine/threonine hydroxyl) and prevents the hydrolysis step in the enzymatic reaction. In

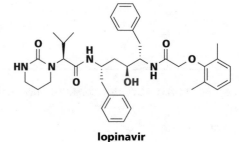

Figure 7.24 Structures of HIV protease inhibitors. Transition-state mimetics found in the HIV drugs darunavir, lopinavir, saquinavir and indinavir are shown in red; vestiges of the original substrate containing Phe-Pro at the scissile bond evident in saquinavir and indinavir are shown in blue.

darunavir

lopinavir

saquinavir

indinavir

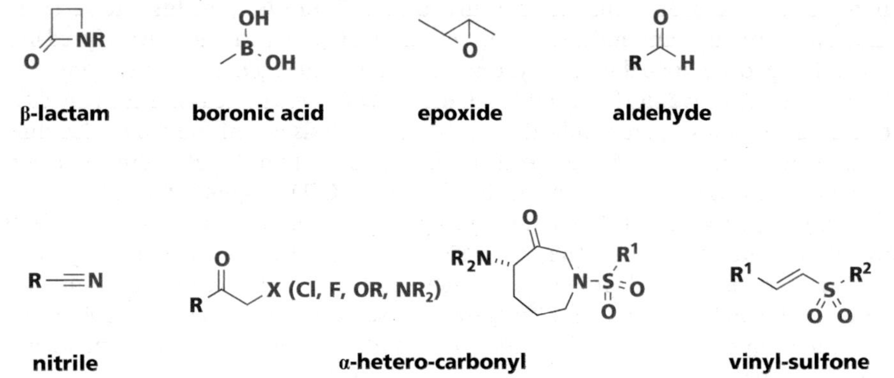

Figure 7.25 Examples of electrophilic warheads (shown in red) incorporated into serine/threonine and cysteine protease inhibitors. All of the functional groups shown are electrophilic warheads that will react with a nucleophilic hydroxyl or thiol found in serine/threonine proteases and cysteine proteases, respectively.

contrast to aspartyl protease inhibitors, most serine/threonine protease inhibitors that act at the active site make a covalent bond to the enzyme. Some of these covalent bonds are reversible (slow tight-binding inhibitors), but most are irreversible. While few approved drugs target **cysteine proteases**, strategies to inhibit them are similar to those used to design drugs to inhibit serine/threonine proteases and include the introduction of a warhead into a substrate-like molecule. Examples of warheads known or reported to generate effective inhibitors include β-lactams, boronic acids, epoxides, aldehydes, nitriles, α-heteroatom carbonyls, and vinyl sulfones (**Figure 7.25**).

Figure 7.26A shows the reaction of penicillin-binding protein (PBP), a serine protease, with its natural substrate, the D-Ala-D-Ala terminus of a peptidoglycan strand in bacterial cell walls. In the presence of penicillin, which contains a reactive β-lactam warhead (**Figure 7.26B**), the active-site serine attacks the electrophilic carbonyl to generate a chemically modified and therefore inhibited protein, thus stopping cell wall biosynthesis. These are covalent irreversible inhibitors.

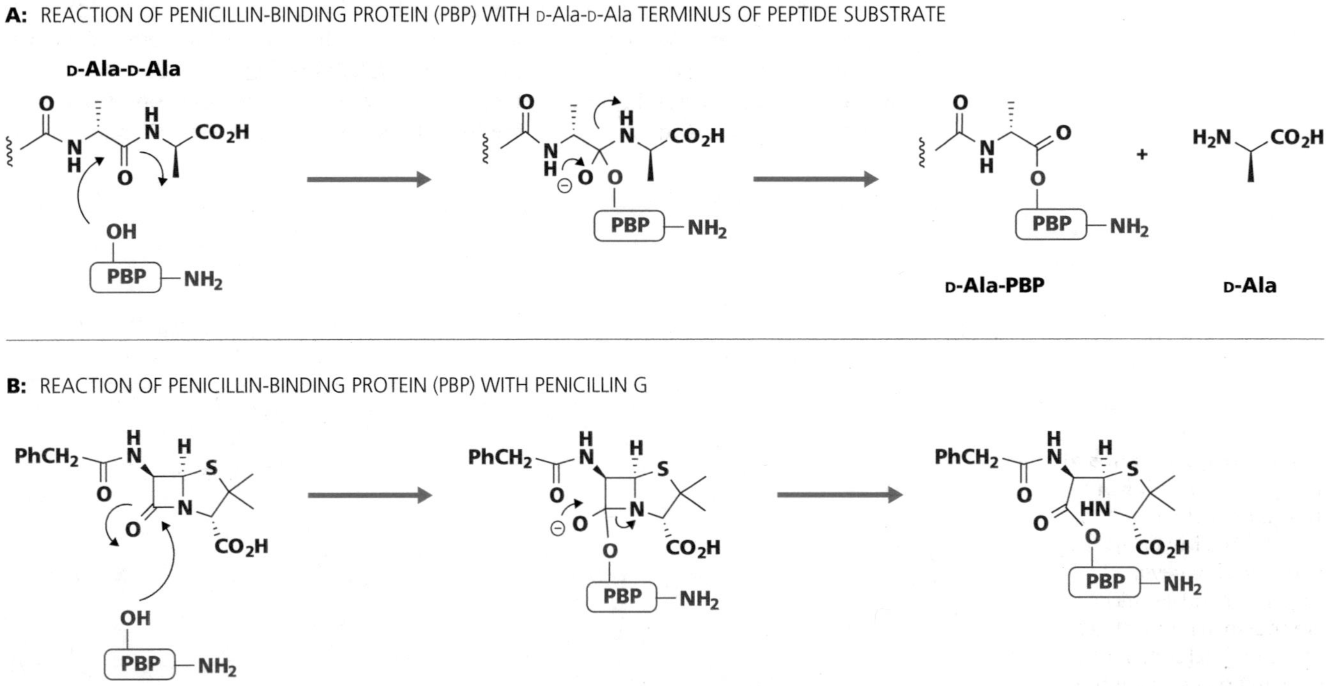

A: REACTION OF PENICILLIN-BINDING PROTEIN (PBP) WITH D-Ala-D-Ala TERMINUS OF PEPTIDE SUBSTRATE

B: REACTION OF PENICILLIN-BINDING PROTEIN (PBP) WITH PENICILLIN G

Figure 7.26 Reactions of penicillin-binding protein. A: Reaction of the serine hydroxyl of penicillin-binding protein (PBP, shown in red) with natural substrate, peptidoglycan terminated in D-Ala-D-Ala. B: Reaction of penicillin-binding protein with penicillin G at the β-lactam carbonyl generates an acylated, inactivated PBP.

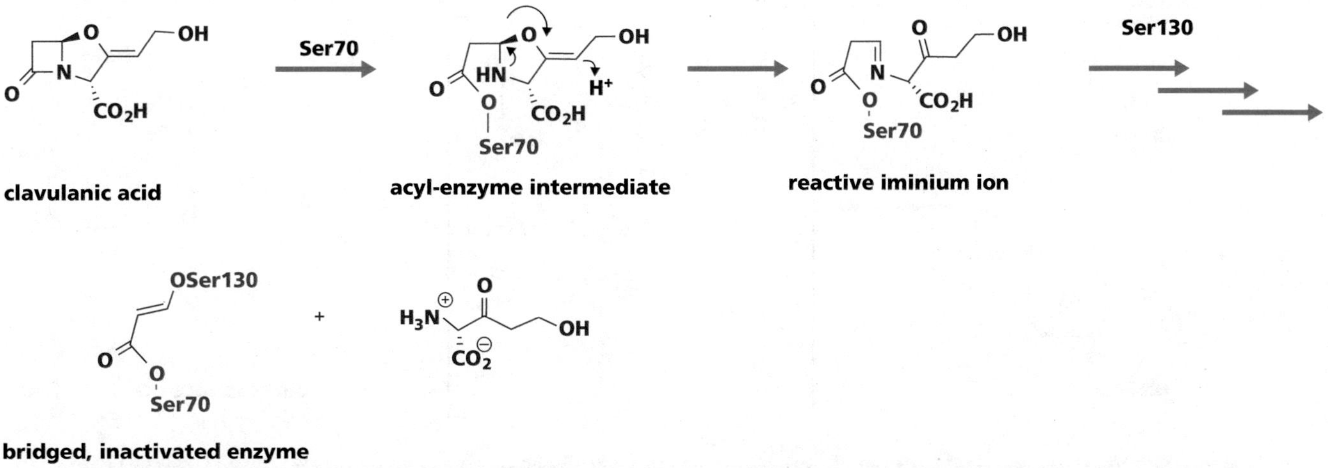

clavulanic acid   acyl-enzyme intermediate   reactive iminium ion

bridged, inactivated enzyme

Figure 7.27 Mechanism of inhibition of β-lactamase by the suicide inhibitor clavulanic acid. Ser70 of β-lactamase adds to the carbonyl in the β-lactam, and the four-membered ring opens, generating an acyl enzyme intermediate. The unstable five-membered ring then opens to give an imine. The imine reacts further with the β-lactamase Ser130, forming a second covalent bond to the enzyme to give a bridged, inactivated enzyme.

Clavulanic acid is another serine protease inhibitor that incorporates the same β-lactam warhead; however, once acted upon by its target, further reaction makes this compound an example of a suicide inhibitor. This natural product does not have antibacterial activity, but it reacts with the penicillin-destroying β-lactamase enzymes. These are serine proteases that evolved from the PBPs as a resistance mechanism towards penicillins, and their substrates are β-lactams. The initial reaction of clavulanic acid with β-lactamases involves addition of a serine hydroxyl (Ser70) to the β-lactam carbonyl of clavulanic acid, followed by ring opening, as in the penicillin mechanism (Figure 7.27). The resultant acyl-enzyme intermediate is unstable and opens to form an imine, the reactive intermediate of a suicide inhibitor. The imine reacts with a second serine (Ser130) in β-lactamase to ultimately give a bridged, inactivated enzyme.

Metalloprotease inhibitors take advantage of not only the structure of the substrate but also the presence of a metal cation at the active site to anchor binding. Inhibitors of angiotensin-converting enzyme (ACE) such as captopril (see Case Study 2 in this chapter) and lisinopril are examples of metalloprotease inhibitors (Figure 7.28). In these cases, the thiol of captopril and the central carboxylic acid of lisinopril bind to zinc in the active site. Other zinc-binding moieties frequently incorporated include hydroxamic acids, phosphonates, and hydantoins, among others.

Overall, inhibition of proteases has been a very successful strategy in drug design, beginning with the introduction of β-lactam antibiotics. The examples included in this chapter cover a few classes of protease inhibitors, but there are many other drugs that work through this mechanism. In many of the most recent examples, structure-based design has been particularly successful. For example, the success of HIV protease inhibitors in treating AIDS led to the investigation of other proteases unique to viruses. This has recently come to fruition with the approval of HCV NS3 protease inhibitors to treat hepatitis C (see Chapter 11).

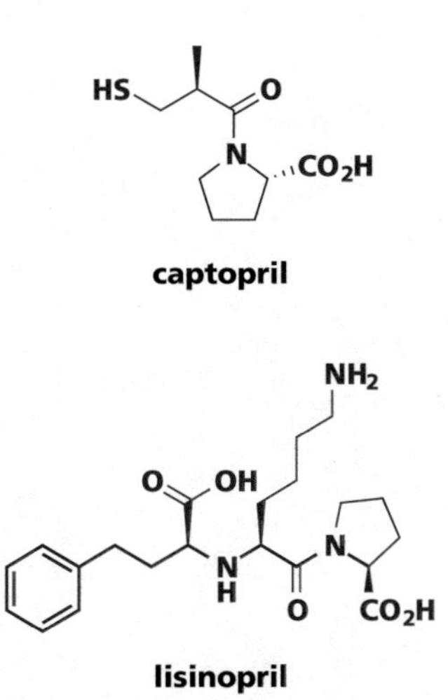

captopril

lisinopril

Figure 7.28 Structures of ACE inhibitors captopril and lisinopril. The thiol of captopril and the carboxylic acid of lisinopril bind to a zinc ion in the active site of the metalloprotease enzyme.

POLYMERASES AND POLYMERASE INHIBITORS

Polymerases are enzymes that catalyze the formation of a phosphodiester bond between two nucleotides, adding the 5′-end of one nucleotide to the 3′-end of a DNA (or RNA) strand, thus elongating the strand (Figure 7.29) and releasing diphosphate. Through a highly complex mechanism involving numerous other enzymes such as topoisomerase, integrase, and helicase, polymerases are essential for nucleic acid replication. Humans use DNA polymerases to replicate and repair DNA, and these as well as other accompanying enzymes are often targets for anti-cancer therapies.

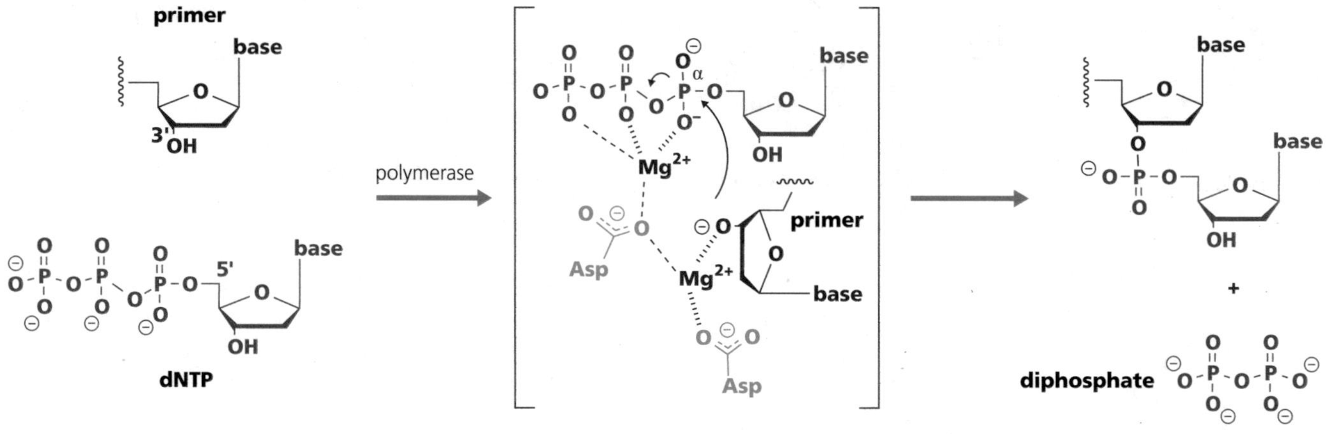

Figure 7.29 Polymerase-catalyzed reaction to form a phosphodiester bond. The phosphodiester bond is formed between a 3′-OH on the primer strand and the α-phosphate of an incoming deoxynucleoside triphosphate to extend the primer strand by one nucleotide. Abbreviated mechanism: a template strand (not shown) directs the identity of the base on the incoming deoxynucleoside triphosphate (dNTP, red) through Watson–Crick base pairing. Two magnesium cations (Mg^{2+}) at the active site coordinate to the incoming triphosphate, the reacting 3′-OH group on the primer terminal (black), and aspartates in the enzyme (blue). Nucleophilic attack of the 3′-O$^-$ on the α-phosphate, followed by release of diphosphate, extends the primer chain by one nucleotide.

Similarly, infectious organisms require polymerase-like enzymes for their replication, and inhibition of these enzymes has been a highly successful therapeutic approach.

Polymerases work through a complex mechanism, abbreviated in Figure 7.29. A template strand of DNA (not shown) serves to direct which of the four nucleoside triphosphates is accepted through Watson–Crick base pairing. The two substrates in the reaction are a primer strand of DNA, which is eventually elongated, and the incoming nucleoside triphosphate (red). Divalent cations (usually magnesium) are also required at the active site; they coordinate with aspartates in the active (blue) and bind to both substrates in order to active them. Formation of the new phosphodiester bond is accompanied by release of diphosphate.

7.6   Inhibitors of polymerases can mimic the substrate or bind at an allosteric site

Drug design for inhibition of RNA and DNA polymerases or their analog, reverse transcriptase used by RNA viruses to make DNA from RNA, has taken a slightly different tack than relying on the characteristics of the active site and preventing substrate binding. In the most successful examples, inhibitors of the HIV reverse transcriptase are **chain terminators** (or **antimetabolites**). A nucleoside-like triphosphate molecule, competing with the natural substrate, is accepted as a substrate of the enzyme and incorporated into the growing nucleic acid chain. The inhibitor, however, does not contain the 3′-hydroxyl group that is required for further elongation, and therefore the growing nucleic acid chain is terminated, effectively inhibiting further activity of the enzyme (Figure 7.30).

Examples of nucleoside reverse transcriptase inhibitors (NRTIs) that inhibit HIV reverse transcriptase through a chain termination mechanism include abacavir, emtricitabine (2′-deoxy-5-fluoro-3′-thiacytidine, FTC), and azidothymidine (AZT), among others (Figure 7.31). All require initial reaction with kinases to form the corresponding triphosphate at the 5′-hydroxyl group, which is the actual enzyme substrate, such as AZT triphosphate. Similar classes of viral polymerase inhibitors, which are nucleoside analogs requiring prior activation to the triphosphate, have been developed for other viruses such as hepatitis C. These will be described in further detail in Chapter 11 on antiviral agents.

A: INCORPORATION OF 2'-DEOXYNUCLEOSIDE TRIPHOSPHATES (dNTPs) INTO GROWING DNA STRAND

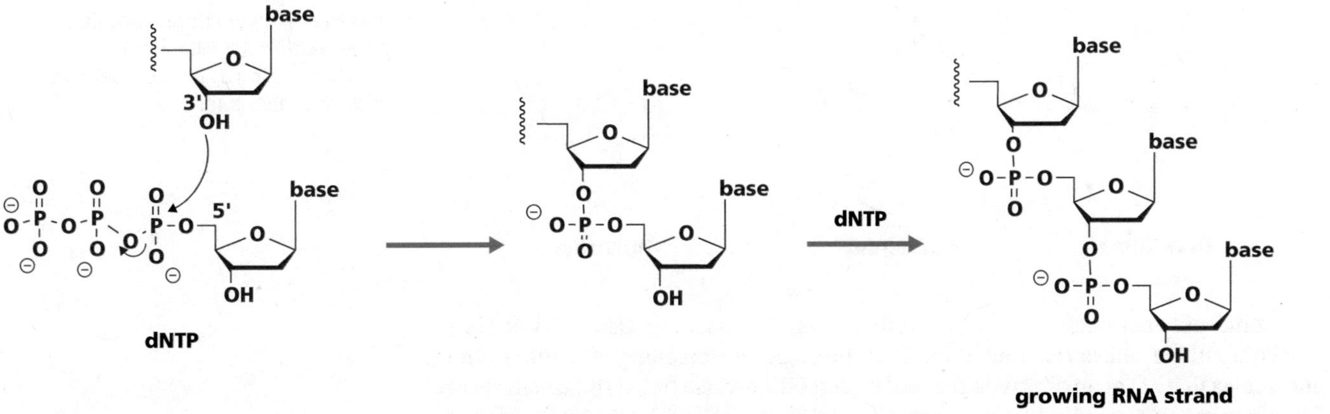

B: CHAIN TERMINATION BY INCORPORATION OF NUCLEOSIDE TRIPHOSPHATE INHIBITOR WITH 3' POSITION BLOCKED

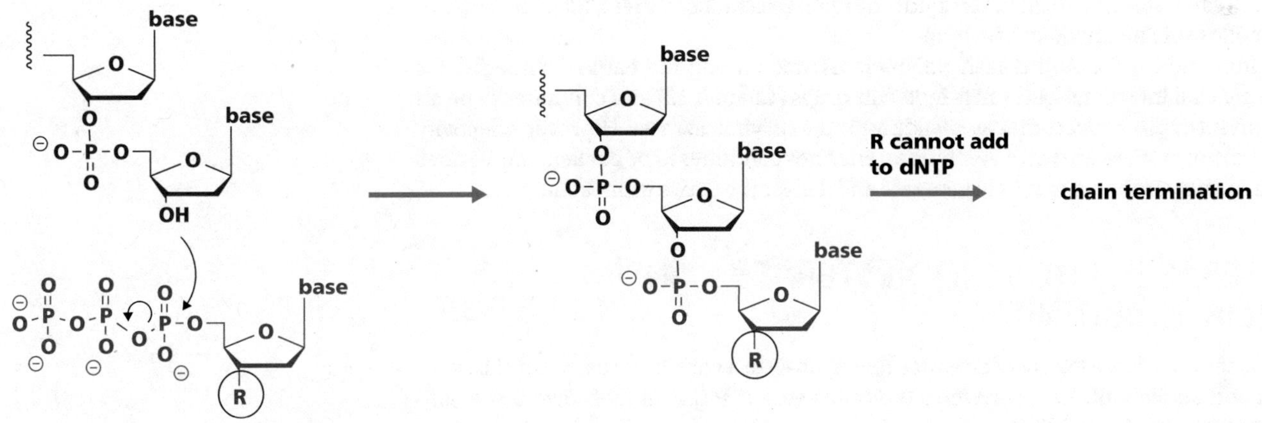

triphosphate of nucleoside inhibitor
(R = H or non-hydroxyl group)

Figure 7.30 Chain termination mechanism, showing incorporation of a nucleoside reverse transcriptase inhibitor (NRTI) into a growing DNA strand. A: The typical process of chain elongation occurs by addition of a 3'-hydroxyl to a 5'-triphosphate. B: Chain terminators work by incorporation of a triphosphate of a nucleoside inhibitor (red) lacking a 3'-hydroxyl group; after its incorporation, chain elongation cannot proceed.

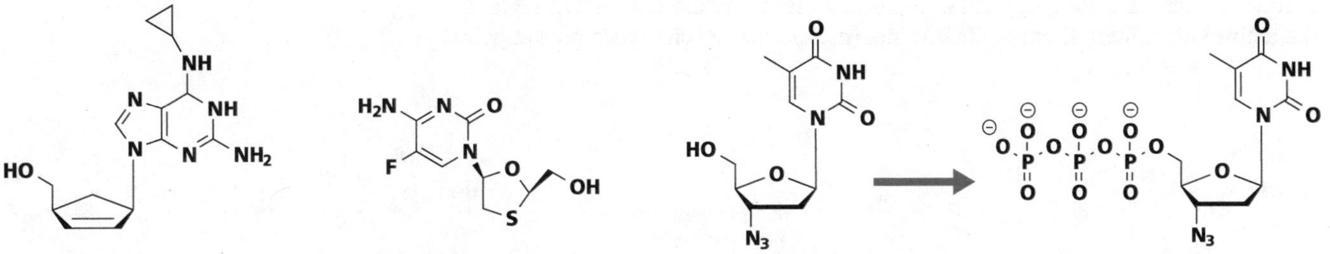

abacavir   emtricitabine   AZT   AZT triphosphate

Figure 7.31 Structures of HIV drugs abacavir, emtricitabine, and AZT. These anti- HIV drugs are converted to the corresponding triphosphates, such as AZT triphosphate, and are substrates for HIV reverse transcriptase; they then act via a chain termination mechanism.

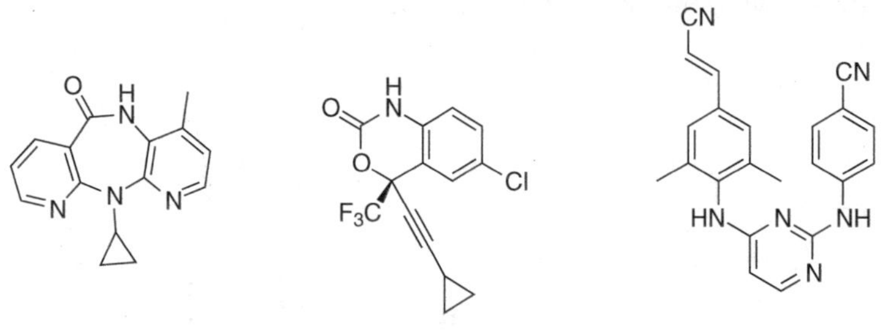

nevirapine   **efavirenz**   **rilpivirine**

Figure 7.32 Structures of nevirapine, efavirenz, and rilpivirine. These anti-HIV drugs are nonnucleoside reverse transcriptase inhibitors (NNRTIs), acting as noncompetitive allosteric inhibitors.

Some polymerases, such as HIV reverse transcriptase, are also susceptible to noncompetitive allosteric inhibition. High-throughput screening identified small molecules that act at an allosteric site and inhibit HIV reverse transcriptase; these are known as nonnucleoside reverse transcriptase inhibitors (NNRTIs). Compounds such as nevirapine, efavirenz, and rilpivirine are noncompetitive inhibitors (Figure 7.32). They bind to a site about 10 Å away from the active site and force a conformational change of the enzyme, making it incompetent for enzymatic activity. Patients (and cells) treated solely with NNRTIs rapidly develop resistance to them, likely because of their allosteric mechanism of action.

Inhibition of DNA and RNA polymerases was among the earliest strategies for treating viral infections with small-molecule drugs (Chapter 12) and continues to be an important approach, in some cases leading to cures of viral diseases. However, selectivity for viral polymerase enzymes over human enzymes continues to be challenging, as does finding an appropriate means to generate and deliver the active triphosphate.

ESTERASES, PHOSPHODIESTERASES, AND THEIR INHIBITORS

Esterases are a large family of enzymes that hydrolyze a carboxylic ester bond into an acid and an alcohol. These enzymes typically contain serine at their active site, and the mechanism is very similar to that of a serine protease. Acetylcholinesterase (see Figure 7.2) is an example of a therapeutically important esterase enzyme. Inhibitors of acetylcholinesterase are used to treat Alzheimer's disease and will be discussed in Chapter 13.

Phosphodiesterases (PDEs) catalyze cleavage of phosphodiester bonds and fall into several categories. Exonucleases and endonucleases cleave phosphodiester linkages on polynucleotide strands of DNA and RNA. However, for therapeutic strategies, the most important class is the cyclic nucleotide PDEs that cleave cAMP or cGMP (Figure 7.33).

The active site of these PDEs has both a nucleotide recognition pocket (structurally unique in each PDE subtype) and a hydrolysis site. There are designated regions in the active site; among them are the M site (metal ions), Q site (core pocket, which

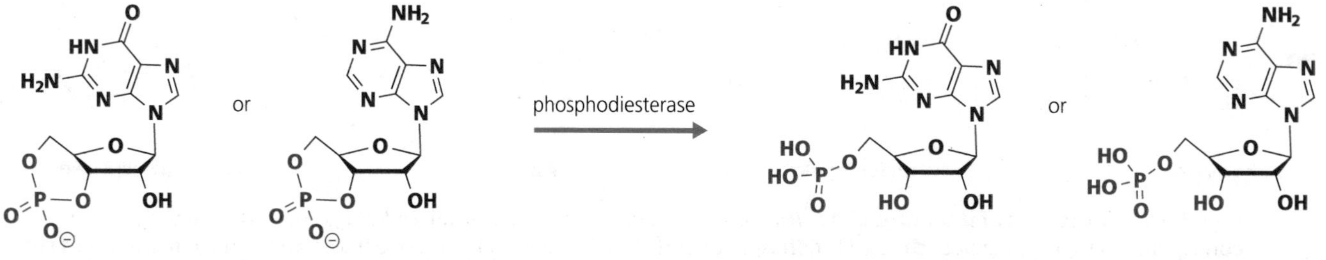

cGMP   **cAMP**   phosphodiesterase   **GMP**   **AMP**

Figure 7.33 Hydrolysis of cGMP or cAMP catalyzed by phosphodiesterase. Phosphodiesterase enzymes generate monophosphates (GMP and AMP) from phosphodiesterases, cGMP and cAMP. The phosphodiester group is shown in red.

likely binds the cyclic nucleotide substrate), and the H site (hydrophobic pocket). The orientation of a specific glutamine (Q453 in **Figure 7.34A**), which forms hydrogen bonds to the purine, is involved in determining whether the PDE is selective for cGMP or cAMP. A mechanism for hydrolysis has been elucidated from X-ray crystal structures, as shown in **Figure 7.34B** for PDE9.

During hydrolysis, two metal ions (M1 and M2) coordinate to a water molecule, deprotonating it (W0), and they also form a complex with the phosphodiester while the activated nucleophilic hydroxide adds to the phosphorus atom in the phosphodiester group. Both Glu423 (E423) and His252 (H252) are involved in acid–base catalysis. A pentavalent enzyme · substrate complex forms, which proceeds to the tetravalent enzyme · product complex upon cleavage of the 3′-O–P bond. Addition of water hydrolyzes the complex to give GMP. During catalysis, a hydrophobic clamp in the H region, composed of Phe and Leu residues, interacts with the nucleobase of the substrate, and the amide of a conserved glutamine (Q453) forms hydrogen bonds to either adenine or guanine.

A: STEREODIAGRAM OF X-RAY STRUCTURE OF PDE9 (GREEN) COMPLEXED WITH cGMP (PURPLE)

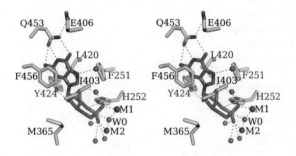

B: MECHANISM OF HYDROLYSIS OF cGMP IN ENZYME ACTIVE SITE

Figure 7.34 X-ray structure of cGMP in the active site of PDE9. A: Stereodiagram of X-ray structure of PDE9 (green) complexed with cGMP (purple). M1 (Zn^{2+}) and M2 (Mg^{2+}) form a complex with a water molecule (W0) in the hydrolysis center; Q453 recognizes the guanine nucleobase . B: Hydrolysis mechanism showing acid–base catalysis by Glu423, His252, and water (shown as OH$^-$) complexed to metal ions M1 and M2 in the M-site. The metal ions form a complex with the cyclic phosphate and deliver the nucleophilic water to give the E · S complex; cleavage of the 3′-O–P bond gives the E · P complex; and addition of water affords the hydrolyzed GMP. Gln453 forms H-bonds with the nucleobase, and Phe456 and Leu420 residues in the H-site, among others, engage in hydrophobic interactions with it. (From Liu S, Mansour MN, Dillman KS et al. [2008] *Proc Natl Acad Sci USA* 105:13309–13314. With permission from National Academy of Sciences.)

There are 11 subtypes of cyclic nucleotide PDEs, some of which cleave both cAMP and cGMP and some of which are selective. Phosphodiesterases 4, 7, and 8 are selective for cAMP, while PDEs 6 and 9 are selective for cGMP. Since cAMP and cGMP are important second messengers and have many roles in physiological processes, increasing their levels by inhibiting their degradation via PDE inhibition can have profound effects.

7.7 Inhibitors of phosphodiesterases treat cardiovascular disease, respiratory disease, and erectile dysfunction

Drug discovery targeting PDEs has focused on subtype selectivity, since global inhibition would generate numerous undesirable side effects. Selective PDE inhibitors are used to treat heart failure (PDE3), chronic obstructive pulmonary disease (COPD) (PDE4), and erectile dysfunction (PDE5). PDE inhibitors were found in the 1970s by phenotypic screening campaigns searching for compounds that increased heart muscle contraction, as an improvement over the cardiac glycosides digoxin and digoxigenin (see Chapter 1). At that time, diuretics and cardiac glycosides were the first line therapy used to treat heart failure, in spite of their very narrow therapeutic index. Scientists at Sterling-Winthrop initiated a search for alternatives and phenotypic screening for positive inotropic activity (increasing heart muscle contraction) identified bipyridines as promising hits. Amrinone (now called inamrinone) was effective in increasing heart contraction and had no adverse effects in animal studies (**Figure 7.35**).

At the time of its discovery (1978), amrinone's mechanism of action was unknown, but several years later it was found to be a selective PDE3 inhibitor. Inhibition of PDE3, which is found in cardiac muscle, results in an increase of intracellular cAMP levels. This effect then results in increased intracellular calcium levels, which promotes contraction of cardiac muscle and vasodilation of vascular smooth muscle.

Later clinical trials of inamrinone revealed side effects such as thrombocytopenia, fever, and anemia after long-term use. Analogs such as milrinone have fewer side effects. A number of other analogs have been investigated and led to drugs such as enoximone, as well as the pyridazinones meribendan and pimobendan, which are all competitive reversible inhibitors. A pharmacophore model (Figure 7.35), proposed in the 1980s, has a dipolar region, corresponding to the carbonyl of active compounds,

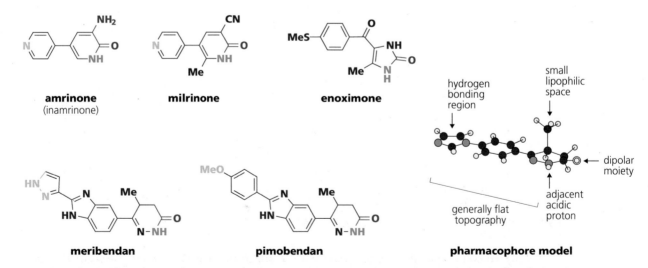

Figure 7.35 Structures of PDE3 inhibitors with pharmacophore model. Structures of amrinone, milrinone, enoximone, meribendan, and pimobendan are depicted. The pharmacophore model contains a dipolar region, corresponding to the carbonyl of active compounds, with an adjacent acidic proton, corresponding to the amide N-H. In the model, there is an area for a small lipophilic group (occupied by methyl groups in meribendan and pimobendan) and a planar-like linker joins these features to a hydrogen-bonding region. Common dipolar regions of drugs are shown in red, acidic proton is in blue, and hydrogen-bonding (or S-bonding) regions are shown in green. (From Bristol JA, Sircar I, Moos WH et al. [1984] *J Med Chem* 27:1099–1101. With permission from American Chemical Society.)

with an adjacent acidic proton. There is also a small lipophilic area; these are linked to a hydrogen-bonding (or S-bonding region) through a mostly planar surface. All of these features are found in the more recent PDE3 inhibitors.

Inhibitors of PDE4, primarily expressed in inflammatory and immune cells, have been developed to treat chronic obstructive pulmonary disease (COPD), a disease that affects over 200 million people. Asthma also affects another 300 million, and together these diseases are an enormous burden on the health care system. The natural product theophylline (found in cocoa beans) (**Figure 7.36**) has been used to treat asthma since the 1920s. It is a nonselective PDE inhibitor, with additional activity as an adenosine receptor antagonist. Its side effects include increased heart contractions and blood pressure, as well as nausea. Newer selective PDE4 inhibitors were based on the compound rolipram, originally investigated at Schering Plough as an antidepressant on the basis of its downstream effect of reducing levels of cAMP in the brain. Rolipram was later found to be a selective PDE4 inhibitor, and analogs such as piclamilast and roflumilast (see Figure 7.36A) were developed to treat COPD.

The development of rolipram was discontinued during its clinical trials due to adverse effects such as nausea and vomiting. According to a docking model, rolipram binds in the active site of PDE4, as seen in Figure 7.36B. Multiple H-bonds in the binding model include ones between the pyrrolidinone carbonyl and the hydroxyl

A: STRUCTURES OF PDE4 INHIBITORS

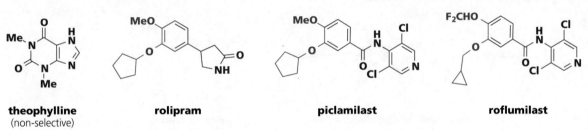

| theophylline (non-selective) | rolipram | piclamilast | roflumilast |

B: MODEL OF ROLIPRAM (BLUE) BOUND IN PDE4 ACTIVE SITE

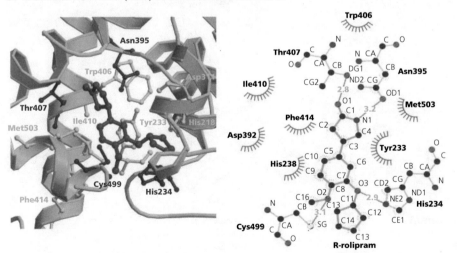

LEFT:

red = side chains that form hydrogen bonds
green = side chains that may form hydrophobic interactions

RIGHT:

schematic of interactions

Figure 7.36 Structures of PDE4 inhibitors and model of binding. A: Structures of theophylline (nonselective inhibitor) and the selective inhibitors rolipram, piclamilast, and roflumilast (dialkoxy catechol in red). B: Left: Model of selective PDE4 inhibitor rolipram bound in PDE4 active site. Key interactions include H-bonds from pyrrolidinone carbonyl to Thr407 hydroxyl, pyrrolidinone nitrogen to Asn395, methoxy oxygen to Cys499, and cyclopentyl ether oxygen to His234 (residues that participate in H-bonds in red); hydrophobic interactions include Tyr233, Phe414, and His238 with the core of rolipram (residues participating in hydrophobic interactions in green. Right: Schematic of specific interactions: rolipram in blue, H-bonding residues in yellow and hydrophobic residues in red. (From Dym O, Xenarios I, Ke H & Colicelli J [2002] *Mol Pharmacol* 61:20–25. With permission from American Society for Pharmacology and Experimental Therapeutics.)

group of Thr407, the pyrrolidinone nitrogen and Asn395, the methoxy oxygen and Cys499, and the cyclopentyl ether oxygen and His234. The core of rolipram can make hydrophobic interactions with Tyr233, Phe414, and His238. Rolipram also interacts with a second binding site in the enzyme (not shown), and binding to that additional site is believed to be responsible for the side effects. Later analogs maintain the important 3,4-dialkoxycatechol of rolipram, which forms two key hydrogen bonds to PDE4, but lack the pyrrolidinone. The 3,5-dichloropyridines piclamilast and roflumilast were based on replacement of the pyrrolidinone with a pyridine isostere, and while piclamilast was discontinued, roflumilast is used clinically.

Inhibitors of PDE5 were originally developed at Pfizer to treat cardiovascular disorders such as angina and hypertension. PDE5 is found in lungs, platelets, and smooth muscle, as well as in the corpus cavernosum (penile tissue). Drug discovery efforts at Pfizer were based on a report in 1975 on zaprinast, a weak and nonselective PDE inhibitor that had been prepared as an anti-allergy medicine. A number of 2-alkoxyphenyl heterocycles were investigated, with the pyrazolo[4,3-*d*]pyrimidin-7-one series showing good selectivity for PDE5. Improvement of the initial lead was based on the rationale that the heterocycle resembled the guanine base of cGMP, and therefore adding a larger group at the 3-position would occupy the pocket in PDE filled by the ribose of cGMP (**Figure 7.37**). This approach led to the 3-propyl analog

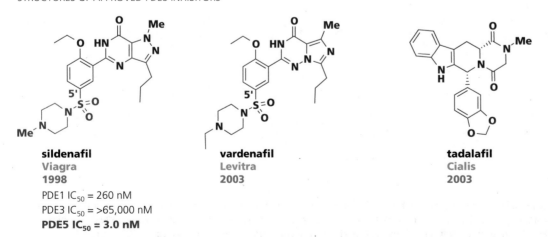

INITIAL PYRAZOLO[4,3-*d*]PYRIMIDIN-7-ONE ANALOGS OF ZAPRINAST

zaprinast
1975
(non-selective)
PDE1 IC$_{50}$ = 9400 nM
PDE3 IC$_{50}$ = >100 μM
PDE5 IC$_{50}$ = 2000 nM

pyrazolo[4,3,-*d*]pyrimidin-7-one
(sildenafil lead: selective for PDE5)
PDE1 IC$_{50}$ = 3300 nM
PDE3 IC$_{50}$ = >100 μM
PDE5 IC$_{50}$ = 330 nM

3-propyl analog
(improved potency)
PDE1 IC$_{50}$ = 790 nM
PDE3 IC$_{50}$ = >100 μM
PDE5 IC$_{50}$ = 27 nM

STRUCTURES OF APPROVED PDE5 INHIBITORS

sildenafil
Viagra
1998
PDE1 IC$_{50}$ = 260 nM
PDE3 IC$_{50}$ = >65,000 nM
PDE5 IC$_{50}$ = 3.0 nM

vardenafil
Levitra
2003

tadalafil
Cialis
2003

Figure 7.37 Lead development of sildenafil and other PDE5 inhibitors. Zaprinast, a nonselective hit, was modified, which led to the pyrazolo[4,3-*d*]pyrimidin-7-one as a more selective lead; progression to the 3-propyl analog was based on mimicking the ribose of cGMP (regions changed in each are colored red). Further modification by adding the piperazinyl sulfonamide led to sildenafil. Current PDE5 drugs include the structurally related sildenafil and vardenafil, as well as tadalafil.

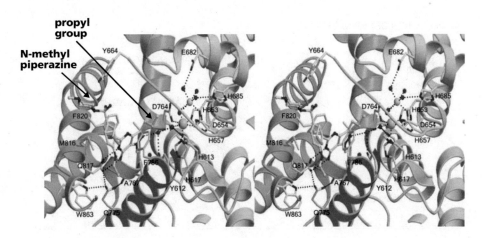

Figure 7.38 Stereodiagram of X-ray structure of sildenafil bound in PDE5. The amide within the heterocycle H-bonds to the glutamine Q817, and the propyl group sits in the same site as the ribose of cGMP. Hydrophobic interactions include Phe786 with the ethoxyphenyl and Phe820 (pi-stacking) with the heterocyclic core. Sildenafil is shown in yellow, metal ions zinc (tan) and magnesium (green) are depicted as spheres. (From Sung B-J, Hwang KY, Jeon YH et al. [2003] *Nature* 425:98–102. With permission from Macmillan Publishers Limited.)

with improved PDE5 selectivity and high binding affinity. This analog was then further modified by addition of the piperazinyl sulfonamide to afford sildenafil.

While the initial focus on this series was a search for compounds to treat angina and hypertension, their activity as a treatment for male erectile dysfunction, based on clinical observations, refocused the therapeutic use. Sildenafil received FDA approval in 1998, and later PDE5 inhibitors vardenafil and tadalafil were approved in 2003. While vardenafil is similar in structure to sildenafil, tadalafil was based on a series of hydantoin PDE5 inhibitors discovered at GlaxoSmithKline.

An X-ray structure of sildenafil bound in PDE5 is shown in **Figure 7.38**. As proposed in the design, the 3-propyl group sits in the same binding site as the ribose of cGMP. Additional interactions include binding of the *N*-methylpiperazine to Tyr664, which contributes to PDE5 selectivity, and hydrophobic interactions in the H region between the ethoxyphenyl group and Phe786, and other hydrophobic side chains. The amide of the heterocycle hydrogen-bonds to Gln817. Similar binding interactions are seen in X-ray structures of tadalafil and vardenafil and are important to maintain in the design of these competitive reversible inhibitors.

In summary, selective inhibitors of PDE are used to treat a variety of conditions. Although early drugs such as amrinone and theophylline were discovered using phenotypic assays, more recent drugs have been discovered by a combination of screening for enzyme inhibition and structure-based drug design.

OXIDOREDUCTASES, CYCLOOXYGENASES, AND INHIBITORS

Numerous enzymes catalyze oxidation and reduction reactions, and the oxidoreductase enzymes are one example. These enzymes act on diverse substrates, but the unifying feature of this family is transfer of electrons and/or hydrogens from one molecule to another. These enzymes rely on diverse mechanisms, such as oxidases that use molecular oxygen as a hydrogen or electron acceptor or dehydrogenases that transfer hydrogen from a substrate to an enzyme system. Conversely, reductases may transfer hydrogens to a substrate. These enzymes may rely on coenzymes such as dihydronicotinamide adenine dinucleotide phosphate (NADPH) or flavin adenine dinucleotide (FAD) for hydrogen transfer. For example, in the folic acid biosynthesis pathway, dihydrofolate reductase (DHFR) catalyzes the addition of two hydrogens to dihydrofolate, resulting in tetrahydrofolate, and uses NADPH as a co-factor and the source of one of the hydrogen atoms (**Figure 7.39A**). Inhibition of this pathway is important in both cancer and antibacterial chemotherapy, and will be described in later chapters.

Two other examples of oxidoreductase-catalyzed reactions are the NADPH-dependent reduction of testosterone (**Figure 7.39B**) and the oxidative aromatization of testosterone to estrogen (**Figure 7.39C**). While the 5-alpha reductase enzyme proceeds through a mechanism similar to DHFR, the aromatase enzyme is a

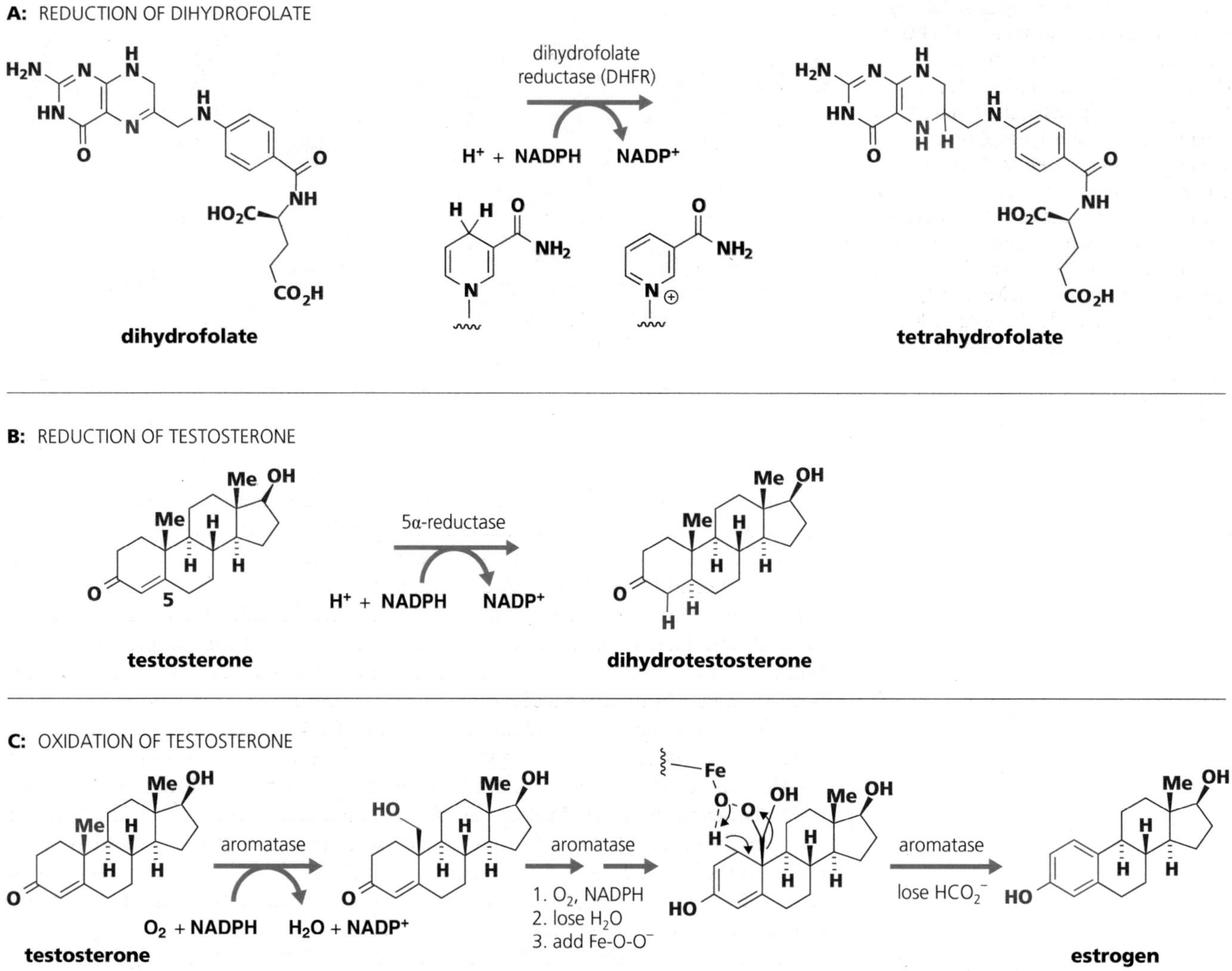

A: REDUCTION OF DIHYDROFOLATE

dihydrofolate

tetrahydrofolate

B: REDUCTION OF TESTOSTERONE

testosterone

dihydrotestosterone

C: OXIDATION OF TESTOSTERONE

testosterone

estrogen

Figure 7.39 Three examples of reactions catalyzed by oxidoreductases. A: Dihydrofolate is reduced to tetrahydrofolate by dihydrofolate reductase, by transfer of two hydrogens (red); one of which is donated by the conversion of NADPH to NADP$^+$. B: Testosterone is reduced to dihydrotestosterone by 5α-reductase, by transfer of hydrogens to C4/C5. This reaction also requires NADPH to be converted to NADP$^+$ as a source of one of the H atoms. C: Testosterone is oxidized by aromatase to estrogen in several steps, involving oxidation of a methyl group to an alcohol, further oxidation to the acetal and then to the aldehyde; this is followed by iron-catalyzed removal of hydrogen and loss of carbon dioxide.

heme-dependent cytochrome P450 that uses molecular oxygen as an oxidant in a complex five-step mechanism.

While there are many diverse therapeutic effects of inhibition of these enzymes, the diverse substrates, coenzymes, and mechanisms used by this class of enzymes make it difficult to generalize specific medicinal chemistry strategies that have been applied. Therefore, two specific examples are discussed in the following sections.

7.8   Inhibitors of HMG-CoA reductase are used to lower cholesterol levels

The early, rate-determining step in the biosynthesis of cholesterol is the conversion of 3-hydroxy-3-methylglutaryl-CoA (HMG-CoA) to mevalonate, which is in equilibrium with its cyclic form, mevalonolactone. The reduction is catalyzed by NADPH-dependent HMG-CoA reductase, which adds hydrogen atoms in two steps (**Figure 7.40**).

On the basis of evidence that buildup of cholesterol is a risk factor for cardiovascular disease, a number of organizations developed inhibitors of the rate-determining step in cholesterol biosynthesis. While a series of ester analogs of HMG-CoA were found to be weak HMG-CoA reductase inhibitors, more success was found with screening

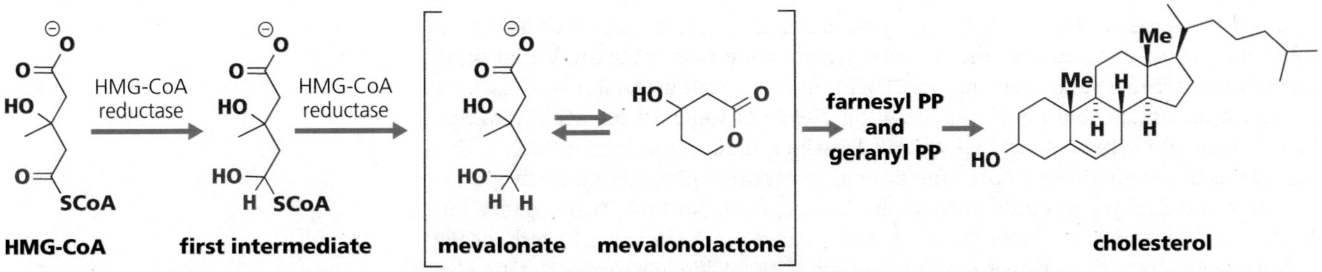

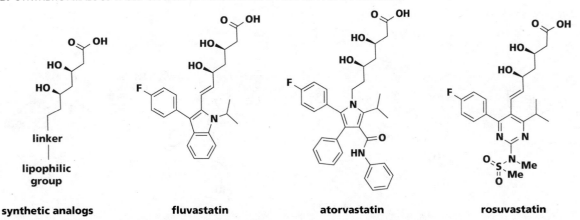

Figure 7.40 Formation of mevalonate, catalyzed by HMG-CoA reductase. This reaction is the rate-determining step in cholesterol biosynthesis. Two hydrogens are added sequentially to give mevalonate, the precursor to farnesyl pyrophosphate (PP) and geranyl PP, which are precursors to cholesterol (reaction site in red).

microbial broths, and compactin was reported by two separate groups (at Beecham Pharmaceuticals and at Sankyo Research Laboratories) in 1976 (**Figure 7.41A**). The ring-opened form of the lactone can be viewed as a transition-state analog of the first reduction step.

Researchers at Merck discovered a close structural analog, mevinolin (lovastatin), in 1978 that contained a 3α-methyl group on the bicyclic core. Both mevinolin and compactin showed excellent efficacy in lowering low-density lipoprotein (LDL) cholesterol with no apparent side effects (at low doses) and mevinolin /lovastatin

A: STRUCTURES BASED ON THE NATURAL PRODUCT COMPACTIN

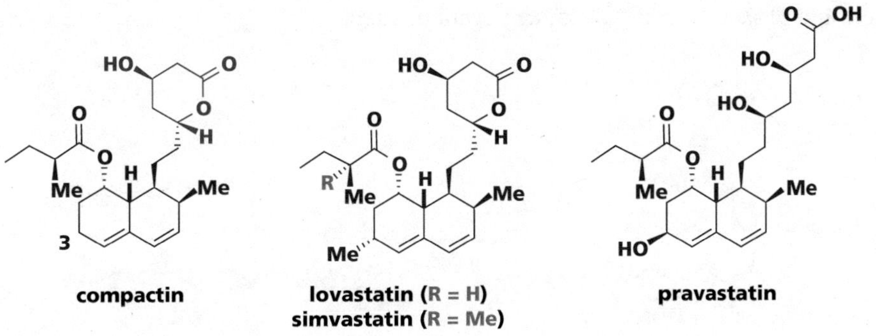

compactin

lovastatin (R = H)
simvastatin (R = Me)

pravastatin

B: SYNTHETIC ANALOGS BASED ON LINKING THE δ-HYDROXY ACID TO A LIPOPHILIC GROUP

linker

lipophilic
group

synthetic analogs

fluvastatin

atorvastatin

rosuvastatin

Figure 7.41 Structures of HMG-CoA reductase inhibitors. A: Structures of compactin, lovastatin, simvastatin and pravastatin, the structural feature in compactin that mimics the transition state when in ring-open form is shown in red. B: Model of HMG-CoA reductase inhibitors and synthetic derivatives. Fluvastatin, atorvastatin, and rosuvastatin. All can be mapped to linking a mevalonate moiety (δ-hydroxy acid) to a lipophilic group. Other common structural features include a 4-fluorophenyl group that occupies the same site as the butyric acid in compactin, a heterocycle that mimics the decalin unit in compactin, and an isopropyl group.

received FDA approval in 1987. A semisynthetic analog, simvastatin, was approved soon after, as was pravastatin, the 3-hydroxy metabolite of compactin. While these compounds, termed statins, are natural or semisynthetic products, later analogs were based on an understanding of the structural elements required for activity, which include a dihydroxyheptanoate moiety linked to a lipophilic group (**Figure 7.41B**). This model was based on a number of synthetic analogs reported in the literature by groups at Merck and Sankyo. The indole analog fluvastatin, from Novartis, was approved in 1994, and at Pfizer and Shionogi, other heterocycles were chosen as synthetically accessible linkers and a series of analogs were synthesized, leading to atorvastatin also known as Lipitor (pyrrole linker) and rosuvastatin (pyrazine linker). These synthetic compounds all have in common a dihydroxyheptanoate mimic of mevalonate, an aryl linker replacing the decalin, a small lipophilic group (isopropyl), and a 4-fluorophenyl group that is proposed to occupy the same space as the butyric ester of compactin. The statins, first introduced in 1987, are the leading treatment for reduction of LDL cholesterol. For a time, Lipitor was the top-selling drug in the United States.

7.9 Inhibitors of cyclooxygenase are effective anti-inflammatory drugs

Cyclooxygenase (COX), or prostaglandin-endoperoxide synthase (PTGS), is a heme-associated enzyme that catalyzes the conversion of the fatty acid arachidonic acid to prostaglandin H_2 (PGH_2), as shown in **Figure 7.42**.

PGH_2 is the precursor to all other prostaglandins as well as thromboxane. The prostaglandins mediate multiple physiological effects including inflammation, uterine contraction, and protection of the stomach lining. Thromboxane is derived from prostaglandins in the platelets and plays a role in platelet aggregation. There

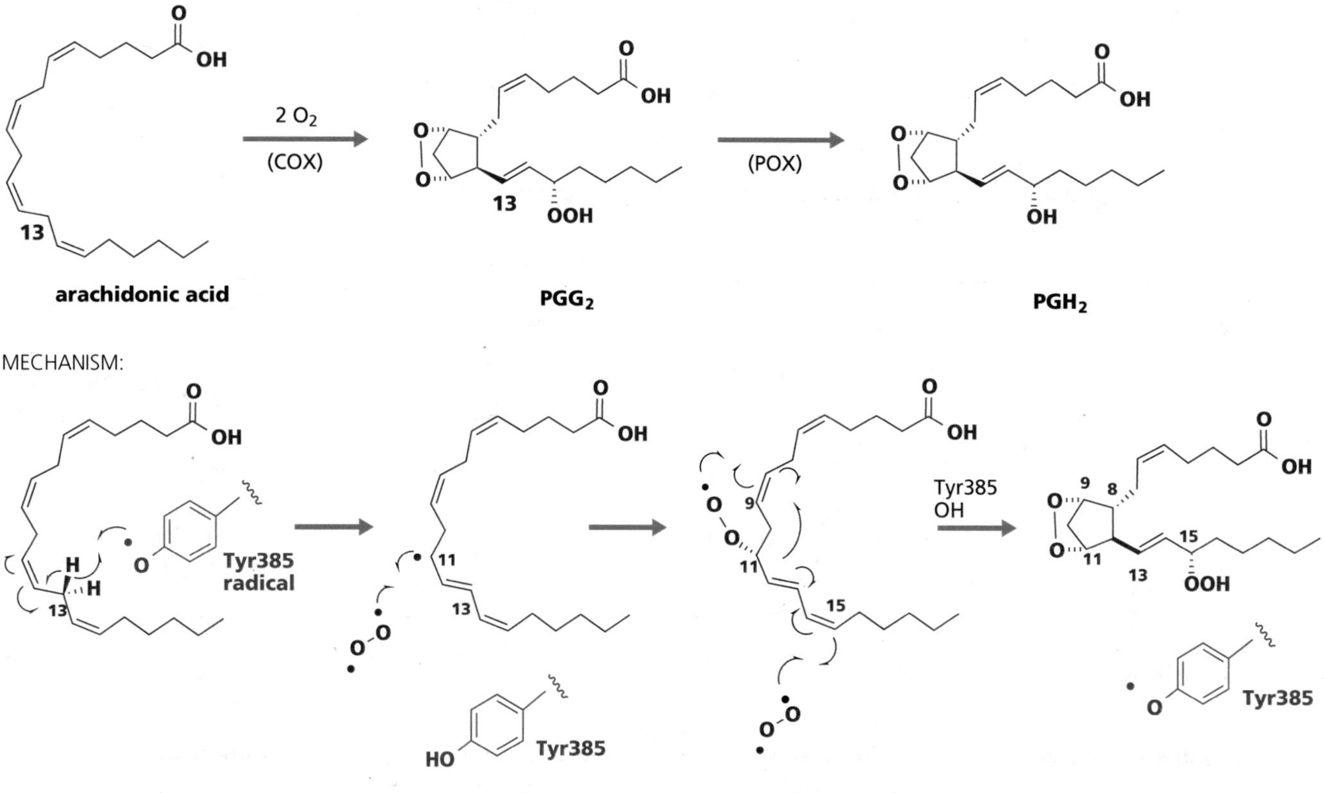

Figure 7.42 Cyclooxygenase catalyzed conversion of arachidonic acid to PGH_2. Cyclooxygenase cyclizes and oxidizes arachidonic acid to form PGG_2, then mediates its reduction to generate PGH_2, a precursor to prostaglandins and thromboxane. The oxidation and cyclization mechanism involves generation of a tyrosyl radical (red) which abstracts a specific H-atom from the substrate., followed by addition of oxygen and then cyclization to an endoperoxide. Addition of oxygen at the C-15 position produces PGG_2 and regenerates the tyrosyl radical.

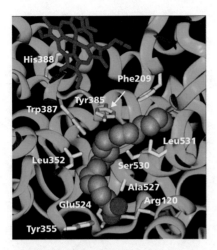

Figure 7.43 X-ray crystal structure of arachidonic acid bound in the active site of COX-1. Arachidonic acid is shown in gray, with the carboxylate oxygens in red; key enzyme residues involved in substrate binding are in yellow; heme unit that generates the initial tyrosyl radical is in red. The carboxylate interactions with Arg120 and Tyr355 are seen at the bottom of the figure. Numerous hydrophobic residues (such as Tyr and Leu) line the binding pocket to accommodate the hydrophobic arachidonic acid chain. Tyr385 is adjacent to the heme moiety and in proximity to the C13 proton. (Adapted from Blobaum AL & Marnett LJ [2007] *J Med Chem* 50:1425–1441. With permission from American Chemical Society.)

are two isoforms of the cyclooxygenase enzyme, COX-1 and COX-2. COX-1 is constitutively active in almost all tissues. The expression of COX-2 is more limited. It is produced at a consistent level in some tissues, such as brain and kidney, but in many tissues it is up-regulated in response to inflammatory events such as cytokine production. In both isoforms, there are two components to the catalytic site: the cyclooxygenase (COX) function converts the substrate to prostaglandin G_2 (PGG_2), and the heme-associated peroxidase (POX) completes the conversion from PGG_2 to PGH_2. The mechanism of the COX reaction is shown in Figure 7.42. Electron transfer from a tyrosine to the heme in COX initiates formation of a tyrosyl radical (Tyr385), which abstracts the 13-pro-(S) hydrogen of the substrate. Addition of molecular oxygen to this species gives an 11-peroxy radical, which cyclizes and adds oxygen at the C-15 position to generate PGG_2. PGG_2 then diffuses to the POX site and is reduced to PGH_2 (not shown).

The membrane-bound enzyme is a homodimer of two 70 kDa subunits, and the catalytic site is at the end of a deep hydrophobic binding pocket. Important binding interactions between the protein and substrate include ionic interactions between the carboxylic acid of the substrate and Arg120 and hydrogen-bonding between the acid and Tyr355. The remaining interactions are hydrophobic, with the substrate aligning in the hydrophobic pocket to orient the C-13 hydrogen near the Tyr385 radical as shown in **Figure 7.43**.

Inhibitors of COX (both isoforms 1 and 2) are used as anti-inflammatory drugs and comprise the family known as nonsteroidal anti-inflammatory drugs (NSAIDs). The oldest member of this family is aspirin; it has been in use as a single agent since the late 1800s, but its medicinal properties have been known for thousands of years as a constituent of willow bark (see Chapter 1). Others include arylacetic acids, such as flufenamic acid, and arylpropionic acids, such as ibuprofen and naproxen, (**Figure 7.44A**). All of these inhibit both isoforms of the enzyme and are reversible competitive inhibitors, with the exception of aspirin. Aspirin irreversibly acetylates Ser530 in the enzyme's binding pocket. This mechanism leads to the use of low doses of aspirin as an anti-thrombotic due to irreversible inhibition of COX in platelets. Since platelets cannot form new enzyme, they are inhibited for the lifetime of the platelet, resulting in lowered production of thromboxane A2, which then inhibits platelet aggregation.

Some prostaglandins have a protective role in the stomach lining, and side effects of the nonselective NSAIDS, since they reduce the production of prostaglandins, include increased incidence of ulcers. Because of this, when the COX-2 isoform was identified in 1991, there was significant effort put into developing selective COX-2 inhibitors based on the rationale that inhibition of the widely distributed COX-1 by the nonselective inhibitors was responsible for their gastrointestinal side effects. One key difference in the two isoforms is a change from Ile523 in COX-1 to the smaller Val523 in COX-2, as revealed in the X-ray crystal structures of the two isoforms (shown in **Figure 7.44B**). This small change reveals an additional binding pocket (blue), allowing for selectivity in drugs that contain a group that can occupy it.

The first selective COX-2 inhibitor reported was an experimental compound from DuPont Merck, known as DuP-697. This compound had a lower incidence of formation of stomach ulcers in animal models and lent credence to the value of selective inhibition. This diaryl heterocycle was a derivative of two older anti-inflammatory compounds, phenylbutazone and oxaprozin. Other compounds in this class include the first COX-2 selective inhibitor to be marketed, rofecoxib (Vioxx), approved by the FDA in 1999, soon followed by celecoxib and valdecoxib. All have in common two aromatic rings on adjacent sites on a central scaffold and a sulfonamide or methylsulfone substituent on one of the phenyl rings that extends into the selectivity pocket. While effective, and with a lower incidence of gastrointestinal side effects, a higher incidence of cardiovascular events such as heart attack and stroke was observed. This side effect has led to the withdrawal of most of the COX-2 selective inhibitors, with only celecoxib still on the market.

While there are other examples of drugs acting at oxidative and reductive enzymes, the two classes described here comprise two of the most successful examples of drug design. As stated previously, the mechanisms of the specific enzymes within this class vary more widely than other classes like the proteases and kinases. As such, general

A: INHIBITORS OF COX THAT ACT AS ANTI-INFLAMMATORY DRUGS

inhibitors of COX-1 and COX-2

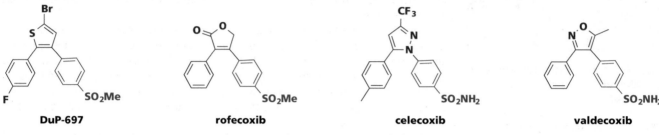

aspirin   flufenamic acid   ibuprofen   naproxen

selective COX-2 inhibitors (portion binding in selectivity pocket in red)

DuP-697   rofecoxib   celecoxib   valdecoxib

B: X-RAY STRUCTURE SHOWING BINDING POCKETS OF COX-1 AND COX-2

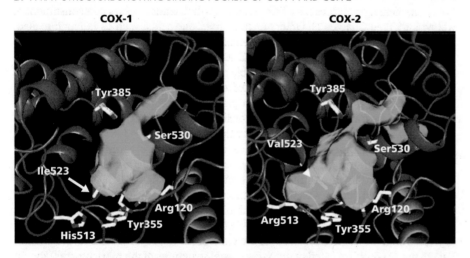

COX-1   COX-2

Figure 7.44 Structures of NSAIDs that are COX inhibitors and X-ray structures of COX-1 and COX-2. A: Structures of NSAIDs that act as COX inhibitors. Aspirin, flufenamic acid, ibuprofen, and naproxen act at both COX-1 and COX-2; DuP-697, rofecoxib, celecoxib and valdecoxib are representatives of selective COX-2 inhibitors. Substituted phenyl groups that instill selectivity are highlighted in red. B: X-ray structures of active sites of COX-1 and COX-2. Binding pockets are shown in blue. The change of an Ile523 in COX-1 to Val523 in COX-2 opens the selectivity pocket (to left of Val523), where the aryl groups (red) in the selective inhibitors bind. (Part B adapted from Blobaum AL & Marnett LJ [2007] *J Med Chem* 50:1425–1441. With permission from American Chemical Society.)

strategies for drug design are not possible, and most often relies on understanding the specific action of the target enzyme.

SUMMARY

There are numerous enzymes, each carrying out specific reactions through unique mechanisms. Likewise, there are numerous enzyme modulators that are effective drugs that work via various mechanisms and target multiple therapeutic indications. In fact, approximately 10% of all drugs act as kinase inhibitors, with the percentage that inhibit any enzyme likely reaching the 30–40% range. While the scope of all of these possibilities cannot be covered in this text, there are several recurrent themes. First, enzymes are considered druggable targets. Their mechanisms are usually well-understood and can be studied by various methods. Small-molecule modulators of enzymes can be readily characterized by kinetics as well as by biophysical measurements. While a number of important drugs that work through enzyme inhibition were discovered via phenotypic screening, more modern approaches rely on a detailed knowledge of the enzyme's mechanism, using the principles of medicinal chemistry and structure-based drug design. The importance of enzymes as drug targets, and the success at developing drugs targeting them is reflected in the observation that as of 2017, kinases and proteases make up approximately 10% of the drug targets, whereas in 2016, that number was a mere 2%.

CASE STUDY 1   DISCOVERY OF THE PROTEIN TYROSINE KINASE INHIBITOR IMATINIB

Imatinib, an inhibitor of the kinase Bcr-Abl, is considered a breakthrough therapy. After its introduction, survival from chronic myelogenous leukemia (CML) reached normal life expectancy, while prior treatment was typically a bone marrow transplant for the few eligible patients and a 30% five-year survival rate. The example of imatinib highlights the power of basic scientific discoveries in cancer biology coupled with medicinal chemistry and iterative rational drug design.

In the 1970s, researchers identified a specific genetic abnormality in patients diagnosed with CML: a reciprocal translocation between two chromosomes that results in the Philadelphia chromosome. This finding was the first that showed a direct connection between genetic changes and cancer. The protein product of the abnormal gene, Bcr-Abl, is a tyrosine kinase with constitutive, increased activity compared to the non-transformed gene product, and was shown to be essential for cellular transformation in CML. By inhibiting Bcr-Abl, a kinase that is not present in untransformed cells, a drug would be possible that was highly specific for cancer cells containing the Philadelphia chromosome.

The starting point for the drug discovery program was the phenylaminopyrimidine core (Figure 7.45), identified in a screen for inhibitors of a related kinase, protein kinase C (PKC). This scaffold exhibited *in vitro* activity against several different kinases including PKC, possessed good lead-like properties, and was amenable to further synthetic chemistry elaboration.

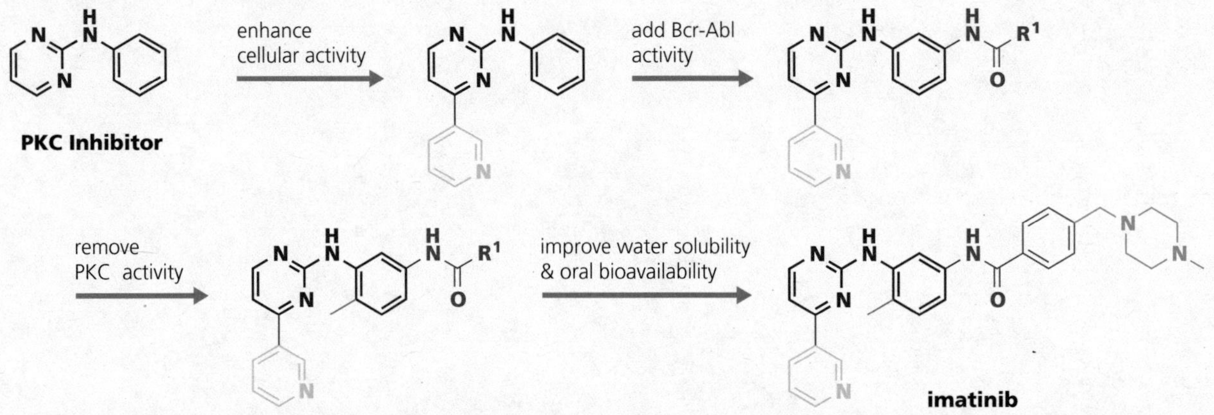

Figure 7.45 Structures in the development of imatinib. The PKC inhibitor (black) was elaborated by adding a 3-pyridyl group (green), which enhanced cellular activity. Addition of an amide group (red) broadened activity to include Bcr-Abl, while selectivity for Bcr-Abl over PKC was achieved by addition of a 6-methyl group (pink). Addition of the N-methylpiperazine moiety (blue) improved bioavailability and led to imatinib.

Incorporation of a 3-pyridyl group (green) onto the scaffold enhanced the cellular PKC activity. A key finding was that further elaboration to include an amide group (red) extended the kinase inhibition profile to Bcr-Abl kinase, while addition of a methyl group (pink) at the 6-position of the diaminophenyl group abolished the PKC activity but retained Bcr-Abl potency. At this stage, potent selective inhibitors were in hand; however, pharmaceutical properties such as solubility and toxicity were of concern. To address those issues, a methylene-N-methylpiperazine moiety (shown in blue) was incorporated. The rationale for addition of this group included using the polar N-methylpiperazine to improve solubility and incorporating a methylene between the piperazine and phenyl group to avoid a potentially mutagenic aniline functionality.

The imatinib–Bcr-Abl co-crystal structure shows that the molecule binds to the conserved nucleotide-binding pocket when the protein is in the inactive DFG-out conformation, thereby occluding access of the substrate to the active site.

Figure 7.46 Key binding interactions of imatinib. These include an H-bond from the 3-pyridyl nitrogen of imatinib to Met318 NH, an H-bond from the secondary amine of imatinib to the side chain of Thr315 (unique to Bcr-Abl), and H-bonds from the amide carbonyl of imatinib to the backbone of Asp381 and from the amide NH of imatinib to Glu286. (Adapted from Pan X, Dong J, Shi Y et al. [2015] *Org Biomol Chem* 13:7050–7066. With permission from Royal Society of Chemistry.)

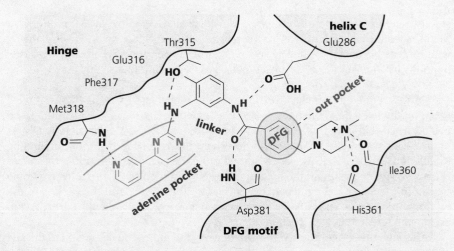

This distinction is the likely root of the high selectivity of imatinib. Some of the key interactions between Bcr-Abl and imatinib are shown in **Figure 7.46**. Some essential interactions that explain potency and selectivity include the following:

- The nitrogen of the pyridine ring makes an H-bond to Met318. This is the same interaction made by adenine N1 in the ATP substrate.

- The secondary amino group makes an H-bond to Thr315; Thr315 is relatively unique to Bcr-Abl. Most other kinases contain a methionine at this site, which is not capable of H-bonding. This interaction provides potency and selectivity for Bcr-Abl.

- Numerous snug van der Waals (hydrophobic) interactions between hydrophobic residues and the aromatic rings of the inhibitor are evident.

- The amide makes H-bonds in the DFG loop to Asp381 and also to Glu286 on helix C.

Since its introduction, imatinib has been shown to inhibit other kinases, despite its original design for selectivity. In addition, resistance toward imatinib has emerged, and this has motivated the design and synthesis of other Bcr-Abl inhibitors.

CASE STUDY 2 DEVELOPMENT OF ENALAPRIL

Discovery of angiotensin-converting enzyme (ACE) inhibitors such as enalapril and captopril is considered the earliest example of successful rational drug design. These drugs can be traced to the 1960s, with John Vane and Sergio Ferreira's discovery of peptide inhibitors of ACE. One of the peptides, teprotide, was isolated from a snake venom (from *Bothrops jararaca*) that had been used in Brazil as an arrow poison and lowered blood pressure. It is a nonapeptide containing a C-terminal proline that was shown to be an inhibitor of ACE. Although it was not orally active, the discovery of the peptide led to the pursuit of orally active analogs for the treatment of high blood pressure. Although no X-ray structure of ACE existed at the time, it was known to be a metalloprotease that cleaved the Phe-His bond of the protein angiotensin I, converting it to angiotensin II. Angiotensin II is the ultimate product of the renin–angiotensin system and is responsible for vasoconstriction and raising blood pressure.

At Merck, the assumption was made that ACE may be similar to carboxypeptidase A, a well-studied zinc metalloprotease, and the initial inhibitor design combined two components: an acid group from benzylsuccinic acid (blue), a known inhibitor of carboxypeptidase A and the C-terminal proline of the teprotide (red). Initial analogs such as the ketoacid and the α-methyl analog gave moderate levels of activity, and the phosphoramide analog was highly active *in vitro* but had low oral bioavailability. At about the same time, Miguel Ondetti and David Cushman at Squibb reported studies leading to captopril, validating the idea of developing ACE inhibitors. At Merck, substitution of CH_2CO_2H for the phosphoramide lead gave an Ala-Pro analog with respectable activity. Adding a second methyl group (dimethyl analog) increased lipophilicity to offset the effect of the polar group, leading to a highly active analog (**Figure 7.47**).

Further refinements included extension of the methyl group to a phenethyl moiety (seen on the left side of the phosphoramide analog in Figure 7.47), which increased activity 1000-fold and provided enalaprilate (**Figure 7.48A**). Enalaprilate itself has poor oral bioavailability and is given as the ester prodrug, enalapril. Important binding interactions (**Figure 7.48B**) were assumed to be the carboxylate binding to Zn^{2+} in the active site. In addition, the methyl group is presumed to fit into a hydrophobic pocket in the S1′ site, the phenylethyl group into the S1 site, and the proline in the hydrophobic S2′ site. The required terminal carboxylate was assumed to participate in an ion–ion interaction with a cation (Figure 7.48).

Although the X-ray structure was unknown at the time of development in the late 1970s, in 2003 a structure was solved, showing the binding interactions of ACE with lisinopril, an ACE inhibitor in which the alanine of enalapril is replaced with a lysine. As proposed, the C-terminal carboxylate forms an ionic interaction with a lysine

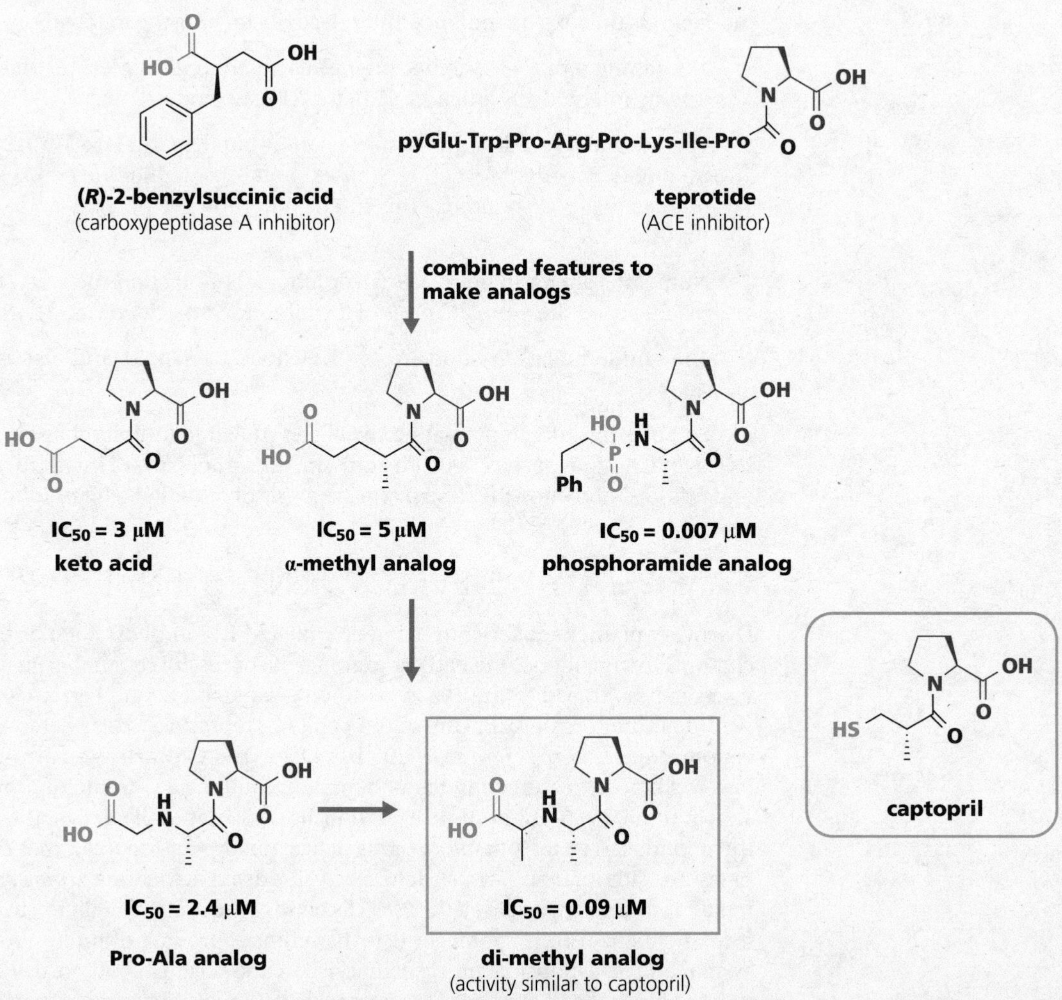

Figure 7.47 Evolution of enalapril. Starting points for the development of enalapril were the snake venom teprotide, which is an ACE inhibitor and (*R*)-2-benzylsuccinic acid, a known carboxypeptide A inhibitor. Features of each, an acid (blue) and proline (red) were combined to give analogs. Of the representatives shown, the phosphoramide analog had good potency but poor bioavailability. Further elaboration by incorporating an amine in the carbon chain was tolerated, and adding a methyl group, afforded a very potent compound (in box). The structure of captopril, another ACE inhibitor is shown for comparison.

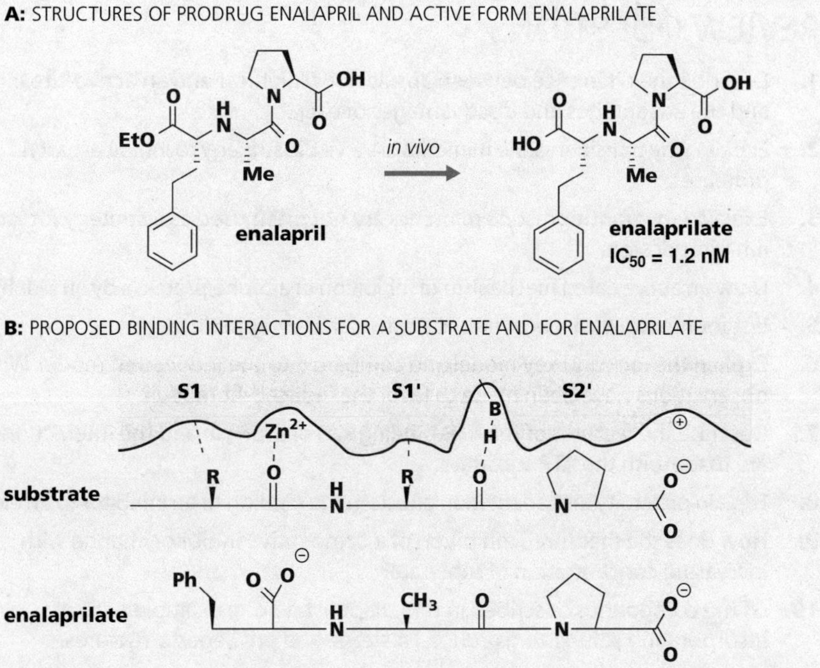

Figure 7.48 Structure of enalapril, enaprilate and representation of enaprilate binding. A: Enalapril is not orally available, so it is delivered as the ethyl ester prodrug. Cleavage of the ester *in vivo* gives the active acid. B: Enaprilate is presumed to mimic the peptide substrate in its binding interactions. Proline binds in the S2' site, methyl in the S1' site, carboxylate in the Zn^{2+} pocket, and phenethyl in the S1 site. In addition the prolyl carbonyl makes an H-bond interaction, in the same manner as the substrate.

A: STRUCTURES OF PRODRUG ENALAPRIL AND ACTIVE FORM ENALAPRILATE

B: PROPOSED BINDING INTERACTIONS FOR A SUBSTRATE AND FOR ENALAPRILATE

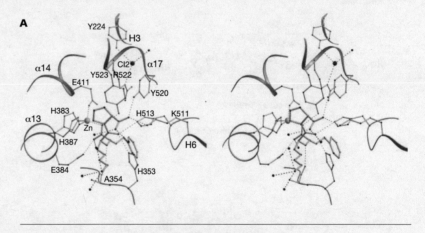

residue (K511), the second carboxylate binds to Zn^{2+}, and the phenyl group sits in the S1 pocket. The lysine side chain of lisinopril corresponds to the methyl of enalapril and fits into the S1' pocket, with the proline ring in the S2' site (**Figure 7.49**).

Since the introduction of captopril in 1981, enalapril in 1985, and lisinopril in 1987, there are currently eight ACE inhibitors on the market, which are widely used to treat hypertension.

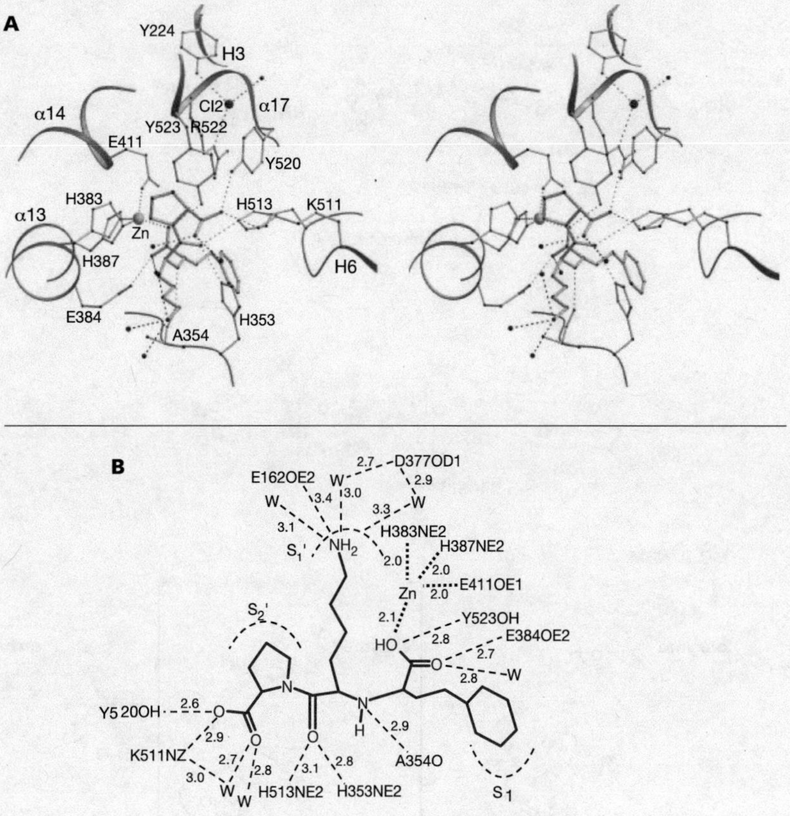

Figure 7.49 Binding of ACE inhibitor lisinopril in ACE. A: Stereodiagram of X-ray structure with lisinopril in yellow and Zn as a green sphere. B: Structure showing specific binding interactions confirming the earlier model where proline binds in the S2' site, lysine in the S1' site, carboxylate in the Zn^{2+} pocket, and the phenyl group in the S1 site. (From Natesh R, Schwager SLU, Sturrock ED & Acharya KR [2003] *Nature* 421:551–554. With permission from Macmillan Publishers Limited.)

REVIEW QUESTIONS

1. Describe the difference between an allosteric inhibitor and an active-site inhibitor and the advantages and disadvantages of each.

2. Explain why transition-state mimetics are a viable strategy to inhibit aspartyl proteases.

3. Explain why transition-state mimetics are not often used as a strategy for kinase inhibitor design.

4. Draw an abbreviated mechanism of inhibition of a serine protease by an aldehyde.

5. List four reasons why enzymes are considered druggable targets.

6. Explain the lock and key model and compare it to the induced-fit model. What observations have been made to favor the induced-fit model?

7. Describe the features of the ATP-binding site of a kinase and the interactions that are made with the ATP substrate.

8. Explain proximity and orientation effects in the binding of an inhibitor to an enzyme.

9. How does the measured inhibition of a competitive inhibitor change with increasing concentration of substrate?

10. Of the compounds described in this chapter, find one example each of incorporating solubilizing groups, isosteres, and privileged structures.

APPLICATION QUESTIONS

1. Hexosaminidase A is an enzyme that hydrolyzes certain carbohydrate residues. The mechanism of the reaction it catalyzes is shown here. Design an inhibitor of this enzyme based on the reaction mechanism. Explain the rationale for your design.

REACTION:

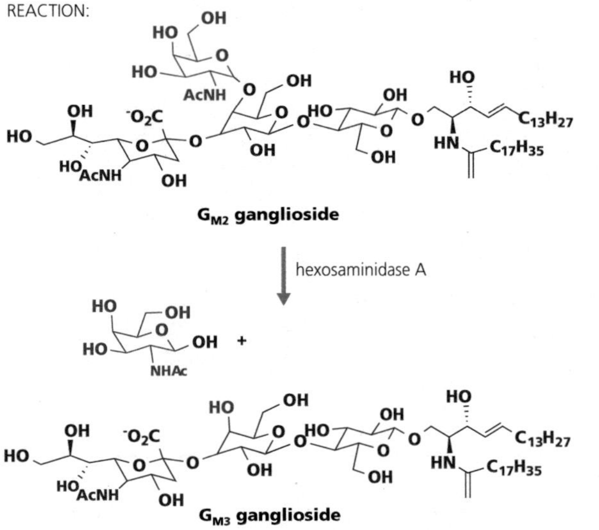

G_{M2} **ganglioside**

hexosaminidase A

G_{M3} **ganglioside**

MECHANISM:

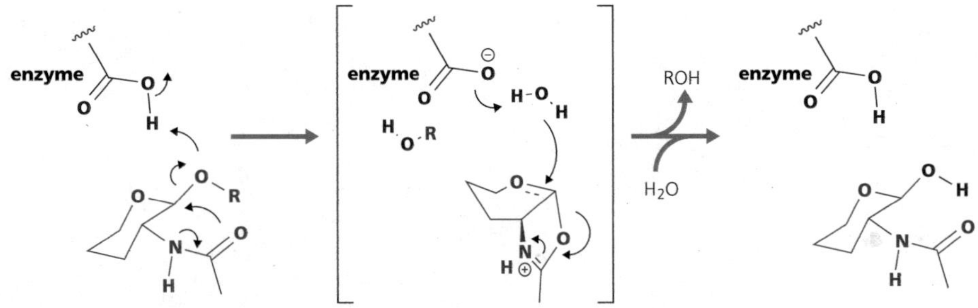

2. Look up the structure of an HIV reverse transcriptase phosphate prodrug. Draw its structure, and explain its mechanism and how it differs from those shown in Figure 7.31.

3. What hit identification strategies can usually be applied to enzyme inhibitor drug discovery? Explain why these strategies can be particularly successful. What are the similarities and differences in approaches to hit identification when working with enzymes versus receptors?

4. A theoretical aspartyl protease cleaves this substrate at the scissile bond shown with the wavy line. Design three inhibitors based on this substrate.

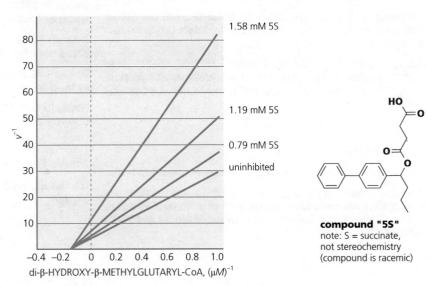

5. Research the structure of staurosporine. What type of enzyme does it inhibit? What are the binding interactions it makes with the target, and compare compounds described in this chapter.

6. Using the PDE3 pharmacophore model in Figure 7.35 and the table of bioisosteres in Chapter 4 (see Tables 4.3 and 4.4), design three compounds that may be PDE3 inhibitors.

7. This plot shows the effects of compound **5S** on the enzyme HMG-CoA reductase. Compound **5S** was one of a series of early compounds prepared as inhibitors of the enzyme. (From Boots MR, Boots SG, Noble CM & Guyer KE [1973] *J Pharm Sci* 62:952–957. With permission from Wiley Periodicals Inc. and American Pharmacists Association.)

What is the name of this type of plot? Is the inhibitor competitive or noncompetitive? What portions of **5S** correspond to the model for synthetic analogs of statins (see Figure 7.41)?

8. A number of the drugs described in this chapter contain fluorine atoms. Identify three of them, and on the basis of the concepts in Chapter 4, hypothesize what role the fluorine may be playing in these molecules.

9. Apply Lipinski rules to Lipitor, indinavir, Gleevec, and sildanafil. Do they comply? (Online tools can be used to calculate log P.)

FURTHER READING

General references

Koshland DE (1994) The key-lock theory and the induced fit theory. *Angew Chem, Int Ed* 33:2375–2378.

Robertson JG (2005) Mechanistic basis of enzyme-targeted drugs. *Biochemistry* 44:5561–5571.

Kinases

Ubersax JA & Ferrell JE (2007) Mechanisms of specificity in protein phosphorylation. *Nat Rev Mol Cell Biol* 8:530–541.

Zhang J, Yang PL & Gray NS (2009) Targeting cancer with small molecule kinase inhibitors. *Nat Rev Cancer* 9:28–39.

Nobele MEM, Endicott JA & Jonson LN (2004) Protein kinase inhibitors: Insights into drug design from structure. *Science* 303:1800–1805.

Shuai K & Liu B (2003) Regulation of JAK-STAT signaling in the immune system. *Nat Rev Immun* 3:900–911.

Mocsai A, Ruland J & Tybulewicz VLJ (2010) The SYK tyrosine kinase: a crucial player in diverse biological functions. *Nat Rev Immun* 10:387–402.

Clark JD, Flanagan ME & Telliez J-B (2014) Discovery and development of Janus kinase (JAK) inhibitors for inflammatory diseases. *J Med Chem* 57:5023–5038.

Proteases

Erez E, Fass D & Bibi E (2009) How intramembrane proteases bury hydrolytic reactions in the membrane. *Nature* 459:371–378.

Hernandez AA & Roush WR (2002) Recent advances in the design, synthesis and selection of cysteine protease inhibitors. *Curr Opin Chem Biol* 6:459–465.

Njoroge FG, Chen KS, Shih N-Y & Piwinski JJ (2008) Challenges in modern drug discovery: A case study of boceprevir, an HCV protease inhibitor for the treatment of hepatitis C virus infection. *Acc Chem Res* 41:50–59.

Polymerases

Steitz TA (1998) A mechanism for all polymerases. *Nature* 391:231–232.

Esposito F, Corona A & Tramontano E (2012) HIV-1 reverse transcriptase still remains a new drug target: structure, function, classical inhibitors, and new inhibitors with innovative mechanisms, of actions. *Mol Biol Int* 2012:586401.

Imatinib

Capdeville R, Buchdunger W, Zimmermann J & Matter A (2002) Glivec (STI571, Imatinib) A rationally developed, targeted anticancer drug. *Nat Rev Drug Discovery* 1:493.

Schindler T, Bornmann W, Pellicena P et al. (2000) Structural mechanism for STI-571 inhibition of Abelson tyrosine kinase. *Science* 289:1938–1942.

Enalapril

Smith CG & Vane JR (2003) The discovery of captopril. *FASEB J* 17:788–789.

Patchett AA (1993) Excursions in drug discovery. *J Med Chem* 36:2051–2058.

Natesh R, Schwager SLU, Sturrock ED & Acharya KR (2003) Crystal structure of the human angiotensin-converting enzyme–lisinopril complex. *Nature* 421:551–554.

Phosphodiesterases

Manallack DT, Hughes RA & Thompson PE (2005) The next generation of phosphodiesterase inhibitors: structural clues to ligand and substrate selectivity of phosphodiesterases. *J Med Chem* 48:3449–3462.

Spina D (2008) PDE4 inhibitors: current status. *Br J Pharmacol* 155:308–315.

Rotella D (2002) Phosphodiesterase 5 inhibitors: current status and potential applications. *Nat Rev Drug Discovery* 1:674–685.

Oxidoreductases

Tolbert JA (2003) Lovastatin and beyond: the history of the HMG-CoA reductase inhibitors. *Nat Rev Drug Discovery* 2:517–526.

Roth BD (2002) The discovery and development of atorvastatin, a potent novel hypolipidemic agent. *Prog Med Chem* 40:1–22.

Blobaum AL & Marnett LJ (2007) Structural and functional basis of cyclooxygenase inhibition. *J Med Chem* 50:1425–1441.

Flower RJ (2003) The development of COX2 inhibitors. *Nat Rev Drug Discovery* 2:179–191.

Media links

U.S. FDA approved protein kinase inhibitors: http://www.brimr.org/PKI/PKIs.htm

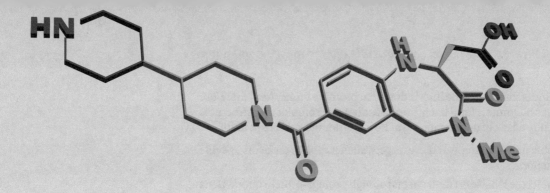

Protein–protein and lipid structure interactions as drug targets

8

LEARNING OBJECTIVES

- Understand why atypical drug targets, such as protein–protein interactions and lipid structures, are more challenging than traditional receptor and enzyme targets.
- Gain familiarity with the general strategies used for hit identification for these targets.
- Understand several design strategies and concepts that have been successfully applied to find modulators of protein–protein interactions.
- Identify several different mechanisms by which small molecules can modulate protein–protein interactions.
- Learn examples of drugs that work by interrupting or mimicking protein–protein interactions and by interacting with lipids and cell membranes.

Receptors and enzymes constitute the majority of small-molecule drug targets. This focus may, in part, be due to the fact that many of these proteins' functions rely on binding of small molecule natural ligands and substrates. In these cases, drug design and discovery efforts can model drugs after those small molecules. Additionally, as discussed in Chapters 6 and 7, the three-dimensional structures of receptors and enzymes have inherent features that make their function amenable to modulation by small molecules. However, receptors and enzymes are responsible for only a fraction of the physiological processes that can be modulated in order to mediate disease states. Many others are mediated by interactions between two proteins. These interactions also offer an opportunity for intervention by small molecules, as do lipids, which perform an essential function in maintaining cell and membrane-bound protein structure and can also act as signaling molecules. However, neither protein–protein interactions nor lipid interactions are common drug targets despite the fact that they play a pivotal role in virtually all physiological processes, such as cell adhesion, cell division, transport of molecules, maintenance of cell structure and morphology, and signaling. In fact, these types of targets are often considered undruggable due to several factors:

- Binding between macromolecules, that mediate physiological effects, often occur at interfaces that are relatively flat and have large surface areas, which do not favor specific binding of a small druglike molecule.

- There is poor understanding of the interactions that promote binary (and therefore selective) versus oligomeric (and likely promiscuous) macromolecular structures and consequently a lack of understanding of how to promote or disrupt them.

- The hydrophobic nature of some of these targets, such as lipids, disfavors specific binding interactions.

Of the small molecules that exert their effects through protein–protein interactions or interactions with lipids in cell membranes, many are natural products (or are derived from natural products), but their mechanisms were determined only after their downstream biological effects were characterized. However, modern medicinal chemistry efforts are now actively focusing on this untapped area, and there are a number of notable successes. **Table 8.1** includes representative examples of such drugs. Treating these atypical targets as one class is not possible, since they constitute diverse macromolecular structures such as monomeric proteins involved in signaling, oligomeric protein assemblies that are part of specific cellular structures, and lipids that constitute cell membranes. Accordingly, the mechanisms by which drugs affect these systems are equally varied and include small molecules that stabilize or destabilize a multicomponent structure, drugs that interfere with binding between two proteins, and compounds that mediate pore formation in membranes. Developing drugs that interrupt protein–protein interactions is a rapidly advancing area of drug design, while targeting lipids by design is still in its infancy.

Methods to measure small molecules that interact with atypical protein targets, like those used for receptors (see Chapter 6), rely on evaluation of binding as a primary assay. When the macromolecule is isolable, common methods to detect binding of the small molecule, or a tagged derivative, include those that measure effects related to differences in size or other physical characteristics between the bound complex and unbound constituents. Fluorescence-based assays, such as fluorescence polarization (FP) and FRET, and enzyme-linked immunosorbent assays (ELISA) detect changes in luminescence or fluorescence upon binding of the small molecule to a tagged protein. Other methods that do not require significant manipulation of one of the binding partners include surface plasmon resonance (SPR), thermal shift assays, isothermal calorimetry, and nuclear magnetic resonance spectroscopy (NMR). Data from these methods can provide dissociation constants (K_d) to measure binding affinity. In some cases, structure determination of the small molecule–macromolecule complex to identify the binding interactions and binding site can be accomplished by NMR, X-ray

Table 8.1   Examples of drugs that affect protein-protein and lipid structure interactions, their specific targets, mechanism of action and therapeutic use.

Macromolecular target	Target type	Mechanism of action	Drug	Indication
transthyretin	protein	Stabilizes correctly folded tetramer, shifts equilibrium away from misfolded monomer	tafamidis	transthyretin familial amyloid polyneuropathy
tubulin	protein	Destabilizes protein oligomer	colchicine, vincristine	cancer
tubulin	protein	Stabilizes protein oligomer	paclitaxel, ixabepilone	cancer
calcineurin	protein	Binds to cyclophilin, complex inhibits enzymatic activity of calcineurin	cyclosporin	anti-rejection therapy
glycoprotein IIb/IIIa	protein	inhibits protein–protein interaction	tirofiban	cardiovascular disease
CCR5	protein receptor	inhibits protein–protein interaction	maraviroc	HIV
fungal ergosterol	lipid	sequesters lipids and/or forms pores	amphotericin, nystatin	fungal infection
bacterial cell membranes	lipids	disrupts lipid membrane	daptomycin	bacterial infection

crystallography, and cryo-electron microscopy. As with receptors, binding does not always translate to biological effects, and additional assays to evaluate downstream consequences are also necessary.

Drugs that interfere with lipid structure and membranes are more challenging to directly evaluate, since the membrane is not a single entity, but a fluid structure. One example of a detection method is atomic force microscopy (AFM) that visualizes changes in the cell surface. Phenotypic assays are also included in the compounds' characterization to determine whether interference in lipid structure has a physiological effect.

PROTEIN–PROTEIN INTERACTIONS AS DRUG TARGETS

Numerous physiological processes are mediated by interactions between two or more proteins, termed **protein–protein interactions** (PPIs). Enzymes and nuclear receptors are regulated by their interactions with other proteins, and GPCRs bind to G proteins as part of the signal transduction process. In addition, many proteins that are not classified as either enzymes or receptors interact with themselves (homodimers) or with other proteins (heterodimers) to initiate or terminate a biological response or even to form a large macromolecular complex that exerts a distinct physiological effect. This process is further complicated by the multiple roles and interactions that can often be attributed to just one protein and by the fact that many of these interactions are transient and context-dependent, occurring only under specific conditions and in specific cellular locations.

Efforts to delineate PPIs have led to databases of the **interactome**, a map of the network of molecular interactions within a particular cell or organism. **Figure 8.1** is one representation of a portion of the human interactome, where each colored circle represents a specific protein and each line indicates an interaction between two proteins.

In Figure 8.1, one can see a vast number of known proteins and an enormous number of interactions, as exemplified by the many overlapping lines. In fact, it has been estimated that, among human proteins, as many as 650,000 binary protein interactions are involved in normal physiological events, but only a fraction of these have been carefully documented in such interactome maps. Accordingly, interfering with PPIs has the potential to be a powerful therapeutic strategy when those interactions mediate pathological processes. For example, PPIs are involved in many cellular events associated with cancer, including regulating transcription factors as well as maintaining structural proteins, such as the microtubules that are necessary for cell division. If even half of the mapped PPIs are involved in disease states, then the opportunities for therapeutic intervention significantly dwarf the number of more traditional enzyme and receptor drug targets. It should be noted that PPIs cannot be considered as a target class in the same respect as enzymes and receptors, since each protein component is unique and general strategies applicable to all PPIs are unlikely.

The success of **biologics** attests to the validity of targeting PPIs. These drugs include protein and antibody therapeutics that either inhibit a PPI or supplement one of the protein partners involved in a PPI. One particularly successful area has been the development of protein conjugates that interfere with the interaction between tumor necrosis factor α (TNF α) and TNF receptor that is part of the immune response. One example is Etanercept, a fusion protein genetically engineered by combining genes that produce the TNF receptor and a portion of immunoglobulin G1 (IgG1). Another example of a biologic is the monoclonal antibody adalimumab, which binds to TNF α. In the first case, the excess receptor binds to and sequesters TNF; in the second the antibody binds to and inactivates TNF. Both result in TNF, which initiates inflammatory responses, being essentially removed from circulation. These large molecule biologics are effective in treating inflammatory diseases such as rheumatoid arthritis and Crohn's disease.

Small molecules that interfere with PPIs can be classified according to three designations:

1. Orthosteric binders directly compete with one of the binding partners at the protein-protein binding site.

2. Allosteric regulators bind to a site that is remote from the protein-protein interface, and alter the conformation or dynamic properties of the proteins involved.

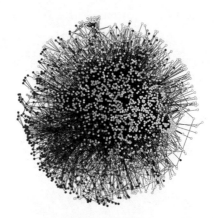

Figure 8.1 Representation of a portion of the human interactome. This map indicates known interactions between proteins. Each colored circle represents one protein; lines between circles represent interactions; In this map, the yellow region represents protein interactions associated with long QT syndrome and the blue region represents protein interactions associated with epilepsy, with the green region where they overlap. (Courtesy of National Institute of General Medical Science, NIH, USA.)

(These first two categories are analogous to those applied to small molecules that interact with receptors.)

3. **Interfacial binders** form a ternary complex with the two protein partners at their interface and lock the proteins in a nonproductive conformation.

One of the more difficult aspects in modulating PPIs with small molecules is the need to cover a large, flat binding interface, as opposed to a small binding pocket typically found in receptors or enzymes. In **Figure 8.2**, a ribbon diagram shows the transcription factor TEAD4 (red) bound to the transcription co-factor Vgll1 (green) and the large, flat extended surface area typical of PPI interfaces (depicted as gray cylinders).

In general, interactions between two proteins are a culmination of many weak interactions over a large surface, with an average area of ~1500 Å². In contrast, the high-affinity binding of a small molecule to an enzyme or receptor relies on several strong interactions in a small, localized binding pocket. That three-dimensional binding pocket allows for the occupying ligand to make contacts in multiple directions, whereas a PPI interface is often only along one dimension. Consequently, molecules that interfere with PPIs have properties distinct from more classical inhibitors of enzymes or receptors. They are typically of higher molecular weight, a characteristic that is not usually considered druglike, and counterintuitively, they possess a greater degree of three-dimensionality. An alternate mechanism by which small molecules modulate PPIs is through binding to allosteric sites. Since protein conformations are dynamic and context-dependent, binding of a small molecule to only one conformation, or under just one set of conditions, may affect the protein's ability to adopt an active conformation and prevent binding to its partner. The protein's dynamic nature may reveal allosteric sites for small-molecule binding that may not be apparent otherwise.

Historically, small-molecule modulators of PPIs were not designed *a priori*. Many that are known today were discovered and developed because they exhibited specific biological activities in downstream or phenotypic assays, such as cell proliferation assays, and their mechanism of interfering with PPIs was determined at a later time. Anti-cancer drugs that bind to tubulin are one such example (see Section 8.3). High-throughput screening has been only modestly successful in identifying hits for this class. The reasons for this vary, but it has been speculated that compound screening libraries are populated with molecules that are more appropriate for traditional enzyme and receptor targets and therefore contain few structures that might inhibit PPIs. In order to address this issue, an active effort to design and synthesize small-molecule libraries that exhibit the known characteristics of PPI modulators for inclusion in screening decks has been a priority. Additionally, high-throughput screening of natural products or natural product-inspired analogs has experienced renewed interest. One PPI hit identification screening strategy that has seen particular success is fragment-based screening (see Chapter 2). Direct binding of a small low-affinity fragment to one of the protein partners is detected by methods such as SPR, NMR, MS, or X-ray crystallography. Further optimization generates small molecules that inhibit protein–protein interactions with very high affinity. When feasible, structure-based design has also been a successful approach.

As a reminder, PPIs and their inhibitors are not a single category in the sense that enzymes, GPCRs, ion channels, and nuclear receptors are; therefore, successful general strategies for hit identification are unlikely. The following sections highlight some specific examples of small-molecule inhibitors of PPIs.

8.1   One strategy to prevent binding between two proteins is to mimic one of the protein partners

When binding between two proteins contributes to a disease state, inhibitors of the PPI are sought. A small molecule that binds to either protein and prevents its interaction with its partner is one common approach. Examples of this approach have been developed by use of several different strategies, including generating peptide mimetics, identifying hits from high-throughput screening, and designing molecules based on a known ligand. The structure-based design approach to identifying PPI

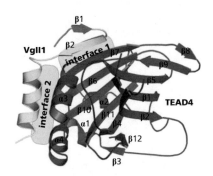

Figure 8.2 Ribbon diagram representation of the interface between two proteins, highlighting a typical flat and extended PPI binding surface. Transcription co-factor Vgll1 is shown in green, transcription factor TEAD4 is shown in red, and the interfaces between the two are depicted as gray cylinders. Interface 1 occurs between two β-sheets (β2 of Vgll1 and β7 of TEAD4), while interface 2 forms between the α-helix of Vgll1 and two α-helices (α3 and α4) of TEAD4. (From Pobbati AV, Chan SW, Lee I et al. [2012] *Structure* 20:1135–1140. With permission from Elsevier.)

modulators involves mimicking one of the binding partners by understanding its structure and conformation and the interactions it makes at the binding interface.

The α-helix is one common protein secondary structure motif, accounting for perhaps over 30% of protein secondary structures, and it is frequently observed at PPI binding interfaces. The precise nature of the interactions varies widely. In the simplest cases, only one face of a relatively short span of the α-helix is involved in recognition; in others, the interface involves multiple faces of the helix over longer stretches, and still others rely on multiple helices interacting with the single binding partner. An α-helix is a right-handed coiled conformation where every peptide backbone N-H makes a hydrogen bond with the carbonyl in the backbone four residues before it. This arrangement results in every third or fourth amino acid side chain being displayed above one another, so that the α-helix can be divided into distinct faces on each turn of the helix (**Figure 8.3A**). Since the overall shape of the scaffold is the same, and differs only in the identity of the side chains displayed, general strategies to mimic α-helices that can compete with the native α-helix partner for binding may be broadly applicable for inhibitor or even agonist design for interactions mediated by α-helices (**Figure 8.3B**).

The earliest and simplest efforts to design mimetics of α-helices relied on modifying an appropriate peptide fragment so that it adopts and maintains the active α-helical secondary structure. To do so, the general concept of conformational constraint (Chapter 4.13) was applied by cyclizing the peptide termini, cyclizing side chains by forming disulfides and lactams. Not unexpectedly, these compounds suffered from the poor druglike properties common to peptides, such as metabolic instability and poor absorption. More recently, stapled peptides, which are short fragments of α-helical peptides constrained by a hydrocarbon bridge between the ends of the helix (see Chapter 4), have seen some success. In many cases, a ring-closing metathesis reaction is applied to cyclize the peptide (**Figure 8.4**). Incorporation of non-native amino acids, particularly those containing an α,α-disubstitution pattern, and further optimization can provide enhanced helicity and protease stability as well as improved cellular uptake compared to native peptides.

In one example, the binding between an α-helix of the tumor suppressor p53 and its negative regulators, murine double minute-2 and -X (MDM2 and MDMX), was targeted. This tumor suppressor has been called "the guardian of the human genome", and controls cellular response to DNA damage. In certain cancers, MDM2 and MDMX (the human versions) are overexpressed and suppress p53's activity, thereby allowing uncontrolled tumor growth; compounds that inhibit this interaction should

Figure 8.3 Representation of α-helix secondary structure motif. A: (Left) Ribbon diagram of several α-helices of a protein in close proximity; (Center) ball-and-stick model highlighting H-bonds (shown as dotted lines) between backbone N-H and carbonyl groups (side chain not shown); (Right) helix showing side chains (yellow) aligned and extending from helix. B: Model of binding between two proteins mediated by an α-helix interface, and schematic of a small-molecule mimic of an α–helix, mimicking the binding of protein 1 to protein 2. (B, adapted from Azzarito V, Long K, Murphy NS & Wilson AJ [2013] *Nat Chem* 5:161–173. With permission from Macmillan Publishers Limited.)

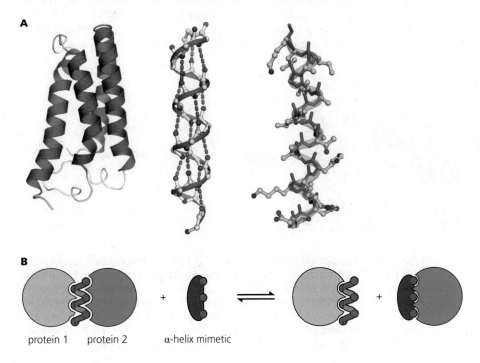

A

B

protein 1   protein 2   α-helix mimetic

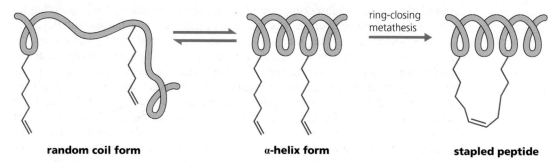

random coil form   **α-helix form**   **stapled peptide**

Figure 8.4 Representation of stapled peptide formation. A properly designed linear peptide containing olefinic side chains can adopt an α-helical conformation, which brings the olefinic side chains in close enough proximity that a ring-closing metathesis reaction will generate the conformationally constrained α-helix stapled peptide.

restore the repressive activity of p53 and slow cancer growth. Stapled peptides were designed which mimicked p53's binding interface with MDM2/MDMX, and bound to them with high affinity and prevented MDM2/MDX from binding to p53, thereby restoring and enhancing p53 tumor suppressor activity. The stapled peptide ATSP-7041 (**Figure 8.5**) was the result of an optimization effort based on linear and cyclic peptides that contained key amino acid residues (Phe, Trp, and Leu) found on the p53 binding surface. It retains the Phe and Trp residues (shown in blue) and replaces the leucine residue with a cyclobutane amino acid (Cba, also shown in blue).

ATSP-7041 exhibits high binding affinity to both MDM2 and MDMX ($K_i = 0.9$ and 7 nM, respectively). The stapled peptide was found to be highly helical, as designed. It exhibited favorable PK properties, was efficacious in *in vivo* models, and served as the basis of additional compounds such as ALRN-6924, which has progressed to clinical trials as an anti-tumor drug. X-ray crystallography of ATSP-7041 bound to MDMX (see Figure 8.5) indicated that the essential Phe, Trp, and Cba residues were indeed bound as expected; however, additional binding interactions from a tyrosine residue side chain and with the hydrocarbon staple were also evident and probably contributed to the high binding affinity.

The stapled peptide strategy has numerous potential applications: for example, stapled peptides can be designed that inhibit a PPI or act as an agonist by binding to a protein partner and propagating downstream events. Reports of effective stapled peptides span therapeutic applications in cancer, infectious diseases, metabolic diseases, and neurology. Several other stapled peptides are undergoing clinical trials, though none have yet been approved by regulatory agencies.

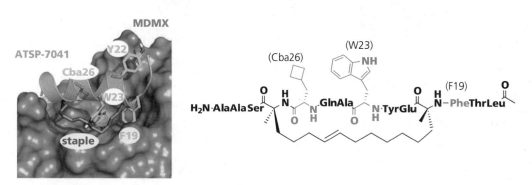

Figure 8.5 Structure of stapled peptide ATSP-7041. Left: X-ray structure of ATSP-7041 bound to MDMX. Helix is shown in brown, the staple is depicted in orange, and side-chain residues (F, W, and Cba) making key contacts are shown in green. Tyrosine 22 also makes significant contacts to the protein. Right: Chemical structure of ATSP-7041, with key residues F19, W23, and Cba26 (a cyclobutane amino acid) shown in blue. (Left, from Chang YS, Graves B, Guerlavais V et al. [2013] *Proc Natl Acad Sci USA* 110:E3445–E3454. With permission from National Academy of Sciences.)

More recently, it has been appreciated that while PPI interfaces may be large, a small subset of residues, or **hot spots**, often contributes disproportionately to binding energies. This is indeed the case for binding of p53 to its negative regulators: the sites on MDM2 and MDMX occupied by the Phe19, Trp23 and Leu26 residues of p53 are considered hot spots. When hot spots are part of the binding interface, there is an increased chance of success in identifying small-molecule modulators of PPIs, since the competing ligand does not need to span such a large area. In fact, a high-throughput screen to identify inhibitors of the interaction between p53 and MDM2 led to one of the early examples of potent small-molecule PPI inhibitors.

The nutlins (named for Nutley inhibitor), reported by workers at Hoffmann-LaRoche, are a series of small-molecule inhibitors of MDM2s binding to p53. These *cis*-imidazolines were the result of an optimization effort that started from a hit identified from a high-throughput screen, and they are considered one of the first examples of highly potent PPI inhibitors developed from traditional screening. X-ray crystallography showed that, when bound to MDM2, the *cis*-imidazoline scaffold (blue) mimics the α-helical backbone of the p53 peptide and orients the substituents so they occupy the binding sites normally filled by the key Phe, Trp, and Leu triad. In the overlay of nutlin-2 (multicolor) and the p53 peptide (backbone = green) containing the hot-spot residues (red) shown in **Figure 8.6**, one bromophenyl of nutlin-2 mimics the the Leu of p53, another overlaps with Trp side chain, and the ethyl ether occupies the same site as Phe.

Since the report of the nutlins, additional small-molecule inhibitors of MDM2 that work by mimicking the p53 helix have been reported. **Figure 8.7** illustrates a few representative scaffolds of MDM2 inhibitors that have advanced to clinical trials. Research on the nutlins led to idasanutlin, which has shown promising results against solid tumors and leukemias. AMG 232 is also in clinical trials, and is a compound developed at Amgen using a combination of high-throughput screening to identify a lead, and rational design based on other known inhibitors for optimization. A third example, NVP-CGM097, was developed at Novartis from a hit identified using a virtual screening approach. This compound is being evaluated for its effects against solid tumors. Despite their diverse scaffolds, all of these structures correctly orient the side chains for optimal binding to MDM2. These small-molecule inhibitors of MDM2, many optimized by rational drug design approaches, illustrate that large peptides can indeed be mimicked by small druglike molecules.

Another example of a PPI target that is mediated by only a few amino acids can be seen in the interaction between the proteins fibrinogen and glycoprotein IIb/IIIa (GPIIb/IIIa). This binding event is essential to platelet aggregation, and its inhibition is a viable therapeutic strategy to treat myocardial infarction and stroke. GPIIb/IIIa recognizes the short amino acid sequence arginine-glycine-aspartic acid (Arg-Gly-Asp or RGD) on fibrinogen. By mimicking this sequence of amino acids, compounds that inhibit binding of fibrinogen to GPIIb/IIIa were developed and have found use as anti-platelet agents.

Eptifibatide is a drug that was developed on the basis of inhibiting this PPI. A series of peptides isolated from snake venom, called disintegrins, were known to inhibit platelet aggregation, and most contained the RGD sequence. Screening of

Figure 8.6 Structure of nutlin-2.
Left: Chemical structure of nutlin-2, with cis-imidazoline scaffold in blue. The substituents occupy the same sub-pockets as the hot spot residues in p53: one bromophenyl occupies the Trp subsite, another the Leu subsite, and the ethyl ether side chain occupies the Phe subsite. Right: Overlay of p53 peptide backbone (red) containing Phe, Trp, Leu triad (green) and nutlin-2 (carbon = white, nitrogen = blue, oxygen = red, bromine = brown). The ethyl ether and Phe sidechain occupy the same space; the bromophenyl groups overlay with Trp and Leu sidechains, respectively. (From Vassilev LT, Vu BT, Graves B et al. [2004] *Science* 303:844–846. With permission from AAAS.)

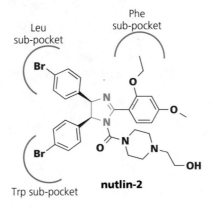
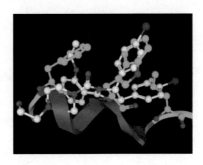

nutlin-2

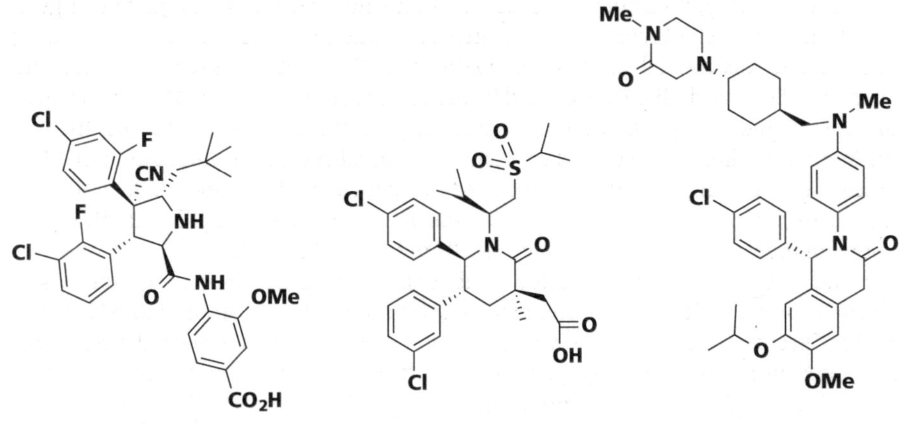

Figure 8.7 Structures of small-molecule inhibitors of p53 binding to MDM2 that have advanced to clinical trials. Idasanutlin was developed from the nutlin leads, while AMG 232 was based on a high-throughput screening lead as well as rational design. NVP-CGM097 was developed from a virtual screening program. Despite containing different scaffolds, all orient their substituents for optimal binding to the hot spot regions of MDM2; all three compounds advanced to clinical trials, and have shown promising results against solid tumors and leukemias.

idasanutlin   **AMG 232**   **NVP-CGM097**

62 snake venoms yielded a 73-amino-acid peptide called barbourin that selectively inhibited binding of GPIIb/IIIa to fibrinogen. Instead of RGD, barbourin contained a KGD sequence, with the basic lysine (K) replacing the arginine (R). Optimization by shortening the peptide and constraining its conformation via cyclization led to eptifibatide (**Figure 8.8**), a heptapeptide containing a disulfide bridge. It is a potent inhibitor of the binding of GPIIb/IIIa to fibrinogen and is approved as an injection to prevent blood clots from forming after certain types of chest pain and heart attack, as well as for patients undergoing coronary angioplasty.

A significant effort to convert the RGD peptide sequence to peptide mimetics with improved druglike characteristics was undertaken by a number of research groups. Isosteric replacement of the polar guanidine and acid groups was a common strategy, as was replacement of the labile peptide bonds. The considerable SAR available indicated that the optimal distance between the acidic and basic functions that correspond to Arg and Asp, respectively, was between 10 and 15 Å, and this information was used to design small-molecule inhibitors, as well as to screen for compounds that adhered to this pharmacophore. Of the many small molecule RGD mimetics that entered clinical trials, only tirofiban (**Figure 8.9**) was approved. The piperidine nitrogen of tirofiban mimics the guanidino group of the RGD sequence, and the tyrosine carboxylic acid replaces the aspartic acid residue. It is proposed that the sulfonamide makes additional interactions with the GPIIb/IIIa protein, not observed in the original disintegrins.

Figure 8.9 also shows a few of the RGD mimetics that advanced to clinical trials but ultimately failed, due to a lack of efficacy as well as slight increases in mortality as compared to placebo. Along with isosteric replacements, design strategies involved mimicking β- or γ-turn secondary structures observed in potent acyclic and cyclic RGD peptides, respectively. Examples include the benzodiazepine analog lotrafiban and the β-turn mimic shown. Efforts to use a prodrug strategy in

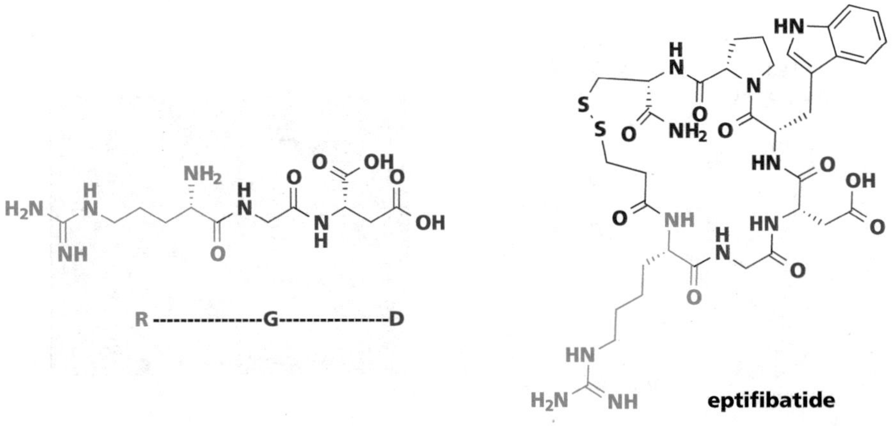

Figure 8.8 Structure of RGD and eptifibatide. Left: RGD, the Arg-Gly-Asp tripeptide present in fibrinogen, is recognized by GPIIb/IIIa. Right: eptifibatide is a constrained macrocyclic peptide that contains the RGD sequence. Blue, red, and purple correspond to R, G, and D residues, respectively.

R --------------G----------------D

eptifibatide

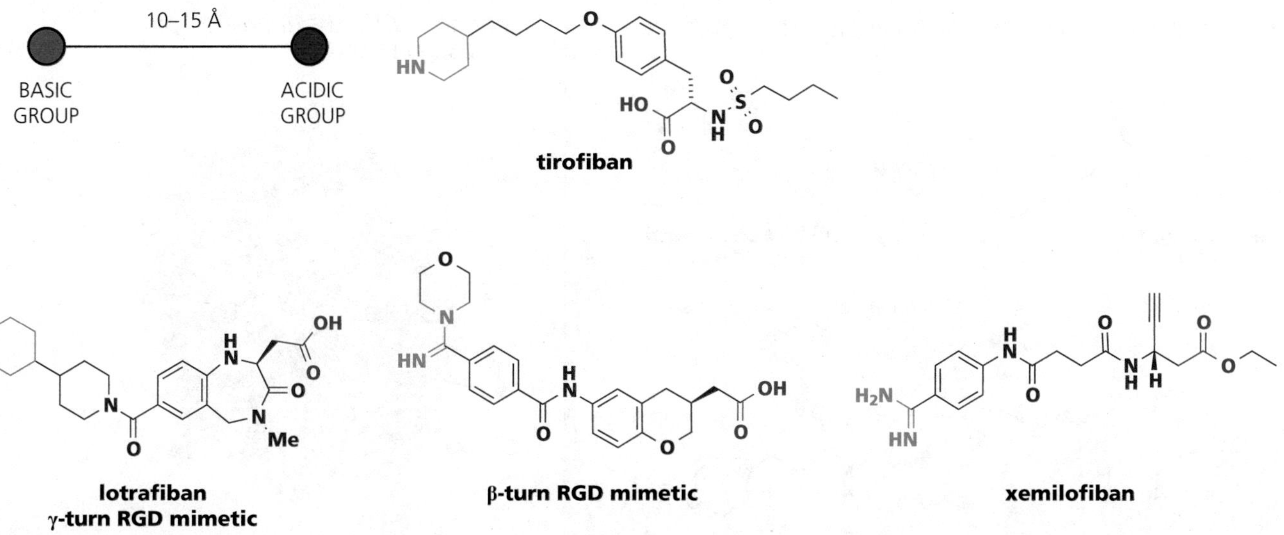

Figure 8.9 Pharmacophore model for GPIIb/IIIa antagonists. Blue denotes basic functionality, and purple denotes acidic functionality. Tirofiban is the only approved peptide mimetic drug in this class. The piperidine (blue) and acid (purple) correspond to the Arg and Asp side chains in fibrinogen. Other representative structures of inhibitors that are RGD mimetics include lotrafiban, a beta-turn mimic, and the prodrug ethyl ester xemilofiban. In each of these, blue indicates the basic group and purple the acidic group of the pharmacophore.

order to generate orally available molecules have also been also described, with the ethyl ester xemilofiban as one example that progressed to clinical trials but did not receive approval.

The development of compounds that bind to BCL-X$_L$ and BCL-2 represent a third example of small molecules blocking protein–protein interactions at their interface. These two proteins are anti-apoptotic and important for the survival of certain cancer cells. It was rationalized that small molecules that interacted with BCL-X$_L$ and its homologs and prevented their binding to their natural partners would inhibit their pro-survival effects, and be potential anti-cancer agents. In a fragment-based screen, researchers at Abbott used NMR to identify low molecular weight compounds that bound to BCL-X$_L$ at two distinct sites, later identified as the P2 and P4 sites, albeit with very low affinity. Linking of these fragments, a biphenyl acid and a biphenyl alcohol, together and further optimization eventually led to navitoclax, an inhibitor of both BCL-X$_L$ and BCL-2 binding to their protein partners. The thiophenyl fragment occupies the same site the original biphenyl alcohol hit did (P4), and the chloro-cyclohexenylphenyl occupies the same site as the biphenyl acid hit (P2). Navitoclax advanced to clinical trials for small-cell lung cancers (**Figure 8.10A**) but was dropped due to an unforeseen side effect of thrombocytopenia, linked to its inhibition of BCL-X$_L$. The similar drug venetoclax, selective for BCL-2, was then advanced and received FDA approval for leukemia in 2016 as the first BCL-2 inhibitor (**Figure 8.10C**). The success of this project has been partially attributed to the fact that the protein interface between BCL-X$_L$ and its partners is smaller than other protein–protein interfaces (~600 Å^2) and consists of a deep hydrophobic groove of about 20 Å where small molecules can bind. This groove has two sites, P2 and P4, that bind its protein partners. An X-ray structure of navitoclax shows that two portions of the molecule bind in those P2 and P4 hydrophobic sites (**Figure 8.10B**).

These examples highlight two general strategies for identifying inhibitors of PPIs. First, by understanding the local conformation and structure of the binding interface, scaffolds can be designed that correctly orient side chains for efficient binding with the protein partner. This approach is applicable not only to α-helices but also to other types of protein secondary structures such as β-turns. Second, the concept of hot spots explains that there are certain segments of some PPI interfaces that contribute to binding more so than others. In these circumstances, identifying small molecule inhibitors of the PPI is much more likely. These interfaces are characterized by hydrophobicity as well as size, shape, and depth. Considerable efforts are under way to accurately identify hot spots by computational methods in order to expedite PPI drug design. Given the diverse nature of PPIs and the interactions that contribute to disease states, a variety of different strategies to modulate these interactions are possible. Some of these strategies have led to approved drugs, while some are still in the earliest stages of discovery.

A: FRAGMENTS AND LINKED OPTIMIZED STRUCTURE OF NAVITOCLAX

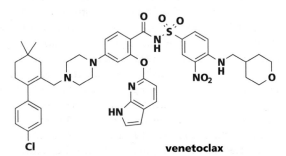

first site ligand
$K_D = 0.3$ mM

second site ligand
$K_D = 6$ mM

Link, optimize

navitoclax
$K_D = <1$ nM

B: X-RAY STRUCTURE OF NAVITOCLAX BOUND TO BCL-2

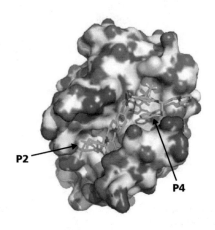

P2

P4

thiophenyl binds in hydrophobic pocket P4;
1-chloro-4-cyclohexenyl aryl binds in
hydrophobic pocket P2

C: STRUCTURE OF BCL-2 SELECTIVE INHIBITOR VENETOCLAX

venetoclax

Figure 8.10 PPI inhibitors of BCL-X$_L$ identified by fragment-based screening. A: Two low-affinity fragments, a biphenyl acid and a biphenyl alcohol, that bind to distinct sites of BCL-X$_L$ were identified by NMR. Linking the two and extensive further optimization generated navitoclax (portions derived from fragments depicted in red and linker in blue) are shown. B: X-ray crystal structure of navitoclax bound in hydrophobic cleft; thiophenyl binds in pocket P4 and chloro,cyclohexenyl aryl binds in pocket P2. C: Structure of FDA-approved BCL-2 inhibitor venetoclax. (B, adapted from Souers AJ, Leverson JD, Boghaert ER et al. [2013] *Nat Med* 19:202–210. With permission from Macmillan Publishers Limited.)

8.2   Modulators of protein–protein interactions may change the equilibrium of a multiprotein complex, and examples of such are valuable anti-cancer agents

When several proteins bind transiently in order to modulate a pharmacological effect, small molecules that either stabilize or destabilize the complex can be used to prolong the effect (stabilize), reduce the effect (destabilize), or merely change the equilibrium. The most notable small molecule examples in this category are those that modulate tubulin polymerization. Tubulins, which exist in two forms, α and β, are spherical proteins that interact to form a heterodimer, that also contains two molecules of GTP. The heterodimers interact further in a head-to-tail orientation to form a long protein fiber called a protofilament that undergoes further elongation by polymerization, eventually leading to a pipelike structure called a microtubule. Microtubules are not static structures but are under active states of polymerization and de-polymerization, and this process is highly regulated by accessory proteins (**Figure 8.11A**). In the depolymerization process, protofilaments curve and peel off from the straight microtubule, releasing heterodimers. Two general classes of small molecule modulators are known: those that destabilize the polymer, leading to excessive depolymerization, and those that stabilize the polymer, thereby preventing depolymerization. These small molecules are thought to mimic the accessory proteins that regulate the polymerization/depolymerization process. Multiple binding sites for small molecules on tubulin have been characterized, and structural studies illustrate how these molecules disrupt tubulin oligomers.

Figure 8.11 Structure of microtubule and small molecule modulator binding sites. A: Schematic of tubulin polymerization: α-tubulin (yellow) and β-tubulin (blue) form α/β-tubulin heterodimers. Further association of the dimers generates protofilaments (not shown) and eventually microtubules, which depolymerize by curving and then releasing heterodimers. B: Binding sites on α-tubulin (yellow) and β-tubulin (blue) of small-molecule modulators paclitaxel (green, binds to a site on β-tubulin, on the inside surface of the microtubule between adjacent protofilaments), colchicine (magenta, binds deep in the β-tubulin monomer, near its interface with the α-tubulin monomer), and vincristine (blue, binds β-tubulin near GTP). GTP molecules are shown in red/orange. The green line represents the axis of growth of protofilaments (stabilized by paclitaxel); cyan and orange lines represent axes of peeling protofilaments, stabilized by colchicine and vincristine, respectively. (From Stanton RA, Gernert KM, Nettles JH & Aneja R [2011] *Med Res Rev* 31:443–481. With permission from John Wiley & Sons, Inc.)

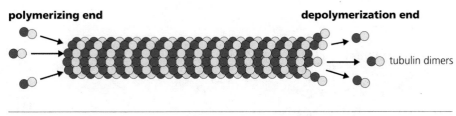

A: STRUCTURE OF MICROTUBULE COMPOSED OF α/β-TUBULIN DIMERS

polymerizing end   depolymerization end

tubulin dimers

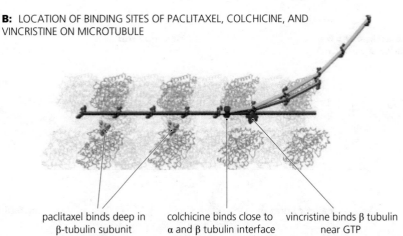

B: LOCATION OF BINDING SITES OF PACLITAXEL, COLCHICINE, AND VINCRISTINE ON MICROTUBULE

paclitaxel binds deep in β-tubulin subunit

colchicine binds close to α and β tubulin interface

vincristine binds β tubulin near GTP

Colchicine (**Figure 8.12**), a natural product derived from the autumn crocus, is a drug used to treat gout. The plant's medicinal effects have been known for many centuries: the Ebers papyrus (ca. 1500 BC) described its use to treat swelling and rheumatism. It binds to the tubulin heterodimer deep in the β-tubulin monomer, near its interface with the α-tubulin monomer (see **Figure 8.11B**). That binding induces kinks in the interface, leading to curved polymers and a preference for depolymerization. Other molecules, such as nocadazole, bind at or near the same site and are frequently used as tools by researchers studying tubulin and cancer biology.

The vinca alkaloids, such as vincristine and vinblastine (**Figure 8.13**), are natural products isolated from the Madagascar periwinkle plant that have been used as anti-cancer agents since the 1960s. Like colchicine, they destabilize tubulin polymers. However, they bind at a distinct interfacial binding site (called the vinca site, see Figure 8.11B) between the α- and β-subunits within a protofilament, and this leads to a curved structure that favors depolymerization. Compounds of diverse structure, some with high complexity, bind at or near the vinca binding site are shown in Figure 8.13 and include hemiasterlin, maytansine, halichondrin and eribulin. This is in contrast to the colchicine binding site: while recognizing multiple scaffolds, that site does not bind compounds of such drastically different structures. A number of compounds that bind and inhibit polymerization or destabilize the polymer have either advanced into clinical trials or are approved drugs. An analog of the natural product hemiasterlin has advanced to clinical trials, an antibody conjugate of maytansine is also being clinically evaluated and a fragment of the natural product halichondrin B (eribulin; see Chapter 1) has been approved to treat certain cancers.

Taxol (paclitaxel), a natural product isolated from the Pacific yew tree, was identified as a highly potent anti-proliferative agent through a government-sponsored natural product screening effort. Its mechanism of stabilizing microtubules rather then destabilizing them, when determined, was unique from others previously known. It binds to a site on β-tubulin (see Figure 8.11B), on the inside surface of the microtubule between adjacent protofilaments, through a large number of H-bonding and hydrophobic interactions. The resultant structures are stabilized and resistant to disassembly. Since the discovery of this mechanism, several other natural products that act in a similar fashion have been identified, such as the epothilones, a family of natural products isolated from a soil bacterium. The epothilones are competitive

MeO · OMe
MeO

MeO

O   NH

O

colchicine

H   O
N   OMe
N

NH
N
O

nocadazole

Figure 8.12 Structures of colchicine and nocadazole. Both compounds bind to tubulin at the same site and inhibit tubulin polymerization.

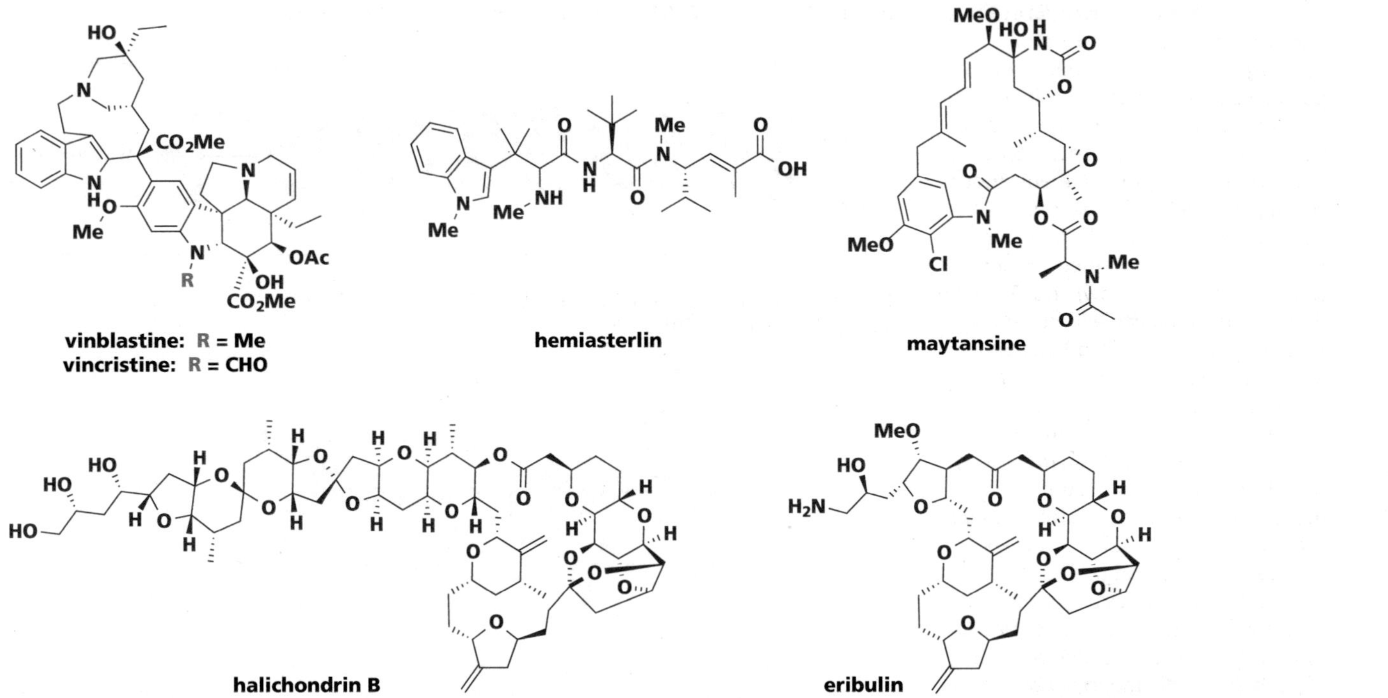

vinblastine: **R = Me**
vincristine: **R = CHO**

hemiasterlin

maytansine

halichondrin B

eribulin

inhibitors of paclitaxel, suggesting that they bind at or near the same site on β-tubulin. Ixabepilone, a semisynthetic derivative of epothilone B, is approved for the treatment of certain cancers, as are Taxol (paclitaxel) and two taxoids, docetaxel and cabazitaxel, which differ primarily in the constitution of the ester side chain (**Figure 8.14**).

Although several high-resolution co-crystal structures of molecules bound to tubulin polymers are available, designing new or improved molecules has primarily relied on developing an understanding of structure–activity relationship studies and developing pharmacophore models. **Figure 8.15** shows one such model that superimposes the diverse structures of taxoids and epothilones, which are believed to bind to the same site.

In this example of a binding model, common structural features of paclitaxel and epothilone B include the *gem*-dimethyl and adjacent alcohol (red), cyclic ethers (oxetane in paclitaxel and epoxide in epothilone B, black), and the H-bond acceptor displayed by the carbonyl oxygen of paclitaxel and alcohol of epothilone B (red). The macrocyclic rings of the two compounds overlap, as do the thiazole side chain of epothilone and the C-2 side chain of the taxane (Figure 8.15B).

However, this area is still controversial, as is the precise bioactive conformation of Taxol. Medicinal chemistry efforts to design improved tubulin stabilizers continues to garner significant interest. For instance, the approved anti-cancer drug ixabepilone is a lactam analog of the natural epothilone B that provides improved metabolic stability compared to the natural product, and many efforts have gone toward modifying taxoids to reduce their tendency to be effluxed. To date, however, the most effective compounds have been very close to the original natural product structure.

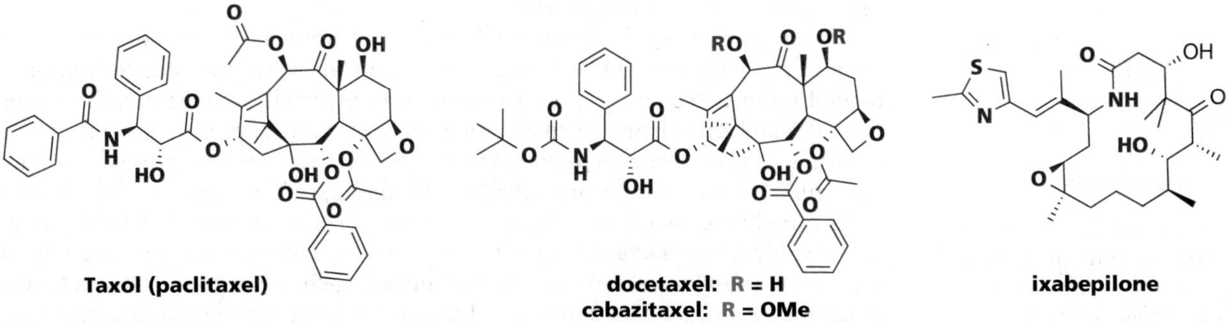

Figure 8.13 Structures of compounds that bind to the vinca binding site and destabilize microtubules. Vincristine, vinblastine, hemiasterlin, maytansine, halichondrin B, and eribulin represent the vastly diverse structures that bind at or near the vinca binding site.

Figure 8.14 Structures of microtubule-stabilizing anti-cancer drugs. Taxol (paclitaxel), docetaxel, cabazitaxel, and ixabepilone are shown. Taxol was the first stabilizing compound identified, and docetaxel and cabazitaxel are close analogs. Ixabepilone is a semi-synthetic analog of epothilone, and is also approved to treat certain cancers.

Taxol (paclitaxel)

docetaxel: **R = H**
cabazitaxel: **R = OMe**

ixabepilone

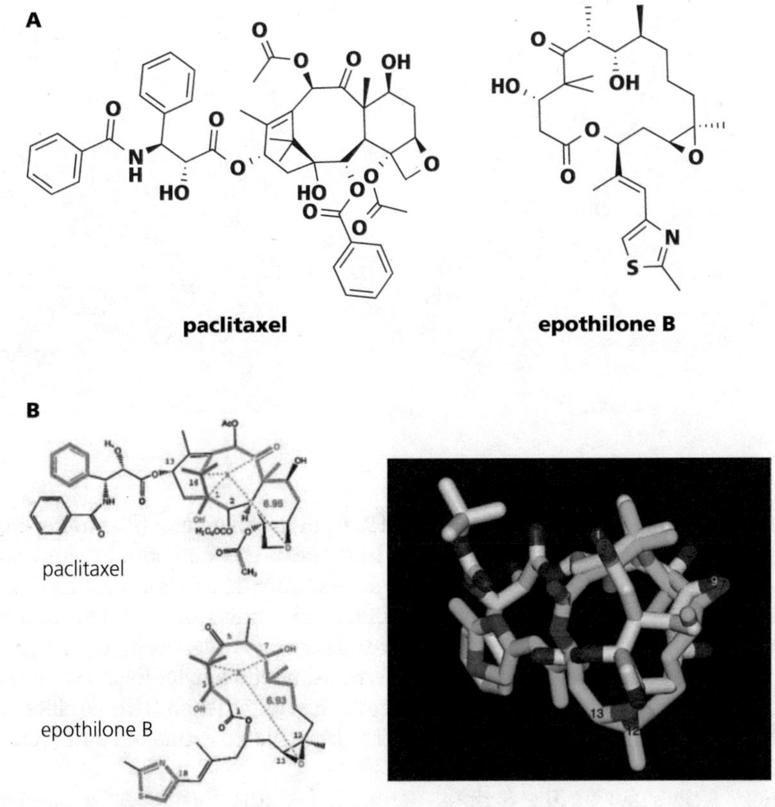

Figure 8.15 Structures of paclitaxel and epothilone B and pharmacophore model. A: Structures of paclitaxel and epothilone B. B: Pharmacophore model of the two molecules, with common structural features (gem-dimethyl with adjacent alcohol, cyclic ether and H-bond acceptor carbonyl and alcohol) shown in red, and X defining the center of the model. Bonds/atoms shown in blue are those that overlap in the model on the right, which is a molecular modeling-derived overlay (paclitaxel in yellow, epothilone B in cyan), showing similar footprint despite different scaffolds. (Adapted from Giannakakou P, Gussio R, Nogales E et al. [2000] *Proc Natl Acad Sci USA* 97:2904–2909. With permission from National Academy of Sciences.)

A

paclitaxel

epothilone B

B

paclitaxel

epothilone B

8.3   Modulators of protein–protein interactions can reduce levels of misactive proteins, and examples are useful to treat rare diseases

Typical drug targets are either overactive or underactive proteins. However, a third possibility is that a protein is misactive. For example, if a protein inappropriately aggregates, it may become pathogenic as the aggregate (gain of function) or incapable of performing its normal function (loss of function). The misfolding of the protein α-synuclein forms fibrils that are components of Lewy bodies found in patients with Parkinson's disease, and misfolding of β-amyloid protein to form amyloid plaques found in the brains of Alzheimer's patients is believed to contribute to the neurodegeneration characteristic of that disease. In instances such as these, a drug discovery strategy is to use a small-molecule PPI modulator to revert the protein to a correctly folded (nonaggregated) conformation or sequester the misactive protein.

Transthyretin (TTR) is a tetrameric protein whose role is to transport certain proteins and hormones. Transthyretin amyloidosis is a rare disease that results from the TTR monomer misfolding and aggregating. Patients first experience degeneration of cardiac tissue and then death within about 10 years of symptom onset. **Figure 8.16** illustrates

Figure 8.16 Equilibrium between various states of TTR tetramers, monomers, and pathogenic aggregates. The functional, ligand-bound tetramer is in equilibrium with the free tetramer as well as folded monomer. When folded monomer becomes denatured, it can misfold and is prone to oligomerization; oligomers form disease-causing aggregates and amyloid fibrils. (Adapted from Johnson SM, Connelly S, Fearns C et al. [2012] *J Mol Biol* 421:185–203. With permission from Elsevier.)

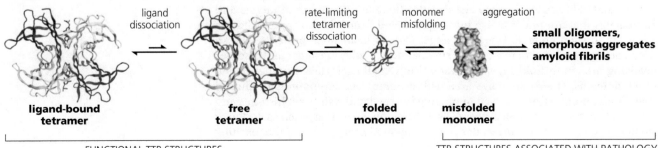

ligand dissociation

rate-limiting tetramer dissociation

monomer misfolding

aggregation

small oligomers, amorphous aggregates amyloid fibrils

ligand-bound tetramer

free tetramer

folded monomer

misfolded monomer

FUNCTIONAL TTR STRUCTURES

TTR STRUCTURES ASSOCIATED WITH PATHOLOGY

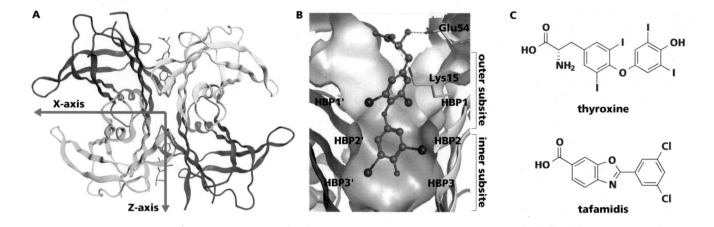

Figure 8.17 Design of molecules to stabilize TTR tetramer. A: X-ray structure of TTR tetramer (each monomer is shown in a different color; two bound molecules of thyroxine are seen at yellow–red and blue–green interfaces. B: Binding site of thyroxine with molecular interactions (HBP = hydrophobic pocket). The inner subsite makes hydrophobic interactions with one aryl ring of thyroxine; the second aryl ring sits in the outer subsite and makes interactions with hydrophobic groups as well as with the adjacent lysine (Lys15), and the terminal amine interacts with a glutamic acid (Glu54). C: Structures of natural ligand thyroxine and drug tafamidis. (Adapted from Johnson SM, Connelly S, Fearns C et al. [2012] *J Mol Biol* 421:185–203. With permission from Elsevier.)

the equilibrium between various states of TTR, from the thyroxine (hormone)-bound tetramer to the misfolded and aggregated monomer. The functional ligand-bound tetramer (left) is the most thermodynamically stable structure and is in equilibrium with the free tetramer as well as with the correctly folded monomer. However, if the monomer is misfolded, it becomes prone to aggregation and generates oligomers, aggregates, and fibrils, which are pathogenic. In many patients, transthyretin amyloidogenesis is caused by mutations in the TTR protein that destabilize the free tetramer, shift the equilibrium to the right, and allow more of the free monomer to be available to misfold and eventually aggregate.

Jeffery Kelly's lab at The Scripps Research Institute developed a strategy to stabilize the properly folded tetramer via binding of a small molecule, thereby shifting the equilibrium away from the misfolded monomer. The TTR tetramer binds the small molecule thyroxine (however, at any given time, only a small percentage of the two thyroxine binding sites on TTR are occupied). The X-ray crystal structure of thyroxine bound to TTR showed thyroxine bound to the inner and outer subsite through multiple hydrophobic and H-bonding interactions, and this structure was used to design molecules that make similar interactions. (**Figure 8.17**). In addition, screening approaches were also employed.

A general feature of all active molecules was the presence of substituted aryl rings connected by a linker. The substituents on the ring occupying the inner subsite make H-bonds with nearby serine residues and/or hydrophobic interactions. Aryl ring substituents in the outer subsite make salt bridges with an adjacent lysine residue as well as hydrophobic interactions that are similar to those made by the iodine atoms in thyroxine (Figure 8.17B). Tafamidis is approved to treat transthryetin-related hereditary amyloidosis. Its dichlorophenyl group sits in the inner subsite, occupying the same site as the terminal di-iodophenyl group in thyroxine. The carboxylic acid makes a water mediated interaction with both the glutamic acid and lysine residues, also seen in the thyroxine-TTR co-structure.

As described above, drugs that work via PPIs are much less common than those that target enzymes or receptors. Despite the challenges, understanding how to design and optimize small molecules that modulate PPIs is an emerging area with considerable success in the last decade. There are a number of targets and approaches that are under active investigation and from which drug candidates are likely to soon emerge. One such target class is heat-shock proteins (HSPs), which are up-regulated in response to stress and have roles in cancer and diseases involving protein misfolding, with several drugs in clinical trials. Another target, bromodomains, is also an active area with a number of compounds in clinical trials. These proteins are involved in binding to acetylated lysines on histones and have a role in proliferation of cancer cells. In addition, new areas, such as design of small molecules that will correct deficient or mutated proteins, is another exciting area of opportunity.

LIPIDS OF CELL MEMBRANES AS DRUG TARGETS

Another atypical drug target is the lipids found in cell membranes. Although they are different from protein–protein interactions, the hydrophobic interactions necessary for membrane integrity, and even for properly maintaining protein structure, can also be affected by drugs. Until recently, lipids and the membrane structures they form were considered inert structural molecules that were devoid of physiological properties. However, today there is a greater appreciation that they can play a significant role in physiological and disease processes. For example, certain lipid structures can sequester proteins and thereby indirectly play a role in cell signaling and protein transport. In addition, lipids can directly bind enzymes and either activate or inactivate them. Therefore by modulating lipids with small molecules, one has the potential to indirectly affect a large number of systems.

Unfortunately, understanding how lipid composition affects membranes and proteins is a very immature field. Consequently, there is not universal agreement on the mechanism of drugs that target lipids, let alone how to design drugs to do so. One reason for this lack of understanding is that few methods are available to study lipid bilayers in their natural setting, primarily because the lipid bilayer is a dynamic supramolecular structure rather than a single molecule with a defined action, such as an enzyme. In most cases, models must be used, and membranes must be reconstituted. Methods such as NMR and specialized microscopy have been used to visualize the changes in membrane structure that result from drug interaction.

8.4   Drugs acting at lipids in membranes act as anti-infective agents

Only a handful of drugs are known to work by modifying the lipid membrane, and they are primarily anti-infective agents. Some of these agents work by disrupting the cell membrane and allowing ions and nutrients to escape, thereby causing cell death. Others bind to lipid components of the cell membrane, such as lipid II of bacterial cell membranes or ergosterol of fungal cell membranes. However, the specific mechanism by which the membrane is disrupted varies, and designing molecules to do so selectively is quite challenging. One example is shown below; other examples can be found in Chapter 12.

Daptomycin (**Figure 8.18**), isolated from cultures of *Streptomyces roseosporus*, is a branched cyclic lipopeptide. The macrocycle is made up of 10 amino acids, and the branch consists of three linked amino acids that terminate with a decanoic amide moiety. Of the 13 amino acids that comprise daptomycin, five are unnatural (shown in blue), either in stereochemistry (D rather than L) or in structure (3-methylglutamate and kynurenine). In addition, a four-amino-acid sequence in the ring (DADG, shown in red) is a calcium-binding motif observed in many calcium-binding proteins. Daptomycin is approved to treat Gram-positive skin infections, including those caused by methicillin-resistant *Staphylococcus aureus* (MRSA), and bacteremia. It represents one of only three new classes of antibacterial drugs approved since the 1970s.

Daptomycin targets the Gram-positive bacterial membrane, and its activity requires the presence of Ca^{2+} at physiological concentrations. Its mode of action is still controversial. One hypothesis is that a micellar structure containing multiple monomers is formed in the presence of calcium ions, allowing the daptomycin micelle to approach the bacterial cell wall (see Figure 8.18). Once there, the supramolecular structure dissociates, inserts into the bilayer, and oligomerizes, disrupting the membrane structure and causing efflux of potassium ions, loss of membrane potential, and eventual cell death. However, other models are also favored.

Another example of an anti-infective agent targeting lipids is the antifungal drug amphotericin B (AmB). This polyene macrolide consists of a polar face (displaying polyol), a hydrophobic face (displaying polyene), and a mycosamine unit. Fungi are eukaryotes that use ergosterol to form their cell membranes, as opposed to cholesterol that is used by animals. While it has been proposed for many years that amphotericin B forms pores in fungal cell membranes by making hydrophobic interactions with ergosterol, and forming a macromolecular structure that makes the membrane permeable (**Figure 8.19A**), this model has been supplanted by one in

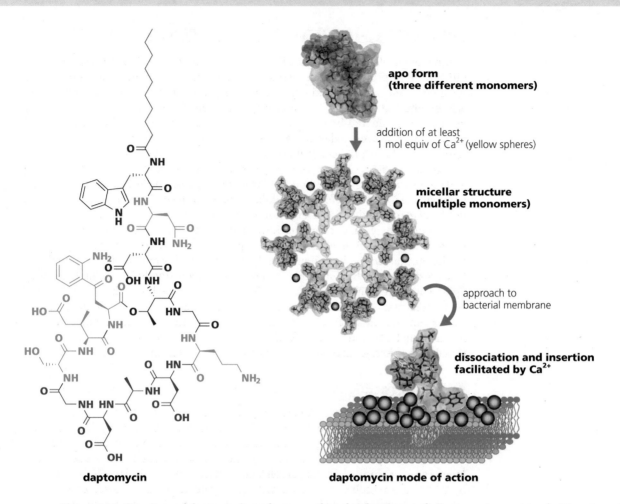

Figure 8.18 Structure of daptomycin and proposed mode of action. Left: Daptomycin consists of a 10-amino acid macrocycle, and pendant acylated tripeptide. Unnatural amino acids are shown in blue, calcium-binding sequence is depicted in red at the bottom and lipophilic tail is shown in magenta at the top. Right: Micellar structure forms in the presence of calcium ions (depicted as yellow spheres), without change in daptomycin's conformation, which favors approach to the cell membrane. Once at the membrane, the supramolecular structure dissociates, daptomycin embeds into the membrane and disrupts it. (B, adapted from Scott WRP, Baek S-B, Jung D et al. [2007] *Biochim Biophys Acta, Biomembr* 1768:3116–3126. With permission from Elsevier.)

which amphotericin B acts by sequestering ergosterol as its primary mechanism, and removing it from the lipid bilayer as seen in **Figure 8.19B**.

Drugs that work by interacting with lipids constitute an evolving area. The few that are known have been identified by phenotypic screening, and their mechanisms were elucidated well after they were discovered. In many cases, their specific mode of action is still being studied and elucidated. However, as more is understood, strategies to design drugs *a priori* to interfere with lipids may be forthcoming. By modulating lipid structure, small-molecule modulators have the potential to affect membrane-bound protein structure, lipid signaling, and cell membrane integrity. While drugs in this class are primarily anti-infective agents, future agents may target central nervous system disorders, cancer, and a wider variety of therapeutic areas.

SUMMARY

While most drug discovery efforts have focused on receptors and enzymes as drug targets, there are many other opportunities. Although there are inherent difficulties in targeting protein–protein interactions and interfering with lipid structures, many natural products have been found to do just that. Drugs such as Taxol and daptomycin are large complex molecules, whose biological effects were identified well before their mechanism of action. While the area of designing small modulators of lipid structures

Figure 8.19 Structures of amphotericin B and ergosterol and proposed mechanisms. A: Amphotericin B (AmB) consists of a macrocyclic polyol that displays a polar and an apolar face (black), with a polar mycosamine unit (blue) appended. Ergosterol (green) is the main constituent of fungal membranes. The polar carbohydrate is proposed to hydrogen-bond (red dashed line) to the alcohol of ergosterol; the polyene has hydrophobic interactions with ergosterol, and the C35-OH (blue) can hydrogen-bond to the polar end of the membrane lipid. B: Two proposed mechanisms based on lipid interaction. The preferred mechanism involves amphotericin B sequestering ergosterol via 1:1 binding. The less favored mechanism requires the ergosterol–amphotericin B complex to form a macromolecular structure that embeds in the membrane, making pores. (Adapted from Gray KC, Palacios DS, Dailey I et al. [2012] *Proc Natl Acad Sci USA* 109:2234–2239. With permission from National Academy of Sciences.)

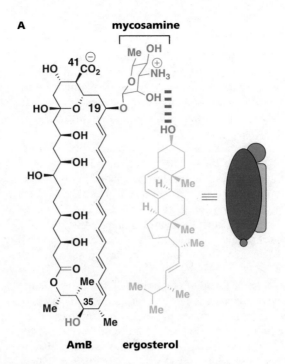

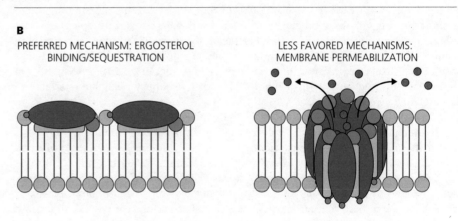

is in its infancy, designing modulators of PPIs is much more advanced. Recent approaches rely on understanding the binding interface and designing molecules that either mimic one of the binding partners or can interact with specific residues at the interface. The use of biophysical techniques such as X-ray crystallography, cryo-electron microscopy, mass spectrometry, and surface plasmon resonance is essential to detect and measure the activity of these small-molecule binders. The importance of protein–protein interactions in pathophysiology makes this area one that will see significant growth in terms of new strategies and approaches, as well as successful drug discovery.

CASE STUDY 1 DISCOVERY OF TAXOL

The discovery and development of Taxol (paclitaxel) highlights the long and arduous process that it sometimes takes to get a drug approved. It involved natural product screening and structure elucidation, careful mechanistic studies that uncovered a unique mechanism of action, total synthesis and semisynthesis efforts to address an issue of limited supply, and eventual agreements between government and industry to move the drug forward.

In 1962, a U.S. Department of Agriculture botanist, Arthur Barclay, working under contract for the U.S. National Cancer Institute (NCI) collected stem and bark samples from the Pacific yew tree (*Taxus brevifolia* Nutt) in Washington state (**Figure 8.20**). Extracts from these samples were found to be cytotoxic to KB cancer cells in a typical assay to predict anti-cancer activity. In 1965, through another NCI contract, a large sample of bark was sent to Monroe E. Wall at the Research Triangle Institute. The isolation and bioactivity of Taxol was reported by Wall and his collaborator, Mansukh Wani, at the 1967 American Chemical Society Meeting, however, its structure was not elucidated until 1971.

Initial enthusiasm for the bioactivity of Taxol and its potential as a drug was not high. Its potency in *in vitro* and *in vivo* leukemia assays was modest, it had very poor solubility in water, and it was only available in small quantities from the bark of the uncommon and slow-growing Pacific yew tree. However, additional *in vivo* testing in B16 melanoma models provided more promising results and led scientists to pursue it further. In 1977, the NCI asked Susan B. Horwitz of Albert Einstein College of Medicine to study the mechanism of Taxol. She received 10 mg of material, and in a short time her lab observed that Taxol-treated cells gave rise to a unique phenotype of highly stable microtubule bundles. Further study revealed a unique mechanism of action: promotion of tubulin polymerization and stabilization of microtubules. Phase I studies of Taxol were initiated in 1984 and phase II studies in 1985, despite significant limitations in drug supply. In 1989 and 1991, positive clinical results in ovarian and breast cancer were reported.

The promising results from clinical trials made solving the supply issue even more urgent. The Pacific yew is a slow-growing conifer found in old-growth forests in the Pacific Northwest. In the late 1980s, the NCI acquired ~120,000 lb of dried Pacific yew bark, which was derived from approximately 7000 trees, and afforded only 18 lb of pure Taxol (0.015% yield). It was estimated that six 100-year old trees were needed to treat one patient, and the relative scarcity of tree bark, as well as the damage that bark removal causes the tree, was a serious concern. A significant effort by a number of synthetic organic chemistry labs around the world focused on developing a scalable synthesis of Taxol to alleviate the supply issue. The problem was eventually solved via semisynthesis. In 1988, Pierre Potier at the Centre National de la Recherche Scientifique (CNRS) in France reported that 10-deacetylbaccatin III was readily available from the needles of a very common shrub called *Taxus baccata* and could be converted to Taxol-like structures. Robert Holton at Florida State University developed an improved method using the general strategy shown in **Figure 8.21**. The key step was acylation of the sterically hindered C13 alcohol with a reactive β-lactam to introduce the side chain.

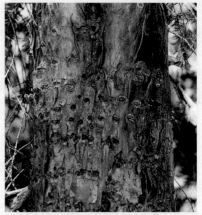

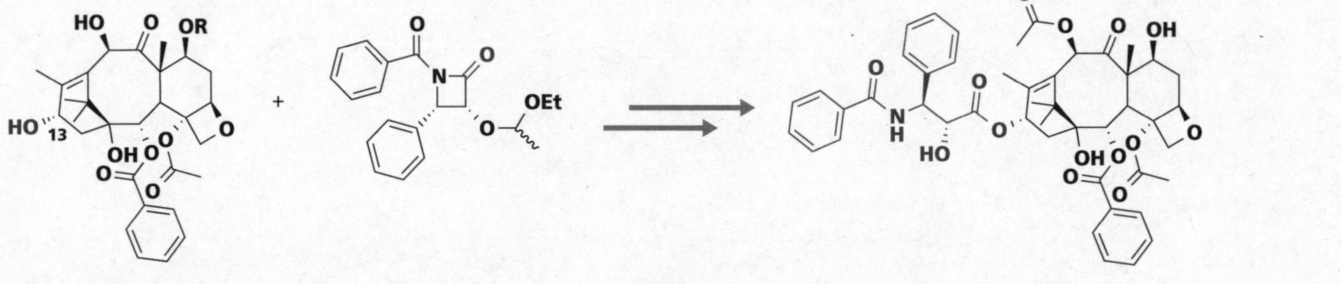

Figure 8.20 Bark of the Pacific yew tree *Taxus brevifolia*. Photo courtesy of Susan McDougall.

Figure 8.21 Key step in taxol semisynthesis. 10-Deacetylbaccatin III was found to be readily available from the needles of a common yew tree, and could be converted to Taxol-like structures. The Taxol side chain was coupled to 10-deacetylbaccatin III, by acylation of the C13 hydroxyl with a β-lactam. The C13 alcohol and the β-lactam carbonyl are shown in red in the starting materials, with the side chain of the coupled product also in red.

10-deacetylbaccatin III: R = H

taxol

The NCI granted a Cooperative Research and Development Agreement (CRADA) to Bristol-Myers Squibb (BMS), and they took over the development of Taxol. The FDA approved Taxol (paclitaxel) on December 29, 1992, 30 years after the extract was first collected, 21 years after the structure was elucidated, and 8 years after the first clinical trials were initiated. Taxol is approved to treat a number of cancers involving solid tumors, including breast, ovarian, bladder, and lung cancers.

Taxol continues to inspire scientific work. The total synthesis of Taxol was reported by a number of academic groups, but its use to provide the quantities needed for development and marketing was never feasible. Analogs of Taxol (docetaxel and cazabitaxel) and other microtubule-stabilizing agents (ixabepilone) are important drugs to treat cancers.

CASE STUDY 2 DISCOVERY OF MARAVIROC

The chemokine receptors CXCR4 and CCR5 are members of a large family of GPCRs that bind to protein ligands (chemokines) and play a role in the immune response. The endogenous ligands for the chemokine receptors are the peptides RANTES, MIP-1α, MIP-1β, and TNF. In addition to their physiological role, in 1999 CCR5 and CXCR4 were identified as essential co-factors for entry of the HIV into T-cells. The glycoprotein gp120, found on the surface of the viral particle, binds to a CD4 molecule on the surface of the host immune cells and then uses either the CCR5 or CXCR4 receptor as a second (co-)receptor. Once the viral particle is bound, it fuses to the cell, releases its genetic materials and infects the cell (**Figure 8.22**).

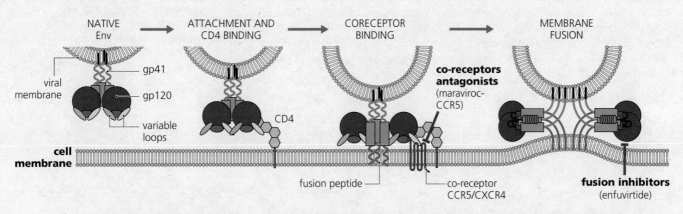

Figure 8.22 Fusion of HIV viral particle. Glycoprotein gp120 (shown in red) binds to a T-cell CD4 receptor (depicted as green hexagons) on the surface of the host T-cell, and then associates with the CCR5 or CXCR4 co-receptor (shown in purple). Fusion of the viral particle, mediated by fusion peptides, and release of viral nucleic acid material into the cell occurs. Maraviroc blocks the protein–protein interaction between gp120 and CCR5 required for fusion. Fusion inhibitors block a later step and prevent the virus from releasing its genetic material into the T-cell. (Adapted from Didigu CA & Doms RW [2012] *Viruses* 4:309–324. With permission from MDPI.)

Validation of the role of CCR5 in HIV infection was based on reports describing individuals who were both healthy and resistant to HIV infection and had a genetic mutation resulting in a lack of the CCR5 receptor. This observation, initially reported in 1996, suggested that compounds that blocked the binding of HIV particles to CXCR4 and CCR5 could be effective anti-HIV agents. Although CXCR4 and CCR5 are GPCRs, the goal was not to prevent the signal transduction they initiate but rather to block binding between gp120 and the chemokine receptor. As such, the target is treated as a PPI rather than a classical receptor.

High-throughput screening in an assay for inhibition of binding of radiolabeled ligand (MIP-1β) to CCR5 led to a series of hits that were filtered on the basis of Lipinski's rules, as well as target affinity and ligand efficiency. This process led to two compounds that were pursued, UK-107543 (**1**) and UK-179645 (**2**), shown in **Figure 8.23**. Both inhibited binding of the natural ligand to CCR5 but had no antiviral activity. Additionally, UK-107543 inhibited CYP450 2D6, which predicted future issues with drug–drug interactions.

Molecular modeling suggested that the pyridine nitrogen in **1** (shown in red) may contribute to CYP inhibition, so it was replaced with the isosteric carbon to give **3**; this modification reduced the CYP inhibition, but increased lipophilicity. Incorporation of an amide, inspired by the structure of **2**, afforded **4**, which had reduced lipophilicity, and now exhibited antiviral activity. Synthesis of both enantiomers of **4** proved that the more potent isomer was the *S*-enantiomer, with 44 times higher inhibition of MIP-1β binding; the *R*-enantiomer showed no measurable antiviral activity, suggesting only the eutomer contributed to the efficacy observed. Further modifications focused on maintaining potency, avoiding hERG liabilities and optimizing permeability. Replacement of the phenyl amide with a tetrahydropyran amide and conformational constraint of the piperidine into a tropane afforded a highly potent compound, with no hERG liabilities but still inadequate PK characteristics. This constrained piperidine modification was predicted to reduce Cyp450 2D6 inhibition due to increased steric hindrance that would remove a key interaction with an aspartic acid residue found in the Cyp enzyme (**Figure 8.24**). The tetrahydropyran group was incorporated as a way to limit hERG liability by adding polar functional groups without limiting permeability.

The tropane analog in Figure 8.24 was shown to be a selective antagonist of CCR5 binding to its chemokine ligands. It was also a potent inhibitor of HIV infection in blood cells and was noncytotoxic. The anti-HIV activity is proposed to result from conformational changes to CCR5 that disrupt interaction with gp120. However, the tropane analog exhibited poor pharmacokinetics, with rapid metabolism and <10% oral availability in dogs. Replacement of the benzimidazole with a triazole reduced both molecular weight and lipophilicity. Further modification of the amide eventually led to UK-427857 (maraviroc), which exhibited potent anti-HIV activity and no CYP or hERG activity (**Figure 8.25**). Although its bioavailability is still somewhat low (23%), it represents an improvement over the benzimidazole series.

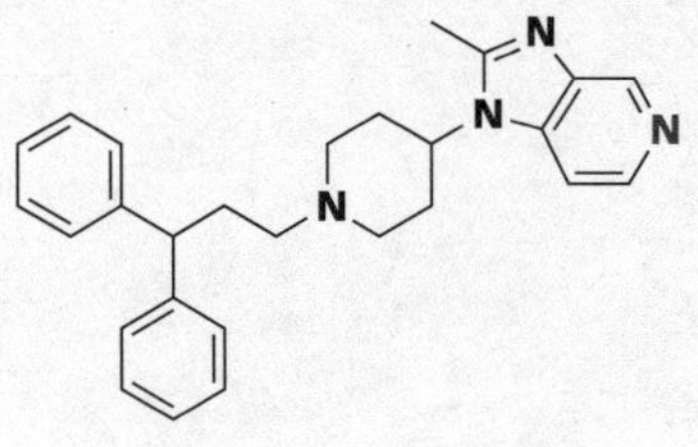

initial hit 1 (UK-107543)

MIP-1β: IC$_{50}$ = 4 nM
no antiviral activity
CYP450 inhibitor

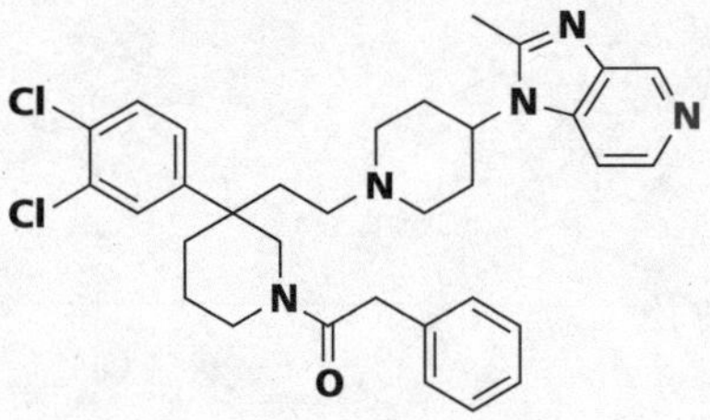

initial hit 2 (UK-179645)

MIP-1β: IC$_{50}$ = 11 nM
no antiviral activity

Figure 8.23 Structures of early hits in maraviroc drug discovery. Compounds **1** and **2** (with the pyridine nitrogen shown in red) both inhibited MIP-1β interaction with CCR5, indicative of binding to CCR5, but they had no anti-HIV activity.

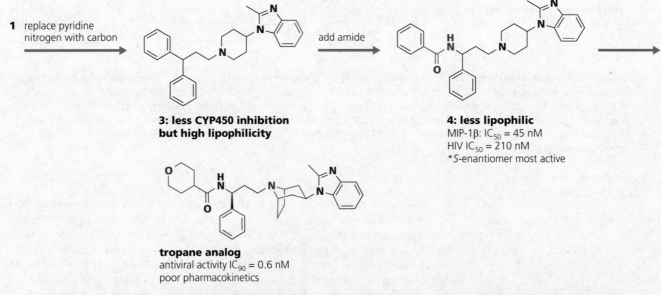

3: less CYP450 inhibition but high lipophilicity

4: less lipophilic
MIP-1β: IC$_{50}$ = 45 nM
HIV IC$_{50}$ = 210 nM
*S-enantiomer most active

tropane analog
antiviral activity IC$_{90}$ = 0.6 nM
poor pharmacokinetics

Figure 8.24 Structures illustrating lead development to give rigid tropane analog. Isosteric replacement of pyridyl nitrogen of **1** with carbon (**3**) reduced CYP450 inhibition, but made the analog too lipophilic. Inserting an amide linkage improved lipophilicity and cell-based anti-HIV activity (**4**), and there was a strong preference for the (S)-enantiomer. Conformational constraint of the piperidine and replacement of phenyl with tetrahydropyran led to a tropane analog, which had improved antiviral activity, but poor pharmacokinetics (changes in each series shown in red).

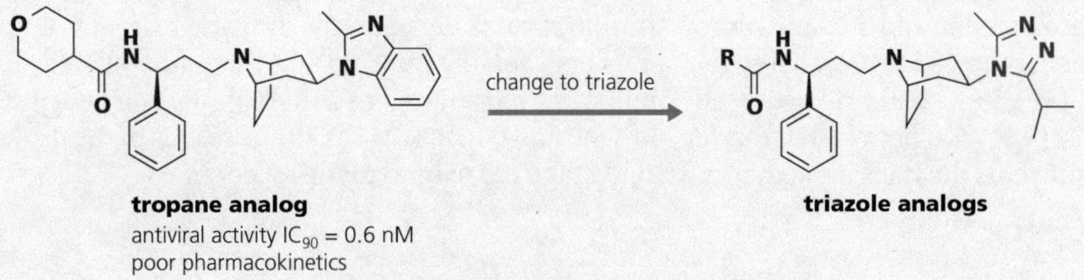

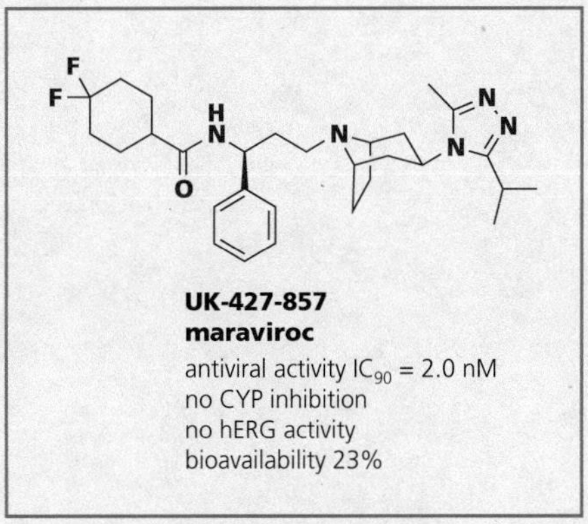

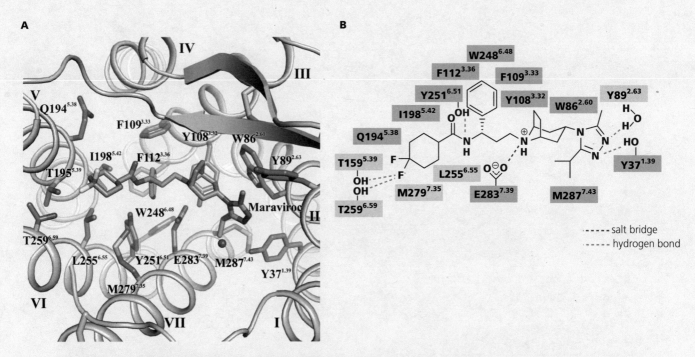

Figure 8.25 Development of maraviroc from tropane analog. Replacement of benzimidazole with a triazole (in red), and varying the amide group R, reduced lipopilicity and improved drug-like features and resulted in maraviroc.

tropane analog
antiviral activity IC_{90} = 0.6 nM
poor pharmacokinetics

change to triazole

triazole analogs

UK-427-857
maraviroc
antiviral activity IC_{90} = 2.0 nM
no CYP inhibition
no hERG activity
bioavailability 23%

Maraviroc was approved by the FDA in 2007 for use in patients infected with HIV. It is interesting to note that an X-ray co-crystal structure of maraviroc and CCR5 was published in 2013, showing that maraviroc binds at an allosteric site on CCR5 rather than the presumptive gp120 binding site (**Figure 8.26**). A number of key interactions

A

B

------ salt bridge
------ hydrogen bond

Figure 8.26 X-ray structure of maraviroc bound to CCR5. A: Maraviroc (depicted in orange) is shown in its binding pocket, away from its originally presumed site of action. B: Structure of maraviroc showing key interactions, including an ion–ion interaction between the tropane nitrogen and aspartate 283 (E283), hydrogen bonds between the fluorine and threonine hydroxyls (T195 and T259), and hydrogen bonding between the triazole and tyrosine 37 and between tyrosine 251 and the amide nitrogen. Residues previously identified by mutagenesis studies as important for binding are in purple squares. (From Tan Q, Zhu Y, Li J et al. [2013] *Science* 341:1387–1390. With permission from AAAS.)

are evident and include an ion–ion interaction between the tropane nitrogen and aspartate 283 (E283), hydrogen bonds between the fluorine and threonine hydroxyls (T195 and T259), and hydrogen bonding between nitrogens in the triazole and tyrosine 37 (Y37) and between the amide nitrogen and tyrosine 251 (Y251). Binding of the drug prevents the helix movements needed for gp120 to bind to the receptor.

REVIEW QUESTIONS

1. Explain why some drug targets (such as enzymes and receptors) are more druggable than others.

2. Describe three biophysical methods that can be used to detect binding between a small molecule and a protein.

3. What are the features of protein–protein interfaces?

4. Name two hit identification strategies that have been particularly successful in identifying modulators of PPIs.

5. Define hot spots and their importance in drug discovery.

6. Explain why drug design to target lipids is particularly challenging.

7. Define an interfacial binder.

8. On the basis of the examples in this chapter, identify at least two compounds that incorporate the medicinal chemistry concepts of conformational constraint and at least two that contain a privileged structure.

9. Explain the concept of stapling a peptide.

10. Compare the structures of ergosterol and cholesterol. What are the differences?

ergosterol

cholesterol

APPLICATION QUESTIONS

1. Research an example of a β-turn mimetic reported in the literature. Draw the structure and compare it to the peptide secondary structure.

2. Research one of the emerging PPI targets in Section 8.3. Describe how small-molecule modulators were identified, and draw their structures.

3. Research the magainins. Describe their structure and mechanism of action.

4. Design three different mimics of RGD (see Figure 8.9) that incorporate isosteres for the acid group.

5. Research other natural products, not mentioned in this chapter, that bind to tubulin. Pick one and draw its structure. Is it a stabilizer or destabilizer? Is its binding site known?

6. Tacrolimus (or FK506) and cyclosporin are important drugs used to prevent transplant rejection. They have very complex mechanisms of action that involve protein–protein interactions. Choose one and research its structure and general mechanism of action.

7. Review the structure of amphotericin B. Does it obey Lipinski's rules? For log*P*, use a program such as ChemDraw to generate a calculated value.

8. Review the MDM2 inhibitor structures in Figure 8.7. Orient them to propose how they share a common pharmacophore. Propose a pharmacophore that is consistent with this orientation.

9. Give one example of a small-molecule drug that is an interfacial binder.

FURTHER READING

Protein–protein interactions

Bonetta L (2010) Interactome under construction. *Nature* 468:851–854.

Pobbati AV, Chan SW, Lee I et al. (2012) Structural and functional similarity between the Vgll1-TEAD and the YAP-TEAD complexes. *Structure* 20:1135–1140.

Arkin M, Tang Y & Wells JA (2014) Small-molecule inhibitors of protein–protein interactions: progressing toward the reality. *Chem Biol* 21:1102–1114.

Scott DE, Bayly AR, Abell C et al. (2016) Small molecules, big targets: drug discovery faces the protein-protein interaction challenge. *Nature Rev Drug Disc* 15: 533–550.

Fry DC (2012) Small-molecule inhibitors of protein–protein interactions: How to mimic a protein partner. *Curr Pharm Des* 18:4679–4684.

Jin L, Wang W & Fang G (2014) Targeting protein–protein interaction by small molecules. *Annu Rev Pharmacol Toxicol* 54:435–456.

Petros AM, Dinges J, Augeri DJ et al. (2006) Discovery of a potent inhibitor of the antiapoptotic protein Bcl-xL from NMR and parallel synthesis. *J Med Chem* 49:656–663.

Azzarito V, Long K, Murphy NS & Wilson AJ (2013) Inhibition of α-helix-mediated protein–protein interactions using designed molecules. *Nat Chem* 5:161–173.

Wilder PT, Charpentier TH & Weber DJ (2007) Hydrocarbon-stapled helices: a novel approach for blocking protein–protein interactions. *ChemMedChem* 2:1149–1151.

Walensky LD & Bird GH (2014) Hydrocarbon-stapled peptides: principles, practice, and progress. *J Med Chem* 57:6275–6288.

Vassilev LT, Vu BT, Graves B et al. (2004) In vivo activation of the p53 pathway by small-molecule antagonists of MDM2. *Science* 303:844–846.

Tubulin modulators

Stanton RA, Gernert KM, Nettles JH & Aneja R (2011) Drugs that target dynamic microtubules: a new molecular perspective. *Med Res Rev* 31:443–481.

Dumontet C & Jordan MA (2010) Microtubule-binding agents: a dynamic field of cancer therapeutics. *Nat Rev Drug Discovery* 9:790–803.

He L, Jagtap PG, Kingston DGI et al. (2000) A common pharmacophore for taxol and the epothilones based on the biological activity of a taxane molecule lacking a C-13 side chain. *Biochemistry* 39:3972–3978.

RGD mimetics

Andronati SA, Karaseva TL & Krysko AA (2004) Peptidomimetics-antagonists of the fibrinogen receptors: molecular design, structures, properties and therapeutic applications. *Curr Med Chem* 11:1183–1211.

Transthyretin

Johnson SM, Connelly S, Fearns C et al. (2012) The transthyretin amyloidoses: from delineating the molecular mechanism of aggregation linked to anthology to a regulatory-agency-approved drug. *J Mol Biol* 421:185–203.

Penchala SC, Connelly S, Wang Y et al. (2013) AG10 inhibits amyloidogenesis and cellular toxicity of the familial amyloid cardiomyopathy-associated V122I transthyretin. *Proc Natl Acad Sci USA* 110:9992–9997.

Johnson SM, Wiseman RL, Sekimina Y et al. (2005) Native state kinetic stabilization as a strategy to ameliorate protein misfolding diseases: a focus on the transthyretin amyloidosis. *Acc Chem Res* 38:911– 921.

Taxol

Oberlies NH & Kroll DJ (2004) Camptothecin and taxol: historic achievements in natural products. *J Nat Prod* 67:129–135.

Horwitz SB (2004) Personal recollections on the early development of taxol. *J Nat Prod* 67:136–138.

Kingston DGI (2001) Taxol, a molecule for all seasons. *Chem Commun:* 867–880.

Borman S (2007) Drugs from academia. *Chem Eng News* 85:42–46.

https://www.acs.org/content/acs/en/education/whatischemistry/landmarks/camptothecintaxol.html

Maraviroc

Palani A & Tagat JR (2006) Discovery and development of small-molecule chemokine coreceptor CCR5 antagonists. *J Med Chem* 49:2851–2857

Wood A & Armour D (2005) The discovery of the CCR5 receptor antagonist, UK-427,857, a new agent for the treatment of HIV infection and AIDS. *Prog Med Chem* 43:239–271.

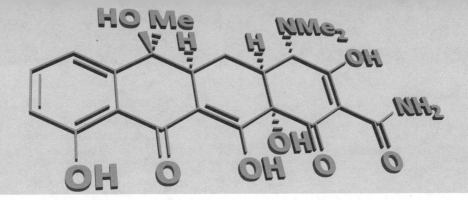

DNA and RNA as drug targets

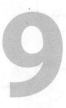

9

LEARNING OBJECTIVES

- Explain the rationale for targeting DNA and RNA.
- Name and describe the various ways small molecules can make noncovalent interactions with DNA.
- Identify several different mechanisms by which small molecules can cause modifications to nucleic acids.
- Describe how antisense oligonucleotides work.
- Learn examples of drugs that work by targeting DNA and RNA.

Deoxyribonucleic acid (DNA) and ribonucleic acid (RNA) are macromolecular polymers, each made up of four different nucleotides linked through 3′–5′ phosphodiester linkages (**Figure 9.1A**). The individual monomers that make up DNA are 2-deoxynucleotides that contain the nucleobases adenine (A), guanine (G), thymine (T), and cytidine (C). RNA monomers contain the bases adenine, guanine, uracil (U), and cytidine.

A DNA duplex consists of two polymers linked at the 3′ and 5′ positions, which are held together by noncovalent interactions between specific nucleobases (A-T and G-C; Watson–Crick pairing, shown in **Figure 9.1B**) in an anti-parallel fashion, forming a double helix. The base pairs are on the interior of the double helix, and the sugar–phosphate backbone sits on the exterior. B-DNA is considered the most relevant form of DNA; it displays two distinct grooves, a deep minor groove and a shallow major groove (**Figure 9.2A**). Rather than double-stranded helices, RNA is often found as a single strand. It can self-associate with self-complementary regions after folding back on itself and form secondary structures with hairpin loops and bulges and into a double helix, usually in the A-form (**Figure 9.2B**). This is a shorter, wider form of a double helix with a deep narrow major groove and a wide shallow minor groove.

Although the structural difference at the molecular level between RNA and DNA is only in the substitution of uracil for thymine and an additional hydroxyl group in the furanose ring, as can be seen in Figure 9.1A, this translates to significant differences in secondary and tertiary structure. There are also significant differences in the function of the two oligonucleotides. The function of DNA is to maintain and transmit genetic information, either to a daughter cell or to RNA (transcription). It is located in the nucleus, where it is typically bound to proteins called histones. The primary role of RNA is to direct the synthesis of proteins on the ribosome (translation). There are several forms involved in this process: messenger RNA (mRNA) is transcribed from

A: STRUCTURE OF DNA AND RNA

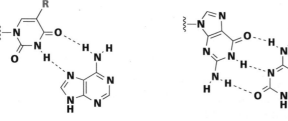

B: BASE PAIRING IN DNA AND RNA

thymine-adenine pair R = methyl
uracil-adenine pair R = H

guanine-cytosine pair

Figure 9.1 Backbone structure and base pairing of DNA and RNA. A: DNA and RNA segments containing the four individual nucleobases adenine, thymine (green)/uracil (red), guanine, and cytosine. B: Watson–Crick base pairing between adenine and thymine (R = Me)/uracil (R = H) and between cytosine and guanine.

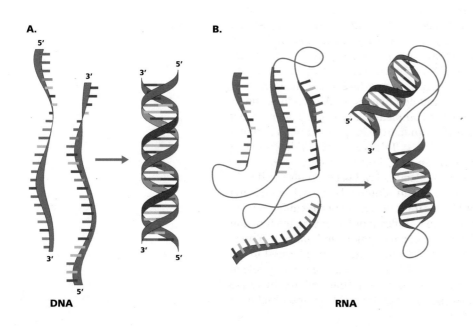

Figure 9.2 Macromolecular structures of DNA and RNA. A: DNA molecules exist in pairs (red and gray strands) with complementary sequences that enable the two molecules to form a continuous anti-parallel double helix. B: RNA molecules frequently exist as single strands that contain self-complementary regions. In this diagram, the segments colored red contain sequences that are complementary to sequences colored gray. The RNA molecule self assembles and adopts a conformation that forms two double helices. For both DNA and RNA, each colored projection on each strand represents a specific nucleobase. (From Kuriyan J, Konforti B & Wemmer D [2012] The Molecules of Life: Physical and Chemical Principles. Garland Science.)

DNA and carries genetic information into the cytoplasm; transfer RNA (tRNA) moves to the ribosome and carries the three-base code for each amino acid needed for protein synthesis; and ribosomal RNA (rRNA) is part of the ribosome, a protein–RNA complex where protein synthesis is carried out. More recently, even more types and functions of RNA have been identified: ribozymes are RNAs that possess enzymatic activity, and small interfering RNAs (siRNA) are naturally occurring 20–25-nucleotide segments of double-stranded RNA whose typical function is to block gene expression. As such, RNA is essential for protein synthesis and ultimately cell division.

Historically, many compounds that bind to nucleic acids were isolated or derived from natural products. The original compounds, often detected on the basis of their antibacterial and/or anti-proliferative effects, were studied and the mechanism of action was determined later. Since DNA and RNA are conserved across all living species, it is not surprising that various organisms have evolved small molecules that bind to nucleic acids as a defense mechanism. Other agents that bind to DNA have more nefarious origins (vide infra), and their beneficial effects were based on clinical observations. More recently, scientists have been developing methods to design compounds that bind with high affinity and high selectivity to specific sequences of DNA and RNA.

Methods to measure the effects of molecules that bind to DNA rely on biophysical techniques such as surface plasmon resonance (SPR), electrophoretic mobility shift assays (EMSA), and melting-temperature assays. These assays, in the broadest terms, detect differences in size or stability between the duplex DNA and a small molecule bound to duplex DNA. Other techniques use spectroscopic changes that occur upon binding, such as fluorescence competition assays. These may rely on changes in fluorescence of an external probe that binds to DNA. Identical or similar assays are also used to detect small-molecule binding to RNA. Secondary assays used to measure downstream events that reflect changes to DNA, such as protein synthesis and cell proliferation, are similar to those previously described.

Small molecules that interact with DNA are primarily used to treat disorders that are characterized by uncontrolled growth, primarily cancer. Some of these drugs are also approved to treat autoimmune diseases, which are characterized by proliferation of immune cells. This focus is due to the fundamental role DNA plays in replication. However, the challenges in developing selective DNA-binding agents usually make them second- or third-line therapies in autoimmune diseases where other therapies are available. The current state of medicinal chemistry has not yet evolved to allow design of highly sequence-selective DNA-targeted drugs, and therefore toxicity due to effects on non-target cells is a significant liability. Drugs that target RNA primarily affect protein synthesis, either in bacteria or in humans. Both DNA- and RNA-binding drugs act by a variety of binding mechanisms, and a summary of those mechanisms is given in **Table 9.1**. However, drugs that exclusively target DNA or RNA as their mechanism of action are rare, and most work via multiple effects.

DNA AS A DRUG TARGET

The role of DNA during cell division and proliferation has made directly targeting it a fruitful avenue to identify drugs, particularly anti-cancer agents. Binding to and/or damaging DNA prevents its accurate replication, often causing the processes of cell division and, eventually, cell proliferation to stop. Drugs that work through this mechanism are often highly potent and effective anti-cancer agents. However, these mechanisms are not selective, and significant toxicities due to effects on noncancerous dividing cells, such as those in the gastrointestinal tract or part of the immune system, limit the usefulness of these agents. Furthermore, certain DNA-damaging agents can cause cancer independently, often years after the original treatment. The mechanisms by which drugs damage DNA involve two primary modes of interaction, reversible and irreversible. Reversible, noncovalent binders may either insert between the base pairs (intercalation) or lie in the minor groove or act via a combination of both. Some compounds that work via an irreversible mechanism contain a reactive electrophilic group that alkylates nucleophilic sites on DNA, while others generate a reactive radical

Table 9.1   Examples of drugs directly targeting DNA and RNA, their mechanisms of action, and therapeutic use.

Nucleic acid target	Drug mechanism	Drug	Indication
DNA	intercalation and minor-groove binding	doxorubicin, daunomycin	cancer
		mitoxantrone	cancer, multiple sclerosis
DNA	minor-groove binding	netropsin*	probe
		trabectedin	cancer
DNA	alkylation	chlorambucil, cisplatin, thiotepa	cancer
DNA	strand cleavage	bleomycin, calicheamicin (as antibody conjugate)	cancer
RNA	rRNA binding	tetracycline	acne, bacterial infections
		erythromycin	bacterial infections
RNA	antisense	mipomersen	familial hypercholesterolemia

*Indicates a research compound.

that abstracts hydrogen atoms from the furanose ring in DNA, ultimately leading to chemical modification of the DNA strand.

9.1   Intercalation is one of the main mechanisms by which small molecules interact with DNA

Drugs that bind to DNA reversibly act directly on DNA through two main mechanisms: intercalation and groove binding. **Intercalators**, typically planar aromatic molecules, insert between the DNA base pairs via π-stacking and additional hydrophobic and electrostatic interactions (**Figure 9.3A**). The antibiotic proflavine, with its planar tricyclic aromatic system, is a prototypical intercalator. This type of binding is nonspecific with respect to the DNA sequence but has a preference for GC-rich regions. Larger molecules with appropriate polar appendages may make additional interactions with the grooves of the DNA duplex. When they make interactions in both the major and minor grooves, like the anthracycline nogalamycin does, they are termed **threading intercalators** (**Figure 9.3B,C**). The aglycon of nogalamycin intercalates between the base pairs, the carbohydrate moiety (nogalose) sits in the minor groove, and the bicyclic acetal lies in the major groove.

Once bound, intercalators produce significant distortion of the DNA structure, resulting in extended bond lengths and unwinding of the helix. This change in structure affects the stability of the duplex, prevents DNA's template function, and disrupts binding and recognition by certain DNA processing enzymes such as topoisomerase, all leading to an inability to replicate the genetic material. Tuning the activity of intercalators so they are only effective in cancerous or proliferating cells has been challenging, and this difficulty limits the usefulness of agents that act solely though this mechanism.

Several natural products that are approved for use in certain cancers work through an intercalation mechanism. The planar aromatic phenoxazone ring system of dactino-mycin (also known as actinomycin D) intercalates between G-C base pairs, and the peptide side chains make H-bonds on the outside of the helix (**Figure 9.4A**). As seen in **Figure 9.4B**, an X-ray structure of the complex between dactinomycin and a segment of

A: INTERCALATOR EXAMPLE   **B:** THREADING INTERCALATOR EXAMPLE   **C:** X-RAY STRUCTURE OF NOGALAMYCIN BOUND TO DOUBLE-STRANDED DNA

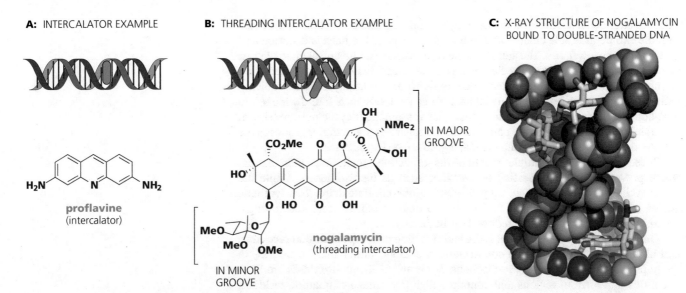

Figure 9.3 Schematic of DNA intercalators and threading intercalators, with examples of each. Red and gray represent two strands of the DNA helix; the blue bar represents a small-molecule binder. A: Intercalators (blue) bind between the base pairs (black) of the DNA helix. Proflavine, with a planar aromatic structure, is a prototypical intercalator. B: Threading intercalators (blue) bind between base pairs (black) but also bind to the minor and major grooves of the helix. Nogalamycin is an example of a threading intercalator, with the carbohydrate binding to the minor groove, and the bicyclic acetal binding to the major groove. C: X-ray structure of two molecules of nogalamycin (shown in stick format) bound to a short sequence of DNA helix. The planar moiety can be seen intercalated between base pairs at the bottom of the figure, with other portions of the molecule bound to helix grooves. (C, from Van Vranken D & Weiss GA [2012] Introduction to Bioorganic Chemistry and Chemical Biology. Garland Science.)

A: STRUCTURES OF INTERCALATING ANTI-CANCER DRUGS

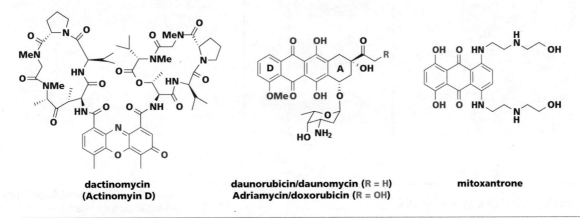

**dactinomycin
(Actinomyin D)**   **daunorubicin/daunomycin (R = H)
Adriamycin/doxorubicin (R = OH)**   **mitoxantrone**

B: STRUCTURE OF DACTINOMYCIN BOUND IN A FRAGMENT OF DNA

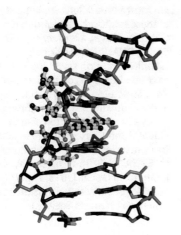

Figure 9.4 Examples of compounds that intercalate into double-stranded DNA. A: Structures of dactinomycin/actinomycin D and of anthracyclines (daunorubicin/daunomycin, Adriamycin/doxorubicin, and mitoxantrone). Planar aromatic regions that intercalate are shown in red. B: X-ray structure of dactinomycin (shown in cyan) bound in DNA double-strand helix. The aromatic core intercalates between base pairs, and peptide side chains bind to the minor groove, resulting in distortion of the helix and unwinding. (B, from Zlatanova & van Holde K [2015] Molecular Biology: Structure and Dynamics of Genomes and Proteomes, Garland Science.)

a double-stranded DNA helix shows the drug intercalating into the middle of the helix, with the two peptide side chains lying in the minor groove. The helix is distorted and unwound at the lower end. The anthracyclines are a class of archetypical intercalators: planar polycyclic aromatic molecules with positive ionizable groups appended. Two members of this class, daunorubicin (daunomycin) and Adriamycin (doxorubicin), both natural products isolated from soil bacteria in the 1960s, have found wide use to treat both solid tumors and leukemias. Their planar aromatic tricyclic portion (shown in red) intercalates between base pairs, the amino sugar lies in the minor groove of the helix, and the D-ring protrudes into the major groove (see Figure 9.4A).

These drugs have multiple mechanisms of action, including intercalation, which prevents further processing by enzymes such as topoisomerase. While the anthracyclines are widely used, they exhibit serious cardiotoxicity. The synthetic analog mitoxantrone (see Figure 9.4A), used to treat certain cancers and multiple sclerosis, has similar activity but reduced cardiotoxicity.

One current avenue of research is the identification of compounds that recognize and bind to specific uncommon conformations of DNA, rather than to B-DNA, in the hope that they will be less promiscuous. For example, G-quadruplexes are DNA structures that form in regions that contain a high percentage of guanine residues. They are composed of multiple sets of four G-residues (tetrads) stabilized by the presence of cations that become stacked upon each other (**Figure 9.5A**). An example

A: STRUCTURE OF QUADRUPLEX DNA: G-RICH REGIONS FORM TETRADS THAT CAN STACK

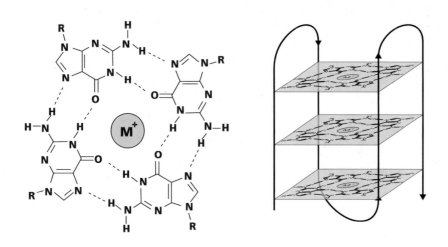

B: LIGAND BOUND IN GROOVE OF QUADRUPLEX DNA

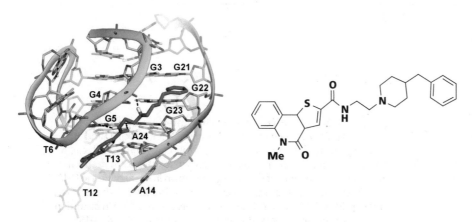

Figure 9.5 Structure of G-quadruplex DNA and bound ligand. A: Hydrogen bonding between four guanosine residues and coordination with a metal ion form a tetrad (left); multiple sets of these tetrads stack (right) to form G-quadruplexes, a tertiary conformation of DNA. B: On the right is a ligand identified through screening that binds to G-quadruplexes; on the left is an X-ray structure showing its binding in the G-quadruplex region through groove-binding and intercalation. Individual G and T base pairs are indicated. (A, from Iridos/Wikimedia Commons/CC BY-SA 2.5. B, from Di Leva FS, Zizza P, Cingolani C et al. [2013] *J Med Chem* 56:9646–9654. With permission from American Chemical Society.)

of a ligand identified by screening is shown in **Figure 9.5B** bound into a G-quadruplex region through intercalation and groove binding.

These G-quadruplex structures are found at regions of DNA near telomeres and oncogene promoters, suggesting they play a regulatory role in cell proliferation and cancer. For example, stabilization of the G-quadruplex in telomeres inhibits telomerase, an enzyme required for the growth of most cancers. While this avenue of research has not yet led to drugs or drug candidates, the strategy to identify compounds that bind to very specific DNA sequences or structures is likely to be an active area of research in the future.

9.2 Drugs may bind in the minor groove of DNA through reversible noncovalent interactions

As noted above, many drugs that intercalate may also contain moieties that make additional contacts with the minor groove. Compounds that act primarily through such minor-groove interactions are known as **DNA groove binders**. As a class, DNA groove binders sit in one of the two grooves of the DNA duplex. While many proteins interact with DNA through binding in the major groove, small molecules usually bind in the narrower yet deeper minor groove. Minor-groove binders typically adopt a crescent shape that is complementary to the minor groove and contain flat, heterocyclic rings between flexible linkers. Specific interactions between the groove binder and DNA often occur at A-T rich regions and include H-bonding with accessible lone pairs of atoms on base pairs in the floor of the minor groove as well as hydrophobic interactions with thymidine methyl groups, and non-polar H-atoms as seen in **Figure 9.6A**. Other points of contact include electrostatic and hydrophobic interactions with the sugar–phosphate backbone. Natural products such as netropsin, distamycin, and trabectedin are examples of minor-groove binders (**Figure 9.6B**). The polyheterocyclic amides netropsin and distamycin form crescent-shaped structures that fit into the minor groove of DNA, as seen in **Figure 9.6C**. When a second molecule of distamycin binds, the groove is significantly distorted.

Compared to intercalators, minor-groove binders generally exhibit greater affinity and can exhibit some sequence specificity. The natural products netropsin and distamycin prefer AT-rich regions of DNA. Many analogs of these have been studied in attempts to develop sequence-specific drugs. For example, Peter Dervan at CalTech has developed rules to predict sequence-specific recognition for various polyamide scaffolds (imidazole, pyrrole, and hydroxypyrrole). According to these rules, an imidazole–pyrrole pair recognizes a G-C sequence, while a hydroxypyrrole–pyrrole pair recognizes a T-A sequence. Studies such as these give insight into the design of sequence-specific minor-groove binders. In spite of many efforts, no approved drugs work solely through minor-groove binding. However, binding to the minor groove of DNA is one aspect of the mechanism of a number of anti-cancer drugs. Trabectedin is one approved drug that binds in the minor groove with a preference for CGG sequences, but it also alkylates the exocyclic amine (N2) of guanine. The potential for designing sequence-specific DNA binders offers opportunities to design drugs that treat genetic disorders that are defined by certain DNA sequences, as opposed to targeting all DNA.

9.3 Drugs that interact with DNA by irreversible mechanisms are anti-cancer agents

In addition to molecules that bind to DNA through reversible noncovalent inter-actions, a number of drugs work by making covalent bonds to DNA. These are known as **DNA alkylating agents**. Despite their significant toxicities, compounds such as these continue to be used for anti-cancer therapy. In general, they contain, or generate upon bioactivation, a highly reactive electrophile that reacts with nucleophilic sites

A: SITES ON A-T AND T-A PAIRS IN THE MINOR GROOVE IN THE FLOOR OF DNA

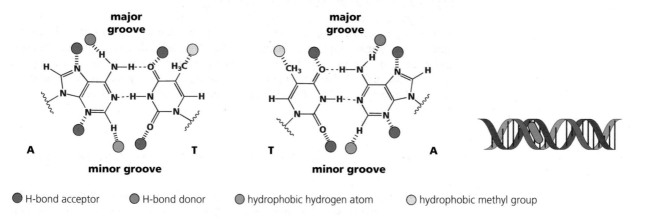

● H-bond acceptor   ● H-bond donor   ● hydrophobic hydrogen atom   ○ hydrophobic methyl group

B: EXAMPLES OF MINOR-GROOVE BINDERS

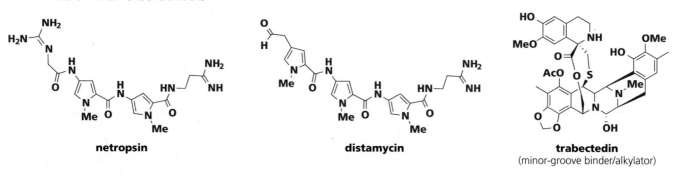

netropsin   **distamycin**   **trabectedin**
                                                      (minor-groove binder/alkylator)

C: X-RAY STRUCTURES OF DISTAMYCIN BOUND IN MINOR GROOVE OF DNA

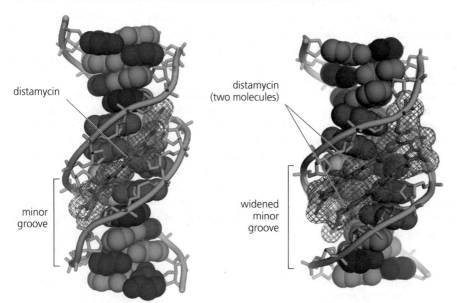

distamycin

distamycin
(two molecules)

minor
groove

widened
minor
groove

Figure 9.6 Structures of minor-groove binders and points of interaction. A: Sites on A-T and T-A base pairs available for interactions with minor groove binders. Colors indicate specific types of interactions: H-bond acceptor (pink); H-bond donor (blue); hydrophobic methyl group (yellow), and non-polar H-atom (gray). Diagram on right shows a compound (blue) seated in the minor groove of DNA. B: Structures of minor-groove binders netropsin, distamycin, and trabectedin. C: X-ray structures showing binding of one or two molecules of distamycin (hashed space filling purple) in AT-rich regions (red and green spheres). Binding of a second molecule of distamycin results in widening of the minor groove. (A and C, from Kuriyan J, Konforti B & Wemmer D [2012] The Molecules of Life: Physical and Chemical Principles. Garland Science.)

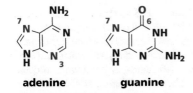

Figure 9.7 Nucleophilic sites on adenine and guanine. Nucleophilic sites (N3 and N7 in adenine; N7 and O6 in guanine;) are marked in red.

on DNA. Modification of N7 of guanine is common, as is alkylation at N3 and N7 of adenine and O6 of guanine (**Figure 9.7**).

With **bis-alkylating agents**, a second reaction on a neighboring base also occurs to cross-link the bases. The linkages can occur between two bases on the same strand (intrastrand) or between two bases on opposite strands (interstrand). Once chemically modified, either by mono- or bis-alkylation, the DNA is incompetent as a template. At that point it is often recognized as damaged and degraded, or it may not be accepted as a substrate by the enzymes required for replication. Regardless of the mechanism, cell division and proliferation is arrested. Alkylating agents are known to alkylate other biomolecules such as proteins, and therefore they are usually quite toxic. Classes of DNA alkylators can be characterized by their electrophiles, and representative examples are shown in **Table 9.2**.

Nitrogen mustards, triazines, and nitrosoureas, through a complex series of biotransformations, generate highly reactive intermediates, such as aziridinium ions from nitrogen mustards and diazonium ions from triazines and nitrosoureas. The nitrogen mustards, of which chlorambucil is an example, were derived from mustard gas, first used in World War I as a chemical warfare agent (**Figure 9.8**). One result of gas (bis[2-chloroethyl] sulfide) exposure was a lowering of white blood cell counts. This observation led scientists to pursue analogs that might be useful for treating leukemia, based on the rationale that less toxic analogs might be effective in lowering abnormal white blood cell counts. Replacing the sulfur atom with nitrogen led to less toxic analogs, with mechlorethamine being used clinically to treat Hodgkin's lymphoma in the early 1940s.

Table 9.2 Classes of DNA alkylators, the reactive electrophile, reaction product, and select examples of drugs.

Class	Electrophile	Drug example	Reaction product
nitrogen mustards	aziridinium ion 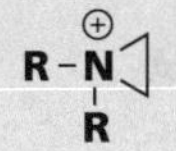	mechlorethamine, chlorambucil, cyclophosphamide	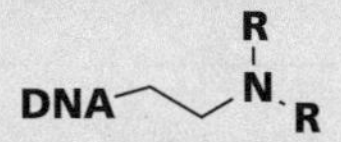 DNA~N(R)~R or DNA~N(R)~DNA 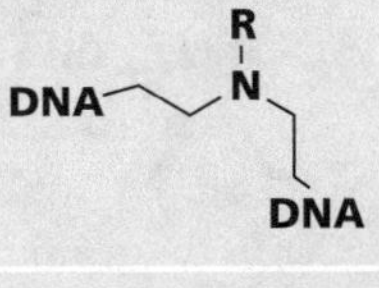
triazines	diazonium ion $R-N{\equiv}N$	dacarbazine	**DNA-R**
nitrosoureas	diazonium ion $R-N{\equiv}N$	carmustine	**DNA-R**
aziridines	aziridine 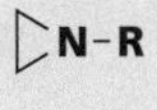	thiotepa	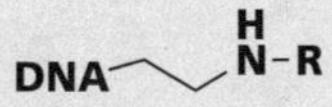 DNA~N(H)~R
sulfonates	methylsulfonate 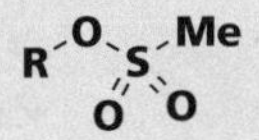	busulfan	**DNA-R**
platins	platinum	cisplatin	**DNA-Pt-DNA**

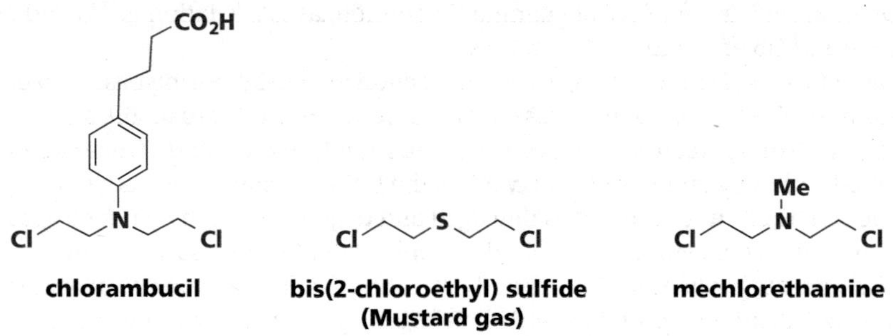

Figure 9.8 Structures of mustards. Chlorambucil is an example of a modern mustard used to treat certain cancers, including leukemias. Bis(2-chloroethyl) sulfide, also known as mustard gas, was used during World War I as nerve gas. In the 1940s, replacement of the sulfur atom with an amine led to a less toxic analog, mechlorethamine, used to treat certain cancers.

chlorambucil

bis(2-chloroethyl) sulfide (Mustard gas)

mechlorethamine

The mechanism of action of cyclophosphamide, a nitrogen mustard prodrug that bis-alkylates DNA, is illustrated in **Figure 9.9**. Bioactivation by cytochrome P450 oxidation and subsequent ring opening affords acrolein and phosphoramide mustard (Figure 9.9A), which then generates the highly reactive aziridinium ion (Figure 9.9B). The aziridinium ion reacts with N7 of a guanine residue in DNA to yield an alkylated derivative. This aziridinium formation process is repeated, and alkylation of a nearby guanine residue generates a cross-linked DNA adduct (Figure 9.9C).

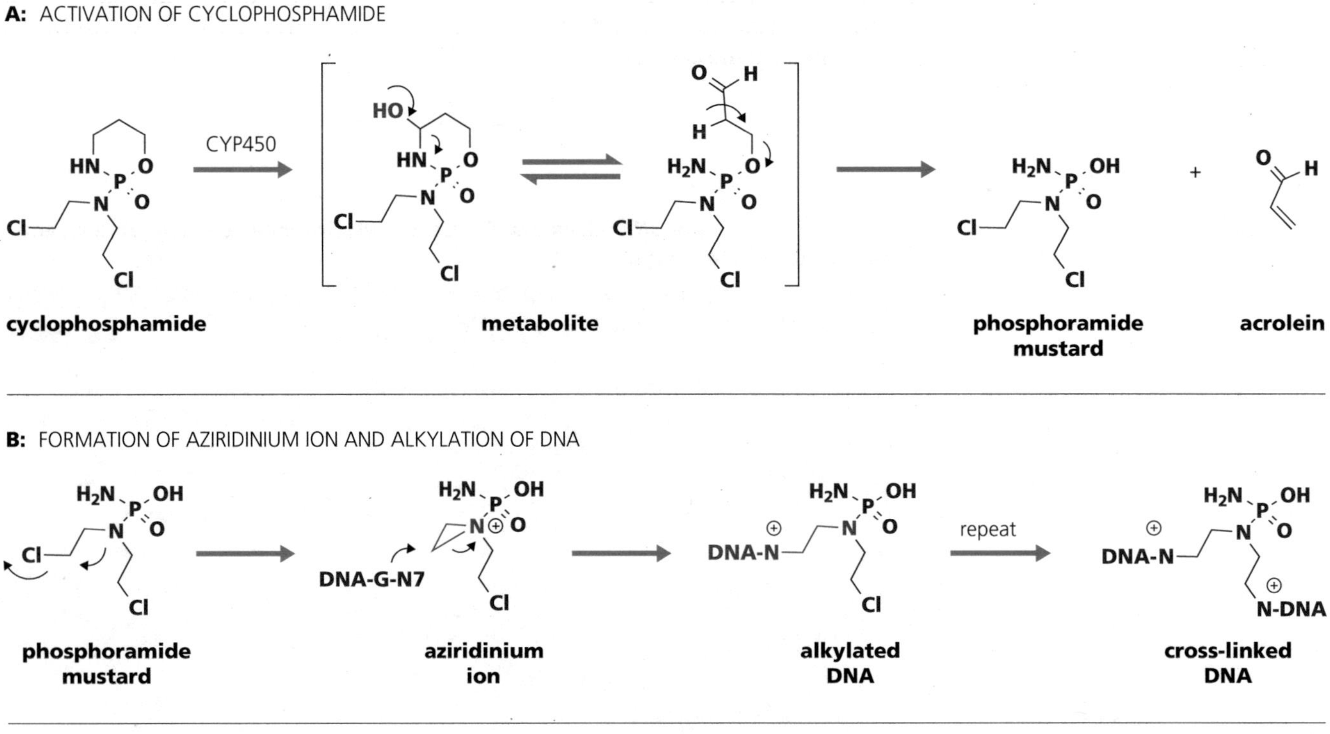

A: ACTIVATION OF CYCLOPHOSPHAMIDE

cyclophosphamide   **metabolite**   **phosphoramide mustard**   **acrolein**

CYP450

B: FORMATION OF AZIRIDINIUM ION AND ALKYLATION OF DNA

phosphoramide mustard   **aziridinium ion**   **alkylated DNA**   **cross-linked DNA**

DNA-G-N7   repeat

C: STRUCTURE OF GUANINE N7 CROSS-LINKED CYCLOPHOSPHAMIDE DNA ADDUCT

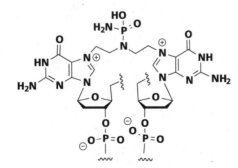

Figure 9.9 Condensed mechanism of action of cyclophosphamide and structure of cross-linked product. A: Cyclophosphamide is oxidized (red) by CYP450 to a metabolite that decomposes to give the reactive phosphoramide mustard and acrolein. B: Phosphoramide mustard then forms the aziridinium ion (red) that alkylates a residue of DNA (usually N7 of guanine). Repeating the sequence gives cross-linked DNA. C: Structure of cross-linked DNA adduct.

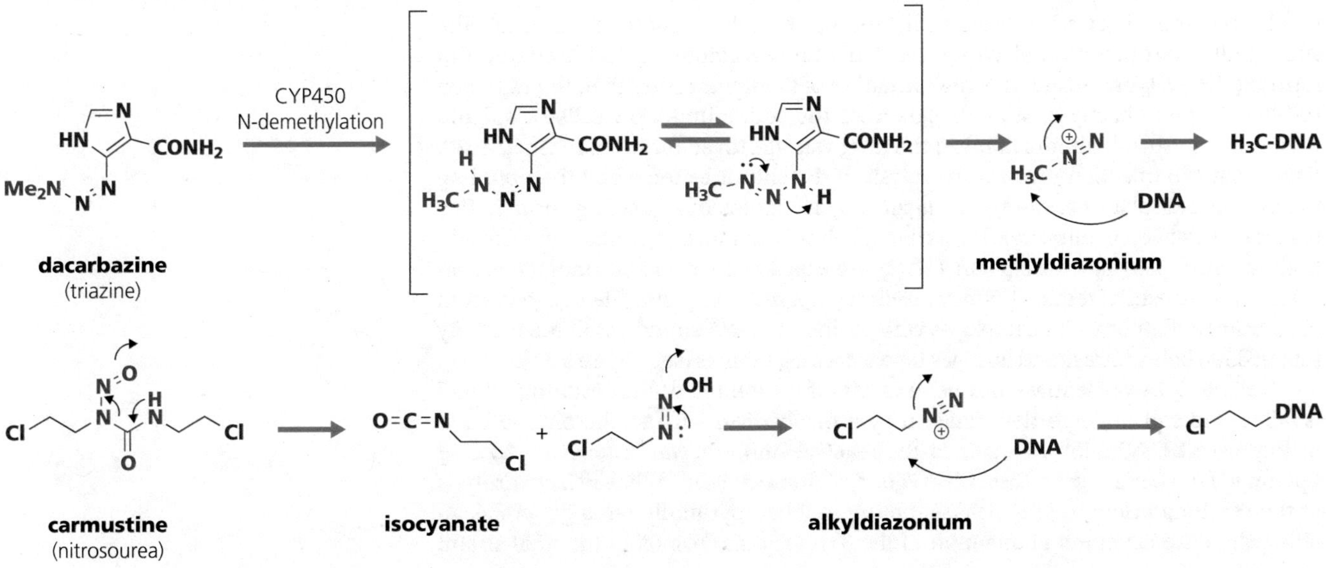

dacarbazine
(triazine)

CYP450
N-demethylation

methyldiazonium

H₃C-DNA

carmustine
(nitrosourea)

isocyanate

alkyldiazonium

DNA

Figure 9.10 Alkylation of DNA by dacarbazine and carmustine. Top: Dacarbazine is N-demethylated *in vivo* to give a product that decomposes to a reactive methyldiazonium ion, which methylates DNA (sites involved in reaction in red). Bottom: Carmustine, a nitrosourea (red), decomposes to an isocyanate and an alkyldiazonium ion; the latter alkylates DNA.

Similarly, dacarbazine (a triazine) and carmustine (a chloroethyl-containing nitrosourea) generate reactive intermediates that alkylate DNA, as shown in **Figure 9.10**. Dacarbazine is first activated by metabolic N-demethylation. The resulting intermediate generates one equivalent of highly reactive methyldiazonium, which reacts with DNA to form a methylated product. The nitrosoureas, exemplified by carmustine, are activated by decomposition to an isocyanate and an alkyldiazonium ion, the latter of which is the alkylating agent.

In contrast, aziridines and sulfonates require no activation for reaction. The requirement for bioactivation by some agents is likely a mechanism by which the drug is protected from reacting with other nucleophiles in the body (e.g., proteins, other biomolecules) and eventually unmasked at the site of action.

While they are technically not alkylating agents, platinum-containing drugs (known as platins) work through a related mechanism. Cisplatin (**Figure 9.11**) was discovered serendipitously in the 1960s as a result of an experiment designed

cisplatin

carboplatin

oxaliplatin

Figure 9.11 Platinum-containing drugs. Top: Structures of cisplatin, carboplatin and oxaliplatin. Bottom: X-ray structure of cisplatin bound to DNA fragment, showing cross-linking. Pt atom = large while ball (Bottom, from Fuertes MA, Alonso C & Perez JM [2003] *Chem Rev* 103:645–662. With permission from American Chemical Society).

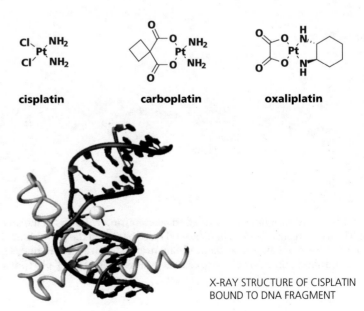

X-RAY STRUCTURE OF CISPLATIN
BOUND TO DNA FRAGMENT

to observe the effect of an electrical current on cell division of bacteria. The supposedly inert platinum electrode reacted with ammonium chloride solution to form $Pt(NH_2)_2Cl_2$ and resulted in the formation of filaments rather than the expected rod-like shape of bacteria. Several years later, the compound, now called cisplatin, was shown to shrink tumors in mice; the drug was approved for human use in 1978. Its mechanism of action involves hydrolysis of the chlorine atoms and then binding to DNA, and displacement of two Pt ligands by N7 atoms of adjacent guanines. This results in formation of intrastrand cross-links, helix distortion, and ultimately cell death. Carboplatin (1989) and oxaliplatin (2002) are considered to be second-generation agents, as they exhibit reduced kidney toxicity compared to cisplatin. These agents form intrastrand and interstrand complexes with purines on DNA strands, with the majority (about 65%) being intrastrand linkages between two guanines (see Figure 9.11).

Once a DNA nucleobase has been alkylated or modified, the resulting adduct is labile and can undergo depurination by a mechanism such as the one outlined in **Figure 9.12**. Addition of water to the reactive iminium ion is followed by ring opening of the heterocyclic base. Cleavage of the furanose ring followed by hydrolysis of the resulting iminium ion releases the ring-opened pyrimidine and generates an aldehyde. Base catalyzed elimination of the 3′-phosphate results in the final strand cleavage.

9.4 Compounds that cleave DNA after binding and generating free radicals are powerful drugs used to treat cancer

As seen in the previous section, drugs that work by alkylating DNA destabilize the duplex and ultimately result in DNA damage. Another mechanism to irreversibly inflict damage onto DNA involves molecules that generate free radicals. DNA **strand**

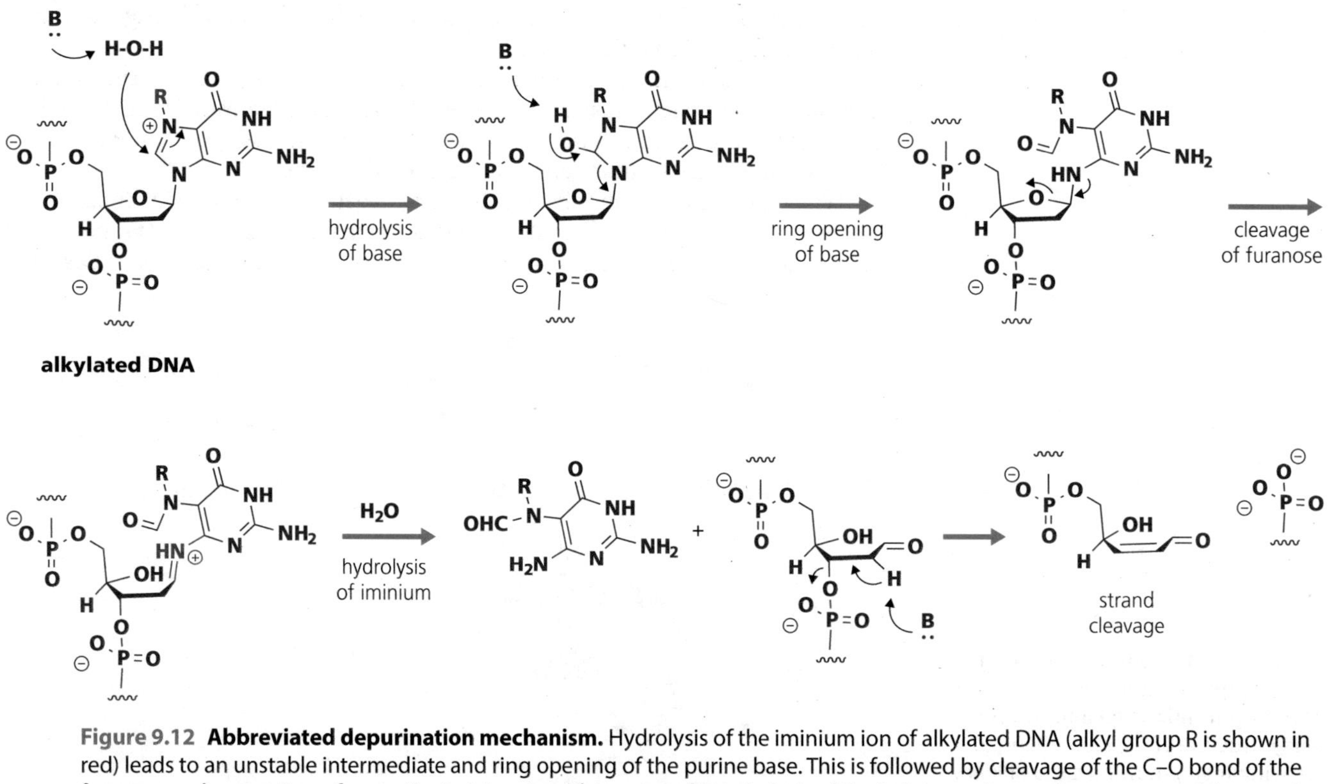

Figure 9.12 Abbreviated depurination mechanism. Hydrolysis of the iminium ion of alkylated DNA (alkyl group R is shown in red) leads to an unstable intermediate and ring opening of the purine base. This is followed by cleavage of the C–O bond of the furanose and generation of a reactive iminium ion (shown in red). Hydrolysis of the iminium releases the remnants of the guanine base and affords an aldehyde. Base catalyzed elimination of the 3′ phosphate results in strand cleavage.

breakers and **nicking agents** are molecules that result in bonds within the DNA duplex being broken. These molecules bind to DNA, often in the minor groove, and generate a free radical. The radical then abstracts a hydrogen atom from the sugar–phosphate backbone, usually at either C4' or C5', leading to a carbon radical, which can react with molecular oxygen. These reactive intermediates react further, ultimately causing the DNA strand to break. While multiple mechanisms have been detected, two examples detailing C4' or C5' hydrogen abstraction, are shown in **Figure 9.13**, each resulting in DNA damage.

These lesions may nick the DNA, cutting one of the strands, or subsequent radical propagation may break both strands. Either situation leads to incomplete duplication, transcription, and translation. Nicking and cleaving agents are usually highly potent, and some exhibit a degree of sequence selectivity due to the need to bind tightly to the DNA duplex. Many are intercalators or minor-groove binders as well as damaging agents.

One DNA strand breaker that is used clinically is bleomycin (BLM), a glycopeptide antibiotic isolated from *Streptomyces verticillus* in the 1960s as its copper complex. BLM operates by generating a radical intermediate after complexation to iron and oxidation by molecular oxygen. The bis(thiazole) moiety of BLM intercalates into DNA, and five nitrogen atoms (shown in red in **Figure 9.14**) as well as molecular oxygen form a complex with iron *in vivo*, generating activated BLM, BLM–Fe(II)–O_2. This activated species generates radicals near the DNA backbone and abstracts either a 4' or a 5' hydrogen.

The enediyne calicheamicin (**Figure 9.15A**), an unusual natural product isolated from soil found in Texas, is another example of a DNA strand breaker.

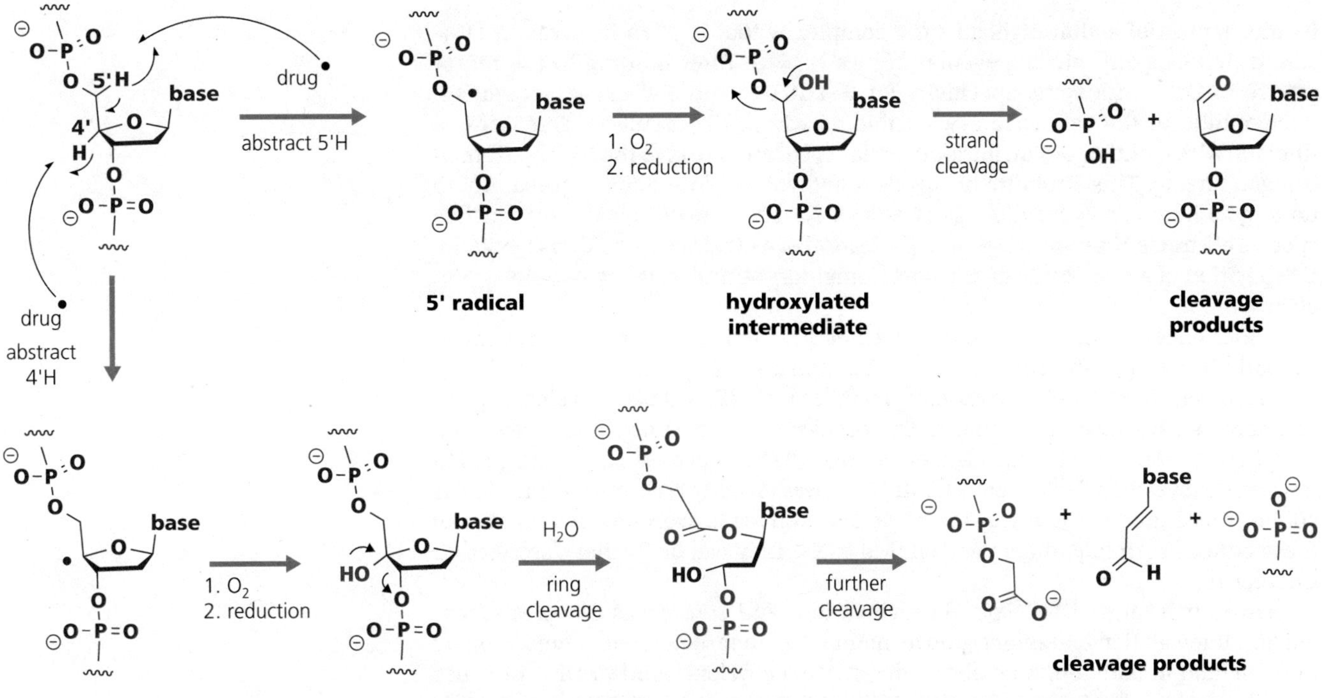

Figure 9.13 Two mechanisms of DNA strand cleavage by radicals. Top: Drug radical abstracts the C5' hydrogen. This secondary radical reacts with molecular oxygen and, after reduction, gives an unstable hydroxylated intermediate (hydroxyl group is shown in red). Elimination of the phosphate generates the cleaved 3' phosphate and an aldehyde, thereby cleaving the strand. Bottom: Drug radical abstracts the C4' hydrogen. This tertiary radical reacts with molecular oxygen and, after reduction, generates the hydroxylated intermediate (hydroxyl group is shown in red). Hydrolysis leads to ring cleavage to generate the ring-opened product. Further cleavage generates a 5'-phosphate (red), a 3' phosphorylated acetate (red) and a nucleobase derivative.

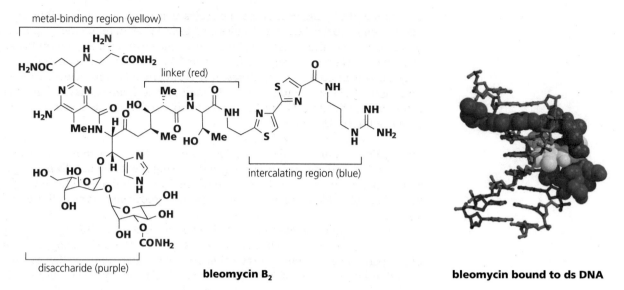

bleomycin B₂

bleomycin bound to ds DNA

Figure 9.14 Structure of bleomycin B₂. Left: Structure of bleomycin with key interacting regions that correspond to the X-ray structure labelled, and five N atoms that chelate to the metal shown in red. Right: X-ray structure of bleomycin bound to DNA duplex (shown in gray ball-and-stick representation). The bis(thiazole) region (blue) intercalates between the base pairs, and a linker (red) orients the metal-binding region (yellow) in the minor groove; the disaccharide (purple) forms additional hydrogen-bonding interactions with the backbone. (Adapted from Goodwin, KD, Lewis MA, Long EC & Georgiadis MM [2008] *Proc Natl Acad Sci USA* 105:5052–5056. With permission from National Academy of Sciences.)

Its mechanism of action highlights the complexity that is often involved in DNA strand breakers and nicking agents (**Figure 9.15B**). After binding to the minor groove of DNA with some specificity for 5′-TCCT-3′ and 5′-TTTT-3′ sequences, nucleophiles in the cell, such as glutathione, add to the trisulfide, generating a thiolate, which undergoes an intramolecular cyclization to give the highly strained bridged analog. This structure brings the enediyne in close enough proximity to undergo a Bergman cyclization, generating a 1,4-benzene diradical. This reactive species abstracts H-atoms from the C5′-position of a cytidine in 5′-TCCT-3′ and the C4′-position of a nucleotide on the complementary strand, causing double-strand cleavage.

Other enediyne natural products, such as neocarzinostatin and dynemicin A, similarly act by generation of a diradical via Bergman-type cyclization (**Figure 9.16**). Unfortunately, their significant toxicity precludes their clinical use as a single agent. Mylotarg, a derivative of calicheamicin conjugated to an antibody directed to a protein on the surface of certain leukemia cells, was used between 2000 and 2010 to treat acute myelogenous leukemia (AML), and was recently reapproved. The area of conjugating antibodies to highly toxic agents continues to evolve, with a number of these entities currently undergoing clinical trials. They will be further described in Chapter 10.

Drugs that target DNA work through various and sometimes complex mechanisms. Intercalation and minor-groove binding are important components to many of them, and in addition, a number either make a covalent bond to DNA or cause strand cleavage. Designing selective inhibitors that will target either a specific DNA sequence or a specific DNA structure remains a challenge, although insights into DNA structure may lead to improved specificity in these types of drugs. The majority of drugs that target DNA are anti-cancer agents, with a few being used to treat serious immune inflammatory disorders such as multiple sclerosis, but they are usually accompanied by significant side effects.

A: STRUCTURE OF CALICHEAMICIN γ1 AND X-RAY STRUCTURE OF DRUG BOUND IN DNA

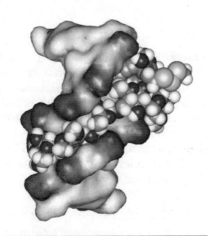

calicheamicin γ1

B: MECHANISM OF ACTIVATION TO DIRADICAL

Nu⁻ → cleavage of trisulfide → **thiolate** → Michael addition of thiolate to enone

bridged analog → Bergman cyclization → **diradical** → DNA → double-strand cleavage

Figure 9.15 Structure and mechanism of action of calicheamicin γ1. A: Structure of calicheamicin γ1, with the enediyne moiety shown in red, and X-ray structure of drug bound in DNA. Carbohydrate binds in the minor groove, with the trisulfide (shown in yellow) accessible to nucleophiles. B: Mechanism of activation of calicheamicin γ1 to generate a diradical. Addition of a nucleophile such as glutathione to the trisulfide generates a thiolate anion, which then undergoes intramolecular Michael addition to the enone. The resultant bridged analog is appropriately oriented to undergo a Bergman cyclization to generate a diradical, which abstracts H-atoms from 4′ and 5′ sites on DNA furanoses, resulting in DNA double-strand cleavage.

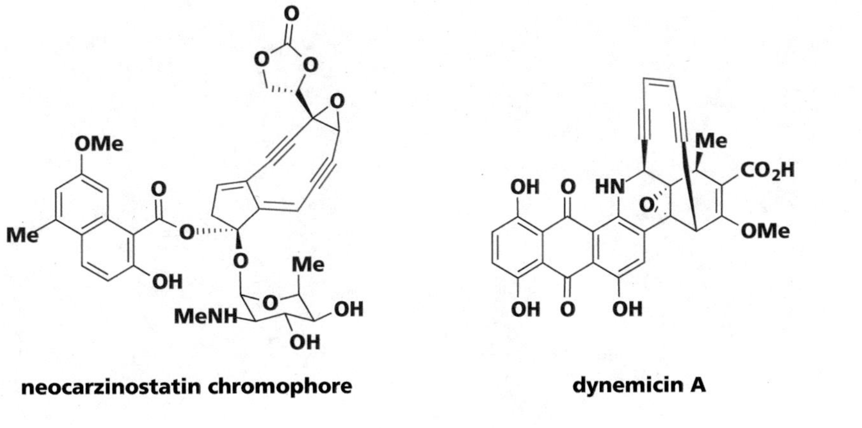

Figure 9.16 Structures of enediyne strand breakers. Neocarzinostatin and dynemicin are other examples of natural products enediynes; enediyne-containing moiety is shown in red.

neocarzinostatin chromophore

dynemicin A

RNA AS A DRUG TARGET

In contrast to DNA-targeted drugs, small molecules that bind directly to RNA are rare. This is surprising since RNA is involved in numerous biological processes, such as protein synthesis and transcriptional regulation, that are likely to be modulated in the disease state, while the function of DNA is more limited. Furthermore, the potential for small molecules to bind directly to RNA and distort its structure, or to disrupt RNA–protein binding events, offers numerous opportunities for drug design. However, to date, success in this arena has been limited to targeting the ribosome with traditional small molecules derived from natural products, and sequence-specific nucleotide drugs called antisense molecules.

9.5   Compounds targeting bacterial ribosomal RNA inhibit protein synthesis and are useful anti-infective agents

Many antibacterial drugs work by interfering with bacterial protein synthesis. While they have distinct binding sites and diverse structures, their common mechanism involves binding to rRNA. Ribosomes are multicomponent complexes that contain both protein and RNA. In bacteria, the 70S ribosome is composed of two parts, the 50S and 30S subunits. In the process of protein synthesis on the ribosome, tRNA carries the three-base code for an amino acid into the A site (acceptance site) of the 30S subunit. One class of antibacterial drugs that binds to rRNA is the tetracyclines (**Figure 9.17**). These drugs interact with the 16S rRNA of the 30S subunit of the bacterial ribosome, and they prevent tRNA from binding at the A site. Several binding sites have been identified, but the highest-affinity site is located in a hydrophobic pocket near the A-site. This pocket is formed by several helices of the rRNA, including helix 34 (H34), H31, H44 and H18. As seen in Figure 9.17, the 1,3-ketone-enol motif on the hydroxyl-rich side of tetracyclines participates in numerous interactions with RNA, mostly to the phosphates in the RNA backbone, including some mediated through coordination

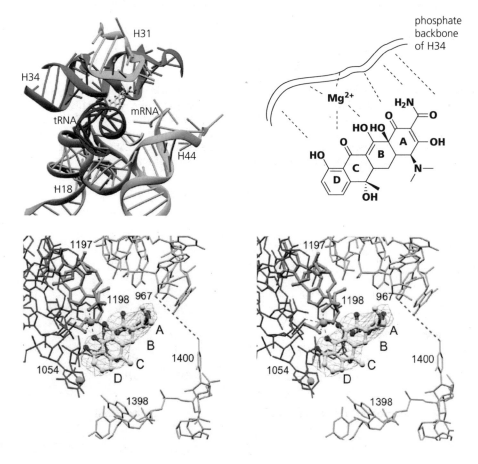

Figure 9.17   Structure of tetracycline bound to rRNA. Top: X-ray structure of tetracycline (yellow) in binding pocket of the A-site, near tRNA (red). Major binding is to helix 34 (H34) (dark blue), with H31 (green), H44 (light blue), and H18 (orange) forming the pocket; structure of tetracycline in same orientation shown on the right with interactions to phosphate backbone of H34 indicated by dotted lines. Mg^{2+} is required for binding, and coordinates to both tetracycline and binding site. (A, B, C, and D rings labeled). Bottom: stereodiagram showing close-up of the binding site, with coordination to Mg^{2+} (orange circle); colors same as above. (From Brodersen DE, Clemons WM Jr, Carter AP et al. [2000] *Cell* 103:1143–1154. With permission from Elsevier).

with an Mg^{2+} ion. It has long been known that an Mg^{2+} ion is required for tetracycline binding, and SAR studies have shown that little variation is tolerated on the side of the molecule that is now known to participate in binding.

Other classes of antibacterial protein synthesis inhibitors that bind to the ribosome include aminoglycosides and erythromycins. These are discussed in detail in Chapter 12.

9.6 Antisense therapies targeting RNA are effective in treating rare diseases and infections

The goal of **antisense therapy** is to block synthesis of proteins resulting from a disease-causing gene or an essential gene from an infectious agent. First, the sequence of a disease-causing gene or a gene essential for an infectious agent's replication is determined. On the basis of that sequence, an oligonucleotide or modified analog with a complementary sequence (thus the term antisense) is synthesized that will bind to the mRNA produced by that gene. Through several different mechanisms, the mRNA is no longer capable of translating the gene into the protein, and its production is turned off. The specific protein the mRNA codes for is not synthesized, thereby effectively inhibiting the protein. This approach is particularly useful in treating disorders caused by a mutant protein, or in treating infections where essential proteins of the infectious agent are targeted.

This approach allows highly precise targeting, since the antisense agents are typically in the range of 20 base pairs, and therefore recognizes very specific sequences of mRNA and also prevents nonspecific binding to other mRNAs. However, this strategy also has some challenges, such as the efficient delivery of the agent to the site of action. While antisense drugs are not quite small molecules, many of the traditional medicinal chemistry principles, such as design of modified analogs for selectivity and physical property optimization, have been applied to the discovery and development of these agents.

All antisense oligonucleotides bind to RNA, and their activity can be divided into two mechanisms: cleavage-dependent or occupation-only (**Figure 9.18**). The majority of antisense therapeutic agents approved and in clinical development work through the **cleavage-dependent mechanism**, with most relying on the action of the enzyme **RNase H** (Figure 9.18, right). This endonuclease normally mediates cleavage of the 3′-O–phosphate bond in RNA–DNA heteroduplexes and cleaves the RNA strand, releasing intact DNA. In the case of antisense molecules, RNase H recognizes the RNA–antisense duplex, cleaves the portion of the RNA sense strand bound to the antisense molecule, and releases the intact antisense oligomer and the smaller, remaining RNA strand. Alternatively, this pathway sometimes relies on the enzyme Argonaute 2 (Ago2), which is involved in RNA silencing. Small interfering RNAs (siRNAs) are naturally occurring 20–25-nucleotide segments of double-stranded RNA whose

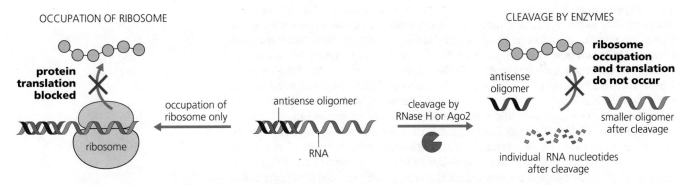

Figure 9.18 Antisense mechanisms. Left: Occupation-only mechanism. Right: Cleavage-dependent mechanism. The antisense oligomer (shown in black) binds to a specific section of RNA, preventing translation to protein. In the cleavage-dependent mechanism (right), either RNase H or Ago2 cleaves the segment of RNA bound to the antisense RNA into individual nucleotides thereby releasing the remaining fragment of RNA and the antisense oligomer. This stops further protein production. In the alternative occupation-only mechanism (left), the antisense oligomer physically blocks entry to the ribosome and translation.

typical function is to interfere in gene expression. Ago2 is similar to RNase H, in that it cleaves the target RNA strand bound to the antisense oligonucleotides, mimicking its endogenous effects on mRNA bound to siRNA .

Antisense oligonucleotides that act by an **occupancy-only mechanism** act by blocking translation (see Figure 9.18, left). They are designed to bind to (or next to) the translation initiation region of an mRNA. In the process, they block movement of the ribosome down the transcript. By either cleavage or occupation-only mechanisms, the overall result is interference with the formation of a specific protein.

In order to design antisense drugs, several issues that plague natural oligonucleotides need to be addressed. These include poor bioavailability, instability due to cleavage by nucleases, and rapid clearance. Additionally, because the oligomers are charged, their cell permeability is poor. Sequence specificity requires that a typical modified oligonucleotide contain between 8 and 50 nucleotides, with most averaging approximately 20 bases; therefore the molecular weights are quite high (~7000). At the same time, the oligomers must display enough of the same structural features in order to be recognized by the complementary RNA strand as well as the relevant enzymes, like RNase H or Ago2. To address all of these requirements, design of antisense therapeutics has included modification of the phosphate backbone and the ribose units as well as the nucleobases.

The first approved antisense drugs, and the dozens of antisense therapeutics undergoing clinical trials, incorporate backbone modifications, with phosphorothioate (PS) being one of the earliest and most widely used replacements for the cleavable phosphodiester linkage. These analogs replace the nonbridging oxygen of the phosphate with sulfur, resulting in compounds with increased stability to nucleases that also elicit RNase H cleavage. Others include N3′ → P5′ thiophosphoramidates, phosphorodiamidates, and peptide nucleic acids (**Figure 9.19A**).

The most widely studied bases are the 5-methylpyrimidines (such as thymine) and the unnatural 5-propynylpyrimidines (**Figure 9.19B**), which exhibit more efficient base stacking, resulting in improved stability of the RNA–oligonucleotide duplex. While duplexes that incorporate the 5-propynyl analogs are even more stable than 5-methyl ones, they are toxic *in vivo*. Examples of modified ribose analogs include the morpholino replacement found in many phosphorodiamidates (Figure 9.19A) and methoxyethyl (MOE)- and fluoro-substituted ribose oligonucleotides (Figure 9.19B). These latter two modifications exhibit increased stability to nucleases and increased affinity to RNA.

The first antisense drug, fomivirsen, was approved in the early 2000s to treat cytomegalovirus infections, although its marketing has been discontinued in the United States. Fomivirsen is a phosphorothioate oligonucleotide containing 21 bases, with no other modifications of the base or backbone. Currently, more complex second-generation antisense drugs are becoming available, such as mipomersen, which is used to treat familial hypercholesterolemia. Mipomersen is described in more detail in Case Study 2 in this chapter. Eteplirsen, approved by the U.S. FDA with some controversy in 2016, targets a mutation found in about 15% of patients with muscular dystrophy. It works by exon skipping, and contains a phosphordiamidate linkage and replaces the ribose sugar with a morpholino group (PMO) (see Figure 9.19A). Another recent drug approved is nusinersen, used to treat spinal muscular atrophy. Many other antisense agents are undergoing clinical trials, including those to treat diseases ranging from Ebola and Marburg viral infections to motor disorders and neurodegenerative diseases such as ALS. It is likely that future antisense therapeutics will have to be similarly optimized with a variety of modifications at multiple sites of the nucleotide.

As seen in Section 9.5, drugs that target RNA directly are far fewer in number than those that target DNA. While several classes of antibacterial drugs have been found to target bacterial ribosomal RNA, these were found from phenotypic screening rather than through rational design. In contrast, antisense drugs are designed to target specific sequences and are optimized for improved physical and pharmaceutical properties. These RNA-targeted agents, (those antibacterials that bind to the ribosome, as well as

A: MODIFIED BACKBONE AND/OR RIBOSE

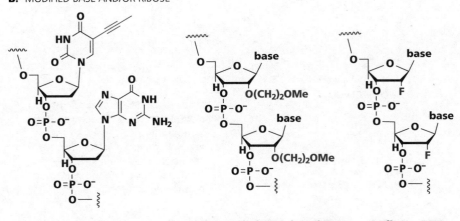

phosphorothioate-DNA (PS)   **thiophosphoramidate-DNA**   **phosphorodiamidate morpholino oligomer (PMO)**   **peptide nucleic acid (PNA)**

B: MODIFIED BASE AND/OR RIBOSE

5'-propynyl-pyrimidines   **2'-methoxyethyl-RNA (MOE)-RNA**   **2'-fluoro-RNA**

Figure 9.19 Structures of modified oligonucleotides.
A: Examples of structures with modified backbones and/or ribose, including phosphorothioate, thiophosphoramidates, phosphorodiamidates, and peptide nucleic acids. B: Examples of structures containing modified bases and/or ribose, such as 5-propynyl thymine, 2'-methoxyethyl and 2'-fluoro analogs. Modified regions are shown in red.

antisense oligonucleotides), affect protein synthesis. Designing selective drugs that will target a specific RNA sequence is just beginning to be successful.

SUMMARY

Approximately 1% of drugs target DNA and RNA, far fewer than those that target receptors, enzymes, and nontraditional targets. Most DNA-targeted drugs are older therapies that are most frequently used to treat cancers. They work through multiple mechanisms, but all require binding to DNA. Some drugs form strong noncovalent interactions, others alkylate DNA, and a third group abstracts radicals from the DNA chain, resulting in breakage of the DNA strand. While still widely used, they all suffer from serious toxicity due to lack of selectivity and specificity. In contrast, antisense therapy targets specific RNA sequences. This approach has been investigated since the late 1990s and has recently come to fruition, with several novel compounds on the market and many in clinical trials for a variety of conditions. Medicinal chemistry strategies to design metabolically stable and permeable oligonucleotides have been an important component to this approach. The potential to design highly selective compounds to target rare genetic disorders is an exciting opportunity for medicinal chemists.

CASE STUDY 1 DOXORUBICIN AND ANALOGS

The first chemotherapy drugs, the nitrogen mustards and folic acid derivatives, were introduced in the 1940s to treat cancer. The realization that drugs rather than surgery alone, could be used to treat cancer spurred the search for novel anti-tumor agents worldwide. At about the same time, with the discovery of penicillin, came the recognition that microbes can produce medicinally active agents. These two findings suggested that natural products, including those from both microbes and plants, might be sources of anti-cancer agents.

The first anthracycline reported was β-rhodomycin II, which contains the fused tetracyclic core common to all anthracycline antibacterial drugs. It was one of a mixture of red compounds isolated from the soil bacterium *Streptomyces purpurascens* in 1951 by H. Brockmann and K. Bauer (**Figure 9.20**). Independently, the C-10-aglycon rhodomycin B was identified in an Indian soil sample by Federico-Maria Arcamone at Farmitalia Research Laboratories, in Italy, in the late 1950s. These red compounds exhibited both antibacterial and anti-tumor activity in preliminary studies but were too toxic in animal models to be pursued as anti-cancer drugs.

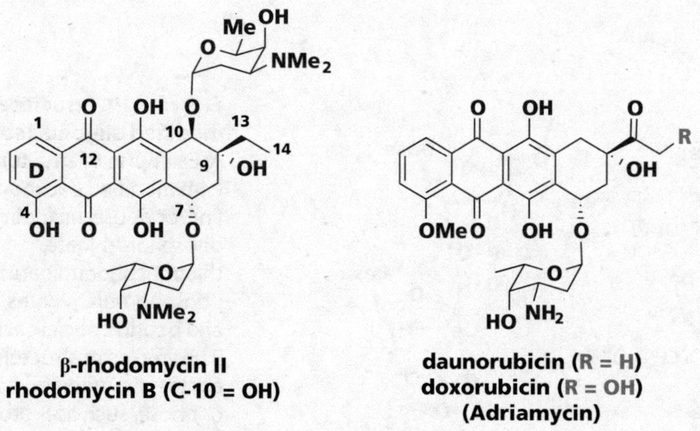

β-rhodomycin II
rhodomycin B (C-10 = OH)

daunorubicin (R = H)
doxorubicin (R = OH)
(Adriamycin)

Figure 9.20 Structures of early anthracyclines. β-rhodomycin II, rhodomycin B, daunorubicin, and doxorubicin. All contain the anthracycline-defining fused tetracyclic core, with the D ring and numbering scheme indicated.

In the early 1960s, the first clinically useful anti-tumor anthracycline was isolated independently at Farmitalia and Rhone-Poulenc. Daunomycin was derived from an Italian soil sample found near Castel del Monte that contained the microorganism *Streptomyces peucetius*. Farmitalia named the compound they isolated daunomycin, derived from the word Daunii, the name of a pre-Roman tribe. A group at Rhone-Poulenc isolated the same compound and named it rubidomycin, from the word rubis, for ruby. Both groups began preclinical testing and determined that they were working with the same compound, which was renamed daunorubicin. The compound proceeded rapidly to clinical trials, where it exhibited excellent activity against leukemias but also showed significant cardiotoxicity. This side effect results in irreversible damage to the heart muscle with long-term use. Despite this liability, daunorubicin became an important anti-cancer drug. The Farmitalia group induced mutations into the microbe used to produce daunorubicin, creating a variant strain that produced a new compound, doxorubicin (also known as Adriamycin), the C-14 hydroxy analog of daunorubicin (see Figure 9.20). It entered clinical trials in 1968 and was approved in the United States in 1974.

Although there is only one change between daunorubicin and doxorubicin, replacement of a hydrogen at C-14 with a hydroxyl group, the anti-tumor spectrum for doxorubicin includes a variety of carcinomas and sarcomas for which daunorubicin is ineffective. The success of doxorubicin led to a search for additional analogs with broader profiles and reduced cardiotoxicity. Most analogs are variants at the C-14 position, the amino sugar (daunosamine), or the terminal aromatic D ring.

Syntheses of over 1000 anthracyclines have been reported, with only a few exhibiting an anti-tumor and toxicity profile that would allow advancement into the clinic. The carbohydrate analogs epirubicin, and esorubicin were synthesized at Farmitalia (**Figure 9.21**). Epirubicin has only one change from doxorubicin: inversion of the 4'-hydroxyl on the carbohydrate from the axial to the equatorial isomer. It has the same anti-tumor profile but reduced cardiotoxicity, which may be attributed to changes in metabolism and elimination. Esorubicin, lacking the hydroxyl on the carbohydrate, is even less cardiotoxic. A possible explanation is that it does not generate oxygen-containing radicals, which may contribute to cardiotoxicity. Amrubicin and valrubicin are newer carbohydrate analogs that were approved in the early 2000s. Amrubicin contains a simplified carbohydrate, replaces the C-9 hydroxyl with an amine, and contains an unsubstituted D ring. Valrubicin is a semisynthetic analog derivatized with ester and amides. D-ring analogs include idarubicin, a close analog of daunorubicin in which the C-4-position in the D ring is unsubstituted, and carminomycin, the C-4-OH analog of doxorubicin. One advantage of both idarubicin and carminomycin is increased oral availability.

A: ANALOGS OF DOXORUBICIN

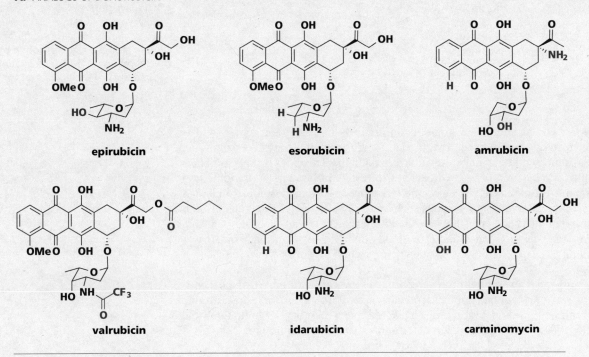

epirubicin

esorubicin

amrubicin

valrubicin

idarubicin

carminomycin

B: NATURAL PRODUCT NOGALAMYCIN AND ANALOG MENOGARIL

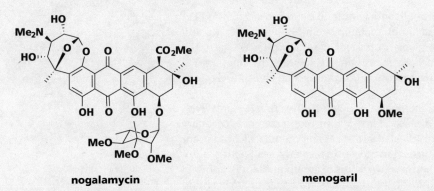

nogalamycin

menogaril

Figure 9.21 Structures of anthracyclines. A. Structures of synthetic and semi-synthetic analogs of daunorubin and daunomycin. Epirubicin, esorubicin, amrubicin, and valrubicin contain modifications in the carbohydrate residue; amrubicin also replaces a hydroxyl group with an amine and eliminates the D-ring hydroxyl group; Idarubicin and carminomycin are modified on the D ring . Structural changes compared to doxorubicin are shown in red. B. Structurally unique natural product anthracyclines nogalamycin, and menogaril. Neither of these compounds is clinically approved.

A related anthracycline natural product, nogalamycin (See section 9.3B,C), isolated from *Streptomyces nogalater*, contains an unusual bicyclic modified D-ring. Menogaril is a synthetic analog of nogalamycin with a simplified A-ring pattern. It is more potent and less cardiotoxic than nogalamycin. Although they are structurally interesting, neither nogalamycin nor menogaril has been approved as a drug.

Mechanisms of action of the anthracyclines include intercalation, topoisomerase II (topo II) inhibition, and radical production. Structure–activity relationships are summarized in **Figure 9.22**.

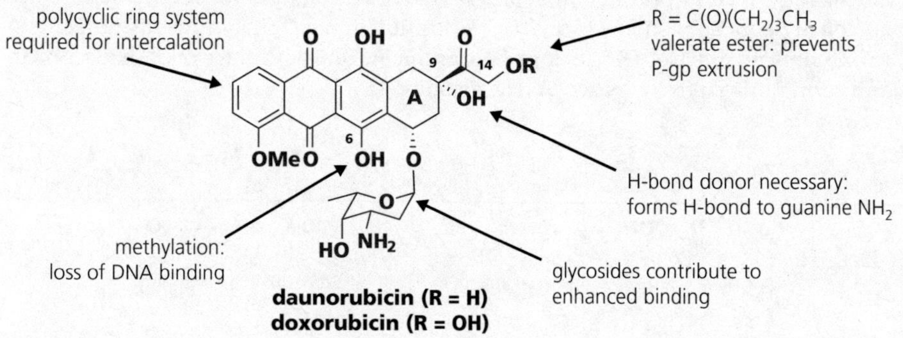

polycyclic ring system
required for intercalation

R = C(O)(CH$_2$)$_3$CH$_3$
valerate ester: prevents
P-gp extrusion

H-bond donor necessary:
forms H-bond to guanine NH$_2$

methylation:
loss of DNA binding

glycosides contribute to
enhanced binding

daunorubicin (R = H)
doxorubicin (R = OH)

Figure 9.22 Structure–activity relationships of doxorubicin analogs. Essential functional groups include a H-bond donor at the C-9 position to bind to the primary amine in guanine amino at the intercalation site, the hydroxyl group at C-6 and the planar polycyclic ring system, The presence of glycosides stabilize DNA binding, with more groups providing tighter binding. Ester groups at C-14 are tolerated and can mitigate P-gp efflux.

The C-9 OH or another hydrogen-bond donor is necessary for activity and is proposed to form a hydrogen bond to guanine 2-amino groups at the intercalation site. The C-9-amino synthetic analog, amrubicin, maintains activity as a topoisomerase II inhibitor. Methylation of the hydroxyl at C-6 results in loss of DNA binding and topoisomerase II-mediated cleavage. One resistance mechanism is efflux mediated by P-glycoprotein (P-gp), and analogs such as the 14-valerate of doxorubicin both increase lipophilicity and prevent P-gp efflux. The glycoside has an effect on stabilizing the DNA–drug complex, and an increase in the number of attached sugars increases the binding to DNA. The polycyclic planar ring system is required for intercalation into DNA.

Doxorubicin is an example of an older drug, discovered in the era when most anti-cancer drugs were identified through screening of natural sources. There are currently several anthracycline anti-cancer drugs marketed, and while there are limitations due to toxicity, they are an important part of the anti-cancer armamentarium.

CASE STUDY 2   DISCOVERY OF MIPOMERSEN

Mipomersen was the second antisense oligonucleotide to be approved by the FDA (2013). It is an inhibitor of the production of apolipoprotein B-100 (apoB-100), and is used to treat hyperlipidemia in patients at risk for cardiovascular disease. The protein apoB-100 is embedded in a lipid membrane of low-density lipoprotein–cholesterol (LDL-C) particles, which have a core of triglyceride and cholesteryl esters. (**Figure 9.23**).

Cardiovascular disease is the leading cause of death in the United States, with one-third of all deaths related to the disease. A major contributing factor is coronary artery disease, which is linked to high levels of LDL-C and apoB-100. Treatment for high levels of LDL-C include the statins, which lower cholesterol levels but are not effective or tolerated in all patients. There are two forms of apolipoprotein B, apoB-48 and apoB-100. ApoB-100 is the form found in lipoproteins synthesized in the liver, and about 85% of apoB-100 synthesized in the body becomes part of LDL particles. A novel approach was proposed to lower levels of apoB-100 by use of antisense oligonucleotides to block production of the protein. The second-generation phosphorothioates had been shown to have good pharmacokinetics, with wide tissue distribution, and were chosen as the basis for the drug.

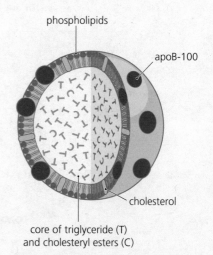

phospholipids

apoB-100

cholesterol

core of triglyceride (T)
and cholesteryl esters (C)

Figure 9.23 Rendition of low density lipoprotein cholesterol particles. The protein apoB-100 is embedded into a lipid membrane that surrounds a core of triglyceride and cholesteryl esters.

The program was initiated at Isis Pharmaceuticals (now named Ionis) in the early 2000s. A number of phosphorothioate 2′-methoxyethyl (MOE) oligonucleotides were prepared, targeting various regions of the apoB-100 gene. Candidate antisense oligomers were evaluated for their ability to reduce levels of apoB-100 mRNA in mouse hepatocytes. Approximately 25% of the oligomers were active, with ISIS 147764 and ISIS 147483 being the most potent, showing 90% inhibition of production of apoB-100 mRNA at 150 nM. ISIS 147764 and ISIS 147483 targeted two different sequences found in the coding region for murine apoB-100:

ISIS 147764: **5′-GTCCC**TGAAGATGTC**AATGC-3′**

ISIS 147483: **5′-ATGTC**AATGCCACAT**GTCCA-3′**

The analogs developed are mixed oligomers. They contain the 2′-MOE-modified furanose only on the ends of the oligomers (shown in boldface type) that flank a sequence containing the natural RNA monomers, creating a gapmer. This strategy avoids the known limitation of using all 2′-modified sugars which results in reduced RNAse H activity, but maintains the benefit of improved nuclease stability. Preclinical studies on ISIS 147764 in mice showed a dose dependent reduction in apoB-100 mRNA as well as reduction of apoB-100, cholesterol, and LDL-C levels. A long half-life of 11-19 days indicated a long duration of action, and there were no adverse toxicological results. Application of the strategy of using mixed oligomers similar to ISIS 147764 led to the inhibitor of human apoB-100, ISIS 301012 (mipomersen).

Mipomersen is a 20 residue antisense molecule that binds to human apoB-100 mRNA (positions 3249–3269) and results in RNase H-mediated degradation of the mRNA, therefore inhibiting translation of the protein. While the entire backbone is phosphorothioate-modified, the specific structure is considered a gapmer since the termini of the sequence are different (modified riboses) from the internal residues (natural ribose). Mipomersen has the following sequence:

G-mC-mC-T-mC-dA-dG-dT-dmC-dT-dG-dmC-dT-dT-dmC-**G-mC-A-mC-mC**

The five terminal bases at each end (shown in boldface type) contain 2′-O-(2-methoxyethyl) riboses, the central core contains deoxyriboses, and all cytidines are methylated at C5 (mC = 5-methylcytidine).

Pharmacokinetic studies showed rapid tissue distribution to the liver and kidney, with slow elimination occurring over weeks. This is a desirable profile and allows for infrequent injections. Metabolism is by endonucleases, resulting in metabolites of 7–14 bases. Since there is no effect on CYP450, mipomersen is potentially free of drug–drug interactions.

Currently, mipomersen is approved as a weekly injection to treat homozygous familial hypercholesterolemia (HoFH), a rare but fatal orphan disease. It is characterized by a mutation in the LDL-C receptor gene that results in highly elevated levels of LDL-C and early death (average life span = 33 years).

REVIEW QUESTIONS

1. Describe two mechanisms by which drugs bind to DNA.

2. Name three classes of DNA alkylators, the electrophiles they generate, and draw the products of their reaction with DNA.

3. Why is alkylated DNA unstable?

4. Which of the compounds shown has characteristics of an intercalator? Explain your answer.

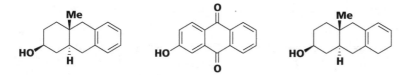

5. Explain why many drugs that directly affect DNA also exhibit significant toxicity.

6. What is the difference between a compound that nicks DNA and a compound that causes strand breakage? Give an example of a DNA strand breaker.

7. Shown is the structure of a sulfur mustard. Draw the mechanism of its reaction with DNA.

8. Briefly describe two methods that are used to detect binding of small molecules to nucleic acids.

9. What are some of the challenges in antisense drug design?

10. Explain why drugs that work by alkylation of DNA are often prodrugs or require bioactivation.

APPLICATION QUESTIONS

1. ISIS 3521 was an antisense oligonucleotide that was in clinical trials for the treatment of lung cancer. Research this compound and answer the following:

(a) What gene is targeted, and why is it targeted?

(b) How is this oligonucleotide chemically modified?

2. Hairpin polyamides, such as those designed and studied by Peter Dervan, bind to DNA with sequence specificity. Research the basic structure, the mechanism of action, and the basis for the sequence specificity.

3. Chromomycin A3 is a natural product that binds to DNA. Research its mechanism of action and the structure of the bound complex.

4. Enediynes all undergo the Bergman cyclization *in vivo* to give diradicals. The mechanism of this cycloaromatization, studied by Robert Bergman in the 1970s, is shown here. Dynemicin A intercalates into DNA, and in one proposed pathway, bioreduction results in ring opening of the epoxide. Then, after attack of a nucleophile, either H_2O or a glutathione (GSH) molecule, it forms an intermediate that undergoes the Bergman cyclization.

dynemicin A

(a) Identify the portion of dynemycin A that would intercalate into DNA.

(b) Draw the product of nucleophilic addition (Intermediate A), write a cyclization mechanism, and draw the resulting diradical.

5. Tumor resistance mechanisms to DNA alkylating agents include activity of DNA repair enzymes. Research two mechanisms for DNA repair of alkylated DNA and work that has been done to circumvent these resistance mechanisms.

6. Research the natural product duocarmycin A. Draw its structure. What is its mechanism of action?

7. Some anti-cancer drugs that target DNA eventually cause cancer themselves. Explain this effect.

8. Compare the structure of phosphorothioate-modified DNA (PS DNA) in Figure 9.19 to the regular DNA backbone. What changes are imparted in PS DNA by introduction of the sulfur?

9. Research the structure of camptothecin. What part of the structure might intercalate?

10. Epirubicin (see Figure 9.21) has a shorter half-life than doxorubicin due to metabolism to the 4′-glucuronide, leading to more rapid clearance. Draw the glucuronide metabolite.

FURTHER READING

DNA drugs

Dervan PB (2001) Molecular recognition of DNA by small molecules. *Bioorg Med Chem* 9:2215–2235.

Di Leva FS, Zizza P, Cingolani C et al. (2013) Exploring the chemical space of G-quadruplex binders: discovery of a novel chemotype targeting the human telomeric sequence. *J Med Chem* 56:9646–9654.

Pogozelski WK & Tullius TD (1998) Oxidative strand scission of nucleic acids: routes initiated by hydrogen abstraction from the sugar moiety. *Chem Rev* 98:1089–1107.

Oppenheimer NJ, Rodriguez LO & Hecht SM (1979) Structural studies of "active complex" of bleomycin: assignment of ligands to the ferrous ion in a ferrous–bleomycin–carbon monoxide complex. *Proc Natl Acad Sci USA* 76:5616–5620.

Shinomiya M, Chu W, Carlson RG et al. (1995) Structural, physical, and biological characteristics of RNA–DNA binding agent N8-actinomycin D. *Biochemistry* 34:8481–8491.

Frederick CA, Williams LD, Ughetto G et al. (1990) Structural comparison of anticancer drug–DNA complexes: adriamycin and daunomycin. *Biochemistry* 29:2538–2549.

Kelland L (2007) The resurgence of platinum-based cancer chemotherapy. *Nat Rev Cancer* 7:573–584.

Fuertes MA, Alonso C & Perez JM (2003) Biochemical modulation of cisplatin mechanisms of action: enhancement of antitumor activity and circumvention of drug resistance. *Chem Rev* 103:645– 662.

RNA drugs

Bennett CF & Swayze EE (2010) RNA targeting therapeutics: molecular mechansims of antisense oligonucleotides as a therapeutic platform. *Annu Rev Pharmacol Toxicol* 50:259–293.

Chopra I & Roberts M (2001) Tetracycline antibiotics: mode of action, applications, molecular biology, and epidemiology of bacterial resistance. *Micro and Mol Biol Rev* 65:232–260.

Dias N & Stein CA (2002) Antisense oligonucleotides: basic concepts and mechanisms. *Mol Cancer Ther* 1:347–355.

Actinomycins

Lown JW (1993) Discovery and development of anthracycline antitumour antibiotics. *Chem Soc Rev* 22:165–176.

Weiss TB, Sarosy G, Clagett-Carr K et al. (1986) Anthracycline analogs: the past, present, and future. *Cancer Chemother Pharmacol* 18:185–197.

Mipomersen

Crooke ST & Geary RS (2013) Clinical pharmacological properties of mipomersen (Kynamro), a second generation antisense inhibitor of apolipoprotein B. *Br J Clin Pharmacol* 76:269–276.

Ricotta DN & Frishman W (2012) Mipomersen: a safe and effective antisense therapy adjunct to statins in patients with hypercholesterolemia. *Cardiol Rev* 20:90–95.

Crooke RM, Graham MJ, Lemonidis KM et al. (2005) LDL cholesterol in hyperlipidemic mice without causing hepatic steatosis. *J Lipid Res* 46:872–884.

Yu RZ, Kim T-W, Hong A et al. (2007) Cross-species pharmacokinetic comparison from mouse to man of a second-generation antisense oligonucleotide, ISIS 301012, targeting human apolipoprotein B-100. *Drug Metab Dispos* 35:460–468.

PART III
SELECTED THERAPEUTIC AREAS

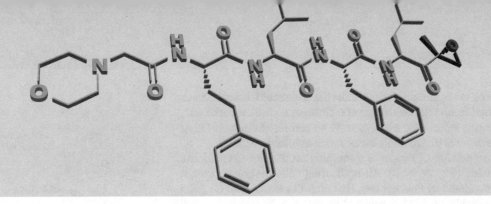

Anti-cancer drugs

10

LEARNING OBJECTIVES

- Explain the genetic changes that underpin the development of cancer.
- Describe why targeting cell division is an effective anti-cancer strategy.
- Understand the mechanism of action of different drugs that target enzymes involved in DNA replication.
- Explain successful strategies for modulating the toxicity of certain anti-cancer agents.
- Identify various approaches to targeting signaling pathways through enzyme inhibition.
- Describe several anti-cancer drugs that work on epigenetic targets.

While there are hundreds of drugs used to treat cancer, it is still the second leading cause of death in the United States, with approximately 600,000 deaths attributed to this disease each year. Each of the >100 types of cancer, usually classified by the origin of the cancerous cell, is quite distinct, as are each one's symptoms, risk factors, outcomes, and mortality rates. However, they are all characterized by the following:

- uncontrolled growth of cells

- invasion and destruction of neighboring tissue

- migration, invasion, and proliferation at a location or organ remote from the primary site (**metastasis**)

- evasion of the immune system

It is commonly believed that multiple successive genetic changes at the cellular level occur to cause cancer. A basic form of this theory was described in the 1950s by Carl Nordling, and it was more explicitly detailed in 1971 by Alfred Knudson. Knudson's **two-hit hypothesis** was a unifying model to explain how a specific cancer (retinoblastoma) developed both in individuals carrying cancer susceptibility genes and those who carried normal genes. In this simplified model, two hits, or two mutations to a gene, are required before cancer develops (**Figure 10.1**). In an individual who inherits a mutant gene at birth, only one rare event (mutation) is required before tumor founder cells develop and cancer results. In individuals who have normal genes, two rare mutations are required. The current view of cancer is that multiple hits or genetic changes within a cell accumulate and allow the cell to acquire the various traits that characterize a cancerous cell. Some avoidable external factors that cause genetic changes include tobacco use, radiation or sunlight exposure, infections, and exposure to certain chemicals. Other genetic changes can be the result of unavoidable factors such as inherited genes.

At the center of the progression of cancer is dysregulation of the cell cycle, the process by which cells divide (**Figure 10.2**). All replicating cells progress through specific stages of a cycle, regulated by checkpoints, that includes the phases G1 (first gap phase), S (DNA synthesis phase), G2 (second gap phase), and M (mitosis or cell division). At checkpoints, a cell will proceed through the next phase of the cycle only if DNA is undamaged and cells are normal. If DNA or cells are abnormal, they are marked for programmed cell death, known as apoptosis.

Genes and the proteins they encode tightly regulate the cell cycle, both positively and negatively. **Proto-oncogenes** are normal genes that promote cell division, while **tumor suppressor genes** oppose it. These genes and their gene products work in concert to ensure that cells replicate appropriately. Most of the uncontrolled cell growth characteristic of cancer occurs as a result of mutation of these proto-oncogenes to form **oncogenes**, which then code for mutant proteins, leading to a loss of control of the cell cycle. Alternatively, mutations to tumor suppressor genes result in loss of function of the encoded proteins that, when functional, block progression through the cycle or promote apoptosis of abnormal cells. Mutations to either oncogenes or tumor suppressor genes lead to dysregulation of the cell cycle and to uncontrolled cell growth and proliferation, the hallmarks of cancer.

Cancer treatment usually involves removal of the tumor by surgery or destruction of the tumor with radiation and/or drug treatment (chemotherapy). Drug treatment may stop cell growth and proliferation directly, or it may stop the signals that promote it. In many cases, therapy involves a combination of these approaches. First-generation cancer drugs were cytotoxic agents that directly targeted the process of DNA synthesis, replication, and cell division. These drugs, working through a variety of mechanisms, are lethal to dividing cells, regardless of whether the cells are cancerous or not. For this reason, the earliest drugs exhibit significant toxicities related to this lack of selectivity, and many of their side effects (such as hair loss, nausea, and immunosuppression) can be directly attributed to their effects on dividing but noncancerous cells.

Facilitating this early phase of cancer drug discovery was the relative ease of identifying potential therapeutics through the use of assays that evaluated a compound's ability to be either **cytostatic** or **cytotoxic**. Cytostatic compounds stop proliferation of cells, while cytotoxic compounds kill the cells. Many drugs were discovered by such phenotypic assays, which are blind to a specific mechanism. In fact, the mechanism of action of these drugs was often understood only after their therapeutic anti-cancer activity was established. Many drugs from this first generation of anti-cancer agents worked by targeting DNA, either its biosynthesis or function, or through direct binding. Others target processes and proteins, such as tubulin, involved in cell division.

Historically, natural products have been a valuable source of anti-cancer drugs. This may be explained by two factors. First, cell-based anti-proliferative and cytotoxicity assays are simple and can be readily applied to track the activity in natural product extracts and the subsequent assay-guided fractionations necessary to isolate purified products. Second, organisms produce such natural products as a defense mechanism; therefore, they are optimized for toxicity and cell permeability, two features essential for anti-cancer activity. Well-known examples of natural product anti-cancer drugs discovered this way include vinblastine, paclitaxel, and doxorubicin (**Figure 10.3**). These compounds and their mechanisms of actions were described in detail in earlier chapters: see Section 8.2, Case Study 1 in Chapter 8, and Case Study 1 in Chapter 9, respectively.

More recently, the field of cancer biology has developed a much deeper understanding of mechanisms that are involved in tumor initiation, progression, and metastasis. As such, cancer drug discovery and medicinal chemistry have undergone a tremendous shift. Finding very potent, broadly anti-proliferative or cytotoxic agents is now considered a less desirable approach to developing cancer drugs. Instead, newer drugs target either oncoproteins or tumor suppressors that have been mutated or cancer-specific changes and processes. In addition, advances in diagnostic tools can identify which patients are most likely to benefit from certain drugs and which have refractory

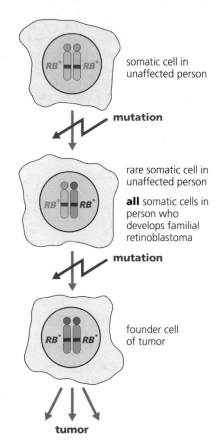

Figure 10.1 Illustration of Knudson's two-hit theory to explain the relationship between hereditary and nonhereditary forms of retinoblastoma. Normal somatic cells carry two undamaged retinoblastoma genes (RB+, shown in blue). Two successive mutations are required to produce a cell that contains a mutated gene (RB*, shown in red) that results in a tumor. In contrast, in an individual with familial retinoblastoma who inherits a damaged gene (RB+, RB*), only one mutation to produce the cancer-causing cell is required. Both individuals develop cancer, but the path to acquiring two hits varies. (Adapted from Strachan R & Read A [2010] Human Molecular Genetics, 4th ed. Garland Science.)

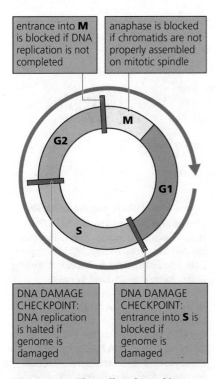

Figure 10.2 The cell cycle and its regulation by checkpoints. Cells enter G1 (first gap) phase, progress to S (synthesis) phase, followed by a shorter G2 phase, and then cell division occurs in M (mitosis) phase. Checkpoints (shown as pink lines) prevent cells with damaged DNA, incomplete replication, or improperly assembled chromatids from progressing to the next phase: these occur toward the end of G1 phase, during S phase, toward the end of G2 phase, and during M phase. (Adapted from Weinberg RA [2013] The Biology of Cancer, 2nd ed. Garland Science.)

Figure 10.3 Structures of vinblastine, paclitaxel, and doxorubicin. These compounds are examples of anti-cancer drugs derived from natural product sources.

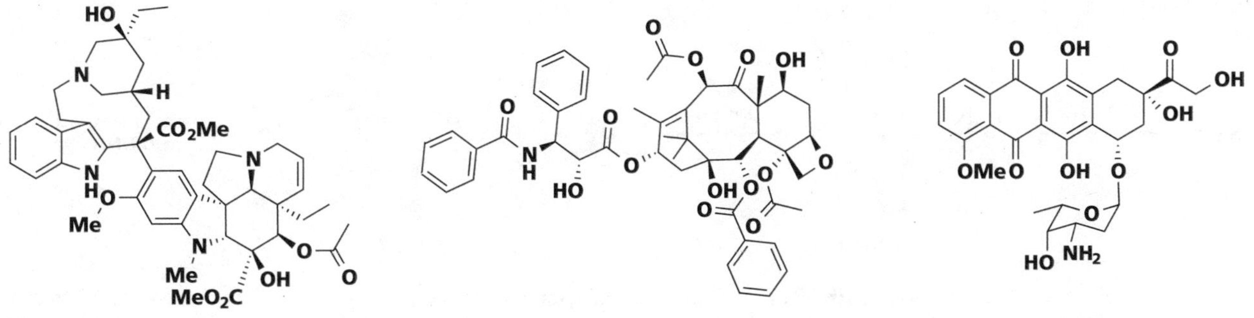

tumors. For example, the characterization of breast tumors as either dependent on (ER-positive) or independent of (ER-negative) the estrogen receptor dictates which treatment is offered and is more likely to be effective. A more recent example of the application of personalized medicine to anti-cancer therapy is the antibody trastuzumab (Herceptin) that is used to treat certain breast and stomach cancers characterized by overexpression of the ERBB2/HER2 oncoprotein. Only patients whose tumors express this genetic marker benefit from treatment with trastuzumab. Finally, an exciting recent example takes advantage of the concept of synthetic lethality. Inhibitors of poly ADP-ribose polymerase (PARP) cause DNA damage that cannot be repaired in tumors containing BRCA mutations. In cells that are not mutated, the effects of PARP can be overcome, making therapy with these drugs only effective in certain tumors.

DRUGS TARGETING DNA REPLICATION AND MITOSIS

Many older anti-cancer agents target either DNA biosynthesis or its replication. As cancer cells are typically rapidly dividing, this approach is often highly effective for various types of cancer and during all stages of cancer. However, these drugs affect all dividing cells, such as immune cells and those lining the intestinal tract. In some cases, this property has been applied for use in nonmalignant disorders. Several are used to treat infectious diseases, where they target the organism's ability to replicate. Autoimmune disorders such as multiple sclerosis and arthritis, which are characterized by the proliferation of immune cells, are also effectively treated with drugs that target DNA synthesis, replication, and cell division. Despite these applications, these drugs have significant toxicities associated with them based on their indiscriminate effects on dividing cells. In addition, their long-term use can itself lead to cancer.

10.1 Drugs may target DNA and DNA processing enzymes such as polymerase and topoisomerase

A variety of mechanisms that target DNA directly and processes that involve DNA have been applied to anti-cancer drug design. Some agents bind to DNA and/or cause lesions in it, thereby making it incompetent for replication. These were described in detail in Chapter 9 and include alkylating agents that damage DNA (such as dacarbazine, cyclophosphamide, and carboplatin); intercalators (for example, daunorubicin, doxorubicin, and mitoxantrone) that bind to the DNA duplex and perturb its three-dimensional structure so that it is not efficiently replicated; and compounds that make lesions in the DNA strand or duplex (like bleomycin and calicheamicin). In general, these compounds are effective, but they cause considerable side effects, such as nausea, bone marrow suppression, and hair loss.

Rather than directly targeting DNA, an alternative cancer drug design strategy is to target DNA processing enzymes. These enzymes use DNA as a substrate or a template to perpetuate the cell's genetic information through replication or transcription into mRNA, and their inhibition results in cell death. Drugs targeting DNA processing enzymes often carry many of the same liabilities as those that directly bind to DNA. However, improvements in safety can sometimes be realized since the processing

vinblastine   **paclitaxel**   **doxorubicin**

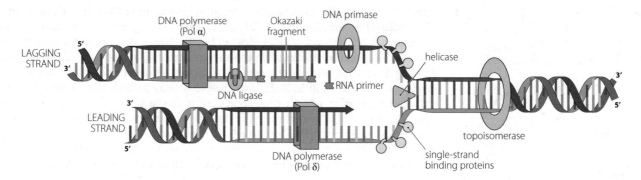

enzymes are active only in replicating cells, while DNA is present in all cells. Some key enzymes involved in DNA replication and processing are polymerases (see Section 7.6), topoisomerases, and helicases. While a thorough discussion of DNA replication is beyond the scope of this text, the basic process is outlined in **Figure 10.4**.

During the process of DNA replication, helicase splits the double strand into two separate template strands, creating the replication fork. The two template strands are replicated in a process catalyzed by polymerase after initiation by primase. Both strands, the leading strand and the lagging strand, are replicated in the 5′–3′ direction. While the leading strand is replicated continuously, the lagging strand is replicated in short pieces, called Okazaki fragments, which are then linked together by DNA ligase. Ahead of the fork, the tension in the supercoiled strand is relieved by topoisomerase. Both polymerase and topoisomerase are targets of current anti-cancer agents.

Polymerases are multienzyme complexes that are responsible for polymerizing DNA. As described in Chapter 7 they catalyze the formation of a phosphodiester bond between a deoxynucleoside triphosphate and a DNA primer, resulting in elongation of the DNA chain. Of the four forms of eukaryotic DNA polymerases known (α, β, γ, and δ), it is believed that DNA polymerase α plays the major role in replication of genomic DNA. Cytarabine (1-β-D-arabinofuranosylcytosine, ara-C) is one of the most widely used DNA polymerase inhibitors (**Figure 10.5A**). An analog of the natural nucleoside deoxycytidine (dC) and the HIV drug dideoxycytidine (ddC), it acts through a mechanism identical

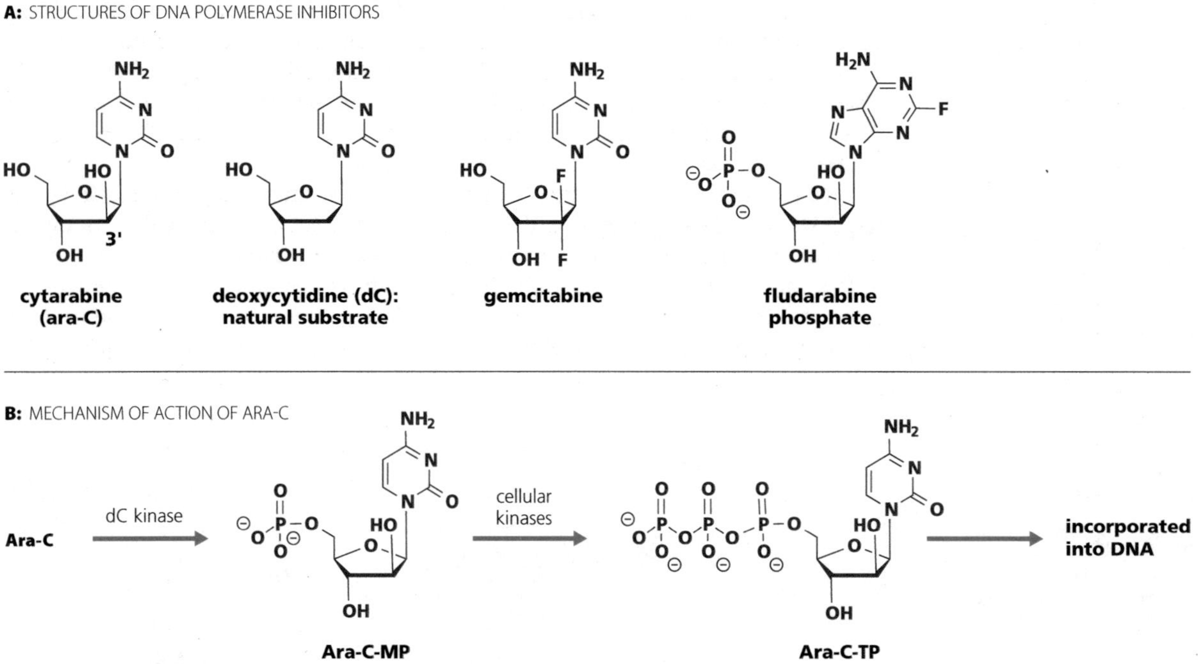

Figure 10.4 DNA replication fork and processing enzymes involved in DNA transcription and replication. Helicase (shown as a green triangle) breaks duplex DNA into single strands, known as leading and lagging strands. DNA primase (shown as a smaller green ring) initiates replication, DNA polymerases, also known as polymerase α and δ (shown as green boxes) catalyze the formation of the new strand, and DNA ligase (shown as a small green oval) links the short Okazaki fragments formed in the lagging strand. Topoisomerase (shown as a larger green ring) relaxes supercoiling of the double strand ahead of the replication fork.

A: STRUCTURES OF DNA POLYMERASE INHIBITORS

cytarabine
(ara-C)

deoxycytidine (dC):
natural substrate

gemcitabine

fludarabine
phosphate

B: MECHANISM OF ACTION OF ARA-C

Ara-C → dC kinase → Ara-C-MP → cellular kinases → Ara-C-TP → **incorporated into DNA**

Figure 10.5 DNA polymerase inhibitors. A: Structures of cytarabine (ara-C), deoxycytidine (dC; the natural substrate), gemcitabine, and fludarabine phosphate. B: Mechanism of action of ara-C: Formation of ara-C-monophosphate (ara-C-MP) is catalyzed by dC kinase; conversion to ara-C triphosphate (ara-C-TP) by cellular kinases is followed by incorporation into DNA.

to that of HIV reverse transcriptase inhibitors as described in Chapters 7 and 11. It is phosphorylated by deoxycytidine kinase to generate its monophosphate (Ara-C-MP), which is converted to the triphosphate (Ara-C-TP) by the action of other cellular kinases (**Figure 10.5B**). The triphosphate competes with the natural substrate, deoxycytidine triphosphate, for binding to DNA polymerase α and incorporation into the growing DNA chain. Once incorporated, chain elongation is terminated; the replicating cancer cells accumulate in the S phase of the cell cycle rather than proceeding through it, and ultimately they die. Gemcitabine (see Figure 10.5A), a fluorinated nucleoside analog, acts by a related mechanism: it is converted to the corresponding triphosphate and incorporated into the growing DNA strand. However, chain termination does not occur immediately but after one additional nucleotide is added. Fludarabine phosphate (see Figure 10.5A) is hydrolyzed to the primary alcohol and then converted to the triphosphate, which inhibits DNA polymerase. Both gemcitabine and fludarabine have additional effects on other DNA processing enzymes, such as ribonucleotide reductase, that contribute to their anti-cancer activity.

The modest numbers of cancer drugs that work through inhibition of DNA polymerase is likely attributed to the lack of selectivity of such drugs. Rational medicinal chemistry approaches to this target are particularly difficult, as they require designing structures that are similar enough to natural substrates to be recognized and phosphorylated by host kinases yet inhibit the DNA polymerase. Furthermore, the triphosphate must effectively compete with the high concentration of natural substrates for binding to the DNA polymerase enzyme, without interfering with the large number of other enzymes and proteins that require nucleosides or nucleotides for their activity. In contrast, antiviral approaches can rely on the significant differences between human and viral kinases that can selectively convert nucleosides to the corresponding nucleotides only in virally infected cells, as well as the differences between human DNA polymerases and viral polymerases. As a result, targeting polymerases is a more common approach to antiviral therapy than anti-cancer therapy (see Chapter 11).

Topoisomerases, enzymes essential for DNA replication, transiently break either one (topoisomerase I) or two (topoisomerase II) DNA strands to allow for unwinding of the helix and replication, and then they re-form (re-ligate) the phosphodiester bond to restore the DNA tertiary structure (**Figure 10.6A**). An abbreviated cleavage mechanism, shown in **Figure 10.6B**, involves reaction of the enzyme with DNA via nucleophilic attack of a tyrosine residue on the DNA phosphodiester bond, and formation of a covalent topoisomerase–DNA complex (called a cleavable complex) at the 5′-phosphate. A number of anti-cancer drugs specifically target topoisomerase, and several others indirectly inhibit the enzyme.

One well-studied class of topoisomerase I inhibitors is the camptothecins. The parent, camptothecin (**Figure 10.7**), is a pentacyclic alkaloid natural product isolated in the early 1960s by Wani and Wall, the same scientists who discovered paclitaxel. It was isolated from the bark of the happy tree, *Camptotheca acuminata*, a plant used in traditional Chinese medicine. Like many other early anti-cancer agents, its mechanism of action was determined well after its anti-cancer effects were described. It acts as an uncompetitive inhibitor, binding to and stabilizing the covalent topoisomerase I–DNA complex after initial strand cleavage. It does not bind to either DNA or topoisomerase alone and is termed a **topoisomerase poison** since it renders the essential topoisomerase I a DNA-damaging agent by virtue of stabilizing its covalent complex with DNA. The result, irreversible DNA strand cleavage, occurs during the S phase of the cell cycle, and blocks progression of the DNA replication fork, leading to cell death by apoptosis.

Camptothecin's insolubility, as well as its limited efficacy, prevented its further development. Therefore, drug design efforts have focused on improving aqueous solubility, increasing lipophilicity to enhance cellular uptake, and/or stabilizing the required but unstable lactone ring. Three synthetic or semisynthetic analogs, topotecan, belotecan, and irinotecan are approved for advanced or recurring cancers, and others are in clinical trials (see Figure 10.7). Topotecan and belotecan have an amine-containing water-solubilizing group, at positions 9 and 7, respectively, that does not affect efficacy. Irinotecan is a water-soluble prodrug; the carbamate is cleaved to deliver the active moiety, SN38. A number of other analogs that address lactone instability are being evaluated clinically. Strategies to do so include incorporation of lipophilic groups (for

A: UNWINDING OF DNA AND RE-LIGATION CATALYZED BY TOPOISOMERASE I

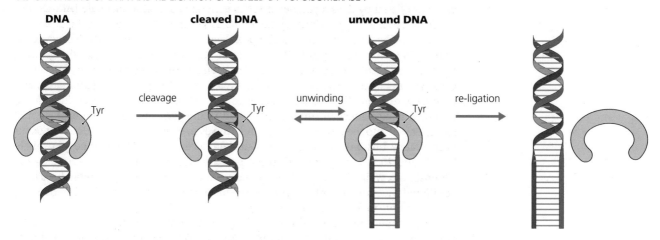

B: ABBREVIATED MECHANISM OF TOPOISOMERASE I-MEDIATED CLEAVAGE OF DNA

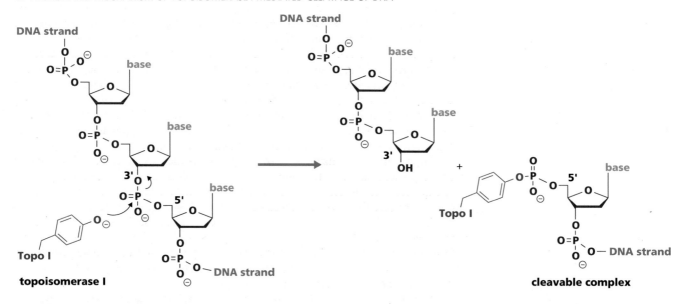

example, silatecan), which sequester the molecule in the lipid bilayer and thereby protect the lactone from hydrolysis, and ring expansion, as in diflomotecan (see Figure 10.7).

The availability of camptothecin analogs (tecans) by isolation, semisynthesis, and total synthesis, as well as X-ray crystallography of DNA–topoisomerase I–drug complexes (**Figure 10.8A**), has generated an excellent understanding of the structure–activity relationships that predict activity and potency. Essential structural features include the pyridone group, the 20S-hydroxyl group, the lactone, and the planarity of the pentacyclic ring system. The rings mimic a DNA base pair and intercalate between the two base pairs that surround the topoisomerase I cleavage site, with carbons 7, 9, and 10 pointed toward the major groove; therefore, modifications (such as those found in the analogs in Figure 10.7) to these regions are tolerated. Specific interactions are highlighted in **Figure 10.8B** and include the following:

- Intercalation of the planar heterocyclic aromatic core between base pairs, with a preference for binding at a site one away (+1) from G-C pair sites.

- A hydrogen bond forms between the 20S-OH group on the E ring and Asp533 of topoisomerase I (the *R*-configuration of the OH group is not appropriately oriented to make the same interaction).

- A salt bridge forms between Asp533 and Arg364, with a hydrogen bond from the Arg364 side chain to the B-ring nitrogen in the minor groove.

Figure 10.6 Mechanism of topoisomerase I-mediated cleavage and unwinding of DNA. A: Overview of DNA unwinding. Once topoisomerase I (shown in blue) binds to double-stranded DNA, a tyrosine residue reacts with DNA and cleaves a phosphodiester bond (shown as a gap in the red strand). The helix unwinds, and then, after replication has taken place, topoisomerase I catalyzes re-ligation of the phosphodiester bond. B: Abbreviated mechanism of cleavage. Addition of tyrosine from topoisomerase I (shown in red) to a phosphodiester bond in DNA (shown in black) results in breaking the phosphodiester bond, and cleavage into two DNA segments. One end of the cleaved DNA strand has a 3'-OH, and the other end, termed the cleavable complex, is bound to topoisomerase I through a 5'-tyrosine phosphate ester.

CAMPTOTHECIN AND ANALOGS WITH IMPROVED SOLUBILITY

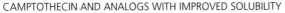

camptothecin　　　　　　**topotecan**　　　　　　**belotecan**

irinotecan
(prodrug)

SN38

CAMPTOTHECIN ANALOGS WITH IMPROVED LACTONE STABILITY

silatecan　　　　　　**diflomotecan**

Figure 10.7 Structures of camptothecin and various analogs and prodrugs with improved solubility and stability. Topotecan, belotecan, and irinotecan are approved to treat certain cancers. The amine groups of topotecan and belotecan improve solubility, as does the amine of the prodrug carbamate ironotecan, which is cleaved *in vivo* to give SN-38. Both silatecan and diflomotecan, which advanced to clinical trials, exhibit improved lactone stability.

Etoposide and teniposide, semisynthetic analogs of the natural product podophyllotoxin (a microtubule binder), are approved anti-cancer agents that act as topoisomerase II poisons and stabilize the DNA–topoisomerase II complex (**Figure 10.9**). While podophyllotoxin binds to tubulin, epimerization at C4 and demethylation at the C4′ ether gives analogs that are topoisomerase poisons. The carbohydrate group, as well as the C and D rings, have been proposed to interact with DNA, while the A, B, and E rings bind to the enzyme. An X-ray crystal structure solved in 2011 of etoposide

A: X-RAY STRUCTURE OF CPT AND TPT BOUND TO TOPISOMERASE
LEFT: SIDE VIEW; RIGHT: TOP VIEW.

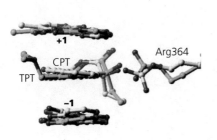

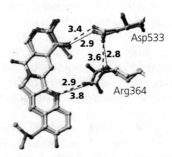

B: SCHEMATIC OF INTERACTIONS BETWEEN CPT AND TOPO I-DNA COMPLEX

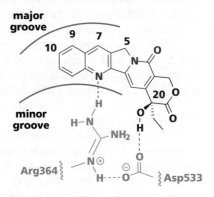

Figure 10.8 Interactions between tecans and topoisomerase I–DNA covalent complex. A: Overlay of X-ray structures of camptothecin (CPT, shown in yellow) and topotecan (TPT, shown in green) bound to topoisomerase I–DNA covalent complex. Left: side view showing intercalation and interaction with Arg364 of protein; Right: top view showing Arg364 and Asp533 interactions with B-ring nitrogen and OH at position 20. B: Schematic of interactions between CPT and topoisomerase I while bound to DNA, including H-bond between 20S-OH and Asp533 and between B-ring N and Arg364 (regions binding to DNA are shown in red; topoisomerase side chains are shown in blue). (Adapted from Staker BL, Feese MD, Cushman M et al. [2005] *J Med Chem* 48:2336–2345. With permission from American Chemical Society.)

STRUCTURES OF PODOPHYLLOTOXIN, ETOPOSIDE, AND TENIPOSIDE

podophyllotoxin
(natural product: binds to tubulin)

etoposide

teniposide

bound to topoisomerase II and a DNA fragment confirmed some of these interactions. In the complex, two molecules of etoposide bind at each cleavage site (four base pairs apart). Rings A–D intercalate between base pairs, while the carbohydrate protrudes into the minor groove of DNA and the E ring into the major groove. The B and E rings also interact with the enzyme, as does the carbohydrate group.

The tecans and etoposides are thought to exclusively target the topoisomerase enzymes. However, other known anti-cancer agents have been reported to poison topoisomerases as one of multiple mechanisms of action. For example, the anthracyclines mitoxantrone and actinomycin (described in Chapter 9 as DNA-binding agents) are reported to poison topoisomerase II. This effect may be secondary and downstream to their intercalating effects, or it may be an additional mechanism through which they act. Bacteria also have an essential enzyme, DNA gyrase, that has topoisomerase activity. It is the target of quinolone antibacterial drugs, an important class of anti-infective agents described in Chapter 12.

10.2 Drugs may target biosynthesis of DNA building blocks

Another strategy that directly targets DNA replication involves inhibiting biosynthesis of the pyrimidine and purine nucleotide building blocks of DNA. The rationale for this approach is that, by limiting access to these building blocks, DNA synthesis is stalled and cancerous cells can no longer proliferate. Of course, as in all strategies that target DNA replication, noncancerous proliferating cells (such as immune cells and those lining the gastrointestinal or GI tract) are also affected, and toxicity results. Compounds that interfere with the biosynthesis of purine and pyrimidine nucleotides by mimicking the natural substrate and acting as enzyme substrates are known as antimetabolites (see Chapter 7). Two general tactics have been especially successful. Targeting folate biosynthesis takes advantage of the fact that folate and its metabolites are required coenzymes for the biosynthesis of purine and thymine nucleotides. A second approach relies on inhibiting enzymes that produce specific nucleotides and results in depletion of that nucleotide and arrest of DNA synthesis. In both cases, the inhibitors are structurally related to the natural co-factor or substrate, and both approaches represent some of the earliest examples of rational drug design.

Folate, also known as vitamin B9, is essential to DNA synthesis, repair, and methylation. It served as the inspiration for one of the earliest anti-cancer drugs, aminopterin, which was first used to treat leukemia patients in 1947 and was marketed in the United States from 1953 to 1964. Folate is obtained from a number of dietary sources, such as spinach and legumes, and is metabolized to a series of derivatives including dihydrofolate, tetrahydrofolate, N^5,N^{10}-methylenetetrahydrofolate, and 5-methyltetrahydrofolate (**Figure 10.10**). Several of these products are required coenzymes for the *de novo* synthesis of purine and thymine nucleotides. Therefore, drugs that inhibit enzymes in the folate pathway, known as **antifolates**, inhibit DNA synthesis by eliminating key coenzymes required for the synthesis of nucleotide building blocks.

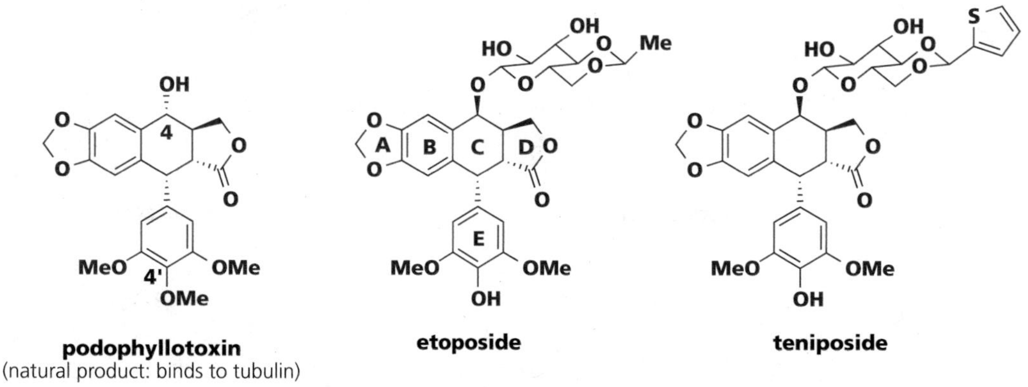

Figure 10.9 Structures of podophyllotoxin and semi-synthetic derivatives that are topoisomerase inhibitors. Podophyllotoxin is a natural product, and binds to tubulin. Etoposide and teniposide are epimerized at C4 and demethylated at C4′ and are topoisomerase inhibitors.

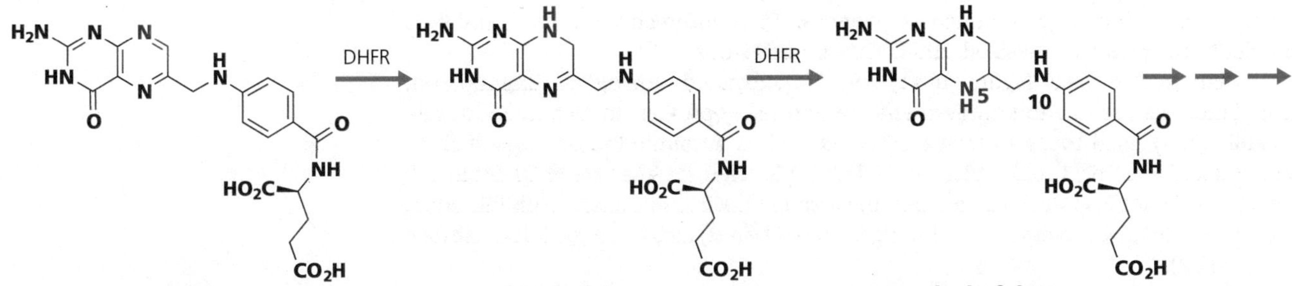

folate   dihydrofolate   tetrahydrofolate

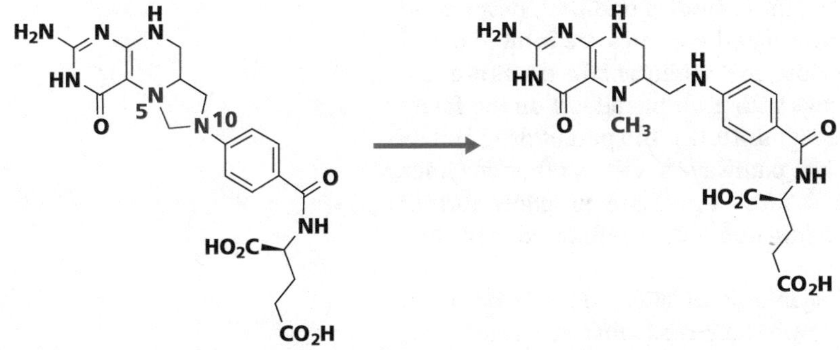

N^5, N^{10}-methylenetetrahydrofolate
coenzyme for thymidylate synthase

5-methyltetrahydrofolate
methylates homocysteine
to form methionine

Figure 10.10 Metabolism of folates.
Folate is reduced to dihydrofolate
and then to tetrahydrofolate; both
reactions are catalyzed by dihydrofolate
reductase (DHFR). Tetrahydrofolate
is converted, in a number of steps, to
N^5,N^{10}-methylenetetrahydrofolate and
then to 5-methyltetrahydrofolate. Both
are coenzymes required for methylation
reactions to biosynthesize nucleotides
and certain amino acids.

Aminopterin (**Figure 10.11**), with a structure similar to that of folate, was
designed on the basis of Sidney Farber's observation that leukemia patients with folate
deficiencies had improved outcomes. Although aminopterin was known to antagonize
production of folate, its actual mechanism of action, inhibition of dihydrofolate
reductase (DHFR), was discovered later. DHFR is one of the enzymes responsible
for folate metabolism; it catalyzes the reduction of folate to dihydrofolate and then
to tetrahydrofolate in two separate steps (see Figure 10.10). Aminopterin therapy
reduces the amount of folate metabolites produced, such as tetrahydrofolate and
N^5,N^{10}-methylenetetrahydrofolate, a coenzyme required by the enzyme thymidylate
synthase (TS). TS is required for the synthesis of thymine nucleotides. By inhibition

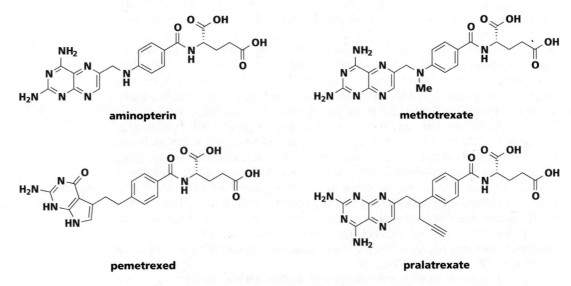

aminopterin   methotrexate

pemetrexed   pralatrexate

Figure 10.11 Structures of inhibitors of folate metabolism. Aminopterin and
methotrexate inhibit DHFR as their primary mechanism; more recently approved
drugs, pemetrexed and pralatrexate, have multiple effects on folate metabolism.

of the production of its required coenzymes, TS is indirectly inhibited, thymine nucleotides are not synthesized, and DNA synthesis stops.

Methotrexate (see Figure 10.11), an N-methylated analog of aminopterin, supplanted its use due to improved efficacy and safety profiles. In fact, methotrexate is still widely used today to treat cancers as well as autoimmune diseases such as rheumatoid arthritis, Crohn's disease, and multiple sclerosis. The role of DHFR in cell proliferation has also been exploited in the area of infectious diseases, with inhibitors of bacterial folate biosynthesis (including bacterial DHFR) also finding clinical use (see Chapter 12).

Significant efforts toward understanding how antifolates work and identifying new DHFR inhibitors as anti-cancer drugs are still underway, despite the fact that the first drugs were invented over 70 years ago. These studies find that, despite the focus on inhibiting one enzyme, various pathways and enzymes are inhibited and an assortment of effects are observed. Furthermore, metabolites of the drugs are also likely to be active. Two recent examples of drugs with multiple effects on the folate pathway are pemetrexed and pralatrexate (see Figure 10.11). The parent drug and its metabolites inhibit several enzymes in the folate pathway as well as other enzymes that use folates as coenzymes. The effects of these drugs are probably further enhanced by their selective uptake or retention into tumor cells compared to healthy cells.

A second approach to inhibiting the biosynthesis of nucleotides is by direct inhibition of the specific enzymes required to produce nucleobases, nucleosides, and nucleotides. Some believe that this strategy offers advantages in efficacy and tolerability that are not possible with broad antifolate approaches, reasoning that folate coenzymes are required for enzymatic reactions other than DNA biosynthesis. The multistep biosynthetic pathway to generate these DNA building blocks requires a series of enzymatic reactions, ultimately leading to the nucleoside triphosphate. Inhibitors often resemble the structure of the natural purine and pyrimidine base and are further modified and activated to the corresponding nucleoside triphosphate to be effective. Not surprisingly, these inhibitors often inhibit multiple enzymes along the pathway and even other enzymes that use nucleotides as substrates, such as DNA polymerase. The following section highlights a few examples of drugs that work primarily through inhibition of purine or pyrimidine biosynthesis.

Fluorouracil (5-FU) is perhaps the mostly widely prescribed inhibitor of nucleotide biosynthesis. It has been used since the 1950s and is effective in a wide array of cancers, particularly colon cancer. Administration of 5-FU results in inhibition of the enzyme thymidylate synthase (TS), which converts deoxyuridine monophosphate (dUMP) to the thymidine analog (dTMP), an intermediate in the eventual synthesis of thymidine triphosphate, dTTP (**Figure 10.12**). The enzyme uses N^5,N^{10}-methylenetetrahydrofolate (partial structure shown in blue) as a coenzyme and as the source of the methyl group introduced at the 5-position of the uridine. 5-FU is converted via the natural biosynthetic pathway to 5-fluoro-2′-deoxyuridine monophosphate (FdUMP) and then, like the natural substrate, it proceeds through the TS reaction pathway, which involves addition of a cysteine residue from TS (shown in red) to the 6-position of the uridine moiety to generate an enolate intermediate (see Figure 10.12). This enolate adds to the reactive methylene group (circled), present in the coenzyme N^5,N^{10}-methylenetetrahydrofolate, to afford a ternary complex. In the case of the natural substrate (where R = H), an elimination reaction occurs, releasing the coenzyme and regenerating the α,β-unsaturated system in the pyrimidine ring (dTMP), now containing the additional methyl group (shown in blue). The monophosphate is further phosphorylated to generate the nucleoside triphosphate, dTTP, which can be incorporated into DNA. However, in the case of the inhibitor adduct (where R = F), elimination is not possible due to the presence of the fluorine atom, and no further reaction of the ternary complex occurs. FdUMP acts as a suicide substrate and inactivates the TS enzyme.

As 5-FU is such an important compound in the anti-cancer arsenal, several prodrugs have been developed that release 5-FU, including capecitabine and tegafur (**Figure 10.13**). The metabolism of these compounds is such that 5-FU is selectively released, either in tumor tissue or in the liver, and therefore these drugs are better

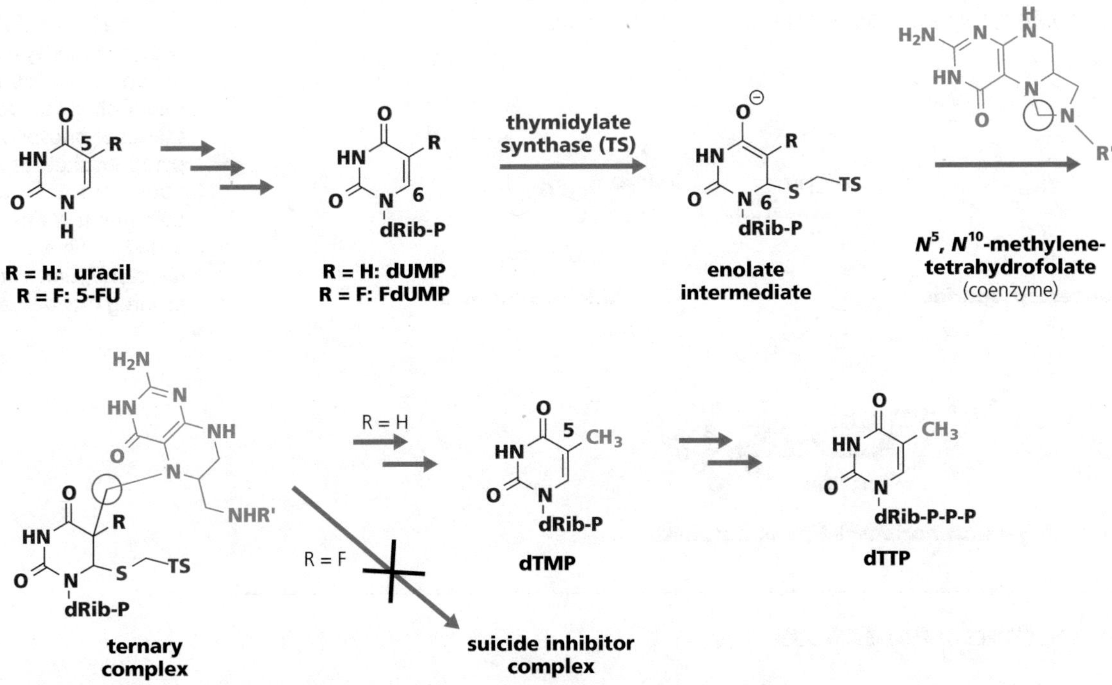

Figure 10.12 Conversion of uracil to dTTP by thymidylate synthase and inhibition by 5-FU. Uracil and 5-FU are converted to their corresponding nucleoside monophosphates, dUMP and dFUMP, respectively (dRib = deoxyribose). Addition of a cysteine of TS (shown in red) to dUMP or FdUMP leads to an enolate intermediate that reacts with N^5,N^{10}-methylenetetrahydrofolate (shown in blue). In the case of dUMP, the ternary complex (R = H) loses a hydrogen atom and eliminates the coenzyme, eventually leading to the methylated product dTMP, which is converted to the nucleoside triphosphate dTTP, which can then be incorporated into DNA. In the case of FdUMP, the presence of the fluorine atom at C5 doesn't allow elimination of the coenzyme from the ternary complex and further reaction is blocked, resulting in suicide inhibition of the enzyme.

tolerated than 5-FU itself. Capecitabine undergoes three separate enzymatic conversions. The first conversion, hydrolysis of the carbamate, occurs in the liver. The second and third conversions, through the enzymes cytidine deaminase and thymidine phosphorylase, occur primarily in tumors. The aminal ether found in tegafur is converted to 5-FU in the liver by cytochrome P450s, and this slow process avoids conversion in the GI tract, making it orally available.

6-Mercaptopurine (**Figure 10.14A**) is another example of an antimetabolite that has found use as an anti-cancer agent. Analogous to 5-FU and the DNA polymerase

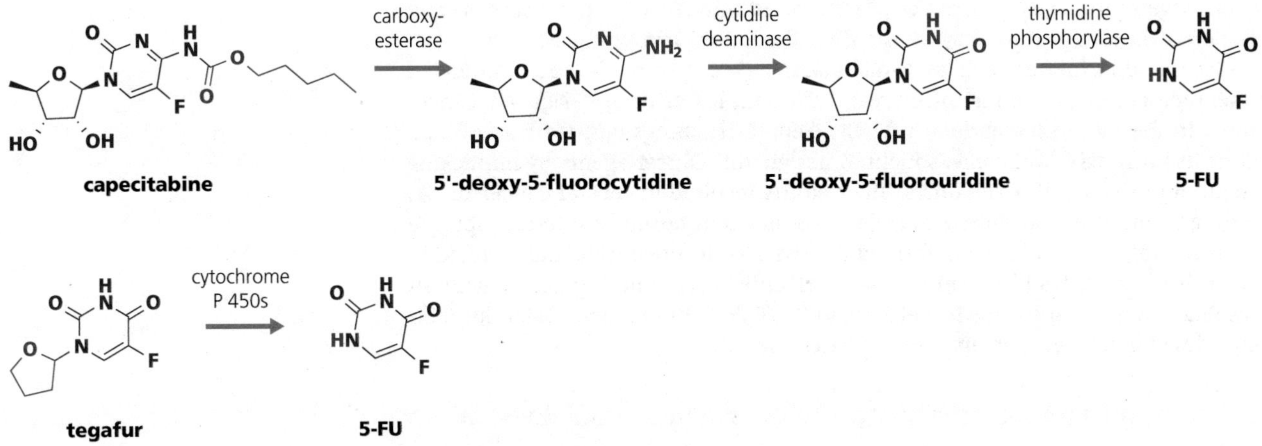

Figure 10.13 Metabolism of 5-FU prodrugs capecitabine and tegafur. Capecitabine is hydrolyzed in the liver by carboxyesterase to 5′-deoxy-5-fluorocytidine. This is then metabolized further by cytidine deaminase in the liver and tumors to 5′-deoxy-5-fluorouridine. The final step to produce 5-FU, catalyzed by thymidine phosphorylase, occurs in tumors. Tegafur is slowly converted to 5-FU in the liver by cytochrome P450s (changes shown in red).

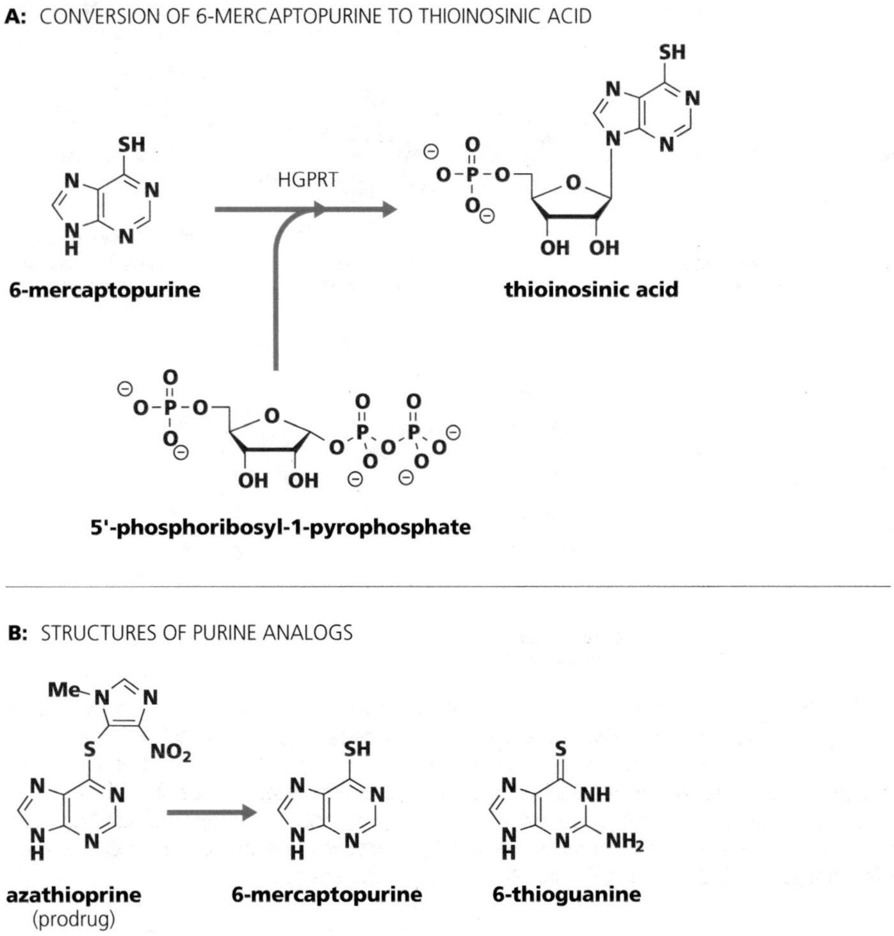

A: CONVERSION OF 6-MERCAPTOPURINE TO THIOINOSINIC ACID

6-mercaptopurine → (HGPRT) → **thioinosinic acid**

5'-phosphoribosyl-1-pyrophosphate

Figure 10.14 Inhibition of purine biosynthesis by antimetabolites.
A: Conversion of 6-mercaptopurine to thioinosinic acid, catalyzed by HGPRT, utilizes 5'-phosphoribosyl -1-pyrophosphate as the source of the ribose unit. B: Structures of drugs that inhibit purine biosynthesis. 6-Thioguanine is related to 6-mercaptopurine, and azathioprine is a prodrug that delivers 6-mercaptopurine.

B: STRUCTURES OF PURINE ANALOGS

azathioprine
(prodrug)   →   **6-mercaptopurine**   **6-thioguanine**

inhibitors described previously (as well as the antiviral reverse transcriptase and polymerase inhibitors described in Chapter 11), the antimetabolite is converted to a nucleotide, which is the active form of the drug. Specifically, 6-mercaptopurine is an analog of adenine, and in a reaction catalyzed by hypoxanthine-guanine phosphoribosyltransferase (HGPRT), it is converted to 6-thioinosinic acid. This molecule inhibits not only HGPRT but also amidophosphoribosyltransferase, both of which are essential enzymes that work very early in the biosynthesis of purine nucleotides. Further metabolism also occurs, as well as inhibition of additional enzyme targets. The end result is the prevention of nucleotide interconversion and inhibition of *de novo* purine biosynthesis, thus disrupting DNA synthesis.

6-Mercaptopurine, as well as 6-thioguanine (see **Figure 10.14B**), a related antimetabolite, represents one of the earliest examples of drug design for cancer therapy. In the late 1940s and early 1950s, George Hitchings and Gertrude Elion, working at Burroughs Wellcome, sought to design anti-cancer agents by mimicking the natural purines and pyrimidines. Their efforts resulted in several cancer drugs, including azathioprine (a prodrug that releases 6-mercaptopurine), 6-mercaptopurine itself, and thioguanine. This work formed the basis for future efforts that resulted in the first drugs for AIDS (for example, AZT). Hitchings and Elion, together with Sir James Black, were awarded the Nobel Prize in Physiology or Medicine 1988 "for their discoveries of important principles for drug treatment."

10.3 Drugs may target structural proteins involved in cell division

During mitosis, structural proteins such as tubulin and its oligomers, microtubules, are responsible for transporting chromosomes to the opposite ends of the cell. Interfering with this process compromises cell division and is an effective strategy to stop cell proliferation. Natural products have been fruitful sources of molecules that interfere with tubulin dynamics, and a number of these have been developed into valuable anti-cancer agents. The structures of these molecules, as well as the mechanisms of action of these modulators of protein–protein interactions, are described in some detail in Chapter 8. The vinca alkaloids vincristine and vinblastine destabilize tubulin polymerization and have been used as anti-cancer agents since the 1960s. Eribulin, a synthetic fragment of the marine natural product halichondrin (see also Chapter 1), was recently approved and works through a similar mechanism. Taxol and epothilone represent anti-cancer drugs that are tubulin stabilizers. To date, three taxoids have been approved to treat certain cancers. The epothilones offer some advantages over taxols due to their resistance to P-glycoprotein efflux and their water solubility. In addition, because their structures are somewhat less complex than taxols, epothilone total synthesis and semisynthetic efforts were more fruitful. These factors contributed to relatively rapid development of the epothilones compared to that of taxol. While certain epothilones are in clinical trials, as of 2017, only the semisynthetic analog ixabepilone is approved as a cancer therapeutic agent. Ixabepilone contains a lactam moiety rather than the lactone found in natural epothilones. This modification confers considerable improvements in pharmaceutical properties, particularly stability, which is a liability of natural epothilones.

10.4 Effects of antitumor compounds may be optimized by targeting delivery systems

In general, drugs that target cell division, regardless of the specific mechanism, tend to be highly effective yet also highly toxic, because they affect all dividing cells rather than only cancer cells. A solution to this issue of selectivity is to direct these agents to cancer cells or to take advantage of characteristics specific to cancer cells. One strategy involves conjugating the compound (known as a payload) though a linker to an antibody that recognizes epitopes selectively expressed on cancer cells (**Figure 10.15**). These are termed **antibody–drug conjugates** (ADCs) and work by first binding to the target antigen on the surface of the cancer cell, then becoming internalized by the cell, and eventually releasing the active small molecule or an active derivative inside the cancer cell, by either degradation of the antibody or cleavage of the linker.

The design and development of ADCs are complicated by numerous factors, including the need to develop tumor-specific antibodies and to study their effects as independent entities, as well as the lack of understanding of how to design optimal linkers. Furthermore, from a medicinal chemistry perspective, considerable understanding of structure–activity relationships on the small-molecule payload is necessary to identify the most effective site for linker attachment, as are synthetic protocols for derivatization under conditions mild enough to maintain the integrity of the antibody.

Gemtuzumab ozogamicin, consisting of the DNA cleaving agent calicheamicin (described in Chapter 9) linked to an anti-CD33 antibody, was the first ADC approved. It was used to treat acute myelogenous leukemia (AML), was voluntarily withdrawn in 2010 but re-introduced in 2017. As of 2017, two other ADCs are available to treat specific cancers. Trastuzumab emtansine (**Figure 10.16**) consists of the HER-2 antibody Herceptin linked to several molecules of mertansine. Herceptin is itself a cancer therapeutic used to treat HER-2-positive breast cancer. Mertansine is an analog of the tubulin-destabilizing agent maytansine, a natural product that underwent clinical trials in the mid-1970s, but was deemed too toxic for further development. Brentuximab vedotin (see Figure 10.16) is an ADC that uses an analog of the natural product auristatin E as the payload, which also targets tubulin dynamics. It is linked to an antibody to CD30 that is expressed on certain lymphoma cells. While only three ADCs are currently approved, many more are in clinical trials. Advances in developing antibodies, and the importance of selectively targeting cancer cells, suggest that this area will continue to grow.

While ADC therapy directly delivers anti-cancer agents to cells expressing specific antigens, other delivery systems may also be used for cytotoxic drugs. Some exploit

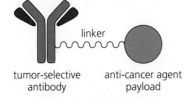

Figure 10.15 General model for antibody–drug conjugate. The ADC consists of a tumor-selective antibody that directs the drug to the tumor, a linker, and an anti-cancer agent or payload that is toxic to the tumor cell.

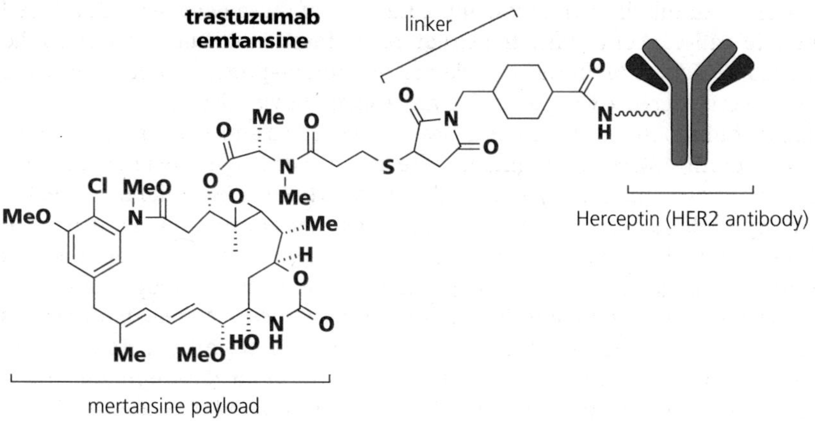

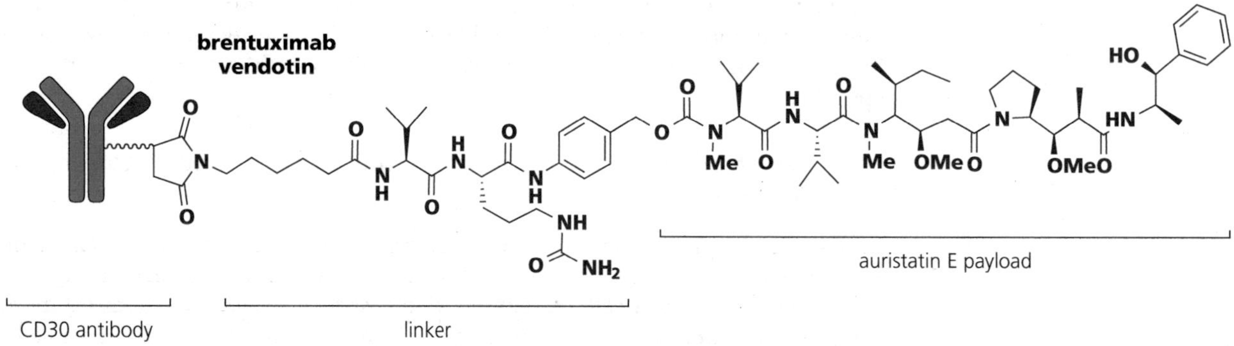

Figure 10.16 Structures of antibody–drug conjugates (ADCs). Trastuzumab emtansine contains the antibody Herceptin (which targets HER2 proteins) and is linked to a derivative of maytansine, a tubulin destabilizer. Brentuximab vendotin contains an antibody to CD30 linked to an auristatin E analog. Antibody, linker and payload are labelled in each.

specific differences between cancer cells and normal cells, such as differences in pH, metabolic environment, and nutritional needs, by incorporating small-molecule moieties that are preferentially taken up by one and not the other. Another approach is the use of micelles and liposomes to carry drugs, improving their pharmacokinetics and reducing toxicity. Liposomes have been used to encapsulate drugs such as doxorubicin and taxol, effectively increasing the concentration of drug that enters the cell. The use of liposomes takes advantage of the differences in vasculature between tumor cells and normal cells. Blood vessels that supply tumors have gaps in the vasculature and are leaky compared to normal vessels, allowing larger particles such as liposomes to selectively enter them.

DRUGS TARGETING ONCOGENES AND SIGNALING PATHWAYS

While macromolecules such as DNA, structural proteins, and enzymes are directly engaged in cell division and proliferation processes, many other proteins, particularly enzymes, are indirectly involved. Through tightly regulated signaling pathways, cell proliferation and survival are turned on and off. Numerous proteins in these pathways, often kinases (see Chapter 7), are positive and negative regulators. However, in cancer the pathway becomes aberrant, and either the growth signal is turned on inappropriately or the signals to stop growth, or for cell death (apoptosis), are missing. In certain cases, these changes have occurred at a genomic level, and the resultant oncogenes or mutant tumor suppressor genes predispose a cell to uncontrolled growth. These cells produce a mutant protein, not found in other cells, that is often hyperactive and insensitive to regulation. In other cases, specific signaling proteins are overexpressed, leading to a similar effect of hyperactivity. The signaling processes are quite complex, with many proteins involved. Some examples include those in the Ras/MAP pathway and the Src/FAK pathway, PI3-kinases, Rho GTPases and protein kinase Cs (PKCs). Many of these involve phosphorylation pathways, and a simplified picture of how mutant proteins in the process affect cell growth is shown

Figure 10.17 Simplified scheme of the effect of mutated proteins on signaling pathways during cell division. Upon receptor activation, proteins in the signaling pathway (depicted as ovals) are activated. In normal cells, these proteins tightly regulate cell division. Mutated proteins lead to aberrant cell division and growth.

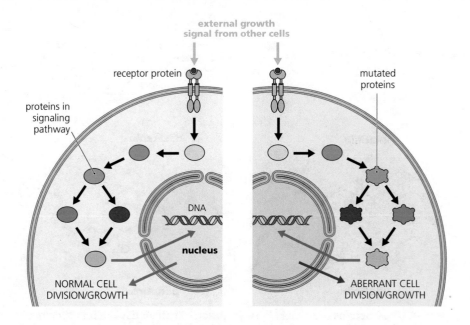

in **Figure 10.17**. In a normal cell, the signal for growth results in a cascade of events, usually kinases phosphorylating other proteins to either activate or deactivate them. Ultimately, certain proteins enter the nucleus to turn on cell division and growth in a highly regulated manner. In aberrant cells, the same pathway is not regulated, and signals to turn on cell division and growth result in a cancer phenotype.

Upon inhibition of these aberrant proteins, the unregulated signaling pathway is attenuated, and the malignant process can be slowed or halted. Furthermore, this approach has the potential to be highly selective for transformations that are involved in certain cancers and lead to fewer side effects. This benefit is in stark contrast to older anti-cancer agents that target all proliferating cells, and exhibit significant, sometimes dangerous side effects.

10.5 Kinase inhibitors target mutant or overexpressed kinases found in cancer cells

As the phosphorylation state often determines whether a protein is active or inactive, kinases (see Chapter 7) play a major role in signal transduction pathways. A number of oncogenes code for kinases, and many more kinases are overexpressed or become mutated in cancers. That role, coupled with their druggability, has made them a frequent target in cancer drug design (see Section 7.4). Finding highly selective kinase inhibitors is challenging due to the highly conserved ATP binding-site domain. On the other hand, identification of hits and leads to initiate drug discovery programs benefits from the existence of numerous kinase scaffolds that have already been developed. This section highlights some examples of drugs that target oncogenes and signaling pathways through kinase inhibition not yet covered. More thorough treatment of the design of kinase inhibitors and several examples of anti-cancer drugs that act through kinase inhibition are found in Section 7.4. In addition, Case Study 1 in Chapter 7 describes the development of imatinib, the first kinase inhibitor of an oncogene product.

As described in Chapter 7, imatinib was the first example of a drug that was designed to inhibit an oncogenic protein. It inhibits Bcr-Abl, a tyrosine kinase that is the product of a mutated gene. This mutation results in high levels of kinase activity essential for the cellular transformation seen in Philadelphia chromosome-positive chronic myelogenous leukemia (CML). Since the introduction of imatinib, resistance toward it has developed, and second-generation Bcr-Abl inhibitors exhibit activity against these mutants. Unlike imatinib, dasatinib (**Figure 10.18**) binds to the DFG-in (active) conformation of the kinase and, as a consequence, is also active against another family of oncogenic kinases called Src. The ability of dasatinib to affect

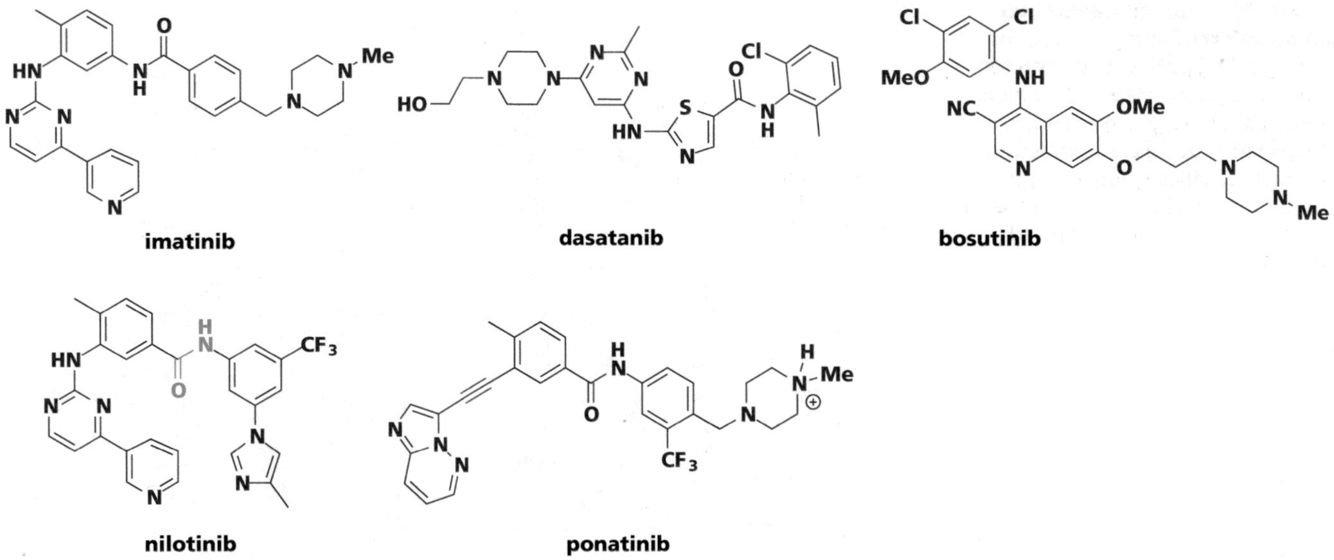

Figure 10.18 Structures of Bcr-Abl kinase inhibitors. Imatinib, dasatanib, bosutinib, nilotinib, and ponatinib are depicted. Imatinib was the first Bcr-Abl inhibitor approved; it binds to the DFG-out conformation. Dasatanib and bosutinib bind to the active DFG-in conformation and therefore exhibit broader kinase inhibition effects. The design of nilotinib, a close structural analog of imatinib, was based on optimizing interactions with the enzyme. The amide (shown in blue) is reversed compared to imatinib. Ponatinib, a DFG-out binder, was designed, by virtue of the alkyne (shown in red), to inhibit native as well as resistant Bcr-Abl kinase.

imatinib-resistant cancers has been attributed to its binding to the active form of the kinase, as well as its ability to bind to multiple conformations of the enzyme. Bosutinib (see Figure 10.18) is also a dual Src and Bcr-Abl inhibitor and binds to the active conformation. It is a member of the quinoline family of kinase inhibitors and originated from screening of a focused library. Nilotinib (see Figure 10.18) is a second-generation Bcr-Abl kinase inhibitor that, like imatinib, binds to the DFG-out (inactive) form of the enzyme. It is a close structural analog of imatinib, and its design was based on optimizing molecular interactions with the enzyme. By reversing the amide (shown in blue) compared to the orientation in imatinib, a more optimal geometry for H-bonds with the kinase was achieved. Dipolar interactions and hydrophobic interactions from the trifluorophenyl group also contribute to improved binding (>10-fold) compared to imatinib.

Ponatinib (see Figure 10.18) was designed to address one of the most common resistance mutations observed after imatinib treatment: replacement of the gatekeeper threonine in the Bcr-Abl ATP-binding region with an isoleucine, known as Bcr-Abl(T315I). Many of the second-generation Bcr-Abl inhibitors make an H-bond to the Thr315 residue and this amino acid change usually results in loss of a key H-bond between these inhibitors and the alcohol of the Thr315 residue, resulting in their being ineffective against this resistant mutant. The substitution also introduces an unfavorable steric clash between the inhibitor and isoleucine's larger alkyl side chain that does not allow access to one of the important hydrophobic binding pockets adjacent to the ATP site. The small linear ethynyl linkage in ponatinib can accommodate the larger isoleucine side chain and also provides favorable entropic considerations by locking the molecule into a favorable binding pose so that it reaches the hydrophobic pocket. Representations of the binding between Bcr-Abl and imatinib, nilotinib, and ponatinib are shown in **Figure 10.19**. These DGF-out binders all occupy the adenine site, a hydrophobic site (occupied by a tolyl group) and the allosteric site revealed in the DFG-out conformation. Common among all three are H-bonds to Met318, Asp381, and Glu286.

The *BRAF* gene, which codes for a serine/threonine kinase, is mutated in numerous cancers. This mutation causes the kinase to become constitutively active and results in an unregulated signal for cell growth. As described in Section 2.11, researchers at Plexxikon used a scaffold-based approach to identify novel fragment-sized molecules (MW < 350) that inhibited several different kinases. The activities of the molecules

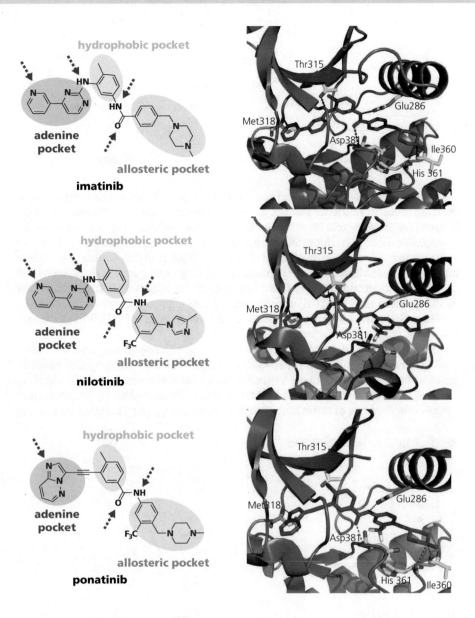

Figure 10.19 X-ray structures of imatinib, nilotinib, and ponatinib showing interactions with Bcr-Abl. All three have components that bind in the adenine, hydrophobic, and allosteric pockets, which are depicted as shaded purple, green, and blue ovals, respectively, in the diagrams on the left; all H-bonds are indicated with dashed red arrows. Key interactions common to all three are an H-bond to Met318 in the adenine site, occupation of a hydrophobic pocket by the tolyl group, H-bonds between the amide linker and residues Glu286 and Asp381, and binding by the side chain deep into the newly revealed allosteric site by the nitrogen heterocycle. The aniline N-H of imatinib and nilotinib make H-bonds to Thr315; this interaction is absent in ponatinib. (Adapted from Wu P, Nielsen TE & Clausen MH [2015] *Trends Pharmacol Sci* 36:422–439. With permission from Elsevier.)

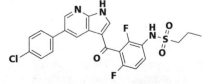

Figure 10.20 Structure of B-Raf inhibitor vemurafenib. Vemurafenib binds to the DFG-in form and inhibits a specific mutant of B-Raf, where a valine is replaced by a glutamic acid.

were validated by X-ray crystallography using available kinase domains. With novel scaffolds that had broad activity against multiple kinases, optimization for inhibition of a specific mutant of B-Raf (V600E) led to vemurafenib (**Figure 10.20**). Vemurafenib binds to the DGF-in form of B-Raf, which is stabilized by the oncogenic mutation, and this characteristic is responsible for its selectivity. It is used to treat metastatic melanomas with the V600E B-Raf mutation.

The epidermal growth factor receptor (EGFR) plays a fundamental role in regulating cell proliferation, differentiation, and survival, as well as in multiple stages of the cancer process such as malignant transformation, uncontrolled cell proliferation, tumor invasion and survival, and metastasis. The clinical success of antibodies to EGFR (for example, cetuximab) provided proof of concept for the potential of small-molecule EGFR inhibitors. EGFR is a receptor tyrosine kinase, and gefitinib and erlotinib (**Figure 10.21**) both inhibit its kinase activity. In this scaffold, the N3 of the quinazoline makes a water-mediated H-bond with the key gatekeeper residue Thr390 in EGFR, while N1 makes an H-bond to the hinge region (see Section 7.4). The ether side chains in both drugs are solvent-exposed and provide improvements in solubility. In the case of gefitinib, the fluoro and chloro substitutions on the phenyl ring afford significant metabolic stability.

The phosphoinositide 3-kinase/mammalian target of rapamycin (PI3K/mTOR) signaling pathway is a highly complex pathway that senses numerous external

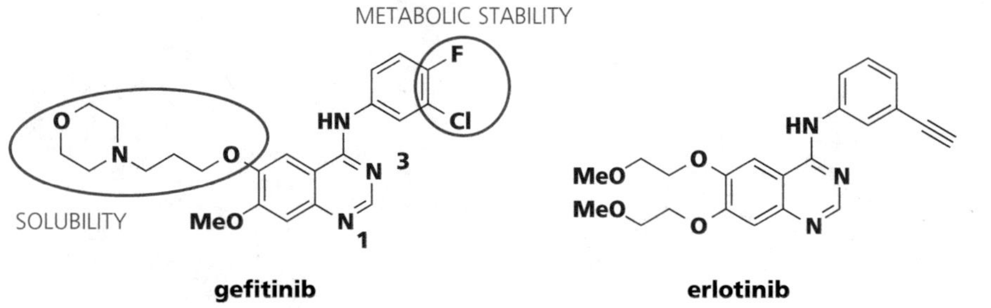

METABOLIC STABILITY

gefitinib

erlotinib

Figure 10.21 Structure of EGFR inhibitors gefitinib and erlotinib. In both molecules, N1 and N3 make H-bonding interactions with the kinase and the ether side chains (circled in gefitinib) afford improvements in solubility. Halogens on the aryl ring in gefinitib (circled) provide improvements metabolic stability.

signals to regulate cell growth and homeostasis. This pathway has evolved to sense the availability of nutrients and put the organism in an anabolic or catabolic state. It therefore plays a role in virtually all cellular functions, and consequently its dysregulation has been implicated in diseases such as diabetes, obesity, and cancer. The network is anchored by several different mTOR proteins, which are serine/threonine kinases. The name mTOR (mammalian target of rapamycin) is derived from the natural product rapamycin (sirolimus), an immunosuppressant used in transplant patients, whose target (mTOR) was determined well after its efficacy was discovered. However, there are proteins both upstream and downstream of mTOR itself that are also viable targets in the pathway.

Temsirolimus and everolimus (**Figure 10.22**) are semisynthetic ester and ether analogs of rapamycin. The ester or ether modification (shown in red) imparts improved physical properties, particularly water solubility. All three work through a similar, unusual mechanism: they bind to a protein called FKBP12, and that macromolecular complex inhibits one of the mTOR proteins. The structural determinants for binding

A: STRUCTURES OF mTOR INHIBITORS

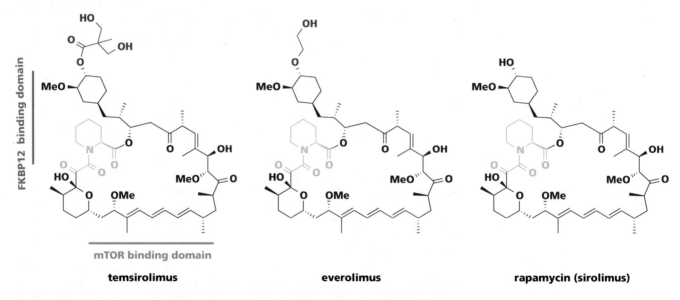

temsirolimus

everolimus

rapamycin (sirolimus)

B: STRUCTURE OF PI3Kδ INHIBITOR IDELALISIB

idelalisib

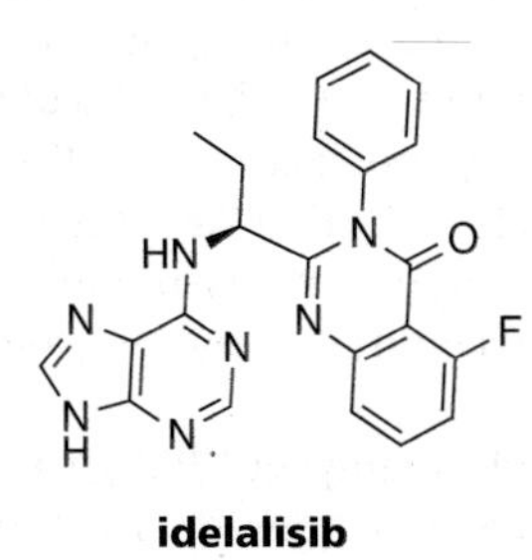

Figure 10.22 Inhibitors of the PI3Kδ /mTOR signaling pathway. A: Structures of temsirolimus and everolimus, which are semisynthetic analogs, and natural product rapamycin. Ester or ether linkages, which impart improved physical properties, are shown in red, and the pipecolic acid—dicarbonyl region, which is essential for binding to FKBP12 is shown in green. A gray line highlights the FKBP12 binding domain and a blue line shows the mTOR binding domain in the temsirolimus structure. B: Structure of PI3Kδ inhibitor idelalisib.

to FKBP12 include the pipecolic acid and dicarbonyl moieties (shown in green). A distinct area of the molecule, the conjugated triene (shown in blue for temsirolimus), binds to mTOR and prevents it from phosphorylating downstream proteins and propagating the signaling cascade.

Idelalisib also inhibits the same signaling pathway but via a more common mechanism. It directly inhibits the enzyme phosphoinositide 3-kinase δ (PI3Kδ). It is an ATP-competitive inhibitor and makes H-bonds to the hinge region, as do other kinase inhibitors. However, its propeller shape forces open a new pocket where the small molecule binds. PI3Kδ is in the identical signaling pathway as mTOR but is upstream of it. While other PI3K inhibitors have advanced to clinical trials, idelalisib is the only FDA-approved inhibitor.

Although compounds like imatinib and vemurafenib were designed to target one oncogenic kinase, subsequent evaluation often finds that other kinases are also inhibited. This characteristic can be a benefit, as these aberrant signaling pathways contain numerous kinases that control cell proliferation and cell survival. Inhibition at multiple nodes may provide multiple points of intervention. Additionally, resistance may be less likely to develop with several different targets being inhibited. However, in these cases a careful balance is required, as kinases are ubiquitous and pan-kinase inhibition is likely to be as toxic as drugs that target DNA or general cell proliferation processes.

Sorafenib (**Figure 10.23**) was designed to be a selective inhibitor of the serine/threonine kinase B-Raf but was also found to be a tyrosine kinase inhibitor. Sunitinib is a highly promiscuous kinase inhibitor. Vandetanib, a quinazoline, inhibits members of the EGFR, VEGFR, and RET tyrosine kinase families. Unlike the others, lapatinib was designed *a priori* to be a nonselective kinase inhibitor that targets both EGFR and HER2, proteins frequently overexpressed in breast cancer.

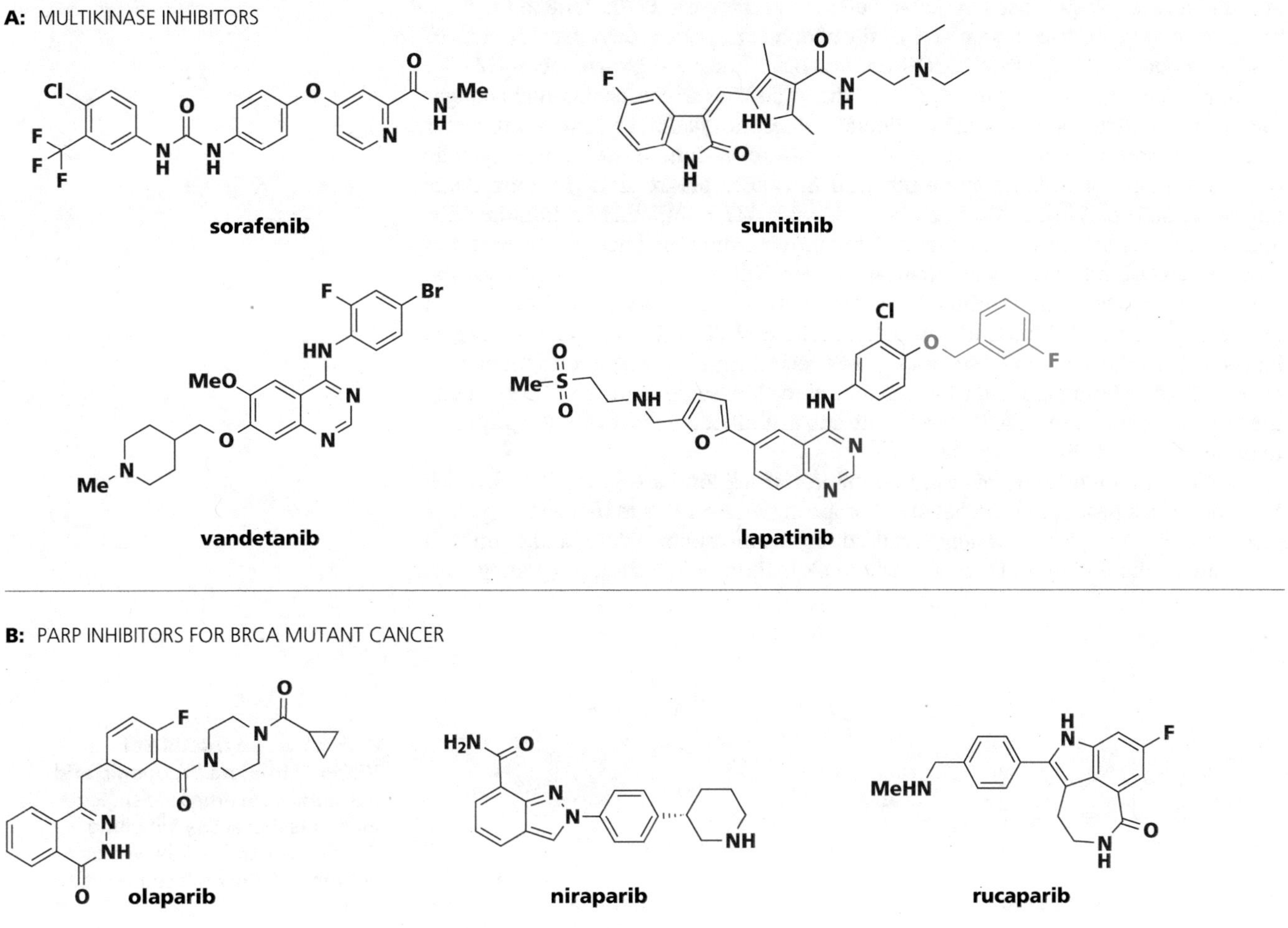

Figure 10.23 Structures of multikinase inhibitors and PARP inhibitors. A: Multikinase inhibitors. Sorafenib, sunitinib, vandetanib, and lapatinib are shown. Unlike the others, lapatinib was specifically designed to exhibit multikinase inhibition. Its quinazoline core (shown in red) imparts EGFR potency, and a benzyloxy moiety (shown in blue) is important for HER2 activity. B: PARP inhibitors for BRCA mutant cancers. PARP is involved in DNA repair and although not mutated in cancers, its inhibitors are effective in cancers with BRCA mutations. The structures of olaparib, niraparib and rucaparib are shown.

A: MULTIKINASE INHIBITORS

sorafenib

sunitinib

vandetanib

lapatinib

B: PARP INHIBITORS FOR BRCA MUTANT CANCER

olaparib

niraparib

rucaparib

The starting point for the design of lapatinib was the quinazoline core (shown in red) found in gefitinib and erlotinib, which imparts potent inhibition of EGFR activity. It was found that replacing the fluoro substituent of gefitinib with a benzyloxy group (shown in blue) provided potent HER2 inhibition while retaining inhibition of EGFR. Lapatinib appears to be highly selective for the two kinases it was designed to inhibit. Future efforts are likely to focus on designing multikinase inhibitors with specific profiles.

A different approach to targeting oncogenes and signaling pathways relies on using inhibitors of poly(ADP-ribose) polymerase (PARP). The PARP enzyme is involved in repair of damaged DNA, and helps to maintain the integrity of the genome. Its inhibition in normal cells can be compensated for by other repair processes. However, in cancer cells containing certain mutations (*BRCA1* and *BRCA2*), the combination of the mutation and PARP inhibition is lethal. This concept is called synthetic lethality, where inhibition of one protein individually does not damage the cell, but in combination causes cell death. *BRCA1* and *BRCA2* are tumor suppressor genes that have a role in activation of DNA repair. Women who inherit these mutated genes are at significant risk for developing breast and/or ovarian cancer and a recent focus of drug development aims to target only cells that have mutated *BRCA* genes. The first PARP inhibitor, olaparib, was approved by the U.S. FDA in 2014. Two others, niraparib and rucaparib, received approval in 2016 and are being used to treat BRCA mutant breast and ovarian cancers.

INHIBITION OF ANGIOGENESIS

Angiogenesis, the formation of new blood vessels from existing ones, is critical to support tumor growth, survival, and metastasis. Once they reach a certain size, tumors require a dedicated blood supply to support their rapid and unregulated growth. The idea of inhibiting angiogenesis as a mechanism to control tumor growth and metastasis was proposed by Judah Folkman in the early 1970s. One of the ways in which angiogenesis is mediated is by the action of peptide growth factors, such as vascular endothelial growth factor (VEGF) and basic fibroblast growth factor (bFGF). Binding of VEGF to its receptor, VEGFR, induces a series of conformational changes that results in activation of its kinase domain. Phosphorylation of various substrates results in initiation of a signal cascade that activates a number of other enzymatic pathways, many of which may be involved in cancer progression. The enzymatic kinase domain of VEGFR has been targeted with ATP-competitive inhibitors. This approach does not target the tumor itself, but the environment it needs to survive and grow. Despite inhibiting a physiological process, VEGFR inhibitors usually exhibit fewer side effects than conventional chemotherapeutics. Currently, a number of marketed kinase inhibitors work through inhibition of VEGFR; however, they all also inhibit at least a few other kinases, and those effects likely also contribute to their anti-cancer efficacy. Sorafenib and sunitinib inhibit the kinase domain of VEGFR, among the other kinases. The efficacy of pazopanib and axitinib has been attributed primarily to inhibition of VEGFR (**Figure 10.24**).

Another example of an angiogenesis inhibitor is thalidomide (**Figure 10.25**), which has a notorious past. It was marketed in Europe in the late 1950s to treat, among other disorders, morning sickness. Sadly, it caused severe limb abnormalities and significant mortality in the children of mothers who took thalidomide during pregnancy. This

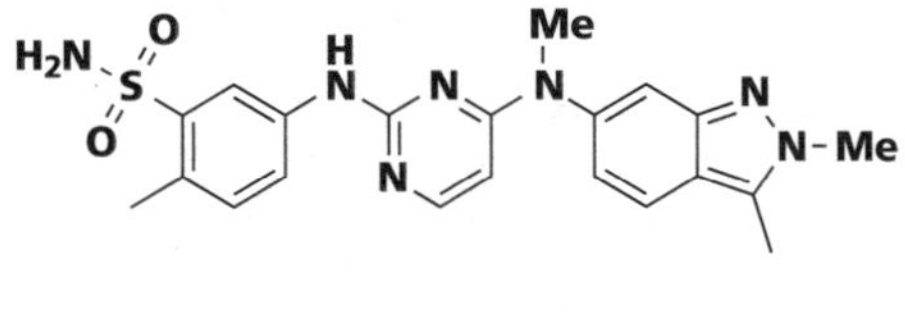

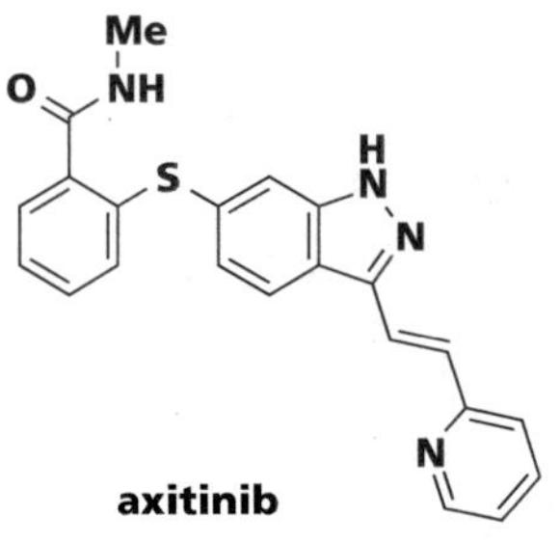

pazopanib

axitinib

Figure 10.24 Structure of VEGFR inhibitors pazopanib and axitinib. Both drugs are angiogenesis inhibitors that act by inhibiting the kinase activity of the vascular endothelial growth factor receptor (VEGFR).

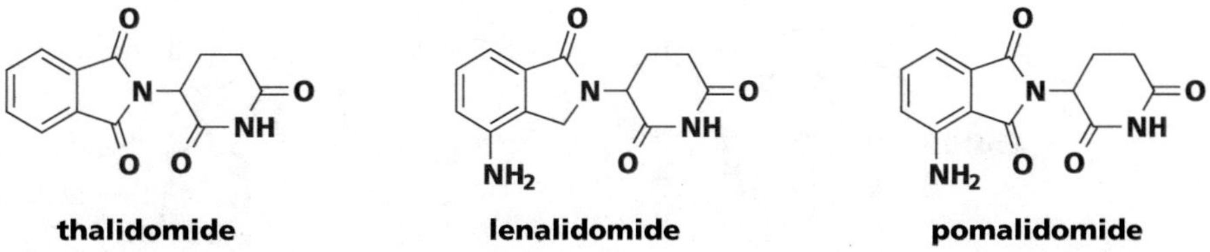

Figure 10.25 Structures of thalidomide, lenalidomide, and pomalidomide. Lenalidomide and pomalidomide are analogs of thalidomide, and all are angiogenesis inhibitors.

thalidomide   **lenalidomide**   **pomalidomide**

tragic example is credited with development of more stringent regulations in government drug approval processes (see Chapter 5). However, thalidomide remained in use to treat inflammatory complications from leprosy. Interest in the effects of thalidomide resurged in the late 1990s with reports of activity against multiple myeloma and other blood cancers, as well as inflammatory diseases. In 2006, it was approved with strict controls in combination with another drug to treat multiple myeloma, and later analogs include lenalidomide and pomalidomide (see Figure 10.25).

These compounds are members of a family of drugs called IMiDs (immuno-modulatory drugs), and they have both anti-inflammatory and anti-angiogenesis effects. Thalidomide and its analogs potently inhibit the growth of new blood vessels; however, the exact mechanism of action is not well understood. Recently, evidence suggests thalidomide's anti-cancer activity is likely due to multiple effects including binding to the protein cereblon, which affects protein homeostasis.

DRUGS TARGETING THE UBIQUITIN–PROTEASOME PATHWAY

The proteasome is a multiprotein complex present in all eukaryotic cells. Its function is to degrade proteins that have been tagged via addition of small proteins called ubiquitin; it is part of a highly complex metabolic process called protein homeostasis that is essential for maintaining cell viability. Proteasome degradation is one mechanism whereby physiological processes, such as cell growth and gene expression, are controlled and regulated. Inhibition of proteasome activity, however, affects normal cells and transformed cells differently. Normal cells usually undergo cell cycle arrest upon proteasome inhibition, whereas cancer cells typically respond by undergoing apoptosis. Exactly why this difference occurs is still being investigated; however, this difference has been exploited by developing proteasome inhibitors as cancer therapeutics.

The proteasome is a cylindrical structure with a catalytic core, where amide hydrolysis is carried out, and a regulatory site that caps both ends of the core and allows recognition of tagged polyubiquinated protein substrates (**Figure 10.26**). The protein is deubiquitinated and enters the proteasome, where it is cleaved, and the peptide fragments are released at the opposite end. Proteins marked for degradation are sequentially processed and cleaved at several sites within the proteasome to eventually generate small peptide fragments with an average length of six amino

Figure 10.26 Protein degradation by 26S proteasome complex. A protein (shown in green) is ubiquitinated (ubiquitin, a small protein, is depicted as orange triangles) and then enters the proteasome (shown as a blue and purple cylinder). Degradation by cleavage of amide bonds releases the protein pieces and ubiquitin for recycling. (Adapted from McDonald RB [2013] Biology of Aging. Garland Science.)

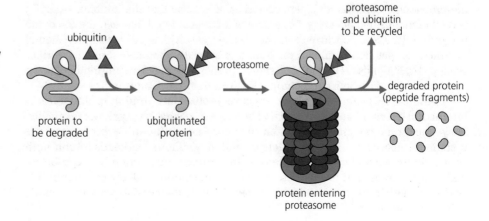

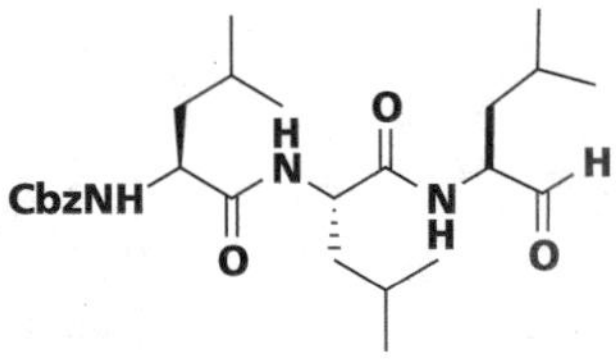

Figure 10.27 Structures of proteasome inhibitors. The warhead portion of each is shown in red. MG132 and bortezomib are reversible inhibitors; carfilzomib and marizomib are irreversible inhibitors.

MG132
(research probe)

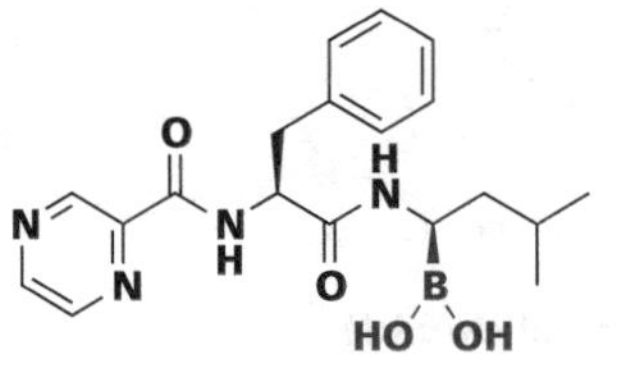

bortezomib
2003

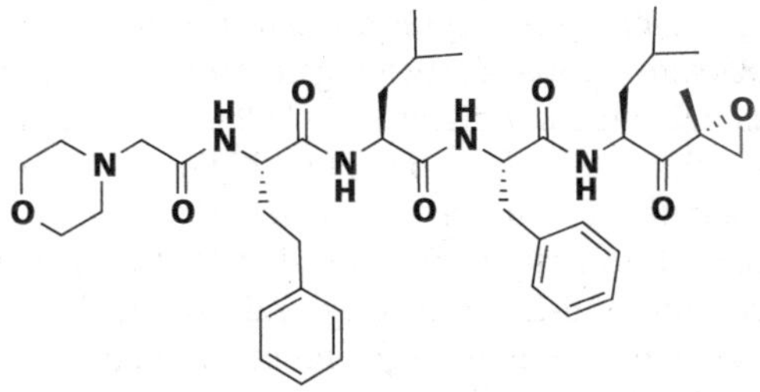

carfilzomib
2012

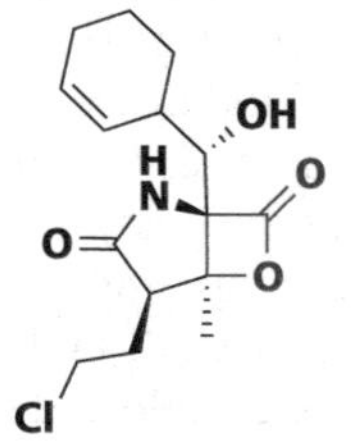

marizomib (clinic)
(salinosporamide A)

acids. The proteasome complex contains multiple proteolytically active sites that are related to serine proteases but contain threonine at the active site. The nucleophilic threonine attacks the scissile amide bond and generates the acyl-enzyme product and one peptide fragment. Hydrolysis of the acyl-enzyme intermediate regenerates the active-site threonine and the second peptide fragment (see Section 7.5 for more details).

The different proteolytic sites within the proteasome exhibit varying substrate specificities, and inhibitors can be generated by applying serine/threonine protease inhibitor design strategies. This approach involves use of a peptidic moiety that binds to the substrate binding site and incorporation of a reactive warhead as described in Section 7.5 to interact with the active-site nucleophile. Aldehydes, vinylsulfones, epoxyketones, and β-lactone warheads have all been incorporated; compounds such as MG132 (**Figure 10.27**) are frequently used as research probes to study the proteasome. In fact, the first proteasome inhibitor approved, bortezomib, was originally used as a probe, but observations of treated cancer cells undergoing apoptosis led to its investigation as an anti-cancer drug.

Bortezomib, which contains the unconventional boronic acid warhead, is a reversible inhibitor of the enzyme (see Figure 10.27). Carfilzomib, the second proteasome inhibitor approved, is based on the natural product epoxomicin and possesses an electrophilic epoxyketone that irreversibly inhibits the enzyme. The natural product salinosporamide A, in clinical trials, has a β-lactone that reacts with the active-site threonine. **Figure 10.28** shows the interactions seen in X-ray co-crystal structures of bortezomib bound to two of the proteolytic sites in the proteasome. Since the proteasome contains multiple active sites, it is likely that the inhibitor occupies several of them simultaneously. Formation of a covalent bond between the threonine hydroxyl and the boronic acid moiety generates a negatively charged boronate tetrahedral intermediate that closely mimics the transition state. The boronate formed is further stabilized by H-bonds to Gly and Thr residues. The peptide residues of the inhibitor make a series of H-bonds to both backbone and side-chain carbonyls and amines.

Boronic acids are particularly effective proteasome inhibitors and form a tetrahedral intermediate with the active-site threonine that is very slowly reversible. They appear to be much more selective for serine/threonine proteases over cysteine proteases. In contrast, aldehyde and vinylsulfone warheads inhibit both serine/threonine and cysteine proteases. The stronger interaction between boron and oxygen, compared to that between boron and sulfur, is likely the root of this selectivity. Other attributes of boronic acids include their resistance to metabolic oxidation and efflux.

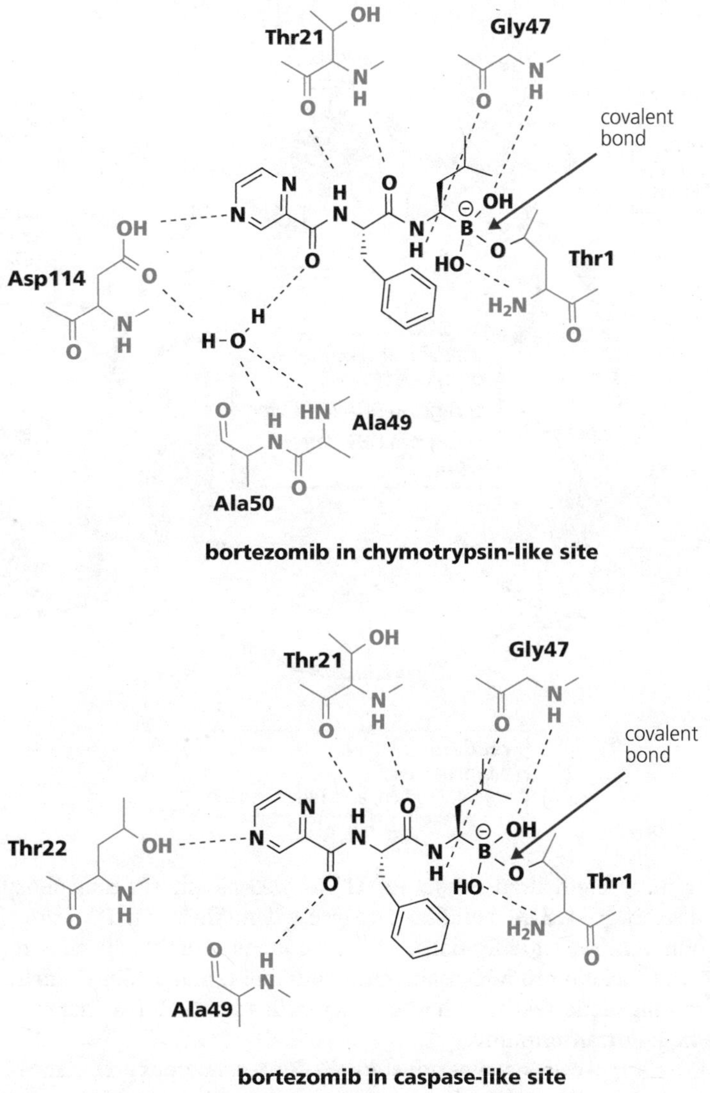

Figure 10.28 Interactions from co-crystal structure of bortezomib bound to two proteasome proteolytic sites. Top: Interactions of bortezomib bound to chymotrypsin-like site. Bottom: Interactions of bortezomib bound to caspase-like site. Both structures show a covalent bond between the threonine1 oxygen and boron atom (arrow), as well as key H-bonds between backbone and side-chain residues (blue) and bortezomib. (From Groll M, Berkers CR, Ploegh HL & Ovaa H [2006] *Structure* 14:451–456. With permission from Elsevier.)

bortezomib in chymotrypsin-like site

bortezomib in caspase-like site

DRUGS TARGETING EPIGENETIC PROCESSES

The term **epigenetics** refers to the carefully controlled chemical reactions that occur on the genome and activate or deactivate gene expression without changing the DNA sequence. These reactions modify DNA itself, as well as the proteins that are involved in compacting DNA in the nucleus, and are heritable. Epigenetic modifications are an important aspect of normal physiological processes that allow control of gene expression; however, an individual's epigenetic profile is dynamic. It will change with age and can be influenced by diet and exposure to toxins, among other external factors. Aberrant epigenetic processes may lead to cancer and autoimmune disorders, as well as other conditions.

In the cell, DNA is packaged in nucleosomes. These are densely packed particles containing DNA and eight units of a small, positively charged protein called histone, which serves to protect and compact the DNA. The DNA chain wraps around the histone octamer 1.65 times and the histone tails extend from the complex, as seen in **Figure 10.29**. The tails typically end in lysine residues; in addition to DNA, these are also sites for modification. When the histone is modified, the process, called chromatin remodeling, exposes the DNA and allows access to the transcription machinery. Some enzymes responsible for these processes are considered epigenetic writers and make a covalent modification. These include enzymes that transfer acetyl groups (histone acetyltransferase, HAT), and methyl groups (histone methyltransferase, HMT, and

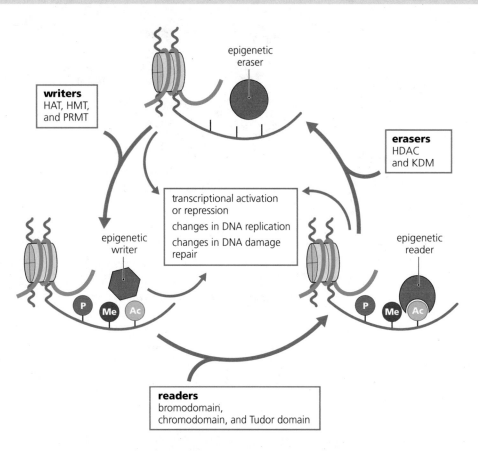

Figure 10.29 Summary of chromatin remodeling. DNA (shown in blue) is wound around histones (orange cylinder) that contain extended tails (shown in orange). Reactions catalyzed by enzymes modify the histone tails to regulate transcriptional activation or repression, DNA replication, and DNA damage repair. Specific reactions of epigenetic writers (HMT, HAT, and PRMT) include methylation (Me), acetylation (Ac), and phosphorylation (P). These changes may be recognized by proteins (such as those containing bromodomains, chromodomains, and Tudor domains) that are epigenetic readers. Epigenetic modifications can be removed by epigenetic erasers such as HDAC and KDM. (Adapted from Falkenberg KJ & Johnstone RW (2014) *Nat Rev Drug Discovery* 13:673–691. With permission from Macmillan Publishers Limited.)

protein arginine methyltransferase, PRMT) as well as kinases that phosphorylate. Histone deacetylase (HDAC) and histone lysine demethylase (KDM) are epigenetic erasers and remove modifications. Other proteins contain specific recognition domains and include bromodomain, chromodomain, and Tudor domain proteins, which are epigenetic readers: they interact with the modified histones or DNA, resulting in gene transcription.

When a normal cell becomes transformed into a cancerous cell, some of the most significant changes are epigenetic ones. Differences in DNA methylation patterns and histone modifications that silence tumor suppressor genes and activate oncogenes are observed. In the context of cancer drug discovery, interfering with the processes of methylation and deacetylation are validated strategies, with others under active investigation.

10.6 Nucleosides with modified bases can act as DNA methyltransferase inhibitors

DNA methyltransferase is an epigenetic writer that modifies the 5-carbon of cytosine at a CG sequence on the DNA backbone. The enzyme uses *S*-adenosylmethionine as a coenzyme and methyl source. As described above, the specific methylation pattern of DNA controls gene expression patterns, and aberrant DNA methylation has been strongly correlated with a number of human cancers. 5-Azacytidine and decitabine (**Figure 10.30**) are nucleoside analogs that contain a common unnatural base, which is the basis of their activity.

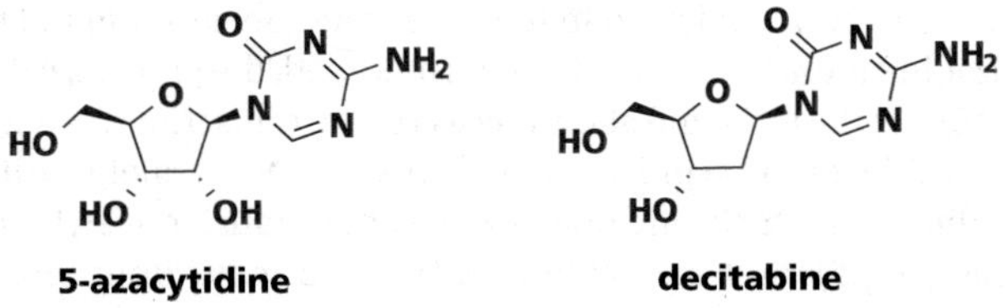

5-azacytidine

decitabine

Figure 10.30 Structures of 5-azacytidine and decitabine. Both compounds contain the same unnatural base, which is the basis of the mechanism of inhibition.

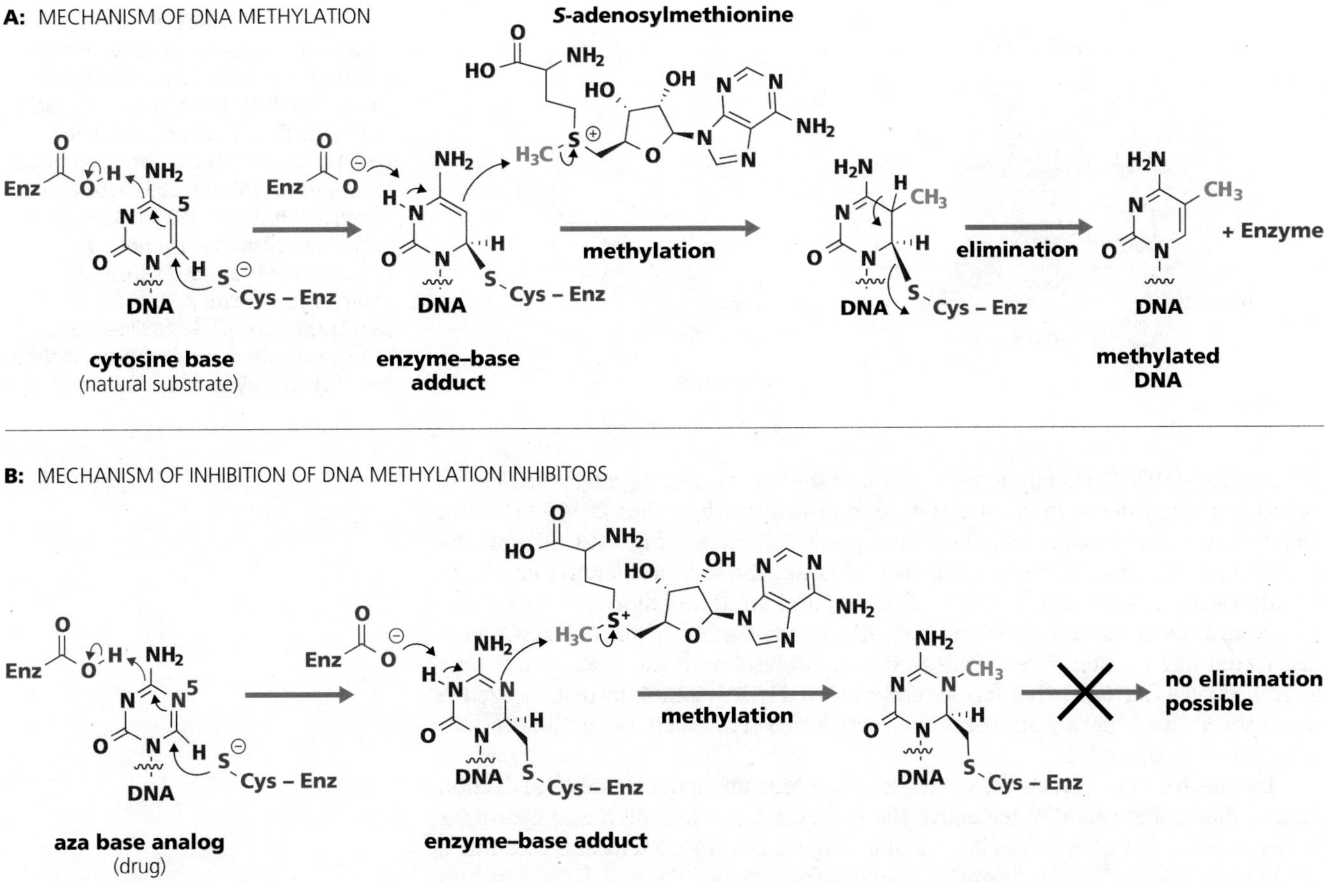

A: MECHANISM OF DNA METHYLATION

B: MECHANISM OF INHIBITION OF DNA METHYLATION INHIBITORS

Figure 10.31 Comparison of the mechanism of DNA methyltransferase with natural substrate and aza analog. A: Mechanism of DNA methylation. A cysteine from the enzyme (red) reacts at the 6-position of the base to generate a reactive enzyme–base adduct. The intermediate reacts with the cosubstrate, *S*-adenosylmethionine to introduce a methyl group at the 5-position. A 1,2-elimination regenerates the enzyme and releases the new methylated base. B: Mechanism of inhibitor of DNA methylation. The unnatural substrate undergoes the same initial reactions to generate the enzyme–base adduct, however the 1,2-elimination is not possible, and the enzyme is irreversibly bound to the inhibitor–DNA complex.

Like most other nucleosides, these analogs are first activated to their corresponding triphosphates. They become incorporated into the host DNA and are substrates for the DNA methyltransferase enzyme. As shown in **Figure 10.31A**, under typical conditions, the cytosine bases in DNA become methylated via methyltransferase enzymes. Addition of a cysteine residue of the enzyme to the 6-position of the base generates an enzyme–base complex. This activated intermediate reacts with the enzyme's cosubstrate, *S*-adenosylmethionine, to transfer a methyl group to the 5-position. In the case of the natural substrate, elimination of the C-5 hydrogen takes place with the enzyme's thiolate as a leaving group to regenerate the active enzyme and the newly methylated DNA. The same initial steps occur when the aza base analog is the substrate (see **Figure 10.31B**), however the final elimination step is not possible. The inhibitor maintains a stable covalent bond with the enzyme, rendering the enzyme ineffective; the damaged DNA is recognized, and signals for the cell's destruction are initiated. This mechanism of inhibition bears some resemblance to inhibitors of thymidylate synthase described in Figure 10.12.

10.7 Histone deacetylase inhibitors bind to zinc in the enzyme's active site

Like DNA, histones are modified by addition or removal of a small group such as acetate, phosphate, or methyl. Gene transcription is regulated by a carefully regulated series of acetylations and deacetylations. Acetylation of the lysine-rich amino-terminal tails of histones is carried out by histone acetyltransferases (HATs), and histone

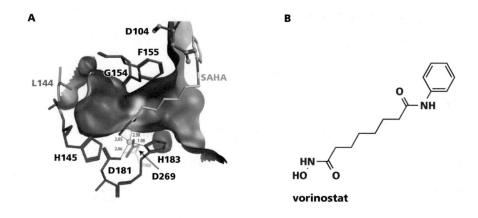

A

D104
F155
G154
L144
SAHA
H145
H183
D181
D269

B

O
NH
HN
HO   O

vorinostat

Figure 10.32 Vorinostat binding to HDAC. A: X-ray structure of vorinostat (SAHA) bound to histone deacetylase-like protein (HDAC2), showing the long narrow enzyme binding pocket and binding to zinc. The zinc ion coordinates to aspartates 181 and 269 (D181 and D269) and histidine 183 (H183) and to the hydroxamide of vorinostat. B: Structure of vorinostat. (A, from Lauffer BEL, Mintzer R, Fong R et al. [2013] *J Biol Chem* 288:26926–26943. With permission from American Society for Biochemistry and Molecular Biology.)

deacetylases (HDACs) catalyze the removal of the same acetate groups (see Figure 10.30). Both enzymes work in concert to appropriately configure the DNA–chromatin complex so that it is competent for transcription. Inhibition of HDACs disrupts the equilibrium, resulting in changes in gene expression and anti-proliferative effects. In addition, HDACs have non-histone substrates, and inhibiting those processes may also contribute to the anti-cancer efficacy. In fact, the first inhibitors of HDACs were discovered due to their potent anti-cancer effects, and their mechanism was only identified later. Currently, there are several approved HDAC inhibitors that are used to treat cancer; those that act on HATs are an active area of research, but inhibitors have not yet been approved.

The mechanism of HDACs is related to that of zinc metalloproteases (see Section 7.5), in that a zinc cation at the active site is required for activation and hydrolysis of the acetate. The active site consists of a long tunnel whose terminal contains a catalytic Zn^{2+}, which is coordinated to a series of aspartic acid and histidine residues that participate in the hydrolysis process. The substrate (or inhibitor) occupies the tunnel and coordinates to the Zn^{2+}. The inhibitor vorinostat (also known as suberanilohydroxamic acid, SAHA) is shown bound to HDAC in **Figure 10.32**.

To date, four HDAC inhibitors, vorinostat, belinostat, panobinostat, and romidepsin (**Figure 10.33**), have been approved to treat cancer. Most conform to a common pharmacophore consisting of a cap structure (shown in red), a linker region (depicted in blue), and a zinc-binding group (shown in green). In vorinostat, belinostat, and panobinostat, the zinc-binding group is a hydroxamic acid. In romidepsin, a disulfide (highlighted in pink) is cleaved *in vivo* to generate the zinc-binding thiol. While there is a large family of HDACs, most of the currently approved inhibitors have

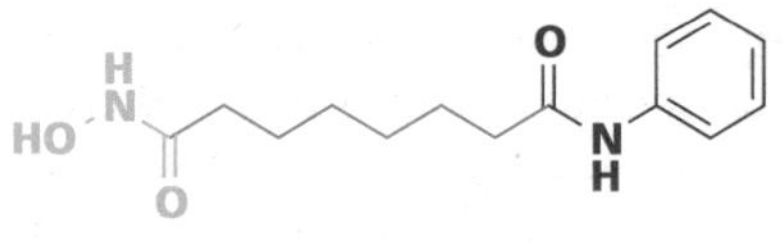

vorinostat

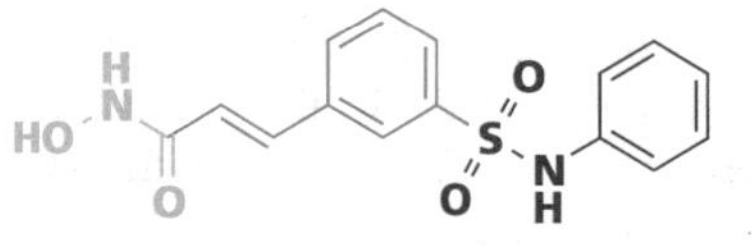

belinostat

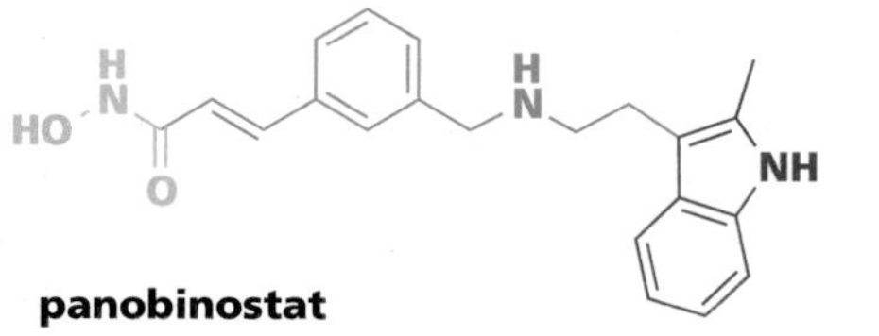

panobinostat

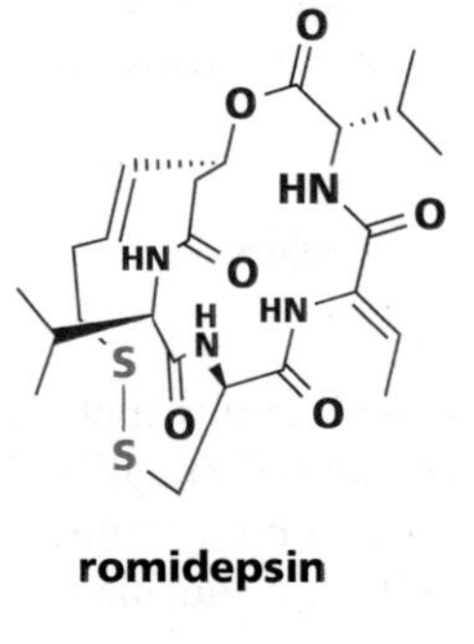

romidepsin

Figure 10.33 Structures of HDAC inhibitors. Common structural features of vorinostat, belinostat, and panobinostat include a cap structure (shown in red), a linker region (depicted in blue), and a Zn^{2+}-binding group (shown in green). The disulfide of romidepsin is highlighted in pink, and upon reduction generates a thiol which binds to the active site Zn^{2+}.

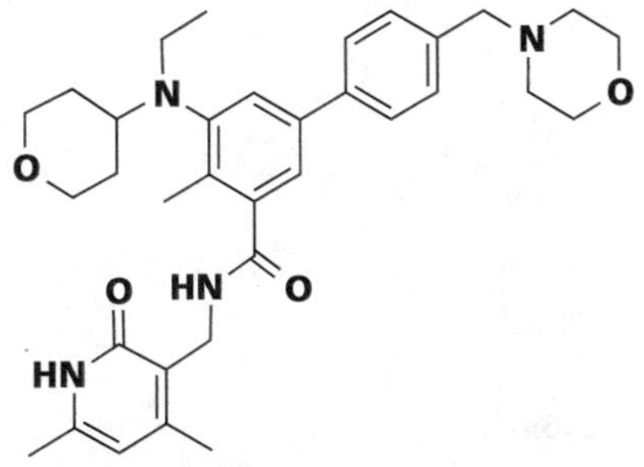

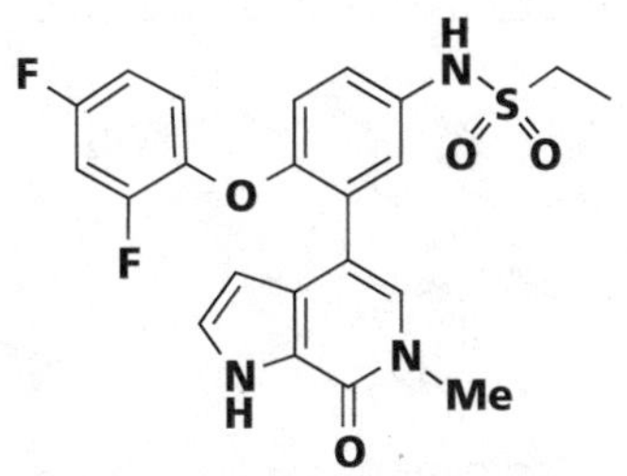

Figure 10.34 Structures of clinical candidates targeting epigenetic processes. Tazemetostat inhibits the histone methyltransferase EZH2, and mivebresib prevents binding between a bromodomain protein and acetylated histones.

tazemetostat

mivebresib

little selectivity for one class over another. The discovery of vorinostat, as well as other HDAC inhibitors, is discussed further in Case Study 1.

While only a few drugs targeting epigenetic processes are approved, work on other epigenetic targets have led to compounds in clinical trials. These include tazemetostat, an inhibitor of the histone methyltransferase EZH2 (an epigenetic writer), and mivebresib (ABBV-075), an inhibitor of the PPI between bromodomain proteins (epigenetic readers) and acetylated histones (**Figure 10.34**).

DRUGS TARGETING HORMONE-DEPENDENT TUMORS

In addition to the above-mentioned aberrant pathways that can drive the malignant process, some tumors require the presence of hormones to proliferate. In these cases, hormone-dependent nuclear receptors (described in Section 6.10) that control gene transcription are dysregulated. For example, some breast cancers grow in response to the female hormone estrogen. When breast cancer patients are first diagnosed, their tumors are categorized by whether they are estrogen receptor positive (ER+) or negative (ER–) to determine whether their growth is responsive to estrogen. This information dictates specific therapy and, often, prognosis.

In the cases of hormone-responsive tumors, one aspect of therapy usually involves reducing or eliminating the amount of receptor signaling. Therapeutically, this is accomplished in two ways: using a receptor antagonist or inhibiting the biosynthesis of the natural ligand. **Figure 10.35** illustrates a few examples of synthetic agents used as anti-cancer agents, their mechanisms of action, and their structures.

Anti-estrogens such as tamoxifen and raloxifene (see Section 6.10) are antagonists of the estrogen receptor and are frequent components of ER+ breast cancer therapy regimens. Other options include reducing amounts of estrogen through the use of biosynthesis inhibitors such as the aromatase inhibitors exemestane, anastrozole, and letrozole. Many prostate cancers respond to similar strategies. For example, abiraterone inhibits biosynthetic pathways to testosterone. Flutamide, bicalutamide, and enzalutamide act as androgen receptor antagonists, blocking the effects of testosterone in prostate cancer.

SUMMARY

Just as there are many biological mechanisms implicated in the development of cancer, there are also many targets for drugs to treat the disease. As of 2017, the U.S. National Cancer Institute lists over 200 chemotherapy agents, and many more if multiple formulations of the same drug or combinations are counted. This number gives some idea of the diversity of compounds that are effective anti-cancer agents. The first chemotherapy drugs were discovered in the 1940s, and until the introduction of kinase inhibitors in the 2000s, many drugs targeted DNA, either directly or by affecting enzymes involved in DNA synthesis. Other early drugs targeted proteins, such as tubulin, that were intimately involved in cell

A: DRUGS TARGETING ER+ BREAST CANCERS

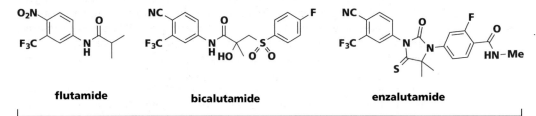

tamoxifen

raloxifene

ESTROGEN RECEPTOR ANTAGONISTS

exemestane

anastrozole

letrozole

ESTROGEN BIOSYNTHESIS INHIBITORS

B: DRUGS TARGETING PROSTATE CANCERS

flutamide

bicalutamide

enzalutamide

ANDROGEN RECEPTOR ANTAGONISTS

abiraterone

TESTOSTERONE BIOSYNTHESIS INHIBITOR

Figure 10.35 Examples of drugs that target hormone-dependent tumors. A: Drugs targeting ER+ breast cancers include estrogen receptor antagonists such as tamoxifen and raloxifene and estrogen biosynthesis inhibitors (exemestane, anastrozole and letrozole). B: Drugs targeting hormone-sensitive prostate cancers include androgen receptor antagonists, flutamide, bicalutamide and enzalutamide; and a testosterone biosynthesis inhibitor abiraterone.

division. The toxicity of these older drugs, due to their limited selectivity, has been mediated more recently by delivery systems, including tumor-directed antibodies, as well as improved formulations. Newer drugs target enzymes and processes that are selective or specific to tumors and lead the way for personalized medicine, where a careful analysis of the patient and the tumor determines the most effective therapy. These small-molecule therapeutic agents include kinase inhibitors, PARP inhibitors, proteasome inhibitors, and drugs that target epigenetic processes, as well as drugs targeting hormone-specific tumors. While it is impossible to cover all anti-tumor drugs in a single chapter, examples of the major classes of drugs and their mechanisms are found here, as well as in Chapter 9.

CASE STUDY 1 DISCOVERY OF VORINOSTAT

Vorinostat, also known as suberanilohydroxamic acid (SAHA) was developed at Columbia University by Ronald Breslow and Paul Marks, based on an observation by Charlotte Friend that cells cultured in high concentrations of the common laboratory solvent dimethyl sulfoxide (DMSO) underwent apoptosis. Examination of other small-molecule polar solvents identified amides such as dimethylformamide (DMF) as having a similar effect. A series of bisamides was prepared, and hexamethylene bisacetamide (HMBA) weakly inhibited the growth of murine erythroleukemia (MEL) cells at 5 mM concentration (Figure 10.36). SAR studies on the chain length showed that the six-carbon linker was optimal, and animal studies with HMBA were initiated. The compound had low toxicity and progressed to phase II clinical trials for acute myelogenous leukemia and myelodysplastic syndrome in 1992. While there were partial remissions in some patients, these were transient, and high doses of the drug were required.

Without knowledge of the target, and based on an assumption that the amides of HMBA may be binding to a metal, the corresponding hydroxamides were synthesized. The analog suberic bis(hydroxamic acid) (SBHA) was twice as potent as the parent bisamide HMBA in causing growth arrest and death of transformed cells. As in the bisamide series, the optimal chain length was found to be six carbons. The next round of optimization came from the decision to maintain one hydroxamide and add a hydrophobic group at the other end. This modification resulted in the synthesis of SAHA in 1996, which was six times more potent than SBHA in cytotoxicity assays. The mechanism of action of these compounds was still unknown at this point; however, a member of the research group, Victoria Richon, noticed the similarity in structure of SAHA to the natural product trichostatin A. Although it had been isolated as an antifungal antibiotic in 1976, trichostatin A was identified as a growth inhibitor in Friend's MEL cells in 1986 and had been identified as an HDAC inhibitor in 1990. In 1998, SAHA was demonstrated to inhibit HDACs at low (50 nM) concentration. This inhibition results in selective apoptosis of transformed (cancer) cells.

In animal models, SAHA inhibited growth of several types of tumors, including prostate, mammary, and neuroblastoma, with little to no toxicity. In addition, SAHA exhibited synergism with other anti-tumor agents such as fludarabine, bortezomib, and imatinib. Sponsored by Columbia University, SAHA entered phase I clinical trials in patients with refractory hematologic and solid tumors and showed little toxicity. At the time, no large pharmaceutical companies were interested in SAHA, due to concerns that the hydroxamic acid moiety might cause toxicity due to nonselective inhibition of Zn^{2+}-containing proteins and enzymes. As a result, the original discoverers formed Aton Pharma, which was then acquired by Merck after promising results from phase II clinical trials. SAHA, now known as vorinostat, received FDA approval in 2006.

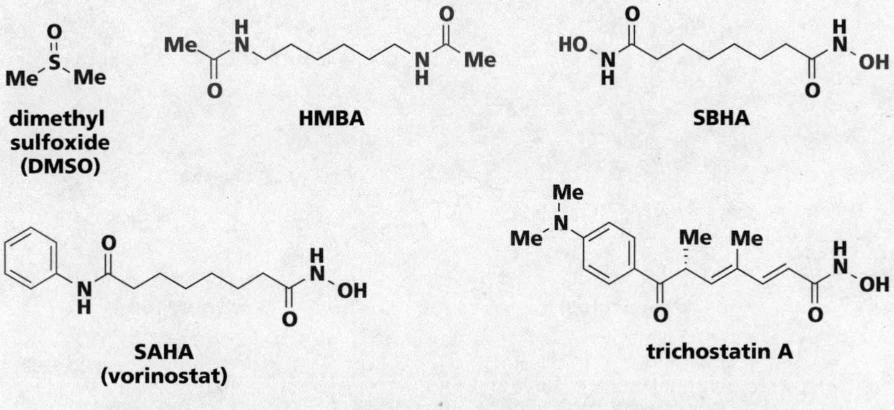

Figure 10.36 **Structures involved in development of vorinostat.** DMSO was the initial lead, and SAR studies identified HMBA, which advanced to clinical trials. Further optimization led to incorporation of hydroxamic acid groups (SBHA) and then desymmetrization to generate SAHA. The structural similarity between SAHA and trichostatin A is shown.

CASE STUDY 2 VISMODEGIB: INHIBITOR OF HEDGEHOG SIGNALING PATHWAY

The hedgehog (Hh) signaling pathway plays a critical role during embryonic development. The natural product cyclopamine was a key tool to understand the role of this pathway (Figure 10.37). Cyclopamine is a teratogenic alkaloid found in the corn lily, and exposure to it prevents the fetal brain from dividing and leads to the development of a single eye. Cyclopamine antagonizes the smoothened (SMO) receptor, which activates the Hh pathway, so cyclopamine indirectly inhibits Hh signaling.

In adults, the hedgehog pathway is also active, and it has been observed that inappropriate activation at a variety of nodes both upstream and downstream of Hh is associated with basal cell carcinoma. As a proof of concept of the potential of small-molecule intervention in the Hh/SMO pathway, cyclopamine was found to inhibit the proliferation of certain cancer cells. However, its poor solubility, limited availability, and structural complexity, as well its chemical instability, led to efforts to find inhibitors of the hedgehog pathway of different chemical classes as potential treatments for cancer. At Genentech, a high-throughput screen identified antagonists of the hedgehog pathway, and benzimidazole 1 was derived from the original hit (Figure 10.38).

Compounds were assayed in a fibroblast cell-based assay using a luciferase reporter gene, where antagonists of the Hh pathway would reduce the signal. While 1 exhibited respectable potency ($IC_{50} = 12$ nM), it exhibited poor pharmaceutical properties, particularly high predicted clearance and low solubility. Synthesis of a series of analogs focused on replacement of the benzimidazole, and SAR studies indicated the requirement for an H-bond acceptor adjacent to the chlorophenyl group. Compound 2, in which a pyridine replaced the benzimidazole, maintained the H-bond acceptor but showed improved solubility as well as improved clearance. Modification of the amide substituent supported the requirement for a lipophilic group at the pyridyl-2-position, such as methyl or chloro, to retain good potency. Further optimization for solubility led to incorporation of a methylsulfone and, eventually, to vismodegib (3). In pharmacokinetic studies, vismodegib exhibited low clearance and high oral exposure. It also showed excellent effects in Hh-dependent tumor animal models. Vismodegib is approved to treat certain metastatic and recurrent basal cell carcinomas.

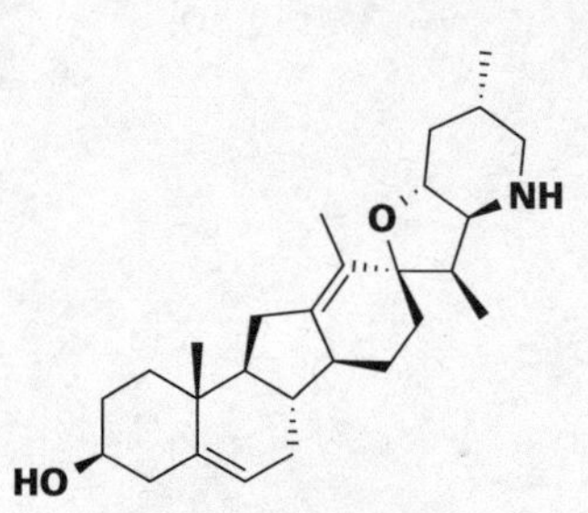

cyclopamine

Figure 10.37 **Structure of cyclopamine.** This teratogenic alkaloid indirectly inhibits the hedgehog signaling pathway.

H-BOND ACCEPTOR REQUIRED

IC_{50} = 12 nM
solubility (pH 1) = 300 μg/mL
solubility (pH 6.5) = 0.3 μg/mL
clearance from microsomes = 9.4 mL/min/kg

1 (lead)

SUBSTITUENT IMPORTANT FOR POTENCY

IMPROVED SOLUBILITY

2 (pyridine analog)

IC_{50} = 42 nM
solubility (pH 1) = 1000 μg/mL
solubility (pH 6.5) = 1.8 μg
clearance from microsomes = 0.6 mL/min/kg/mL

3 (vismodegib)

IC_{50} = 13 nM
solubility (pH 1) = 3,000 μg/mL
solubility (pH 6.5) = 9.5 μg/mL

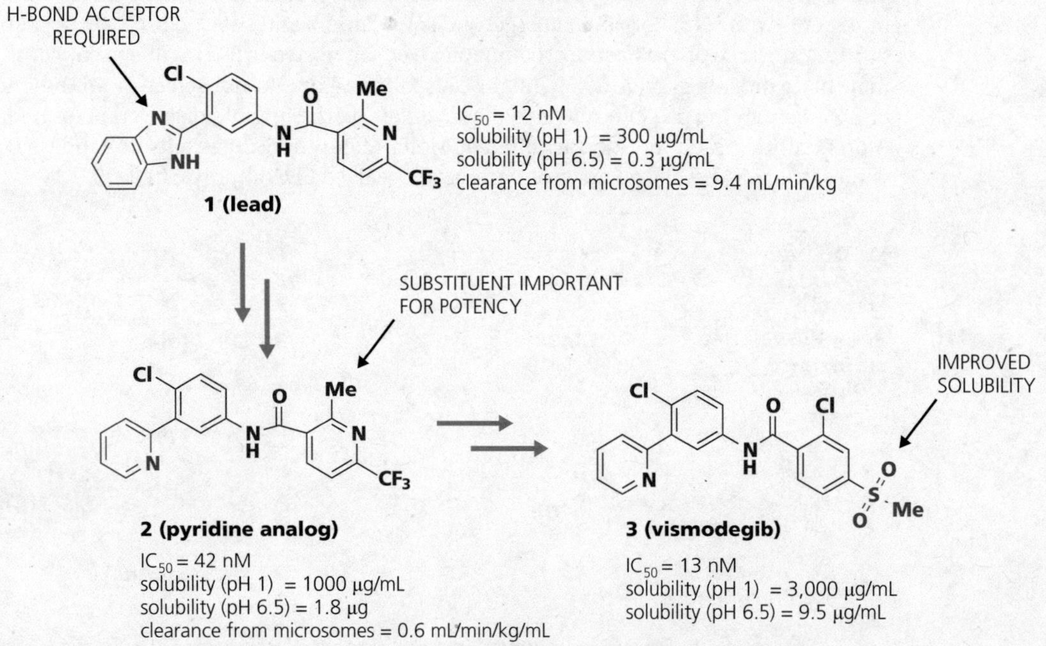

Figure 10.38 **Structures involved in development of vismodegib.** Benzimidazole lead **1** was modified to the pyridine analog **2** (change shown in red) which retained a key H-bond acceptor. This modification improved solubility and predicted clearance. Further optimization led to the incorporaton of a chloro, methylsulfone aryl group found in vismodegib (**3**).

REVIEW QUESTIONS

1. Explain why drugs that target DNA directly are intrinsically more toxic than drugs that target oncogenes.

2. Given the interactions from the X-ray co-crystal structure of bortezemib bound to the proteasome proteolytic site shown in Figure 10.28, draw the expected structure of MG132 bound to the same sites.

3. Several examples in this chapter were developed by use of structure-based design. Name one class that is particularly amenable to this approach and explain why.

4. Explain the importance of the ethynyl moiety in ponatinib.

5. Explain why natural products are a frequent source of cancer drugs. List five different cancer drugs (of at least three different mechanisms) that were derived from natural products and their mechanisms of action.

6. Identify two examples of a suicide inhibitor described in this chapter.

7. Explain why hormone receptor antagonists are useful therapies for certain cancers. Conversely, explain why hormone replacement therapy may be harmful.

8. Explain the mechanism of temsirolimus and everolimus.

9. A number of anti-cancer agents are also used as anti-inflammatory or immunosuppressant agents. Explain why.

10. Review the drug examples in this chapter and find three where an isosteric replacement strategy was used. Draw the structures of the drugs and the original compounds and identify the isosteres.

APPLICATION QUESTIONS

1. Research the drug raltitrexed. Draw its structure and explain its mechanism of action.

2. Hydroxamic acids and thiols are zinc-binding groups found in FDA-approved histone deacetylase inhibitors. Research another zinc-binding group that is found in HDAC inhibitors being evaluated in the research phase.

3. Research antibody–drug conjugates that are in clinical trials. Choose one. What does the antibody target? What is the small-molecule payload, and what is its biological target? Is either component of the ADC an approved drug itself?

4. Crizotinib is a drug that targets an oncogenic fusion protein. Research its structure and its mechanism of action.

5. The compound neocarzinostatin has been used in Japan to treat liver cancer. Research its structure and its mechanism of action.

6. Review the binding of camptothecin to topoisomerase in Figure 10.8. Draw a pharmacophore that is consistent with these interactions, and design a novel compound based on this pharmacophore.

7. Research the mechanism of epoxomicin's reaction with the proteasome's active site threonine. Draw the product of that reaction.

8. Review the examples in this chapter and identify two compounds (targeting different proteins or enzymes) that incorporate functional groups that improved their solubility. Draw the structures with and without the solubilizing groups in ChemDraw (or another program), and calculate the differences in solubility and cLogP for each. How different are the pairs?

9. Review the structures of methotrexate and pralatrexate. Draw a pharmacophore model that is consistent with both. Design two new molecules that will test two different aspects of your pharmacophore.

10. Identify three compounds in this chapter that contain fluorine. From what was described in Chapter 4, the mechanism of action of each chosen drug, and the site of the fluorine, propose the function of fluorine in each molecule.

FURTHER READING

General references

Kamb A, Wee S & Lengauer C (2007) Why is cancer drug discovery so difficult? *Nat Rev Drug Discovery* 6:115–120.

Alberts B, Johnson A, Lewis J et al. (2002) Chapter 23: Cancer. In Molecular Biology of the Cell, 4th ed, pp 1091–1144. Garland Science.

Drugs targeting topoisomerase

Staker BL, Feese MD, Cushman M et al. (2005) Structures of three classes of anticancer agents bound to the human topoisomerase I–DNA covalent complex. *J Med Chem* 48:2336–2345.

Wu C-C, Li T-K, Farh L et al. (2011) Topoisomerase inhibition by the anticancer drug etoposide. *Science* 333:459–462.

Deweese JE & Osheroff N (2009) The DNA cleavage reaction of topoisomerase II: wolf in sheep's clothing. *Nucleic Acids Res* 37:738–748.

Redinbo MR, Stewart L, Kuhn P et al. (1998) Crystal structures of human topoisomerase I in covalent and noncovalent complexes with DNA. *Science* 279:1504–1513.

Drugs targeting microtubules

Jordan MA & Wilson L (2004) Microtubules as a target for anticancer drugs. *Nat Rev Cancer* 4:253–265.

Epigenetics

Blancafort P, Jin J & Frye S (2013) Writing and rewriting the epigenetic code of cancer cells: from engineered proteins to small molecules. *Mol Pharmacol* 83:563–576.

Falkenberg KJ & Johnstone RW (2014) Histone deacetylases and their inhibitors in cancer, neurological diseases and immune disorders. *Nat Rev Drug Discovery* 13:673–691.

Special issue on epigenetics. (2016) *J Med Chem* 59:1247–1654.

Proteasome

Borissenko L & Groll M (2007) 20S Proteasome and its inhibitors: crystallographic knowledge for drug development. *Chem Rev* 107:687–717.

Orlowski RZ & Kuhn DJ (2008) Proteasome inhibitors in cancer therapy: lessons from the first decade. *Clin Cancer Res* 14:1649–1657.

Angiogenesis

Kerbel R & Folkman J (2002) Clinical translation of angiogenesis inhibitors. *Nat Rev Cancer* 2:727–739.

Case studies

Marks PA & Breslow R (2007) Dimethyl sulfoxide to vorinostat: development of this histone deacetylase inhibitor as an anticancer drug. *Nat Biotechnol* 1:84–90.

Meinke PT & Liberator P (2001) Histone deacetylase: a target for antiproliferative and antiprotozoal agents. *Curr Med Chem* 8:211–235.

Robarge KD, Brunton SA, Castanedo GM et al. (2009) GDC-0449-A potent inhibitor of hedgehog pathway. *Bioorg Med Chem Lett* 19:5576–5581.

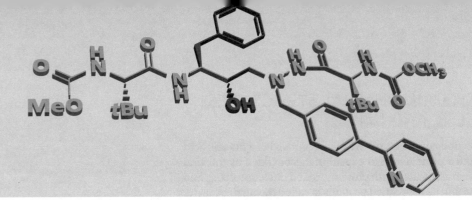

Antiviral and antifungal agents

11

LEARNING OBJECTIVES

- Describe the common points of intervention for antiviral therapy.
- Identify classes of drugs that target viral enzymes involved in nucleic acid replication.
- Understand the medicinal chemistry approaches taken to discover and develop antiviral protease inhibitors.
- Describe drugs that target viral attachment, uncoating, and budding.
- Explain the mechanism of action of antifungal agents.

Both viral and fungal infections lead to diseases and conditions that range from mild, such as the common cold or athlete's foot, to deadly, such as AIDS or systemic fungal infections. Until the mid-1900s, there were no safe drugs to treat either type of infection. Historically, however, certain viral infections such as smallpox and polio have been prevented with vaccines, which, when administered, provoke an immune response so that antibodies are present in case of exposure. Vaccines have been in use since 1798, when Edward Jenner advocated the use of cowpox vaccine to protect against smallpox. Although they are effective against many viruses, for a variety of reasons, vaccines against certain viruses, as well as against fungal infections, have not yet been developed, despite the medical need.

For the instances when vaccines are not available (or not effective), there are a number of approved drugs to treat viral diseases, but far fewer drugs are available to treat fungal infections. These numbers are small, however, when compared to drugs that treat bacterial infections, which are the subject of Chapter 12. There are several reasons for this disparity, but a primary explanation is related to the difference between bacterial, viral, and fungal drug targets and human homologs. Since viruses rely, to varying degrees, on human proteins to replicate, there are only a few viral-specific targets that drugs can affect. The reason for the lack of drugs for fungal infections is different. Fungi are eukaryotic organisms, as are animals. As a result, the potential drug targets for fungi are very similar to the targets found in humans, which leads to difficulties in selectivity. In contrast, prokaryotic bacteria have their own replication machinery, and therefore drug targets are often quite distinct from mammalian targets, making selectivity between human and bacterial targets more readily achievable.

ANTIVIRAL AGENTS: COMMON VIRAL STRUCTURES, REPLICATION PROCESS, AND IMPACT

Structurally, all viruses are infectious particles, or **virions**, composed of a nucleic acid containing the viral genome and a protein coat or capsid that is encoded by the viral genome. The viral genome is often associated with proteins, called nucleoproteins, and the combination of the genome and its associated proteins is called the nucleocapsid. In some viruses, the nucleocapsid is helical and the protein subunits, or protomers, form rigid rods or flexible filaments around the nucleic acid. In other viruses, the protomers are arranged in clusters called capsomeres that form an icosahedral shell, a polygon with 20 equilateral triangular faces and 12 vertices. Some viruses may be spherical, like the influenza virus (**Figure 11.1**). Some viruses, in addition, have an envelope surrounding the nucleocapsid. This envelope is a lipid bilayer that is derived from a modified host cell membrane with an outer layer of glycoproteins derived from the virus; these glycoproteins are involved in determining which specific cells the virus infects.

The nucleic acid contained in the virion can be either single-stranded (ss) or double-stranded (ds) RNA or DNA. It can be configured in either a linear or circular orientation, and the entire genome may be present either on a single nucleic acid molecule or on several segments of nucleic acid. Genomes can also be either (+)-sense, which can be translated immediately into protein, or (–)-sense, which must be first converted to (+)-sense RNA before translation. Since viruses are intracellular parasites, they cannot express their gene products or replicate without the help of a living cell; the specific replication strategy depends on the type of genome in the virus. For example, most DNA viruses replicate in the cell nucleus and use host cell DNA-dependent RNA polymerase to synthesize mRNA. The early proteins translated from the mRNA include viral DNA polymerases that are responsible for ongoing replication of the viral genome. Most RNA viruses replicate in the cytoplasm and have their own polymerases to transcribe RNA into mRNA, since the host cell does not have an enzyme to accomplish this. Retroviruses are a specific type of RNA virus, containing a dimer of two identical (+)-single-stranded RNA molecules. The retroviral reverse transcriptase transcribes the viral RNA into dsDNA (reverse transcription), which is then incorporated into host DNA by the viral enzyme, integrase (integration). Regardless of the strategy used, once mRNA is synthesized, it is translated into viral proteins such as viral kinase and viral DNA polymerase needed for production of viral progeny.

While the exact steps may vary from one virus to another, all viruses follow a general replication cycle of attachment, entry, uncoating, transcription and translation to early (replicative) and late (structural) proteins, replication, virion assembly, budding, and release from the host cell. A detailed process for the life cycle of the influenza virus,

Figure 11.1 Shapes and components of virion structures. Common components are nucleic acid genome (DNA or RNA) enclosed in a protein coat, the capsid. The protein coat can form helical (e.g. tobacco mosaic virus); icosahedral, made up of clusters called capsomers (e.g. adenovirus) and spherical shapes (e.g. influenza virus). Some viruses contain a lipoprotein envelope made up of lipids derived from the host and may have glycoprotein spikes on the surface. The nucleic acid can be present as one strand, or several segmented strands.

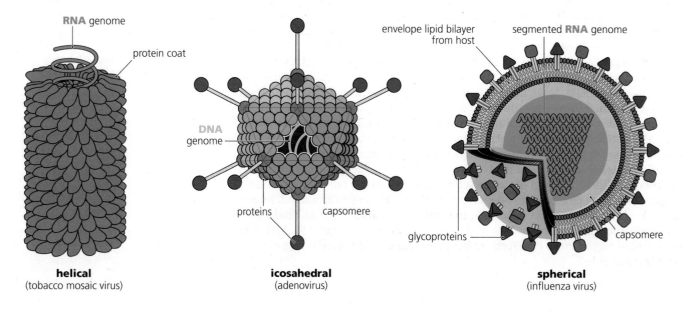

helical
(tobacco mosaic virus)

icosahedral
(adenovirus)

spherical
(influenza virus)

an enveloped ssRNA virus, is illustrated in **Figure 11.2**, with an emphasis on possible points for drug action.

Specific steps in the replication cycle are as follows:

- Attachment: The virion binds to the host cell by interacting with specific host cell-surface receptors.

- Entry: The virion may enter the cell by endocytosis or by fusion with the cell membrane.

- Uncoating: The virion sheds its protein coat to release the viral genome.

- Transcription: Viral nucleic acids are transcribed via mechanisms that are dependent on the specific virus class (DNA, RNA, or retrovirus).

- Translation: Proteins are translated from viral mRNA by use of host machinery.

- Integration: The DNA of some viruses is integrated into host DNA, resulting in that cell becoming permanently infected (not shown).

- Replication: Viral genome is replicated (usually by use of host machinery).

- Virion assembly: New viral particles are packaged.

- Budding and release: New viral particles bud from the infected cell (enveloped viruses) or cause the host cell to burst, releasing viral particles.

- Re-initiation: The process begins again.

Virions can go on to infect other cells but can also exist externally (in the air, in mucus, and in blood) and can infect other individuals. Viruses that are stable in airborne particles, such as influenza, are highly contagious since large numbers of virions are dispersed when an infected individual sneezes or coughs, and others can be infected when they come into contact with a viral particle. Other viruses are spread less easily; for example, those that are transmitted via blood, such as the human immunodeficiency virus (HIV) and hepatitis C virus (HCV). Therapeutic intervention to prevent healthy but at-risk individuals from infection (**prophylaxis**) is a strategy in antiviral drug discovery that focuses on intervening prior to the integration step. For example, it is routinely used when health care workers have an occupational exposure to HIV, to treat pregnant HIV-positive women to prevent transmission to neonates, and in individuals at high risk for HIV infection.

The pathological effects of a viral infection vary greatly. Some viruses, such as rhinoviruses, are relatively harmless and infected individuals recover with no medical treatment. Infection with HCV often causes no acute symptoms but years later can result in very serious disorders such as liver cancer or cirrhosis. Influenza causes

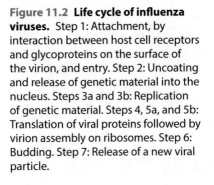

Figure 11.2 Life cycle of influenza viruses. Step 1: Attachment, by interaction between host cell receptors and glycoproteins on the surface of the virion, and entry. Step 2: Uncoating and release of genetic material into the nucleus. Steps 3a and 3b: Replication of genetic material. Steps 4, 5a, and 5b: Translation of viral proteins followed by virion assembly on ribosomes. Step 6: Budding. Step 7: Release of a new viral particle.

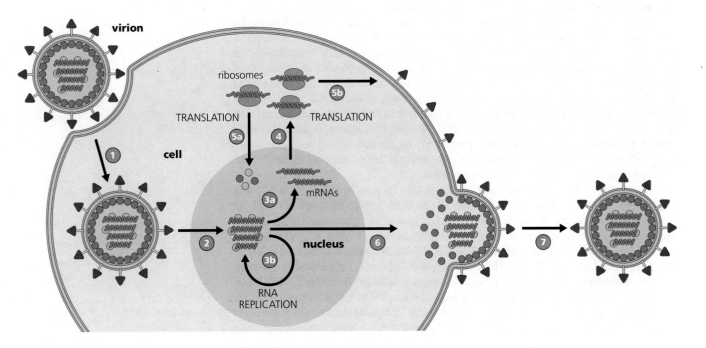

severe acute symptoms that can be deadly in certain patient populations. The specific symptoms of a viral infection depend on the type of cell it targets, the fate of that cell, and the life cycle of the virus. Some infected cells are destroyed by the host immune response; some die because the virus overtakes the cellular machinery; some cells burst and die, releasing virions; and other cells replicate with the virus remaining latent for extended periods of time (years) before the virus reactivates. Some symptoms of a viral infection can be the result of the body's own immune response to the infection (as is the case with the common cold) or because the function of the infected cell is compromised. For example, HIV targets immune cells, and symptoms (immunosuppression) are a consequence of depletion of those cells. The respiratory symptoms of influenza infection reflect that it targets airway epithelial cells.

Untreated viral infection can cause significant mortality and morbidity. During the 1918 influenza pandemic, it is estimated that one-third of the world's population was infected (~500 million) and between 50 and 100 million people died in a single year. While modern versions of influenza are less severe, the potential for a virulent strain spreading rapidly, in a world where transmission is easier than it was in the early 20th century, is high. HIV, the causative agent of acquired immunodeficiency syndrome (AIDS), is a bloodborne pathogen. As of 2016, over 35 million people are living with HIV worldwide, and over 39 million have died since 1981, when AIDS cases were first described. While today HIV infection can be controlled, the life expectancy of an infected individual in the 1980s was less than two years. Globally, 130–150 million individuals are infected with the hepatitis C virus, and >60% will develop chronic liver disease. In the United States, the major cause of liver transplants is HCV infection, and no vaccination is available. Unlike many other diseases such as cancer, which has been known for thousands of years, new viral diseases are continually emerging; therefore, the need to develop new therapies is continual.

ANTIVIRAL DRUG DISCOVERY

While vaccines have been highly effective in preventing and even eradicating certain diseases caused by viruses, in some instances no effective vaccine exists (for example, HIV and HCV), and in other cases such as influenza, infections still occur even though a vaccine is available. Despite the need, small-molecule antiviral drug discovery is a relatively new area. One reason is that, for certain viruses, highly specialized skills, equipment, and laboratories are required to perform even the simplest cell-based assays. Furthermore, animal models that replicate human viral diseases are often inadequate. Therefore, early research in antiviral agents was limited to specialized organizations and laboratories.

Some of the first antiviral drugs were developed in the 1970s at Burroughs Wellcome to treat herpes simplex viruses (HSV). Drugs were characterized using a phenotypic assay (a plaque inhibition assay) that monitored HSV-1 replication in mammalian cells. This success was the result, in part, of the pioneering research of George Hitchings and Gertrude Elion on purines and nucleosides and of the need for drugs to treat genital herpes. The approach used was based on rational design to inhibit fundamental biochemical processes involved in herpesvirus replication and was related to the earlier work of Elion and Hitchings on antimetabolites to treat cancer. The success of this effort, which produced a highly safe, selective, and effective drug called acyclovir, spurred others to pursue antiviral drug discovery and validated the feasibility of targeting **viral-specific proteins**.

These discoveries were followed in the 1980s by massive efforts to identify treatments for AIDS. While the first AIDS drugs were known nucleosides such as azidothymidine (AZT), dideoxycytidine (ddC), and dideoxyinosine (ddI), library screening later identified nonnucleoside inhibitors of the viral enzyme reverse transcriptase, such as nevirapine. The 1988 Nobel Prize in Medicine, awarded to Elion, Hitchings, and James Black, noted that the idea of designing drug molecules that bear structural similarity to natural substances was applied to the design of anti-AIDS drugs.

Investigation of the inhibition of viral proteases has led to many successful drugs, including the transition-state mimetics saquinavir, indinavir, and ritonavir used to treat HIV. These compounds were some of the first drugs whose development was

Table 11.1   Common infectious viruses, select examples of drugs, and their mechanisms of action.

Virus	Category	Family	Drug	Mechanism
herpes simplex virus (HSV-1, HSV-2)	dsDNA	*Herpesviridae*	acyclovir, valacyclovir	polymerase inhibitors
varicella zoster virus (VZV)	dsDNA	*Herpesviridae*	acyclovir, valacyclovir	polymerase inhibitors
cytomegalovirus (CMV)	dsDNA	*Herpesviridae*	ganciclovir	polymerase inhibitor
			fomivirsen (withdrawn)	antisense, early gene products
human immunodeficiency virus (HIV)	ssRNA	*Retroviridae*	azidothymidine, nevirapine	reverse transcriptase inhibitors
			indinavir	protease inhibitor
			maraviroc	entry/fusion inhibitor
			raltegravir	integrase inhibitor
hepatitis C virus (HCV)	ssRNA	*Flaviviridae*	ribavirin	multiple viral and host targets
			sofosbuvir	polymerase inhibitor
			telaprevir	protease inhibitor
			daclatasvir	NS5A inhibitor
hepatitis B virus (HBV)	partial dsDNA	*Hepadnaviridae*	lamivudine, entecavir	polymerase inhibitors
influenza virus	ssRNA	*Orthomyxoviridae*	amantadine	uncoating inhibitor
			oseltamivir, zanamivir	neuraminidase inhibitor

based on iterative structure-based computer-assisted drug design using X-ray crystallography. More recent examples of viral protease inhibitors include the HCV-NS3 protease inhibitors grazoprevir and paritaprevir that are used to treat hepatitis C infections. Novel nucleosides, such as sofosbuvir, to treat HCV have also been developed and are curative when used in combination with other agents. The search for drugs to treat HIV/AIDS and HCV are excellent examples of how basic science research combined with drug discovery efforts allowed the rapid development of drugs to treat or cure a newly identified virus and the disease it causes.

While much of the notable progress in antiviral drugs has been made in the areas of HSV, HIV, and HCV, there are many other successes in treating viral infection. Drugs have been developed to treat influenza and infection by various members of the *Herpesviridae* family, including HSV-1 and HSV-2, varicella zoster virus (VZV), and cytomegalovirus (CMV). These herpesviruses can cause venereal disease and cold sores (HSV), chicken pox and shingles (VZV), and birth defects and retinitis (CMV). The idea of targeting viral-specific enzymes has also been applied to other viral infections, including dengue virus, West Nile virus, and Zika virus. **Table 11.1** contains a representative list of viral diseases for which drugs are available, examples of drugs, and their mechanisms of action.

ANTIVIRAL DRUGS TARGETING VIRAL LIFE CYCLE

While the discovery of antiviral drugs was initially based on a combination of design and phenotypic assays, it has progressed to being based primarily on rational design targeting viral-specific proteins. Some drugs are thus specific for certain viruses, such as HIV protease inhibitors, while others may be effective against a number of different viruses, such as DNA polymerase inhibitors. Whether they target one virus, or several, all antiviral drugs affect a certain point in the viral replication cycle and can be categorized as such.

11.1 Drugs may target viral attachment or entry

There are a few drugs that target viral attachment or entry (in particular, fusion), and they are approved to treat HIV/AIDS. The HIV fusion inhibitors prevent HIV particles from infecting T cells by blocking protein–protein interactions (see Chapter 8). The initial

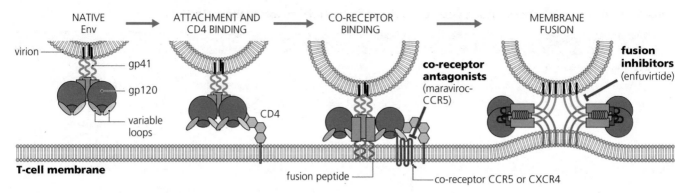

Figure 11.3 Attachment and entry of HIV viral particle into host T-cell and points of intervention. The HIV surface glycoproteins gp120 (depicted in red, with variable loops in orange, pink and yellow) and gp41 (blue lines/green rectangles) mediate attachment and membrane fusion with the target T-cell. Gp120 binds to CD4 receptors (depicted as green hexagons) on the surface of the host T-cell. Conformational changes of variable loops enable binding to a co-receptor (either chemokine receptor CCR5 or CXCR4, shown in purple), with activation of the fusion machinery (orange lines). Once bound, the membranes fuse and the contents of the viral particle enter the cell. Maraviroc, and other co-receptor antagonists block the protein–protein interaction between gp120 and chemokine receptors required for entry. Enfuvirtide binds to a region of gp41 and prevents fusion. (Adapted from Didigu CA & Doms RW [2012] *Viruses* 4:309–324. With permission from MDPI.)

steps of infection by HIV are shown in **Figure 11.3**. The HIV envelope glycoprotein, on the surface of the virion, consists of two subunits, gp120 and gp41. Binding between the virion and the target T-cell is mediated by the interaction between CD4 proteins in the surface of the T-cells and gp120. The glycoprotein then undergoes a series of conformational changes and binds to a co-receptor, a chemokine receptor (usually CCR5, but sometimes CXCR4). Ultimately, the membranes fuse, and the contents of the virion enter the T-cell.

One approach to blocking attachment or entry is to interrupt the interaction between the chemokine co-receptors and gp120. These chemokines are G protein-coupled receptors, and entry inhibitors block their binding to gp120. The first lead in the development of this type of inhibitor was a peptide based on the chemokine's natural ligand, the protein RANTES, although those leads did not result in viable drugs. Other small molecules were developed from screening programs, and have resulted in marketed drugs (see Case Study 2 in Chapter 8 for a discussion of maraviroc). Currently, maraviroc is the only approved drug that works via this mechanism of blocking interaction between gp120 and co-receptors; however, several others, including cenicriviroc and vicriviroc (in combination), progressed to clinical trials for HIV infection (**Figure 11.4**).

Another approach to block HIV entry into cells led to enfuvirtide, which is a synthetic 36-amino-acid peptide. The peptide binds to gp41, preventing it from adopting the specific conformation that is necessary for membrane fusion to occur.

Figure 11.4 Structures of gp120–chemokine antagonists. Maraviroc was approved to treat AIDS in 2007; cenicriviroc and vicriviroc advanced to clinical trials, but were discontinued for AIDS treatment. These compounds originated from hits identified from independent library screening campaigns.

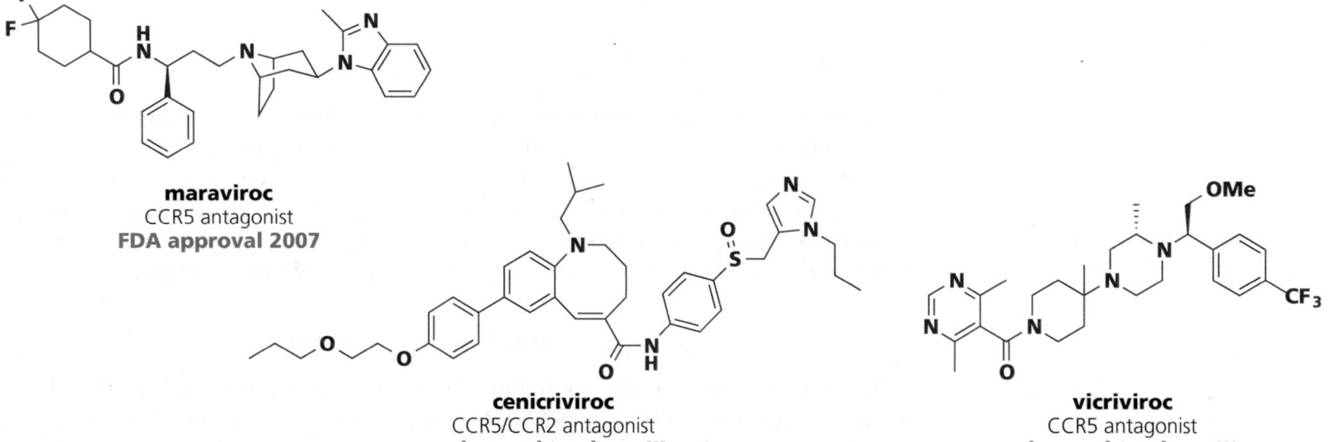

maraviroc
CCR5 antagonist
FDA approval 2007

cenicriviroc
CCR5/CCR2 antagonist
advanced to phase III

vicriviroc
CCR5 antagonist
advanced to phase III

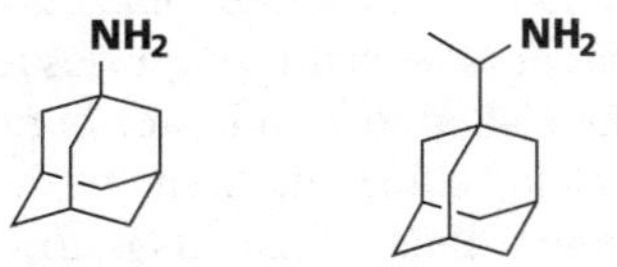

Figure 11.5 Structures of amantadine and rimantadine, and X-ray co-structure. Left: Structures of amantadine and rimantadine. Right: X-ray crystal structure of amantadine bound in the M2 channel. Protons pass through the channel to allow uncoating, and amantadine (shown in orange) physically blocks the pore of the ion channel; mutations at Ser31, His37, and Trp41 confer resistance to amantadine. (Left, from Das K, Aramini JM, Ma L-C et al. [2010] *Nat Struct Mol Biol* 17:530–538. With permission from Macmillan Publishers Limited.)

amantadine   rimantadine

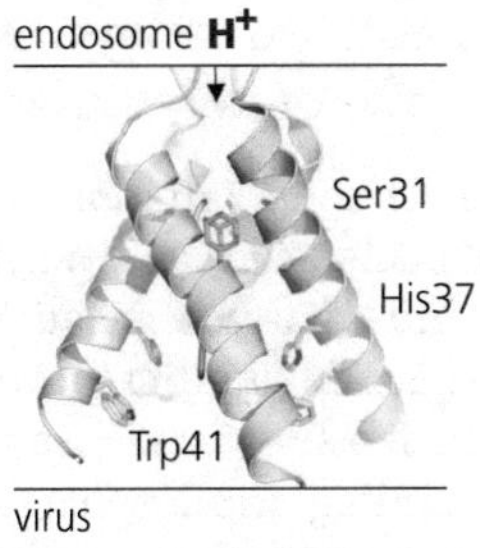

amantadine (orange)
bound in M2 channel

11.2 Drugs may target uncoating of viral particles

The uncoating process varies among viruses and is complex, but inhibiting it is a viable therapeutic approach. To date, the only uncoating inhibitors approved are amantadine and rimantadine, and their effectiveness is poor. Amantadine (**Figure 11.5**) was found to have antiviral activity against the influenza A virus in 1963 and was approved for that use in the United States in 1966. The mechanism of action of amantadine and rimantadine involves binding to the viral M2 protein. This proton ion channel is specific to influenza A viruses and is involved in the early stage of uncoating.

The viral M2 ion channel is a homotetrameric channel, and an influx of protons acidifies the interior of viruses trapped in endosomes, allowing the virus to dissociate and uncoat. Several X-ray and NMR structures of amantadine bound in the channel have been solved. Two of the structures place amantadine in the pore, essentially physically blocking the channel, as seen in the X-ray structure in Figure 11.5. Drug resistance is conferred by mutations to Ser31, His37, and Trp41. Side effects of amantadine and rimantadine, possibly caused by inhibition of host ion channels, as well as viral resistance have significantly limited use of these drugs, although there has been renewed interest in their effects against avian flu.

Another example of antiviral agents that block uncoating is based on a phenyl ether scaffold. A series of small molecules was investigated in the 1980s to treat rhinoviruses, the causative agent for the common cold. They were developed around the advanced analog disoxaril, which was in turn evolved from a lead compound called arildone (**Figure 11.6**).

Screening at Sterling-Winthrop identified arildone as a compound with some activity against the poliovirus, and lead optimization led to disoxaril, which had activity against several rhinovirus serotypes. Its mechanism involves binding to a hydrophobic cleft on the viral capsid that prevents uncoating of the virus. The most advanced compound in the series, pleconaril, exhibited oral activity in mice infected with enteroviruses and rhinoviruses. Pleconaril entered clinical trials but was ultimately rejected as an oral drug due to safety issues and low efficacy.

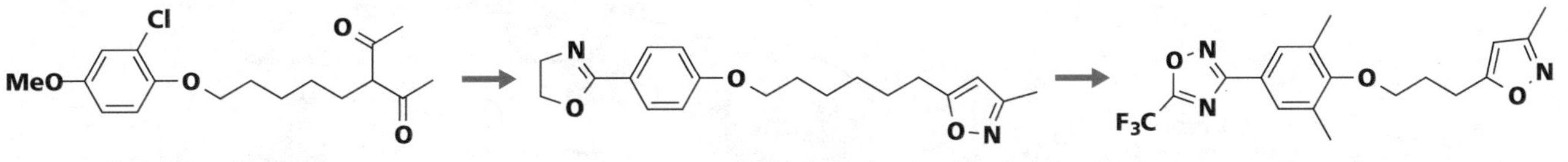

arildone (lead)   disoxaril   pleconaril

Figure 11.6 Structures of rhinovirus uncoating inhibitors. Arildone was identified as a compound with activity against poliovirus. Optimization led to disoxaril, which exhibited activity against rhinoviruses. Further optimization generated pleconaril, which advanced to clinical trials for the treatment of the common cold.

11.3   Many antiviral drugs inhibit transcription by targeting the active site of polymerases

As outlined in Chapter 7 in more detail, kinases can catalyze phosphorylation of the 5′-position of nucleosides, and polymerases or reverse transcriptases recognize these nucleotides, and catalyze formation of the 3′–5′ phosphodiester bond between the incoming nucleotide and the growing nucleic acid chain. Some of the first antiviral drugs were nucleosides or nucleoside mimics; they utilize this pathway to generate their corresponding triphosphates. These antimetabolites are recognized by the polymerase and then incorporated into the growing viral DNA chain. This results in chain termination, and stops replication, as summarized in **Figure 11.7**. Points of structural modification of the nucleosides include the base and the ribose unit. Virtually all the early nucleoside antiviral agents maintain the 5′-hydroxyl group, and many are 2′- or 3′-deoxy analogs of naturally occurring nucleosides.

The earliest nucleoside antiviral drug, idoxuridine, containing a modified base, (**Figure 11.8A**) was approved in 1962. It was synthesized by William Prusoff as a potential anti-cancer agent, as were many antiviral nucleosides. It is used topically to treat HSV eye infections but its utility is limited by cardiotoxicity. Another nucleoside with a modified base is ribavirin, which was first synthesized in the 1970s. While it has broad-spectrum antiviral activity and was used in the 1980s to treat respiratory syncytial virus (RSV), since the 1990s it has been used in combination with α-interferon to treat HCV infection. Recently, it has been supplanted by more effective drugs. However, ribavirin's mechanism is not well understood and appears to be more complex than solely polymerase inhibition.

The approval of idoxuridine was followed several years later by the approval of vidarabine (Figure 11.8B), an arabinose analog of adenosine that has activity against HSV and VSV. Its discovery can be traced to the 1950s, when spongothymidine and spongouridine were isolated from a Caribbean sponge by Werner Bergmann. Both natural products differ from thymidine and uridine at the 2′-stereogenic center, by having the arabinose rather than the ribose configuration. Although modified bases had been prepared prior to this, activity of these compounds as polymerase inhibitors or antiviral agents gave the first indication that modification of the carbohydrate could also lead to active analogs. This idea was the basis for the synthetic analog vidarabine, as well as cytarabine (arabinocytosine), which entered clinical use in the 1960s.

While the earliest synthetic nucleosides either lacked the 2′-hydroxyl group or had inverted configurations, further modification of the carbohydrate by opening the ring generated acyclic nucleosides, an important structural motif. Compounds such as these were originally investigated not as antiviral agents but as substrates for adenosine deaminase, an enzyme in the purine biosynthesis pathway that converts adenosine to inosine. During these studies, it was found that, of the three hydroxyl groups present on ribonucleosides (2′, 3′, and 5′), only the one at the 5′-position was required for recognition by the enzyme. This observation led Howard Schaeffer at SUNY Buffalo to synthesize the acyclic analogs acycloadenosine and acycloguanosine (acyclovir) in 1971, which were substrates for adenosine deaminase (Figure 11.8C).

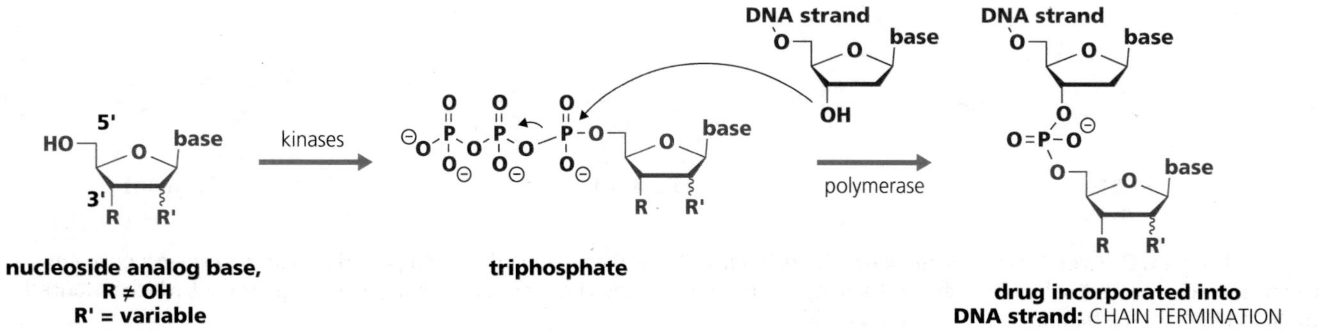

Figure 11.7 Incorporation of nucleoside antiviral drugs into DNA. The 5′-position of the nucleoside analog (red) is phosphorylated to the corresponding triphosphate by kinases. Attack by the 3′-hydroxyl of the DNA strand terminus incorporates the drug into the growing DNA strand. The R substituent cannot participate in subsequent polymerization reactions, therefore chain termination results and replication stops.

nucleoside analog base,
R ≠ OH
R′ = variable

triphosphate

drug incorporated into
DNA strand: CHAIN TERMINATION

A: MODIFIED BASE NUCLEOSIDES

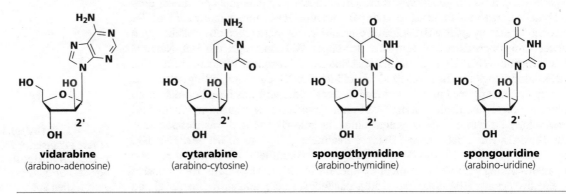

B: ARABINO NUCLEOSIDES

vidarabine
(arabino-adenosine)

cytarabine
(arabino-cytosine)

spongothymidine
(arabino-thymidine)

spongouridine
(arabino-uridine)

C: ACYCLIC NUCLEOSIDES

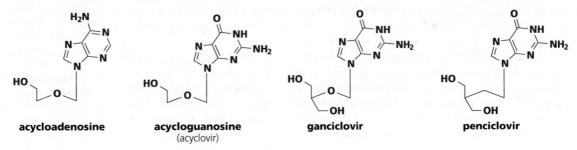

acycloadenosine

acycloguanosine
(acyclovir)

ganciclovir

penciclovir

Figure 11.8 Early cyclic and acylic nucleoside antiviral drugs. A: Idoxuridine, an iodo analog of 2'-deoxyuridine, and ribavirin, a triazole, contain modified bases (modifications are shown in red). B: Vidarabine and cytarabine are arabino analogs based on the natural products spongothymidine and spongouridine (arabino OH configuration is shown in red). C: Acycloadenosine, acycloguanosine (acyclovir), ganciclovir, and penciclovir are acyclic derivatives modified at the carbohydrate moiety.

Acyclovir was then investigated by Elion and Hitchings in 1977; it was found to have antiviral activity against HSV-1 infected cells and little toxicity towards uninfected cells. This selectivity is based on the compound's being selectively monophosphorylated by the virally encoded thymidine kinase, but not by mammalian kinases, and thus being converted to the active triphosphate polymerase substrate only in virally infected cells. As the triphosphate, it also selectively inhibits the viral DNA polymerase over host polymerases. Acyclovir, one of the most successful nucleoside antiviral agents, is used primarily to treat HSV and VZV infections. Other acyclic nucleosides include ganciclovir and penciclovir, which both contain a guanine base.

While the nucleoside drugs developed in the 1970s and early 1980s were successful antiviral agents, none was effective against the HIV infection that leads to AIDS and emerged as a pandemic in the mid-1980s. The first drugs to treat AIDS were not approved until the late 1980s; they were nucleoside analogs that targeted the enzyme reverse transcriptase and are known as nucleoside reverse transcriptase inhibitors or NRTIs. HIV is an RNA-based retrovirus, which relies on its reverse transcriptase (RT) to catalyze transcription of viral RNA to proviral DNA. Reverse transcriptase is a type of polymerase, and its mechanism is described in Chapter 7. In theory, treatment with an RT inhibitor immediately after exposure could prevent the initial formation of viral DNA and thereby prevent permanent infection. Indeed, this rationale is the basis for post-exposure prophylaxis (PEP), which is used to treat individuals who may have been exposed, for example, via occupational exposure to blood of an infected individual. However, RT inhibition is also effective once permanent infection is established, since it will prevent formation of new viral particles. Unlike most host polymerases, however, the HIV RT does not possess a repair function, so that when an error in transcription is made, it persists. The lack of a repair mechanism allows NRTIs to be quite effective. These nucleoside analogs, like those described above, are considered competitive inhibitors/substrates and act at the active site. Despite the availability of X-ray structures of reverse transcriptase, design of inhibitors is often based more on an empirical approach, since the molecule needs to be recognized and acted upon by multiple enzymes (kinases and RT) to be active. The considerable historical work in the area of nucleoside analogs that inhibited related polymerases or other DNA processing enzymes as anti-cancer agents was the basis of much of the earliest work on RT inhibitors.

In 1987, azidothymidine (AZT) became the first approved treatment for HIV/AIDS. (Figure 11.9). It was originally synthesized in the 1960s as a potential anti-cancer drug and had been reported to be active against a retrovirus. It was one of many nucleosides screened for activity against HIV-infected cells. Its development relied on a collaboration between the pharmaceutical company Burroughs Wellcome and the U.S. National Cancer Institute (NCI), based on the historical interest of Burroughs Wellcome in antiviral nucleoside analogs and the specialized capabilities of NCI for antiviral testing and access to patients. The approval of AZT occurred in record time and was based on data from only one clinical trial. The lack of HIV/AIDS animal models, as well as the urgent medical need, allowed a minimal development time. The sole clinical trial was stopped after only 19 weeks when data showed that the treatment group was much healthier than the placebo group, and it was deemed unethical to continue to administer a placebo to patients. Along with AZT, a number of other nucleoside analogs have been found to be effective against HIV: didanosine (ddI), zalcitabine (ddC), and stavudine (d4T) had all been synthesized in the 1960s as potential anti-cancer agents, and were among the earliest drugs approved for the treatment of HIV/AIDS. The enantiomer of the thiosugar analog of zalcitabine, lamivudine, and a base-modified derivative, emtricitabine, are also effective against HIV as well as against hepatitis B infection. Many of these drugs suffer from poor bioavailability and require frequent dosing.

Carbocyclic nucleoside analogs, where the ring oxygen is replaced with a carbon, have also been investigated. Two that have been successful are entecavir and abacavir, which are used to treat chronic hepatitis B and HIV infections, respectively. Lamivudine, emtricitabine, entecavir, and abacavir all contain significant structural modifications to the furanose ring. However, all NRTIs (see Figure 11.9) contain a 5′-hydroxyl group, are activated to the triphosphate, are recognized by RT, and act as chain terminators.

Figure 11.9 HIV nucleoside reverse transcriptase inhibitors and other nucleoside antiviral agents. Structures of NRTIs and the year of their approval are shown. Azidothymidine, didanosine, zalcitabine and stavudine are structurally close to the natural nucleoside with minor modifications on the ribose unit. Lamivudine, emtricitabine, and entecavir contain significant changes to the ribose; abacavir contains a modified base and unsaturated ribose. All compounds retain a 5′-OH group that is phosphorylated and incorporated into the growing nucleic acid chain, resulting in chain termination.

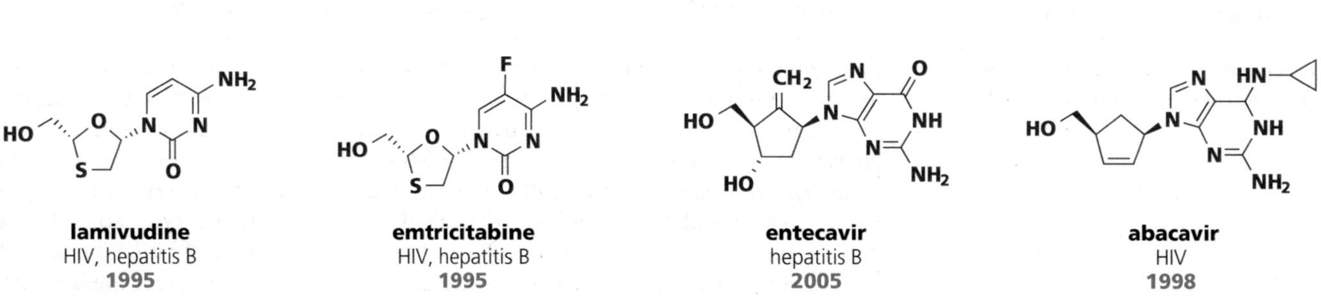

azidothymidine
HIV
1987

didanosine
HIV
1991

zalcitabine
HIV
1992

stavudine
HIV
1994

lamivudine
HIV, hepatitis B
1995

emtricitabine
HIV, hepatitis B
1995

entecavir
hepatitis B
2005

abacavir
HIV
1998

11.4 Prodrugs improve the properties and effectiveness of nucleosides

As shown in Figure 11.7, nucleoside drugs require a complex series of transformations to generate the active triphosphate. This requirement, coupled with some of their physical properties requires high dosing; efforts to overcome the poor bioavailability has led to the application of prodrug strategies. One approach has focused on ester prodrugs of acyclic nucleosides. Valacyclovir, the valine ester of acyclovir, has approximately four-fold better oral bioavailability than acyclovir (**Figure 11.10**) and is used to treat various herpes infections, as is valganciclovir. Famciclovir is a diacetate ester, but is also modified at the base. Hydrolysis of the esters and oxidation of the purine ring generates the acyclic nucleoside penciclovir. Due to its poor oral bioavailability, penciclovir is only used topically, but famciclovir, with 77% oral bioavailability, is used to treat both VZV and HSV infections. In these prodrug examples, the esters are cleaved by host enzymes to reveal the 5′-OH.

In addition to improving oral bioavailability, nucleoside prodrug strategies have also been applied to circumvent the first phosphorylation step on the pathway to the active triphosphate. This step, carried out by kinases, is considered to be the most discriminating, and therefore efforts to design analogs that would bypass it are an active area of research. The monophosphate cannot be administered directly due to its highly charged nature and therefore lack of permeability, as well as its relative instability.

The prodrug sofosbuvir (see Figure 11.10) is approved for the treatment of HCV infections, and its triphosphate inhibits the NS5B protein, which is HCV's viral RNA polymerase. Sofosbuvir is an example of the use of a pronucleotide (ProTide) strategy, developed by Christopher McGuigan. Hydrolysis *in vivo* of the aryloxy

valacyclovir (R = H)
valganciclovir (R = CH₂OH)

acyclovir (R = H)
ganciclovir (R = CH₂OH)

Figure 11.10 Structures of nucleoside prodrugs. Valacyclovir and valganciclovir are valine esters of acyclic nucleosides. Famciclovir, a di-ester, requires oxidation to form the guanine base as well as hydrolysis of the esters to generate penciclovir (ester groups are shown in red). Sofosbuvir is a phosporamidate ester (shown in red) that is hydrolyzed to the monophosphate, thereby bypassing the need for the first slow phosphorylation step.

famciclovir

penciclovir

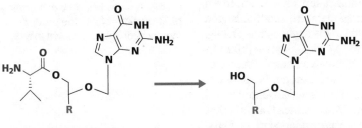

sofosbuvir

sofosbuvir monophosphate

sofosbuvir triphosphate
(active form)

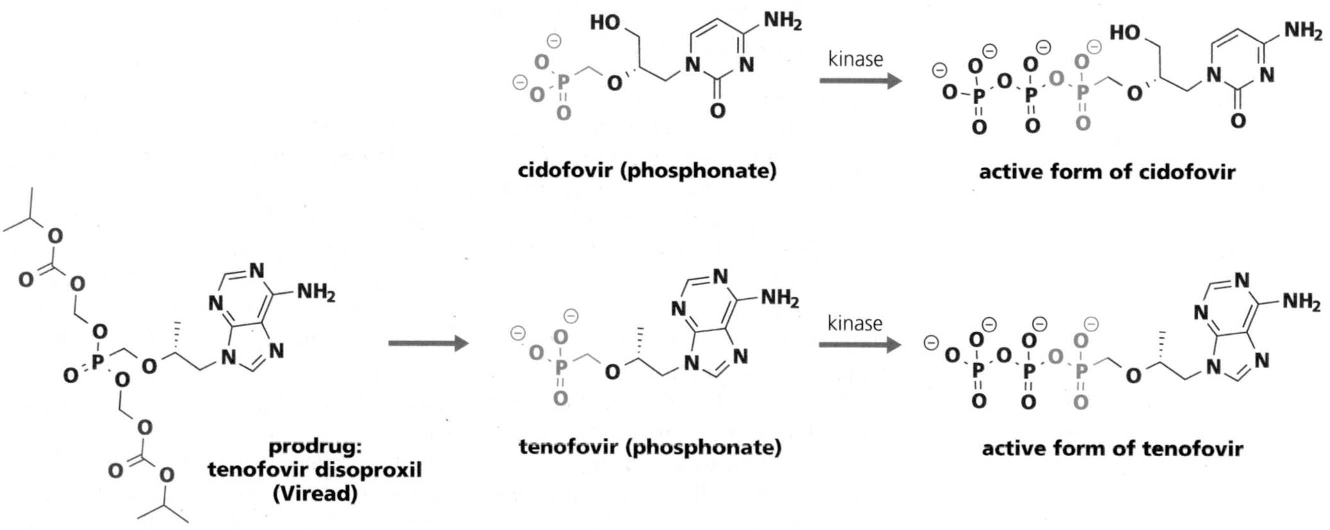

cidofovir (phosphonate)

active form of cidofovir

prodrug:
tenofovir disoproxil
(Viread)

tenofovir (phosphonate)

active form of tenofovir

phosphoramidate triester generates the monophosphate, which is then converted by kinases to the active triphosphate. The enzymes responsible for its activation reside in the liver, the site of HCV infection, and this also contributes to its efficacy. Sofosbuvir was invented at Pharmasset in 2007 and proceeded rapidly to clinical trials in 2010. Its remarkable activity in combination with other HCV drugs (it is curative) led to rapid FDA approval in 2013 to treat hepatitis C infection.

A related strategy incorporates a phosphonate in place of the monophosphate; in addition to bypassing the first kinase step, this modification affords improved stability. The acyclic phosphonate cidofovir, due to its charged nature, is administered intravenously; it is used to treat CMV retinitis. It is converted to the triphosphate analog, which is a substrate for viral DNA polymerase (**Figure 11.11**). Phosphonate prodrugs have also been developed to improve physical properties. Viread is a phosphonate ester prodrug of tenofovir. The esters are cleaved in the gut to generate the monophosphonate, which, unlike the monophosphate, is stable to esterases. This monophosphonate is a substrate for the next two kinases to afford the triphosphate analog, which is an inhibitor of HIV reverse transcriptase (see Figure 11.11). Although it was developed to treat HIV, Viread has also been approved for the treatment of hepatitis B infections.

Figure 11.11 Examples of antiviral nucleoside phosphonates. Cidofovir and tenofovir are nucleoside phosphonates (phosphonate moiety is shown in blue). The phosphonates are more stable than the monophosphate but are still recognized by kinases to generate the active triphosphate analog. Tenofovir disoproxil is an ester prodrug of tenofovir; the prodrug moiety hydrolyzed is shown in red.

11.5 Some HIV drugs that target reverse transcriptase bind at allosteric sites

In addition to being inhibited by nucleosides, HIV reverse transcriptase is also sensitive to allosteric inhibition by nonnucleoside drugs. In the early search for drugs to treat AIDS, many compound libraries were screened for anti-RT activity, leading to hits from unexpected drug classes. Nevirapine is one such example. Screening for inhibitors of RT identified a hit originally synthesized as a potential muscarinic antagonist in the 1960s. The hit was optimized by chemists at Boehringer Ingelheim for potency and physical properties and approved to treat AIDS in 1996. Other nonnucleoside reverse transcriptase inhibitors (NNRTIs) were also developed from screening programs, leading to additional drugs in this class. At Upjohn, 1500 compounds of distinct structural classes in their compound library were chosen for screening based on computational analysis for dissimilarity. Screening against HIV-1 RT led to 100 compounds that were active and, after optimization, to delavirdine. At DuPont, similar screening of their compound library identified an unstable hit that was optimized, resulting in efavirenz. Rapid emergence of resistance to these NNRTIs was noted and was likely due to the molecules acting at an allosteric site that was not essential for enzymatic activity. **Figure 11.12** shows the first-generation NNRTIs that are approved to treat HIV/AIDS.

Efforts to identify second-generation NNRTIs focused on screening and optimizing inhibitors that were active against multiple resistant strains of HIV. The structures of the

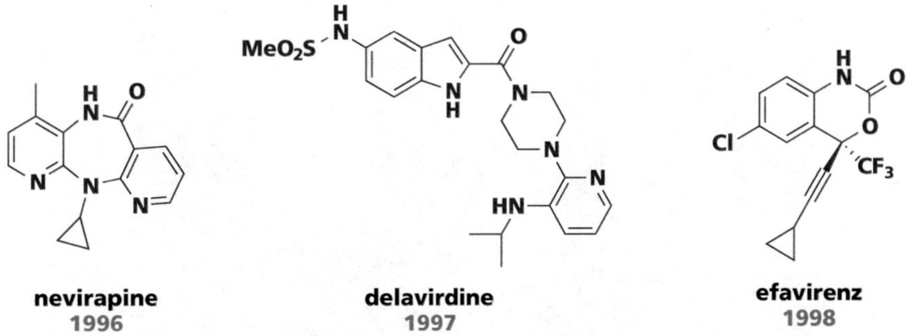

Figure 11.12 Structures of first-generation nonnucleoside reverse transcriptase inhibitors and year of approval. The NNRTIs nevirapine, delavirdine and efavirenz were derived from hits identified from library screening for activity against HIV RT, and act at an allosteric site.

nevirapine
1996

delavirdine
1997

efavirenz
1998

newer NNRTIs, etravirine and rilpivirine, are considerably more flexible than the first-generation compounds (**Figure 11.13**). It is believed that the flexible nature of these compounds allows them to adapt to mutations in the active site while still maintaining their inhibitory effects. These compounds can be traced to early screening efforts at the Rega Institute for Medical Research. They screened 600 compounds from Janssen Pharmaceuticals and identified tetrahydroimidazobenzodiazepinone (TIBO) and related thione analogs as well as α-aminophenylacetamide (α-APA) scaffolds as leads that inhibited replication of HIV-1. Mechanistic studies identified RT as the target of the compounds. One of the TIBO leads was investigated further in a search for compounds with activity against resistant strains, and this effort ultimately resulted in tivirapine, which progressed to clinical trials. The APA leads evolved into etravirine and rilpivirine, approved in 2008 and 2011, respectively (Figure 11.13). The development of rilpivirine from the APA lead is outlined in Case Study 2 in this chapter.

The NNRTIs bind at a common site on the enzyme ~10–15 Å away from the catalytic site, but precisely how they inhibit the enzyme is not well understood. The flexibility and large size of the enzyme (a heterodimer consisting of 66 and 51 kDa subunits), its multiple components, and its relative insolubility have made biophysical studies challenging. X-ray crystallography of HIV RT shows a structure like a right hand, with fingers, a thumb, and a palm region. One common theory is that NNRTIs act as a molecular wedge and lock the thumb region into an open conformation (known as an arthritic thumb) (**Figure 11.14**), resulting in a change in orientation of the catalytic triad at the active site. It should be noted that this hypothesis is still controversial, and exactly how these allosteric modulators result in inhibition is not completely understood.

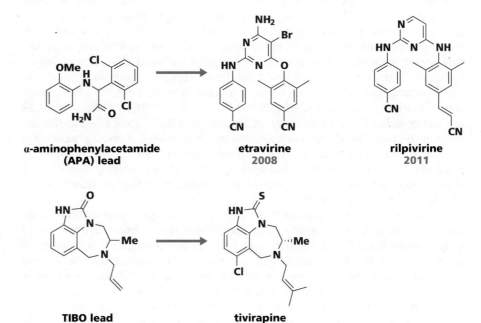

α-aminophenylacetamide
(APA) lead

etravirine
2008

rilpivirine
2011

TIBO lead

tivirapine

Figure 11.13 Second-generation nonnucleoside reverse transcriptase inhibitors. Etravirine and rilpivirine are approved to treat HIV and were derived from an α-aminophenylacetamide (APA) lead. Tivirapine was based on the tetrahydroimidazobenzodiazepinone (TIBO) lead and advanced to clinical trials.

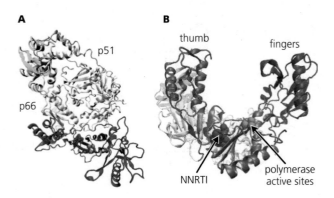

Figure 11.14 Structure of efavirenz bound to HIV RT. A: HIV-1 RT is a heterodimer consisting of p66 (multi-colored) and p51 (light gray) subunits with an RNase H domain (green, not labelled). B: View along HIV-1 RT from the polymerase active site illustrates the resemblance of the p66 subunit to an open hand: the fingers are shown in blue, the palm in dark gray, the thumb in red, the linker in yellow, and the RNase H domain in green. In both figures, the location of the polymerase active-site triad is depicted in orange, and the location of the bound NNRTI efavirenz is shown in magenta. (From Wright DW, Sadiq SK, De Fabritiis G & Coveney PV [2012] *J Am Chem Soc* 134:12885–12888. With permission from American Chemical Society.)

11.6 Viral protease inhibitors have been developed by use of structure-based drug design

One of the most successful applications of structure-based drug design has been the development of HIV protease inhibitors. The role of the protease enzyme (PR) of HIV is to cleave the Gag-Pol fusion protein into smaller functional and structural viral proteins, such as reverse transcriptase and integrase, that are essential for the replication, function, and maturation of infectious viral particles. Sequencing of the HIV genome led to the conclusion that the virus encoded an aspartyl protease (see Section 7.5). Target validation was based on observations that mutating the putative active-site aspartate residues resulted in immature, non-infectious viral particles. Drug discovery was accelerated by the considerable medicinal chemistry expertise accumulated in designing transition-state mimetics (described in Chapter 4) for other aspartyl proteases, such as renin.

Many of the HIV protease inhibitors were designed on the basis of specific cleavage sites that are recognized by the enzyme. Phenylalanine-proline (Phe-Pro) and tyrosine-proline (Tyr-Pro) were two such recognition sites, not commonly cleaved by human proteases. By use of a substrate-like scaffold and incorporation of transition-state mimetics, a series of inhibitors of HIV protease was developed. An X-ray structure of the enzyme was solved in 1989, and it showed a homodimer with C_2 symmetry. This information, combined with knowledge acquired from the design of other aspartyl protease inhibitors, rapidly led to a number of transition-state analogs being advanced as HIV protease inhibitors (**Figure 11.15**). Many of these (such as saquinavir, indinavir, and nelfinavir) retain vestiges of the original Phe-Pro peptide substrate on which the design was based. Some, such as ritonavir and lopinavir, were developed from C_2 symmetrical leads designed to inhibit the enzyme and still retain some of that symmetry, as evidenced by the presence of two benzyl groups flanking the transition-state mimetic. One exception is tipranavir, which was based on hits from high-throughput screening.

Many of the early compounds suffered from very poor oral bioavailability and required frequently administered high doses. These poor pharmaceutical properties are likely due to the molecules' high molecular weights, the presence of multiple peptide bonds, and their highly polar nature. Furthermore, like the reverse transcriptase inhibitors, resistance toward them soon developed. Newer compounds such as tipranavir and darunavir are less prone to the development of resistance.

The broad activity of darunavir against resistant strains is based on a design strategy to maximize interactions with backbone amides rather than side-chain

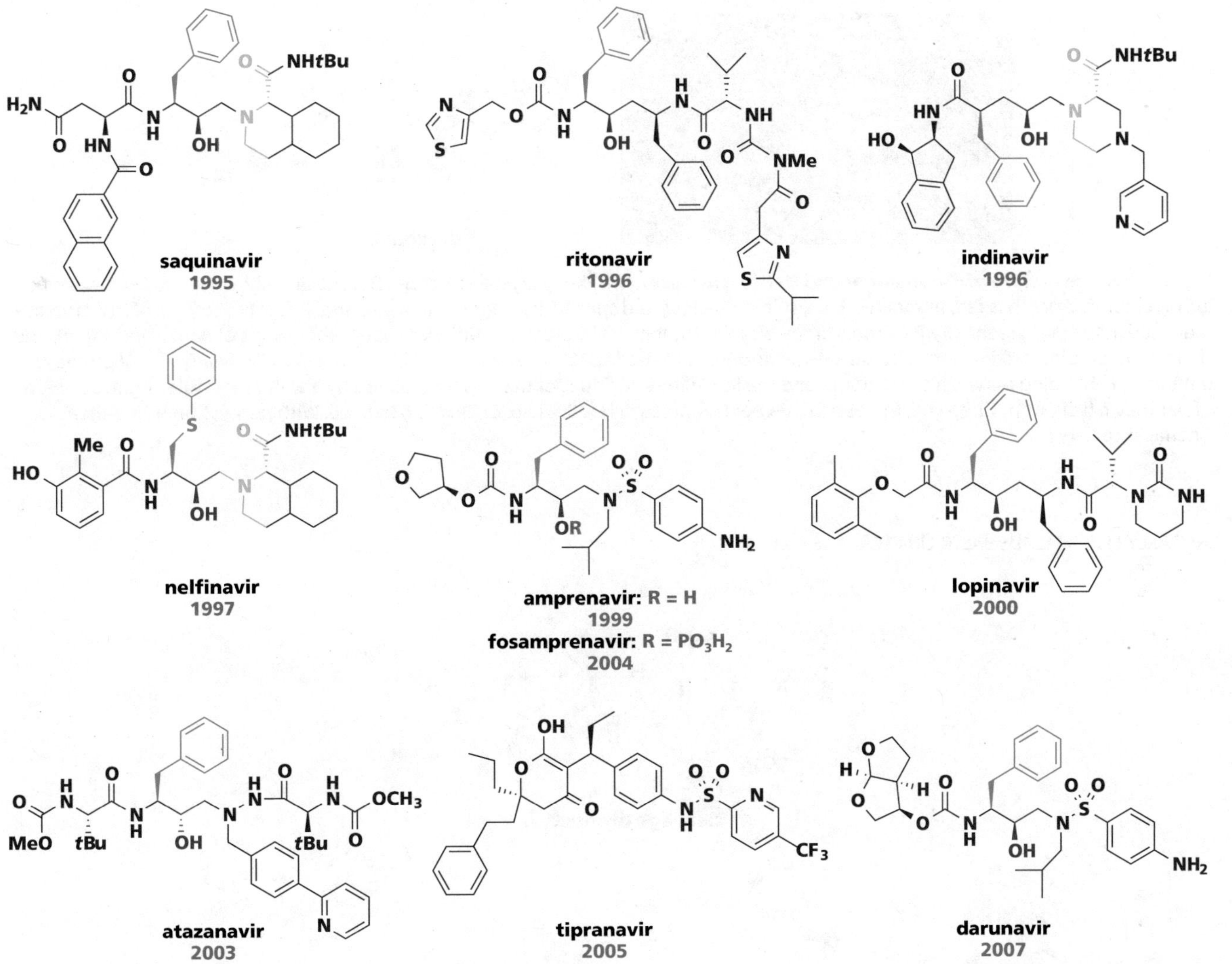

Figure 11.15 Structures of HIV protease inhibitors, in order of date of approval. All except tipranavir contain transition state mimetics (show in red), and are based on mimicking the enzyme's natural substrate (fosamprenavir is a pro-drug of amprenavir). In these cases, structural features of the Phe-Pro cleavage site are evident: Phe mimic in blue, and Pro mimic in green. The symmetry evident in ritonavir and lopinavir reflect the *C2* symmetry of the enzyme. The exception, tipranavir, was evolved from a high throughput screening hit.

moieties. It was known that drug-resistant strains undergo significant reorganization of protein side chains, compared to native strains, but minimal movement in the protein backbone. As predicted, X-ray co-crystal results of darunavir bound to HIV protease showed that the two oxygen atoms in the bicyclic ether group made H-bonds with Asp29 and Asp30 in the main chain (**Figure 11.16**). In addition, polar interactions between the aniline nitrogen of the inhibitor and the amide in the main chain and the carboxylate oxygen of Asp30′ were also observed.

The success of the HIV protease inhibitors has led to the search for inhibitors of other virus-specific proteases. The hepatitis C virus was identified as a unique virus in 1989, and cloning of the HCV genome identified the proteolytic enzyme HCV NS3 as a potential drug target. Lessons learned from drug discovery efforts in the HIV arena have been applied to HCV, with a number of drugs approved. The observation that the NS3 protease was subject to feedback inhibition by two of the N-terminal peptide products led to the design of early peptide leads for enzyme inhibition. One of these is the N-acylated hexapeptide shown in **Figure 11.17A**, which is a cleavage product from proteolysis of the substrate at a cysteine residue. Several peptide analogs of this product were prepared as inhibitors, with two early leads shown in Figure 11.17A. Notably, the tetrapeptide lacking N-terminal residues and containing a vinylcyclopropane replacement for the P1 thiol, was a potent enzyme inhibitor. Modification of these leads ultimately afforded the drugs boceprevir, telaprevir, and asunaprevir (**Figure 11.17B**). Common features based on the original peptide include the P3/P2 core based on the Val-Pro segment.

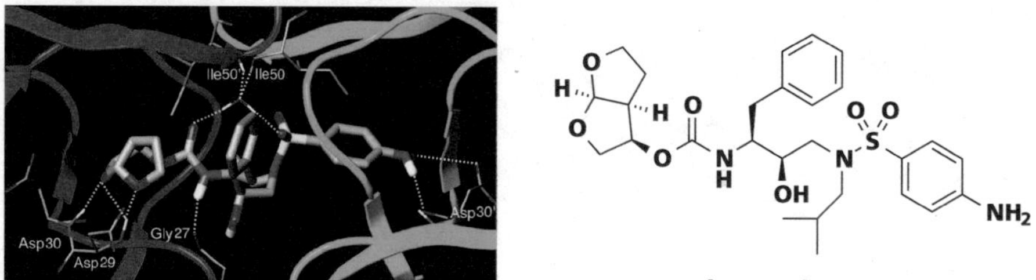

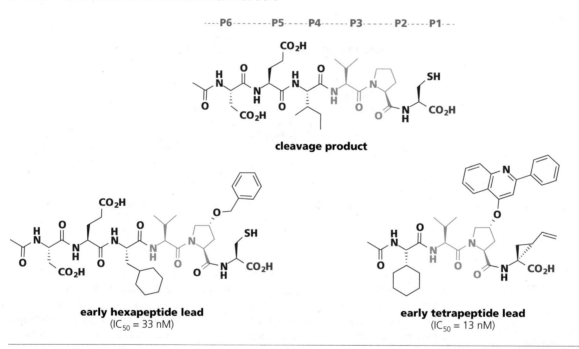

darunavir

Figure 11.16 Structure of darunavir bound to HIV protease. Left: X-ray crystal structure. Darunavir is shown in gray with specific atoms colored: oxygen is red, nitrogen is blue, sulfur is yellow, and specific hydrogens are white. Individual monomers of HIV protease indicated in red and green. Oxygen atoms of the bicyclic ether make interactions with backbone N-H groups of Asp29 and Asp30, and there is an ionic interaction between the aniline nitrogen and the Asp30′ carboxylate and backbone. As with nearly all HIV protease inhibitors, H-bonding between the inhibitor and the Ile50/Ile50′ residues of the flap is mediated by a water molecule. Right: Structure of darunavir. (Left, from Ghosh AK, Chapsal BD, Weber IT & Mitsuya H [2008] *Acc Chem Res* 41:78–86. With permission from American Chemical Society.)

A: EARLY PEPTIDE LEADS BASED ON CLEAVAGE PRODUCTS

cleavage product

early hexapeptide lead
(IC$_{50}$ = 33 nM)

early tetrapeptide lead
(IC$_{50}$ = 13 nM)

B: EARLY DRUGS DEVELOPED FROM MODIFICATION OF PEPTIDE LEADS

boceprevir

telaprevir

asunaprevir

Figure 11.17 Evolution of early HCV NS3 protease inhibitors. A: The peptide was derived from cleavage products of the NS3 protease, which caused feedback inhibition of the enzyme. The hexapeptide and tetrapeptide leads were designed to mimic this cleavage product. B: Modification of the tetrapeptide lead afforded the earliest HCV NS3 protease inhibitors, boceprevir and telaprevir (both now withdrawn), and the later drug asunaprevir (approved in Japan). All maintain versions of the Val-Pro segment found in the original peptides (shown in blue), with the *tert*-butyl group replacing the isopropyl group.

Boceprevir (Merck) and telaprevir (Vertex) were approved in 2011 to treat patients with the G1 genotype of HCV. Both contain a keto-amide warhead, with the active-site serine forming a covalent bond to the ketone (see Section 7.5). Both drugs were given in combination with interferon and ribavirin and were effective in more than half of patients that were nonresponsive to the interferon/ribavirin combination alone. More recent efforts focused on drugs that can be given as a single oral dose without interferon, and these have supplanted telaprevir and boceprevir.

Newer drugs, approved since 2013, such as grazoprevir and the related glecaprevir and voxilaprevir, as well as simeprevir, and paritaprevir, (**Figure 11.18**) were developed by applying conformational constraint strategies to the linear peptides by tethering the binding elements to form a macrocycle (see Section 4.13).

All of these agents are given in combination with other drugs that target HCV-specific proteins. They are distinguished from telaprevir and boceprevir in that they do not require co-administration with interferon to be effective, and have fewer side effects.

Two specific examples of application of the conformational constraint strategy are highlighted in **Figure 11.19**. BILN 2061, developed at Boehringer Ingelheim, was a more potent enzyme inhibitor than the linear tetrapeptide (IC_{50} of 3 nM versus 13 nM for the tetrapeptide, Figure 11.19A) This compound was designed by linking the P1 and P3 regions of the lead, and advanced to clinical trials.

Docking of the linear tetrapeptide into the enzyme active site showed binding of the His528 residue in the protease to the carbonyl of the P4 amide and Gln526 binding to the P2 O-arylquinolone (Figure 11.19A). Because of these important interactions, chemists at Merck proposed to constrain those two binding elements by linking P2 to a truncated P4, as shown in Figure 11.19B. As with the P1–P3 constraint, the P2–P4 constraint developed into a compound with improved enzyme affinity compared to the acyclic peptide; incorporation of a sulfonamide bioisostere ("second series") for the P1 carboxylic acid provided a compound with sub-nanomolar affinity. Optimization occurred by introducing branching of the P3 side chain (to a tert-butyl moiety) and removal of the phenyl substituent on the quinolone. This advanced lead resulted in a compound with similar potency, that achieved high concentration in the target organ (liver).

Figure 11.18 Structures of conformationally constrained macrocyclic HCV NS3 protease inhibitors. Grazoprevir, glecaprevir and voxilaprevir resulted from linking between the P2 and P4 peptide positions; simeprevir and paritapevir are linked between P1 and P3 peptide positions. All contain the sulfonamide bioisostere for the carboxylic acid.

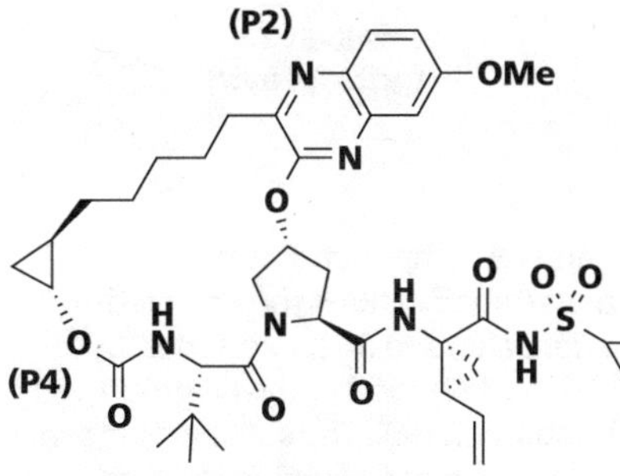

grazoprevir

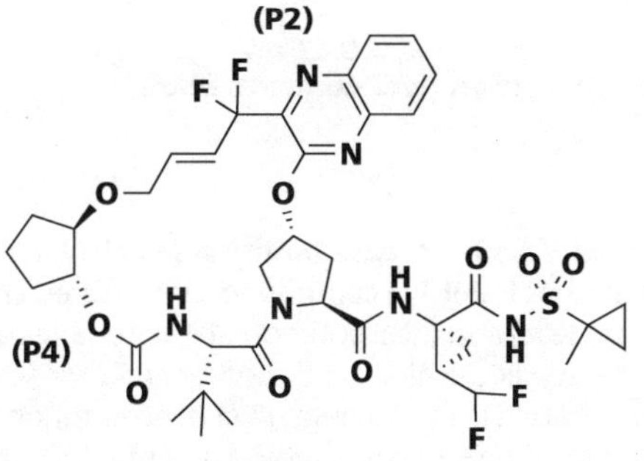

glecaprevir

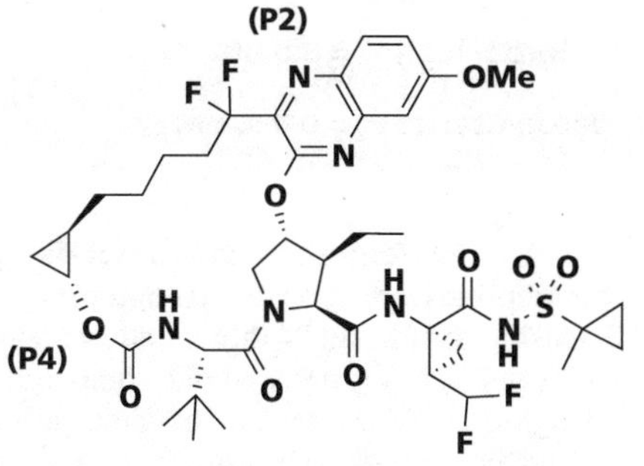

voxilaprevir

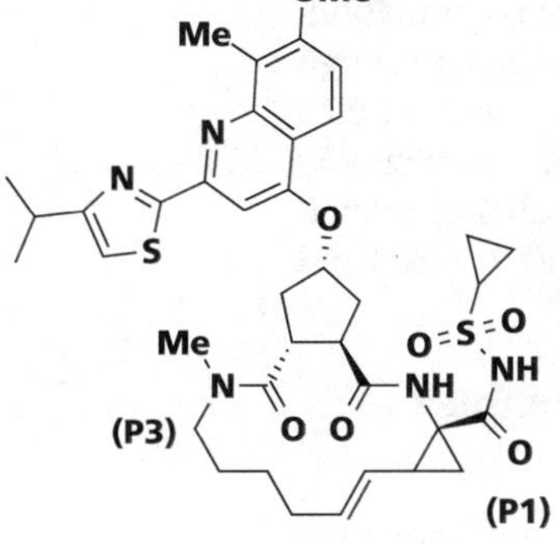

simeprevir

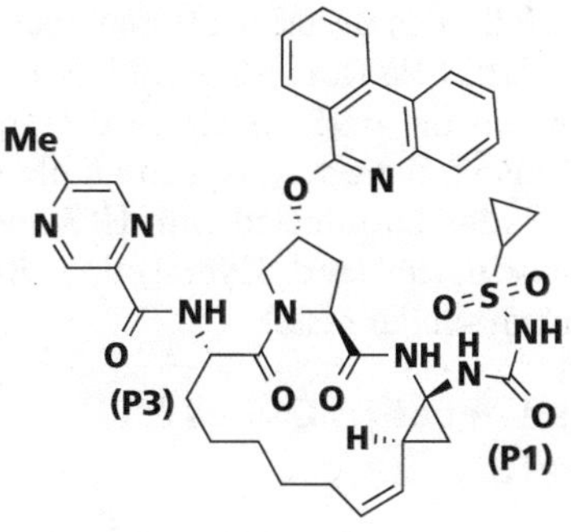

paritaprevir

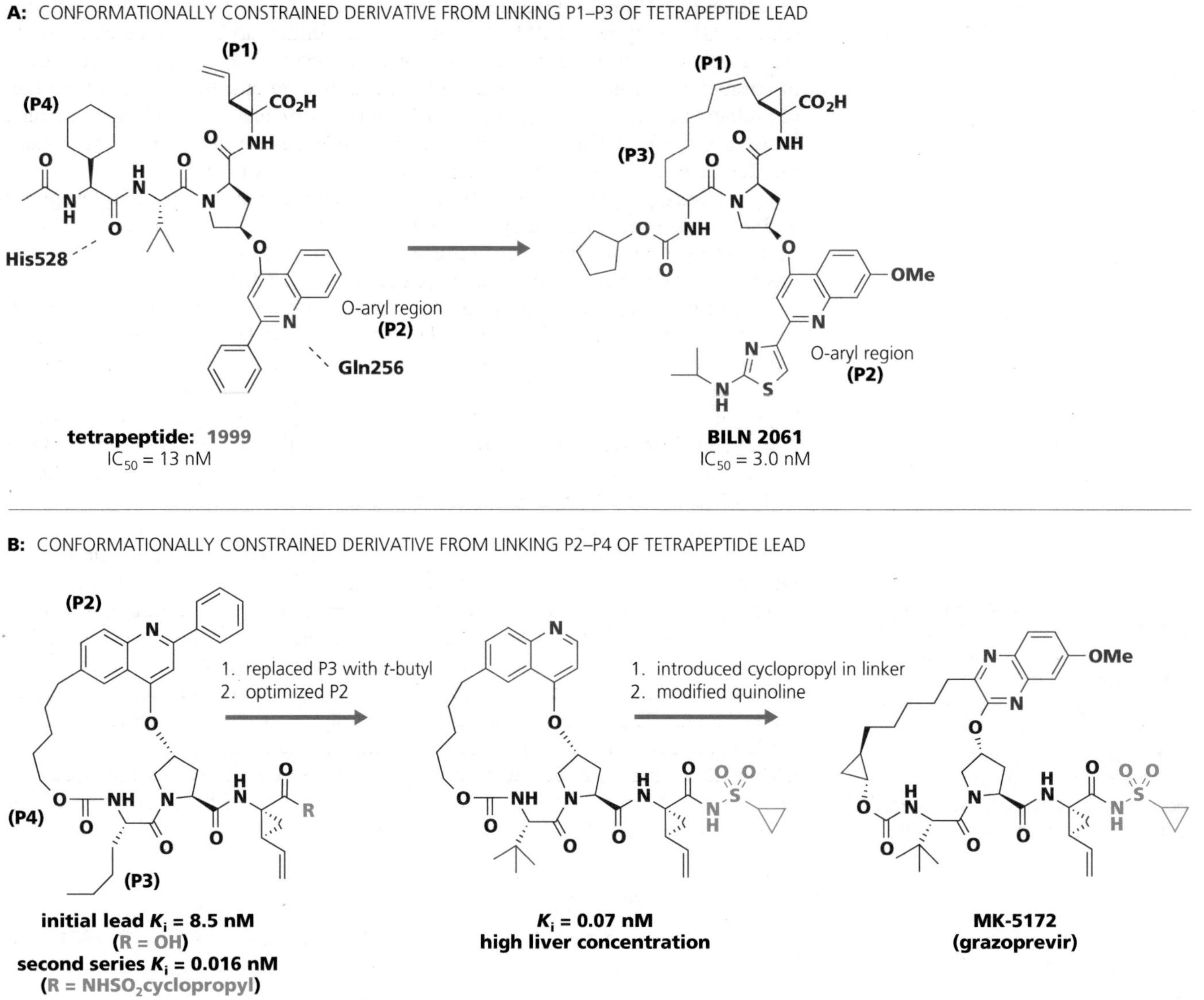

A: CONFORMATIONALLY CONSTRAINED DERIVATIVE FROM LINKING P1–P3 OF TETRAPEPTIDE LEAD

tetrapeptide: 1999
IC_{50} = 13 nM

BILN 2061
IC_{50} = 3.0 nM

B: CONFORMATIONALLY CONSTRAINED DERIVATIVE FROM LINKING P2–P4 OF TETRAPEPTIDE LEAD

1. replaced P3 with *t*-butyl
2. optimized P2

1. introduced cyclopropyl in linker
2. modified quinoline

initial lead K_i = 8.5 nM
(R = OH)
second series K_i = 0.016 nM
(R = NHSO₂cyclopropyl)

K_i = 0.07 nM
high liver concentration

MK-5172
(grazoprevir)

Figure 11.19 Tethering strategy for design of HCV NS3 protease inhibitors. A: Linking the P1 and P3 components of the tetrapeptide lead, upon further optimization, led to BILN 2061, a compound that entered clinical trials (modifications shown in red). B: Linking the P2 and P4 regions afforded an initial lead, and incorporation of a sulfonamide bioisostere afforded a second series, both with significantly greater affinity compared to the acyclic peptide . In the sulfonamide series (in blue), optimization of the P2 group and changing the P3 group to a tert-butyl gave an optimized lead with high liver concentration (modifications in red). The sulfonamide series was further optimized by introduction of a cyclopropyl group in the linker, and quinolone modification, ultimately leading to grazoprevir.

This conformational constraint strategy ultimately led to the development of MK-5172 (grazoprevir), which received FDA approval when used in combination with the NS5A inhibitor MK-8742 (elbasvir, described in the next section). This combination, like other combinations of HCV NS3 and NS5A inhibitors, was awarded breakthrough designation by the FDA, on the basis of phase II results, which showed a 100% decrease in viral load. This co-therapy was also highly effective in the particularly challenging patient population co-infected with HIV and HCV, with 90% of treated patients showing a decrease in viral load. Several other combinations of HCV NS3 and NS5A inhibitors have shown similar results.

11.7   Inhibitors of the hepatitis C virus NS5A replication complex exhibit antiviral activity

In in the early 2000s, a number of organizations initiated high-throughput screening campaigns using cell-based replicon assays to identify inhibitors of viral replication.

Replicons consist of RNA from HCV that is non-infectious but capable of self-replicating in a cell. These cell-based assays allowed screening against the entire virus, rather than specific enzymes, and were an important advance for HCV drug discovery because HCV-infected cells are difficult to grow. This phenotypic screening, using the most prevalent genotypes of hepatitis C infections (GT1a and GT1b), identified compounds whose target was, at first, unknown, but later was determined to be NS5A and led to starting points of an entire class of anti-HCV agents. The eventual identification of HCV NS5A as the target was based on assaying early leads in the development of one of the drugs, daclatasvir, in cells infected with drug-resistant mutant virus (see Case Study 1 in this chapter). The HCV NS5A protein complex is essential for viral replication; however, its specific function is unknown. Daclatasvir, developed at Bristol-Myers Squibb, was approved by the FDA in 2015 (**Figure 11.20**) in combination with sofosbuvir. Several other HCV NS5A inhibitors, including ledipasvir, elbasvir, ombitasvir, velpatasvir, and pibrantasvir, have also been approved, all in combination with other anti-HCV agents.

During the course of discovery of daclatasvir, the importance of symmetry of the molecules was noted. HCV NS5A exists as a symmetrical dimer, and therefore symmetry of inhibitors is most likely related to their binding in the target. Several models of daclatasvir and other inhibitors binding to HCV NS5A have been developed that are based on X-ray structures of a portion of the protein; however, co-crystal structures have yet to be solved. Ledipasvir was optimized with a goal of high potency combined with a long half-life, and both symmetrical and unsymmetrical leads were investigated. An unsymmetrical imidazole/benzimidazole series ultimately led to ledipasvir, the first NS5A inhibitor approved. Elbasvir was elaborated from a hit derived

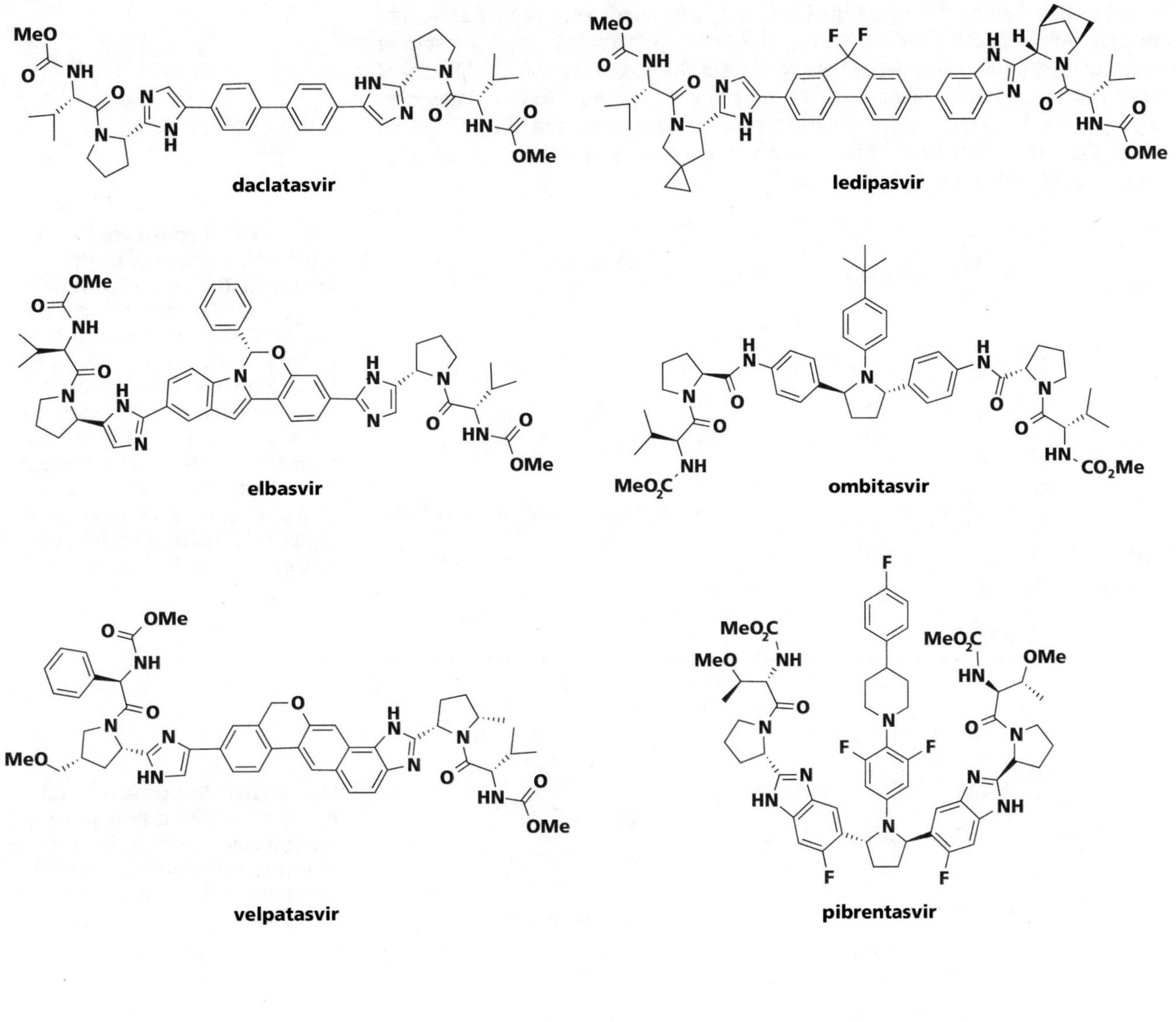

Figure 11.20 Examples of HCV NS5A inhibitors. These drugs inhibit the viral replication complex, and all have elements of symmetry in common. All are administered with other anti-HCV agents. The most recently approved agents, velpatasvir and pibrantasvir are effective against multiple resistant strains of HCV.

daclatasvir

ledipasvir

elbasvir

ombitasvir

velpatasvir

pibrentasvir

from HTS of an in-house library. Ombitasvir was derived from compounds containing chiral pyrrolidines to match the symmetry of the target. Velpatasvir was developed to be a pan-genotype inhibitor, improving on the spectrum of the first generation NS5A inhibitors. Pibrantasvir is highly potent (picomolar) against all of the common HCV genotypes as well as against common resistant mutants. These drugs are used in combination with HCV NS3 protease inhibitors, such as grazoprevir, or the NS5B polymerase inhibitor sofosbuvir. These combinations have revolutionized treatment for hepatitis C infection, which previously relied on a combination of interferon and ribavirin, which was much less effective and had severe side effects.

11.8 Drugs to treat retroviruses may target the viral integrase

Retroviruses, such as HIV, utilize a viral integrase (IN), which catalyzes the incorporation of viral DNA into the host genome through a complex multistep process. The newly synthesized viral DNA (formed by the action of reverse transcriptase) is processed at the 3′-end and forms a pre-integration complex. The complex migrates to the nucleus and is inserted into the host DNA by a metal-mediated transesterification reaction through a mechanism like the one shown in **Figure 11.21**. Two metal cations (M_A and M_B) at the enzyme active site are essential for the reaction and serve to activate and properly orient the nucleophile (3′-hydroxyl group of the viral nucleic acid) as well as to stabilize the pentacoordinate transition state, once formed. Following initial transesterification, the gaps between the viral and host DNA are closed by host polymerases (not shown).

Understanding the role and mechanism of IN suggested that screening for inhibitors of the enzyme might yield hits. For example, at Merck, 250,000 compounds were screened and the hits all contained a diketo function as well as an aromatic moiety. They were characterized as active site inhibitors that were competitive with the host DNA substrate. Other groups identified compounds with similar structural motifs. Optimization of hits led to two drugs: the N-methylpyrimidone raltegravir from Merck and the quinolone-derived elvitegravir from Gilead (**Figure 11.22**). Structural studies indicate that the coplanar oxygen atoms present in raltegravir and elvitegravir coordinate to the two metal (Mg^{2+}) ions in the enzyme active site and also bind to the viral DNA substrate. Like all other modern drug regimens, these compounds are used in combination with other anti-HIV drugs.

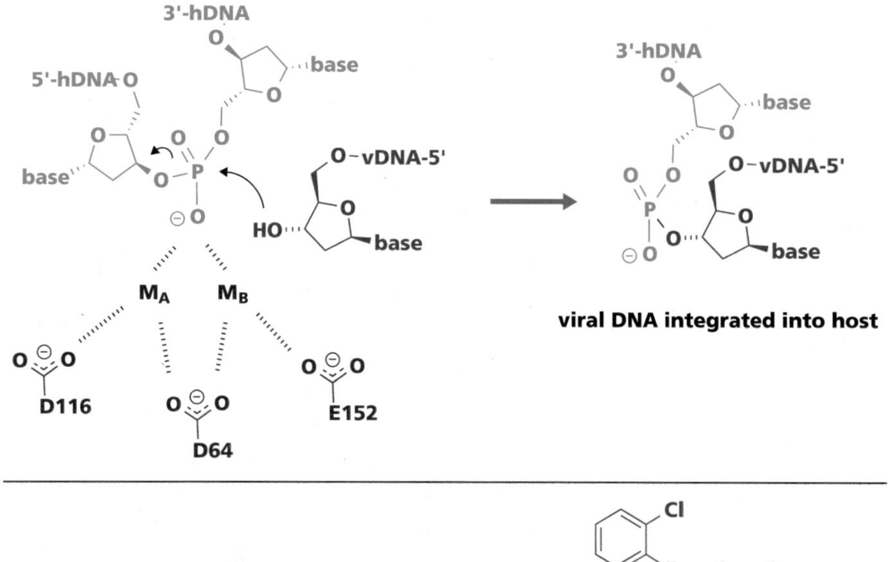

Figure 11.21 Representation of the reaction catalyzed by HIV integrase. The 3′-hydroxyl of viral DNA (vDNA, shown in red) adds to the phosphodiester of the host DNA (hDNA, shown in blue), which is coordinated through two metal ions (M_A and M_B) to acidic side chains of HIV integrase (D116, D64, and E152). The viral DNA becomes integrated into the host DNA after a further round of integration mediated by host polymerases (not shown), and a permanent infection results.

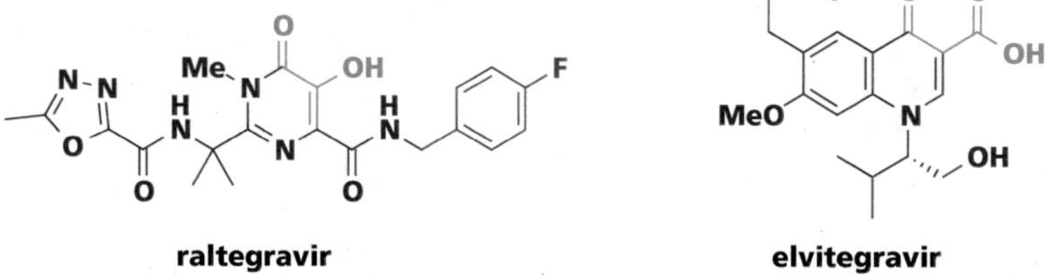

Figure 11.22 Structures of viral integrase inhibitors raltegravir and elvitegravir. Common pharmacophore elements are shown in blue (metal binding) and red (aromatic and hydrophobic).

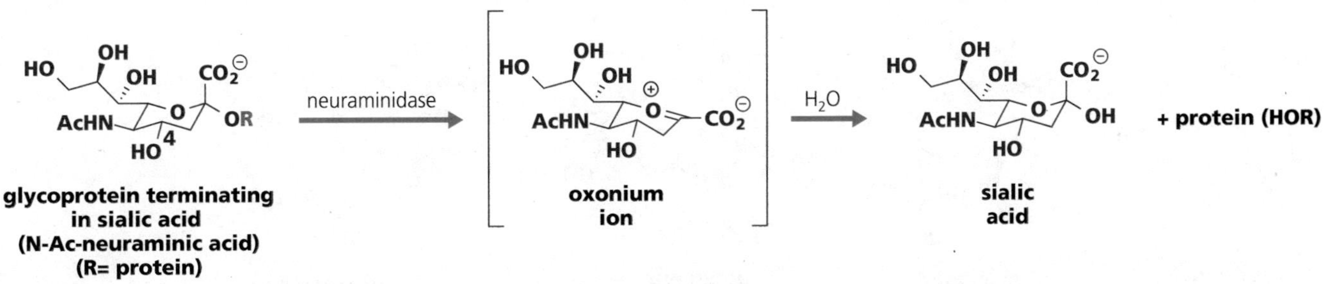

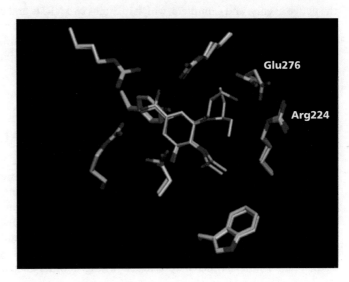

Figure 11.23 Neuraminidase-catalyzed cleavage of sialic acid from glycoprotein. Glycoproteins containing terminal sialic acid (also known as N-Ac-neuraminic acid) are substrates for neuraminidase, which cleaves off the carbohydrate. This abbreviated mechanism shows the intermediate where the pyranose ring develops a positive charge. Hydrolysis of the oxonium ion generates free sialic acid and the processed glycoprotein. Host neuraminidase activity is required for budding by influenza virions.

11.9 Influenza drugs target viral budding

Viral budding is an essential process for a virus to spread from one cell to another, and therefore, targeting this step is a viable therapeutic approach. To date, the only drugs that inhibit this process target influenza virus, an enveloped single-stranded RNA virus. Its viral surface glycoproteins are made up of hemagglutinin (H) and neuraminidase (N), and serotypes are characterized by antibody responses to H and N. For instance, the H5N1 strain causes avian flu, while the seasonal flu is primarily from H1N1, H1N2, and H3N2 variants. While the primary treatment is prevention of infection by vaccination, the most widely used small-molecule drugs are neuraminidase inhibitors. As mentioned earlier, the uncoating inhibitors amantadine and rimantadine (see Figure 11.5) are no longer recommended.

The enzyme neuraminidase is a glycoside hydrolase that cleaves terminal sialic acid (also called *N*-acetylneuraminic acid) residues from glycoproteins (**Figure 11.23**). The mechanism of the cleavage process involves an intermediate oxonium ion where the pyran oxygen holds a positive charge; hydrolysis generates the free sialic acid and the new glycoprotein. Sialic acid-containing glycoproteins are widely distributed on cell surfaces and are recognized by the protein hemagglutinin for attachment of influenza virions. When the new virions are ready to bud from the cell, cleavage of sialic acid residues from cellular glycoproteins facilitates their release. When neuraminidase is inhibited, influenza virions do not bud from cells, and their further spread to new cells is prevented.

The first X-ray crystal structure of a neuraminidase was solved in the early 1980s and led to structure-based drug discovery programs. On the basis of the structure of the active site, it was proposed that an amine or equivalent replacing the C-4 hydroxyl would afford important ionic binding interactions with a glutamate at the active site. Another important interaction is the ionic bond between the carboxylate of the substrate and two arginines of the enzyme. One example of a drug developed on the basis of the enzyme's X-ray structure is oseltamivir (**Figure 11.24**). An early neuraminidase inhibitor, Neu5Ac2en, which is identical to *N*-acetylneuraminic acid except for unsaturation at C2, mimics the intermediate oxonium ion. This compound had some activity in a mouse model of influenza and was a basis for later drugs. Oseltamivir replaces the

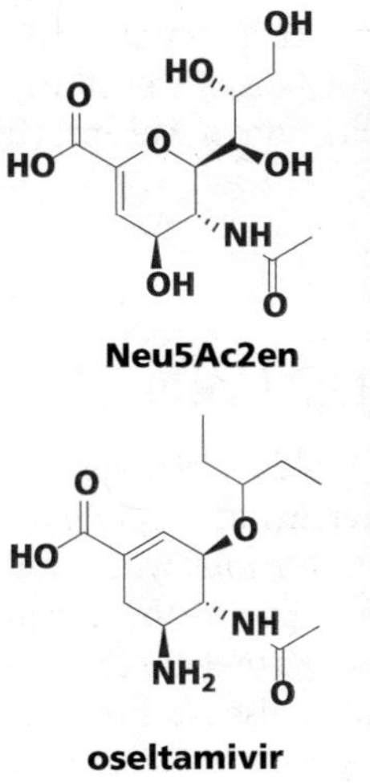

Figure 11.24 Overlay of X-ray structures of oseltamivir and Neu5Ac2en bound to neuraminidase. Oseltamivir (white) and Neu5Ac2en (green) occupy the same binding site. While Neu5Ac2en forms hydrogen bonds to Glu276, oseltamivir does not. In the oseltamivir co-structure, Glu276 reorients to form an ionic interaction with Arg224, exposing a hydrophobic surface that interacts with alkyl ether side chains. (From von Itzstein M [2007] *Nat Rev Drug Discovery* 6:967–974. With permission from Macmillan Publishers Limited.)

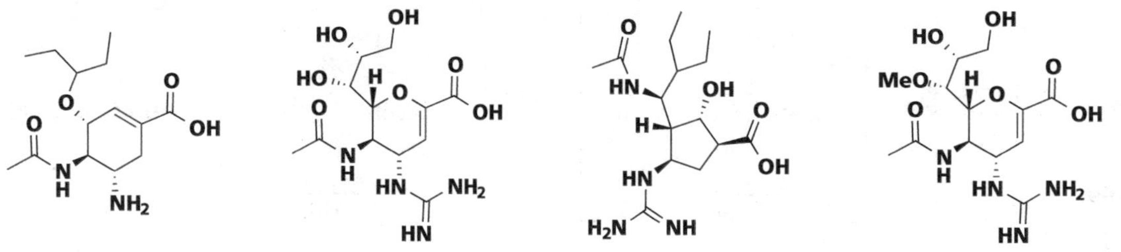

oseltamivir
2003

zanamivir
2003

peramivir
2014

laninamivir
(approved in Japan)

C4 hydroxyl group with an amine and the glycerol side chain with a 3-pentyl ether. While incorporation of the ether eliminated the possibility of hydrogen-bonding to the glutamate residue, reorientation of it exposes a hydrophobic surface that interacts with the alkyl chain of the ether. These interactions can be seen in Figure 11.24.

The drugs oseltamivir and zanamivir are transition-state mimetics (see Section 4.12) of the formation of the pyranosyl cation (oxonium ion), during the neuraminidase catalyzed hydrolysis reaction. Both contain an sp^2 carbon that resembles both the oxonium ion and the twist boat conformation generated in the transition state and seen in X-ray co-structures of sialic acid bound to neuraminidase. Additional neuraminidase inhibitors include the cyclopentane peramivir and laninamivir, which is a methoxy analog of zanamivir and is approved in Japan (**Figure 11.25**). Each structure contains a mimic of the flattened pyranose ring that forms in the transition state; in some cases it is achieved through incorporation of unsaturation and in others through contraction of the ring.

As seen in preceding sections, the life cycle of the virus contains a number of points of intervention for therapeutic agents. While some antiviral agents were developed on the basis of phenotypic screening, a majority were based on rational design. In contrast to anti-cancer drug discovery, the history of small-molecule antiviral drug discovery and medicinal chemistry is much more recent. In part, this is due to the nature of viruses, which can evolve and cause new diseases that spread rapidly. In fact, HIV/AIDS and HCV were virtually unknown prior to the mid-1980s. The ability of viruses to mutate has also encouraged the development of agents that are effective against multiple variants. More commonly, however, multidrug regimens are used that rely on different drugs affecting different points in the viral life cycle in an effort to minimize the development of resistance. Current practice for treating HIV/AIDS, called highly active anti-retroviral therapy (HAART), and HCV uses multiple drugs targeting multiple steps in the viral life cycle. In fact, many of the recently approved therapies are combinations of drugs formulated in one pill in an effort to ease the burden on patients and improve compliance. Examples include Stribild, which combines an integrase inhibitor, two RT inhibitors, and a pharmacokinetic enhancer that improves the bioavailability of the active agents; and Complera, which includes two NRTIs and one NNRTI. Harvoni, a combination of sofosbuvir and ledipasvir, has a cure rate of >90% in certain HCV patient populations. Approvals in 2017 include Vosevi, a combination of sofosbuvir, velpatasvir and the new drug voxilaprevir, and Mavyret, a combination of glecaprevir and pibrentasvir, that requires only 8 weeks of treatment.

Figure 11.25 Structures of the neuraminidase inhibitors used to treat influenza. Approved neuraminidase inhibitors, which are unsaturated at C2 (unsaturation is shown in red) and mimic the oxonium ion (Figure 11.23), except for peramivir which has a contracted cyclopentane ring. Oseltamivir and zanamivir were approved in the early 2000s; peramivir in 2014 and laninamivir is approved in Japan.

ANTIFUNGAL AGENTS: COMMON FUNGAL STRUCTURES, REPLICATION PROCESS, AND IMPACT

Unlike viruses, fungi are eukaryotic organisms; they include molds and yeasts as well as mushrooms. Some of the more common pathogenic fungi include *Aspergillus fumigatus*, *Candida albicans*, *Cryptococcus neoformans*, and *Pneumocystis* and *Histoplasma* species. Local or systemic infections can result from exposure to fungi in the environment (air, surfaces, soil) or from overgrowth of organisms that are present in normal human flora. Exposure alone does not necessarily lead to disease, however symptomatic infection is usually the result of fungal organisms evading host defenses in their target organs, which may be the skin, lung, or other deep tissue sites. Pathology is a result of numerous factors, such as release of toxic or destructive proteins and metabolites by the fungi, competition between fungi and host for nutrients, and host immune response. The specific symptoms associated with a particular fungal infection depend on the location of the infection and the immune status of the patient.

Over the past 50 years, there has been an increase in the number of fungal infections, both topical and systemic. While topical infections such as athlete's foot and thrush are somewhat minor, systemic infections may affect internal organs and are deadly. For example, mortality rates for patients infected with the three most common invasive species are 20–40% for *C. albicans*, 50–90% for *A. fumigatus*, and 20–70% for *C. neoformans*. The increase in invasive fungal infections is due, in part, to an increase in the number of patients who are immunocompromised from chemotherapy, organ transplantation, and certain disorders such as AIDS. In addition, the increased use of indwelling catheters and medical devices provides surfaces on which fungi can grow. Fungal biofilms on hospital surfaces are also a growing problem, mainly due to *C. albicans*.

The recorded history of fungal infections precedes that of bacterial and viral infection. In 1665, thrush (caused by *C. albicans*) was recorded as a fatal disease. In 1835, silkworm disease was attributed to the fungus *Beauveria bassiana*; this report is considered the first time an organism was identified as the cause of a disease. Until the 1940s, fungal infections were treated with nonselective toxic agents such as phenols. The first selective drugs were discovered in the 1940s, with the introduction of the natural product griseofulvin.

Unlike prokaryotic bacteria, or simpler viral particles, fungi are eukaryotes. They range from single-celled organisms like yeasts to multicellular organisms like mushrooms. Their structure is characterized by an outer cell wall composed of chitin, glucose polymers (β-(1,6) and (1,3) glucan polymers), and mannoproteins (proteins linked to mannose residues). The inner cell membrane is composed of phospholipids containing steroid ergosterol, rather than cholesterol, the constituent of animal cell membranes. The internal features of part of a fungal cell are very similar to mammalian cells, with a nucleus, mitochondria and ribosomes, and other cellular structures (**Figure 11.26**).

Figure 11.26 Model of fungal cell structure, with points of drug interaction. The fungal cell wall is composed of an outer layer of mannoproteins covering β-(1,6) and (1,3)-glucan polymers and a layer of chitin over the phospholipid bilayer of the cell membrane, which contains ergosterol. Inside the cell, there are mitochondria, ribosomes, and a nucleus. Points of action of the various drug classes are highlighted in the figure.

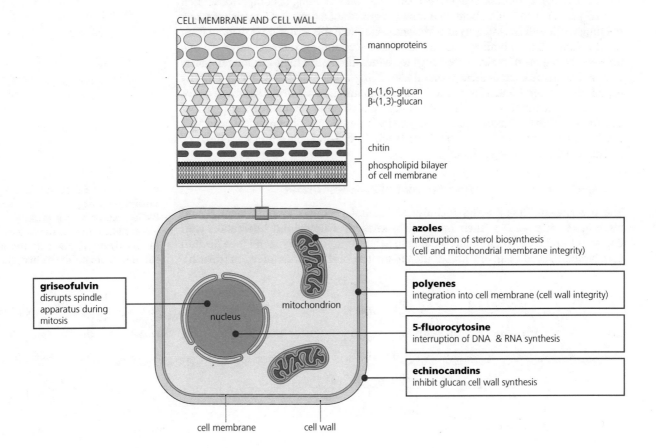

CELL MEMBRANE AND CELL WALL

mannoproteins

β-(1,6)-glucan
β-(1,3)-glucan

chitin

phospholipid bilayer
of cell membrane

azoles
interruption of sterol biosynthesis
(cell and mitochondrial membrane integrity)

polyenes
integration into cell membrane (cell wall integrity)

5-fluorocytosine
interruption of DNA & RNA synthesis

echinocandins
inhibit glucan cell wall synthesis

griseofulvin
disrupts spindle
apparatus during
mitosis

nucleus

mitochondrion

cell membrane   cell wall

Table 11.2   **Examples of small-molecule antifungal drugs and their mechanisms of action.**

Antifungal drug	Mechanism	Representative indication
amphotericin B, Nystatin	binds ergosterol, disrupts membrane integrity	Amphotericin: serious systemic fungal infection Nystatin: (topical) skin & mucosal infections
Ketoconazole, terbinafine itraconazole	inhibits ergosterol biosynthesis, disrupts membrane integrity	Ketoconazole (topical): skin infections (athlete's foot; dandruff) Itraconazole: blastomycosis, histoplasmosis, aspergilossis (in immunocompromised patients); fungal nail infections
griseofulvin, flucytosine	inhibits cell replication	Flucytosine: serious fungal infection caused by candida or cryptococcus Griseofulvin: skin, hair, nail infections
echinocandins	inhibits cell wall synthesis	Aspergillus and candida systemic infections

ANTIFUNGAL DRUG DISCOVERY

While fungal cell structure is similar to that of mammalian cells, there are some enzymes and structures, unique to fungi, that are targeted by antifungal drugs. Most drugs to treat fungal infections have, for the most part, been discovered by phenotypic assays for overall antifungal activity, and elucidation of their mechanisms has identified why they are selective. There are only a few classes of antifungal drugs: polyenes and azoles affect fungal cell membrane integrity, echinocandins affect cell-wall synthesis, 5-fluorocytosine affects DNA and RNA synthesis, and griseofulvin disrupts the spindle apparatus assembled during mitosis (Figure 11.26). **Table 11.2** highlights a few examples of antifungal agents that work via these different mechanisms.

DRUGS TARGETING FUNGI

The discovery of antifungal agents has been based on screening of compounds, often natural products, for their ability to inhibit the growth of a fungus. Many drugs target the fungal cell wall (its integrity and biosynthesis) since this structure is distinct from mammalian cell membranes, and this difference accounts for their selectivity. While the specific targets of many older drugs were identified after their antifungal effects were realized, the current focus is on on identifying small molecules that specifically exploit these targets and others that are unique to fungi. Some drugs are more active against certain fungi, but recent efforts are concentrated on identifying pharmacophores that exhibit broad-spectrum activity. In addition, phenotypic assays that are biased toward specific mechanisms (such as cell-wall biosynthesis, efflux, or resistance) are also being adopted.

11.10   Polyene drugs target the fungal cell membrane

The polyene antifungal drugs include the natural products amphotericin B and nystatin (**Figure 11.27**). Their mechanism involves a lipid–lipid interaction with ergosterol in the cell membrane, leading to sequestration of ergosterol (see Section 8.4). Nystatin, used as an oral preparation to treat an oral *Candida* infection (thrush),

Figure 11.27 Structures of polyene antifungal drugs. Amphotericin B and nystatin, which work by interaction with ergosterol, differ only in their hydroxylation patterns and the saturation of one alkene in nystatin.

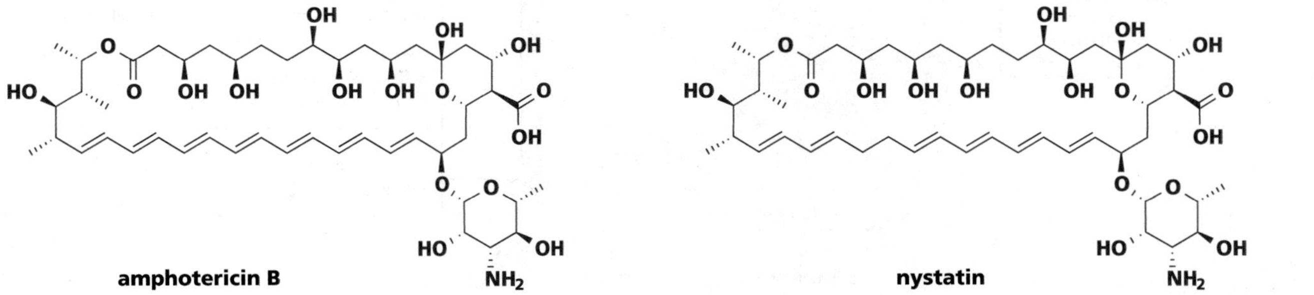

amphotericin B

nystatin

is well-tolerated, However, amphotericin B, used intravenously to treat systemic *Candida* and other fungal infections, often has serious acute and chronic side effects.

Amphotericin B was discovered at Squibb in the 1950s as the result of a natural product screening effort that examined fungal *Streptomyces* strains with the goal of identifying novel compounds that could be used to treat systemic infections. In 1953, an isolate from a Venezuelan soil culture provided amphotericin B, which was potent and could be prepared in a formulation that could be administered intravenously.

Nystatin was also discovered in the early 1950s, by Elizabeth Hazen and Rachel Brown at the New York State Department of Health (hence the name nystatin). The compound was isolated from *Streptomyces noursei* in a soil sample and was patented and licensed to Squibb for development.

11.11 Azoles and allylamines inhibit ergosterol biosynthesis

Like the polyene antifungal compounds, the azole and allylamine class also disrupt the fungal cell membrane, but their mechanism involves inhibiting the synthesis of ergosterol. The biosynthesis of all steroids begins with squalene, which is oxidized to 2,3-oxidosqualene, in a reaction catalyzed by squalene-2,3-epoxidase. Cyclization to lanosterol, the precursor of all steroids, is catalyzed by lanosterol synthase. One step in the conversion of lanosterol to ergosterol is catalyzed by the enzyme sterol 14α-demethylase. The key steps in the transformation from squalene to ergosterol are shown in **Figure 11.28**.

The discovery of azoles in the 1970s was spurred by both an increased incidence of fungal infections and a need for drugs that were less toxic than the available treatments. The earliest imidazole approved, clotrimazole, was identified as having antifungal activity against *Candida* and *Aspergillus* in the late 1960s. It was synthesized at Bayer in Germany by Karl Buchel and marketed in the early 1970s. The drug was much less toxic than amphotericin B and nystatin and could be administered either orally or intravenously. Variations in the aryl substituents led to a number of analogs, including miconazole, ketoconazole, fluconazole, and itraconazole (**Figure 11.29**). These azoles are used to treat *Candida* infections. While ketoconazole is no longer widely used to treat systemic infections, it is present in over-the-counter drugs used to treat mild infections such as athlete's foot, dandruff and jock itch.

More recent antifungal drugs include posaconazole and voriconazole. Posaconazole, approved in 2006, was designed on the basis of tetrahydrofuran-based azoles, which were identified as showing improved activity over the dioxolane itraconazole. Optimization of initial compounds focused on introduction of hydroxyl groups on the periphery to improve the physical properties of the liphophilic parent compounds. This lipophilicity, characteristic of all azoles, makes formulating them into an intravenous delivery system challenging, so design focused on incorporating polarity. Voriconazole was designed to have a broader spectrum of activity compared to fluconazole, based on the observation

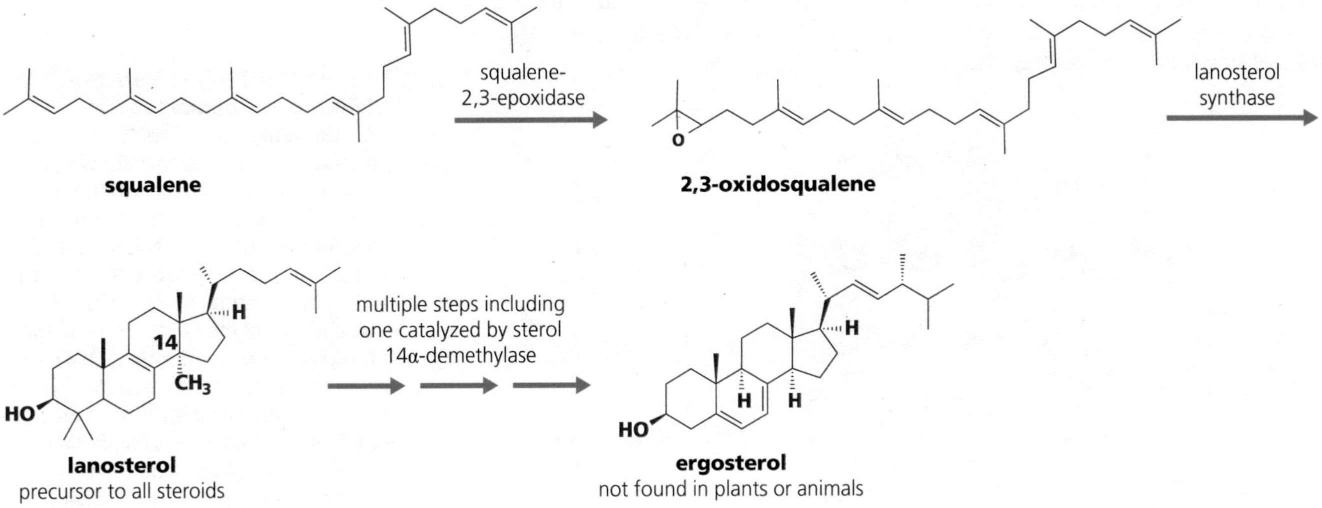

Figure 11.28 Key steps in biosynthesis of ergosterol. The precursor squalene is epoxidized to 2,3-oxidosqualene, in a reaction catalyzed by squalene-2,3-epoxidase. Lanosterol synthase catalyzes the cyclization of the epoxide to lanosterol. Multiple steps, one of which is catalyzed by sterol 14α-demethylase, convert lanosterol to ergosterol.

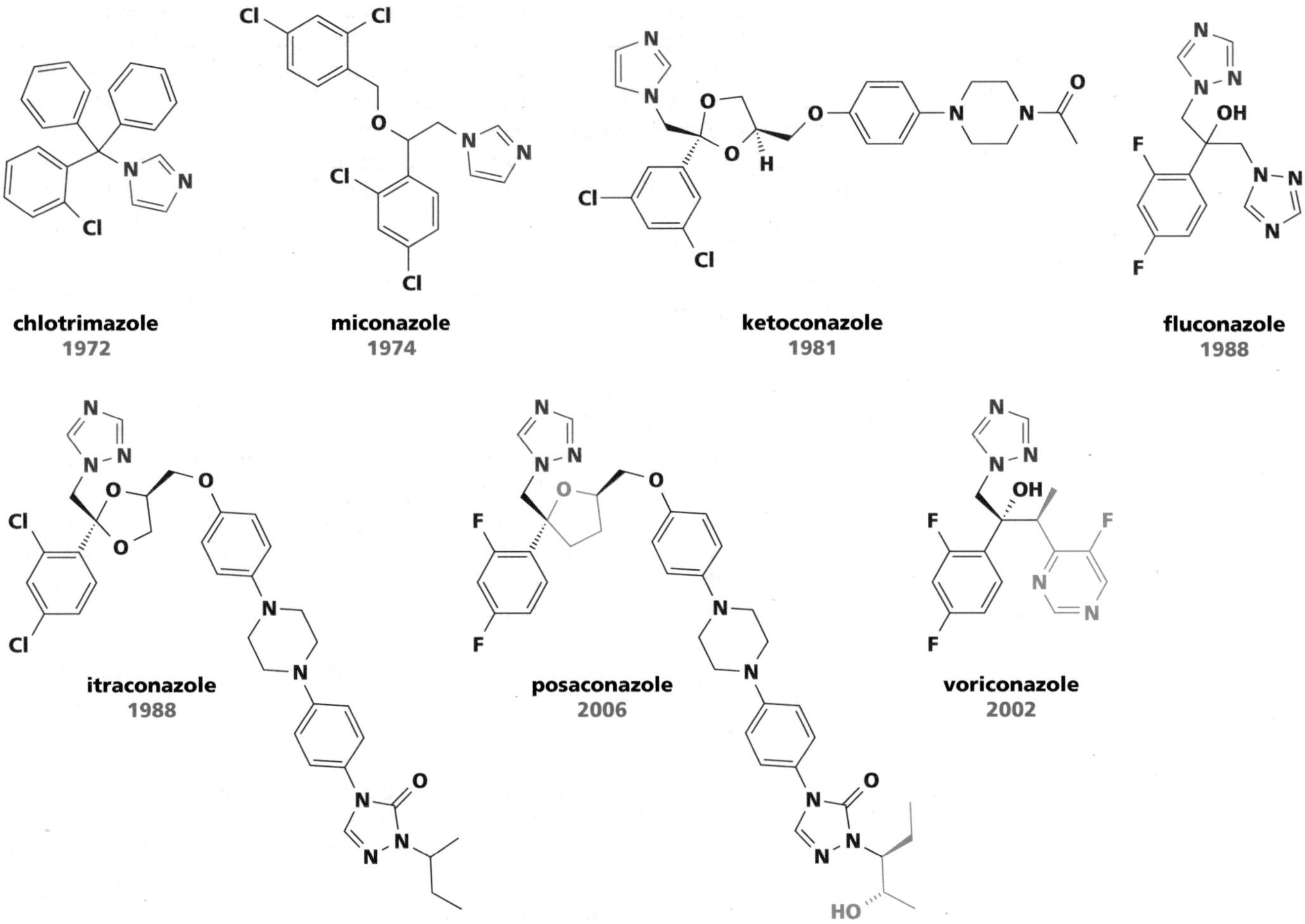

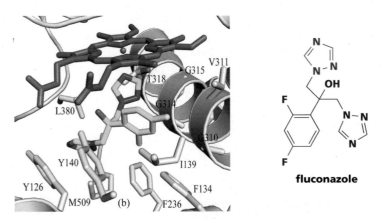

chlortrimazole
1972

miconazole
1974

ketoconazole
1981

fluconazole
1988

itraconazole
1988

posaconazole
2006

voriconazole
2002

that substitution α to one of the triazoles resulted in an increase in potency toward *A. fumigatus*. A series of analogs were prepared that contained α-substitution, as well as replacement of one of the triazoles with a six-membered ring heterocycle. Voriconazole, approved in 2002, has a broader antifungal spectrum than fluconazole.

The azoles are all inhibitors of the enzyme sterol 14α-demethylase. This fungal enzyme, also called CYP51, is an oxidoreductase (see Chapter 7) and a member of the class of P450 enzymes. The same class is found in humans and is responsible for metabolism of xenobiotics, among other activities. Some of the side effects of azoles are due to their activity toward these related human homologs. These enzymes contain a heme group at their active site where the imidazole or triazole nitrogen binds. The relatively lipophilic side chains occupy hydrophobic pockets that are normally occupied by the substrate, as seen in **Figure 11.30**. The availability of X-ray structures of this enzyme has aided drug design.

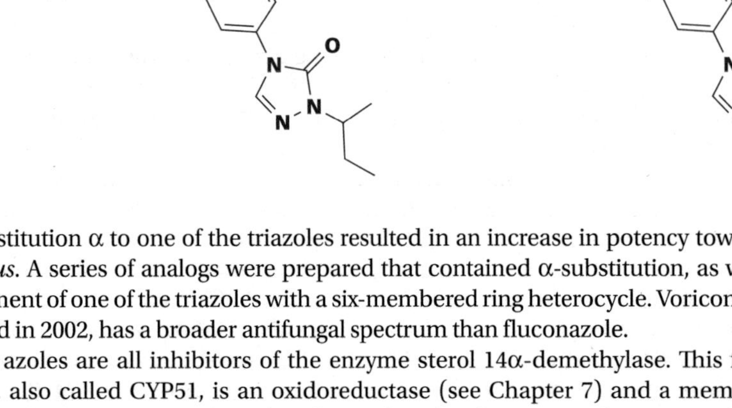

Figure 11.29 Structures of azole antifungal drugs and year of approval. The defining common structural feature, imidazole or triazole, is shown in red. Recent antifungal drugs include posaconazole (modifications compared to itraconazole are shown in blue) and voriconazole (modifications compared to fluconazole are shown in blue).

Figure 11.30 X-ray co-structure of fluconazole bound to sterol 14α-demethylase. In this X-ray co-structure, the protein is shown in gray, with specific residues in the active site labeled, the heme group is in magenta and fluconazole is in cyan. One triazole ring of fluconazole (indicated in red in the structure on the right) interacts with the heme group. The difluorophenyl and second triazole sit in a hydrophobic pocket of the enzyme. (From Sagatova AA, Keniya MV, Wilson RK et al. [2015] *Antimicrob Agents Chemother* 59:4982–4989. With permission from American Society for Microbiology.)

fluconazole

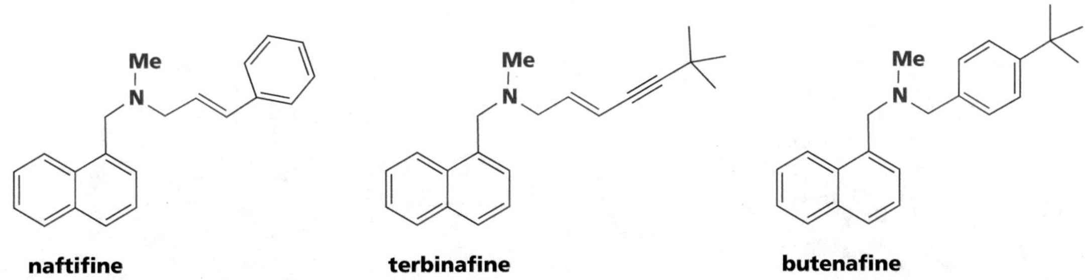

naftifine **terbinafine** **butenafine**

Figure 11.31 Structures of allylamine antifungal drugs. Naftifine was developed from a screening campaign; incorporation of a *tert*-butyl group, as seen in terbinafine and butenafine provided increased potency. The required allylamine common feature is shown in red; these drugs act by inhibition of squalene-2,3-epoxidase.

Another class of drugs, the allylamines, also inhibit the synthesis of ergosterol, but through a different mechanism. These compounds inhibit the enzyme squalene-2,3-epoxidase, which catalyzes the first step in the conversion of squalene to lanosterol (Figure 11.28). These are broad-spectrum topical antifungal agents, which are widely used to treat dermatomycoses (skin and toenail infections). The parent compound, naftifine, was discovered at Sandoz through random screening of their compound library for antifungal activity, and introduced in 1988. This compound was originally isolated as a by-product in a synthetic program directed at synthesizing spironaphthalenes (**Figure 11.31**). The allylamine is a requirement for activity, and incorporation of *tert*-butyl moieties provided terbinafine and butenafine, which are reversible, noncompetitive inhibitors of the enzyme and show improved potency compared to naftifine.

11.12 Some antifungal drugs inhibit cell replication

Griseofulvin, a natural product isolated in 1939 from *Penicillium griseofulvum* was the first antifungal drug marketed (1959), (**Figure 11.32**). It is used as a treatment for ringworm, and although many analogs have been prepared, it is the only drug in its class.

The mechanism of action of griseofulvin is still not completely understood. It has been shown to bind to tubulin and interfere with mitosis. However, the binding affinity is low, and it is possible that its antifungal effect is due to binding to a microtubule-associated protein instead.

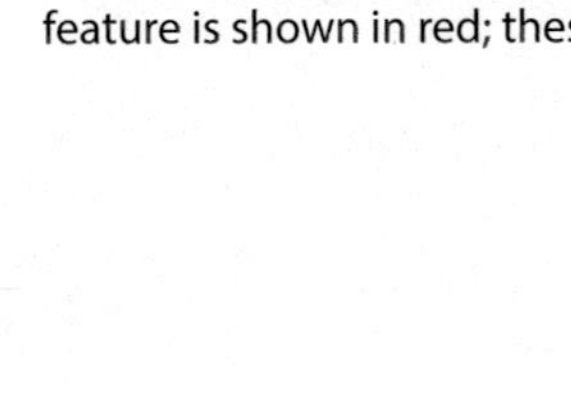

Flucytosine, a derivative of cytosine, was originally synthesized as an antitumor agent, but was inactive. Although, it does not possess antifungal activity either, in fungi it is converted to 5-fluorouracil (5-FU). It is taken up into fungal cells by the action of cytosine permease. Once in the fungal cells, it is converted to 5-FU by cytosine deaminase, an enzyme not found in mammals. Like other nucleosides, 5-FU is converted to the monophosphate (FdUMP) and then to the corresponding triphosphate, which inhibits fungal DNA replication (**Figure 11.33**). Flucytosine is generally used in combination with other antifungal drugs and is limited by toxicity.

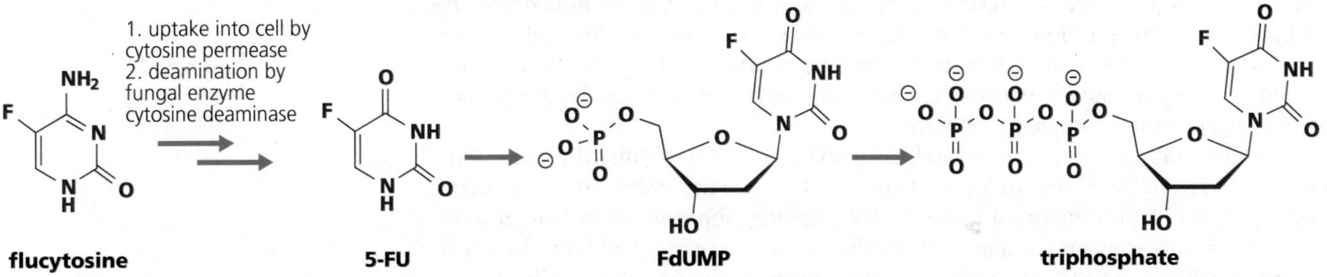

griseofulvin

Figure 11.32 Structure of griseofulvin. Griseofulvin was the first antifungal agent approved. It inhibits mitosis, but its exact mechanism of action is not well understood.

1. uptake into cell by cytosine permease
2. deamination by fungal enzyme cytosine deaminase

flucytosine **5-FU** **FdUMP** **triphosphate**

Figure 11.33 Mechanism of action of flucytosine. Flucytosine, a modified nucleobase, is taken up into fungal cells by cytosine permease. It is converted to 5-FU in fungal cells by the fungal-specific enzyme cytosine deaminase, and then eventually to the triphosphate, which inhibits DNA replication.

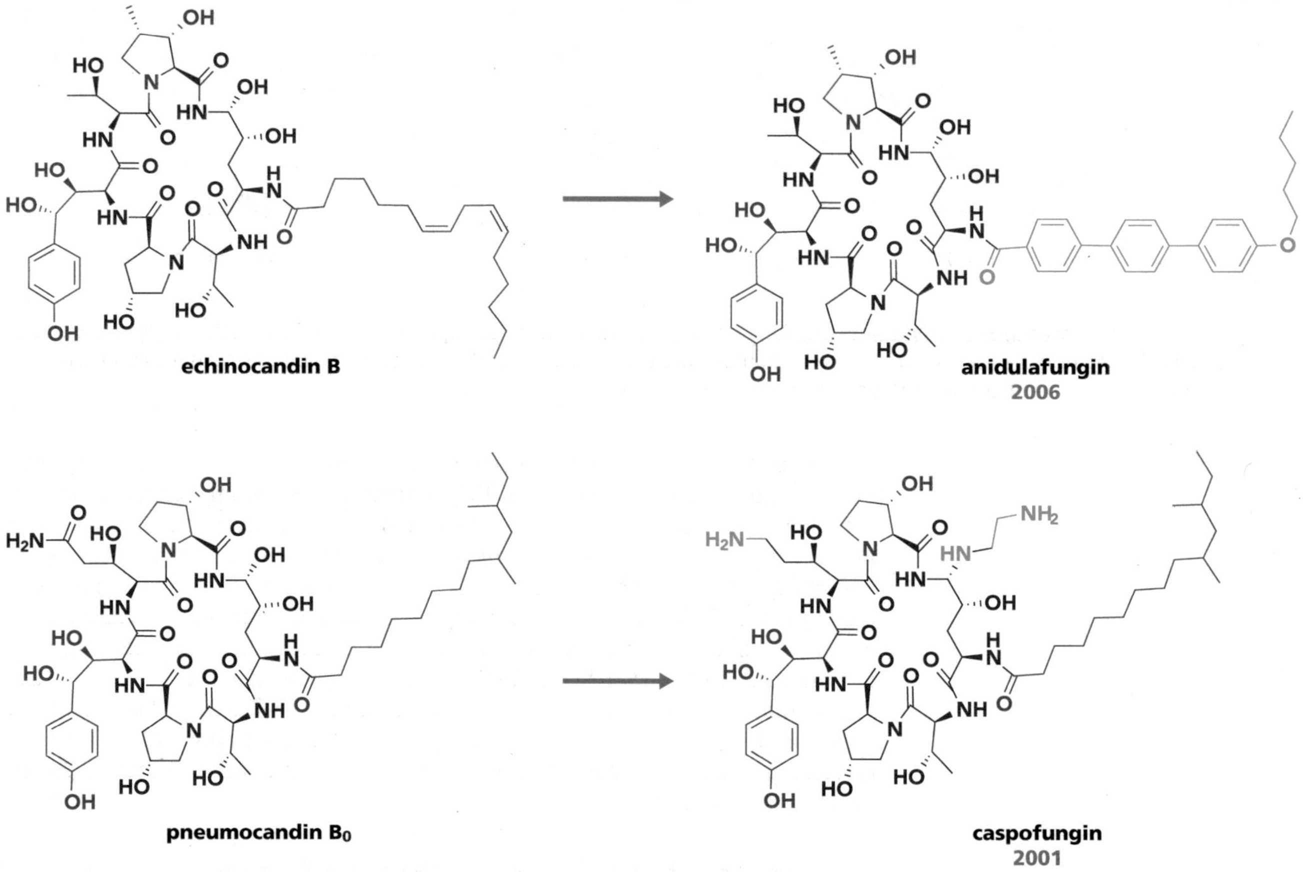

Figure 11.34 Structures of 1,3-β-glucan synthase inhibitors. Natural products echinocandin B and pneumocandins, B_0 are on the left, and approved drugs anidulafungin and caspofungin are on the right. Moieties required for activity are shown in red and semisynthetic changes shown in blue.

11.13 Echinocandins inhibit fungal cell-wall synthesis

The echinocandins are a relatively new class of antifungal drugs. They are naturally occurring cyclic lipopeptides that inhibit fungal cell-wall synthesis. Specifically, they are noncompetitive inhibitors of 1,3-β-glucan synthase, an enzyme involved in the synthesis of the glucan polymers that are found in fungal cell walls. Since this enzyme has no mammalian counterpart, targeting it is expected to be relatively safe. Echinocandin B was isolated in 1974 from an *Aspergillus* strain; a related class, the pneumocandins, were isolated in the 1980s (**Figure 11.34**).

While echinocandin B was found to be too toxic for use, several semisynthetic analogs are now used clinically, including anidulafungin and caspofungin. SAR studies on echinocandin B analogs found that the lipophilic side chain as well as the hydroxlyated L-homotyrosine residue were required for activity. While not crucial, the 3-hydroxy-4-methylproline found in echinocandin B enhanced antifungal activity, and is maintained in anidulafungin. The approved drugs maintained the essential features, incorporating modifications in the lipophilic side chain in anidulafungin and additional of amino groups in caspofungin.

Another target involved in cell wall biosynthesis includes chitin synthase. Chitin is a polymer of N-Ac-glucosamine, and not found in humans. Polymerization occurs by reaction of the 3′-hydroxyl group of the growing polymer chain with uridine diphosphate *N*-acetylglucosamine (UDP-GlcNAc) in a reaction catalyzed by chitin synthase (**Figure 11.35**). The natural product nikkomycin Z is an inhibitor of this enzyme.

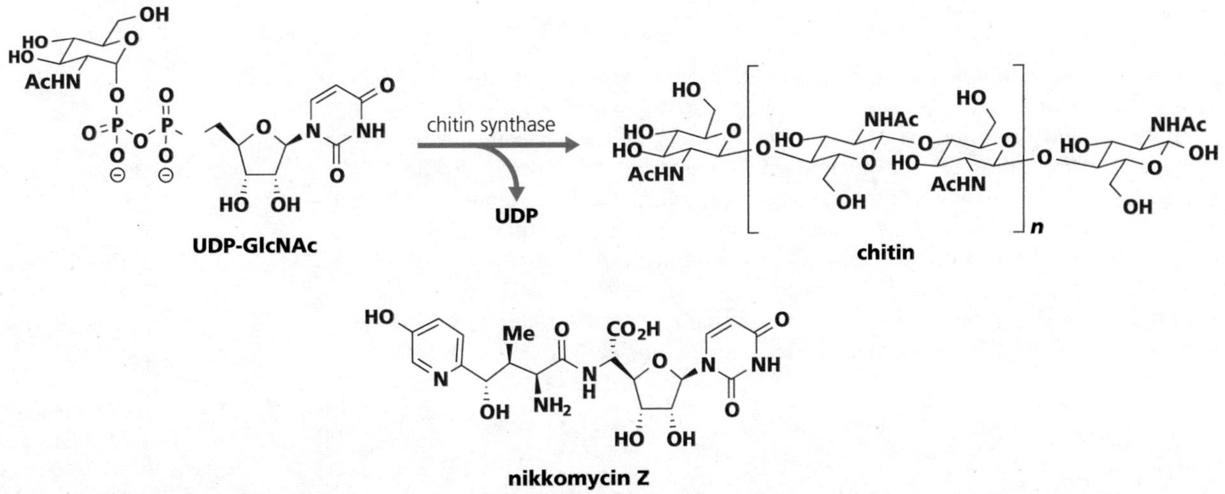

Figure 11.35 Formation of chitin and structure of nikkomycin Z. Chitin synthase is a transferase that catalyzes the addition of an *N*-acetylglucosamine unit (from uridine diphosphate *N*-acetylglucosamine, UDP-GlcNAc) to the chitin polymer. The inhibitor, nikkomycin Z, is structurally similar to the natural substrate.

Nikkomycin Z resembles the enzyme's substrate and has progressed to phase II clinical trials as a treatment for valley fever (coccidioidomycosis). This relatively rare disease is localized in the southwestern United States and Central and South America, and causes respiratory symptoms that can be fatal in immunocompromised patients.

While the number of antifungal drugs lags far behind the number of antiviral drugs, recent efforts in searching for novel antifungal compounds should add to those on the market. Many of these drugs were identified via phenotypic screening. However, in some cases extensive medicinal chemistry optimization afforded improved analogs. For example, the extensive SAR developed around the azole scaffold, as well as an understanding of its binding mode to its enzymatic target, has allowed a more rational approach to drug design that has culminated in new analogs with broad-spectrum activity and improved physical properties. In addition, new screening strategies that specifically target one pathway are leading to new structural leads. These approaches are starting to address the difficulties in developing drugs selective for fungal targets.

SUMMARY

In the past 30 years, much progress has been made in the development of both antiviral and antifungal drugs. The significant advancement in the development of antiviral drugs was directly related to the initial success of drugs to treat herpes in the 1970s and then the massive efforts devoted to the development of drugs to address the AIDS pandemic in the late 1980s. Both library screening and structure-based drug design were used to identify RT inhibitors, HIV protease inhibitors, and fusion inhibitors. Structure-based drug design was also applied to the development of neuraminidase inhibitors that are currently approved to treat influenza. The current therapies for hepatitis C, many of which are curative, also rely on similar strategies: inhibition of viral polymerase and protease.

Antifungal compounds represent a much smaller family of drugs, and initial leads have primarily been identified through screening rather than drug design. With an increase in fungal infections, including dangerous systemic infections, and the identification of specific mechanisms, medicinal chemistry has led to the introduction of improved compounds.

CASE STUDY 1   DISCOVERY OF DACLATASVIR

In a search for compounds to inhibit replication of hepatitis C, scientists at Bristol-Myers Squibb identified BMS-858 from a library screening program. Over 1 million compounds were screened in a high-throughput assay that was specifically designed to identify compounds with a mechanism distinct from NS3 protease and NS5B polymerase inhibition. A screening strategy was used that simultaneously evaluated antiviral activity and selectivity versus human cells. The hit pursued, BMS-858, contains a thiazolidine core and inhibited HCV replication at an EC_{50} of 0.57–1 μM with no cytotoxicity. Exploration of this promising result by synthesis of analogs afforded the lead compound BMS-824, which replaced the carbamate of BMS-858 with an amide and had ~100-fold improvement in potency (**Figure 11.36**).

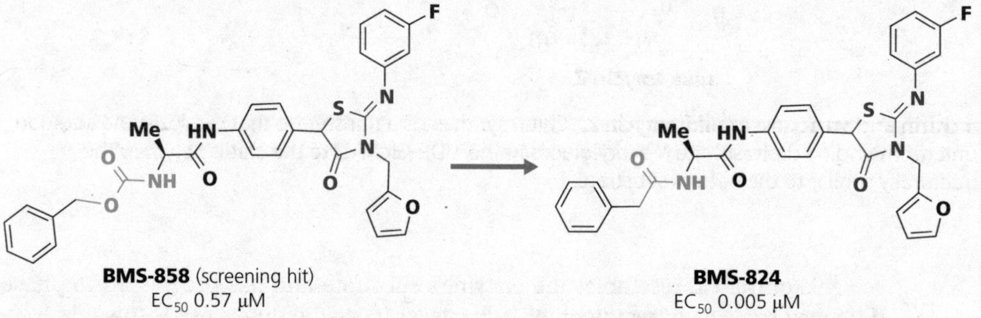

BMS-858 (screening hit)
EC_{50} 0.57 μM

BMS-824
EC_{50} 0.005 μM

Figure 11.36 Structures of hit and early lead compounds in the development of daclatasvir. BMS-858 was identified from a high throughput screen for inhibitors of HCV replication that was biased away from known targets. Further optimization afforded the more potent BMS-824. The thiazolidine core is shown in red, and the change from carbamate (BMS-858) to amide (BMS-824) is shown in blue.

Investigation of the mechanism of BMS-858 indicated that it was inactive against both the HCV NS3 protease and NS5B polymerase. The target was ultimately identified by generating cells that exhibited BMS-858-resistant phenotypes; all had mutations in the N-terminal region of the HCV NS5A replication protein. The antiviral activity of the compound confirmed that this was a new, valid target for HCV drugs.

Despite its potent activity, BMS-824 was found to be unstable in the assay medium. Furthermore, the scaffold is related to rhodanines, which are characterized as PAINS compounds (see Section 2.13). To determine the source of its instability, BMS-824 was incubated in the assay medium. HPLC and bioassay of individual components showed that oxidation/ rearrangement product **1** and a thiourea fragment **2** (**Figure 11.37**)

Figure 11.37 Decomposition products formed during incubation of thiazolidine BMS-824 in assay medium. The major products were inactive compounds **1** and **2**; the minor product **3** was an active symmetrical dimer (a second molecule of BMS-824 is connected as shown). Red indicates the thiazolidine and its associated decomposition products.

BMS-824
EC_{50} = 5 nM

assay medium

assay medium

assay medium

compound 1

compound 2

compound 3: active dimer (symmetrical)
EC_{50} = 0.06 nM

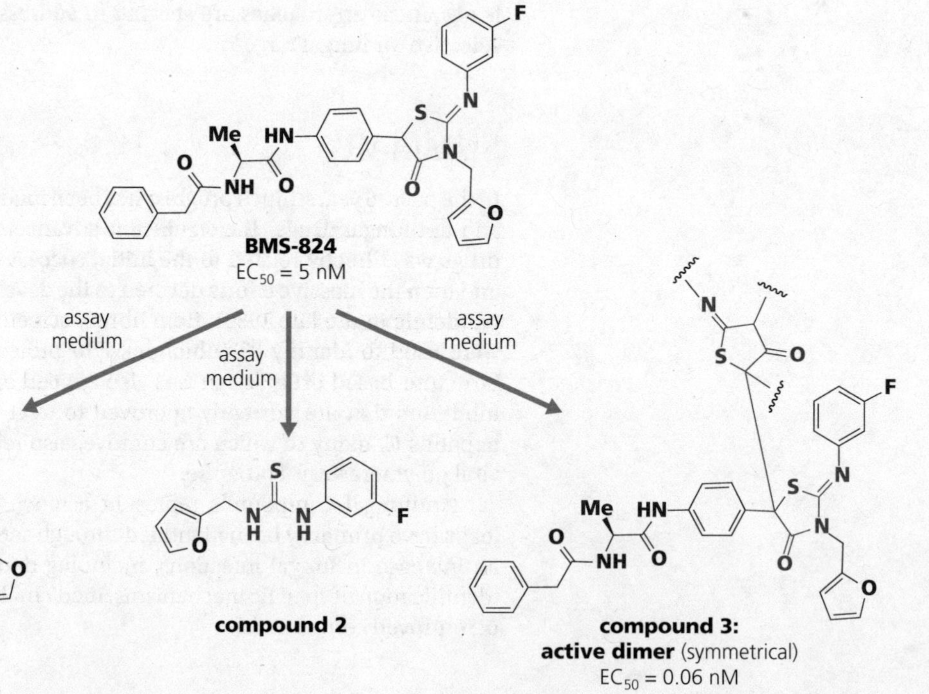

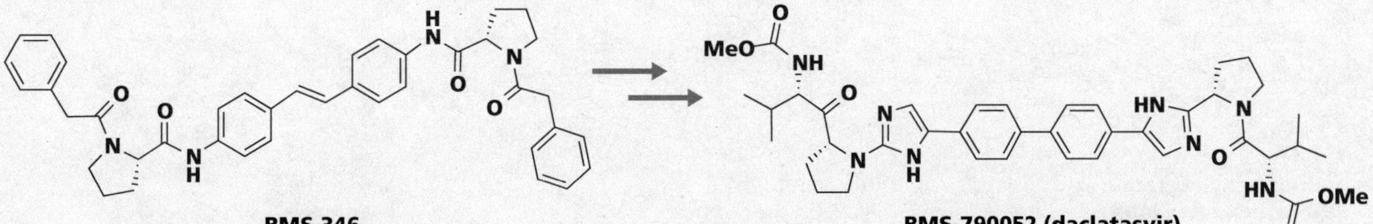

Figure 11.38 Symmetrical analog of active dimer and structure of daclatasvir. Replacement of the unstable thiazolidine with a styrene and further optimization including incorporation of L-proline caps afforded BMS-346. Daclatasvir retains the proline groups, but replaces the styrene with a biphenyl group. It is a highly potent inhibitor of viral replication.

were major decomposition products. Neither was active, but further isolation of minor products identified the dimeric structure **3** to be a very active inhibitor of HCV replication (EC_{50} = 0.06 nM); it was nearly 100-fold more potent than BMS-824.

On the basis of the structure of the active dimeric compound, stable symmetrical analogs were designed, and the unstable thiazolidine was replaced. The stilbene analog BMS-346, with L-proline caps, was the most active, with the corresponding D-proline isomer being completely inactive (**Figure 11.38**). The inhibitor binds in the amino terminus of the HCV NS5A protein, which crystallizes as a dimer. This dimeric structure complements the symmetry of the inhibitors.

The stilbene BMS-346 maintained the potency seen in the thiazolidine dimer, with an EC_{50} of 0.086 nM. Further modifications of the core led to the biphenyl analog BMS-790052 (daclatasvir), with EC_{50} values of 50 pM against the HCV 1a genotype and 9 pM against the 1b genotype. Daclastasvir is orally available and was found to be well-tolerated in phase I clinical trials at doses up to 200 mg. In infected patients, a combination of daclatasvir and sofosbuvir, given as an oral dose once a day, led to a sustained response after 12 weeks of treatment. This combination was approved by the European Union in 2014 and by the U.S. FDA in 2015.

CASE STUDY 2 DISCOVERY OF RILPIVIRINE

In the late 1980s, Janssen Pharmaceuticals initiated a search for compounds to inhibit HIV-1 replication in collaboration with the Rega Institute for Medical Research. A library of 90,000 compounds was screened for their ability to inhibit HIV-1 replication in a cell-based assay, and 2000 hits were chosen applying the additional criteria of low toxicity and lack of off-target effects.

One of the hits identified from the library was the α-aminophenylacetamide (α-APA) R15345 (**Figure 11.39**), which had an EC_{50} of 610 nM in the HIV-1 replication assay, although it was cytotoxic at higher doses. A series of aryl substitutions were investigated, and the nitro analog R18893 had improved potency and lower cytotoxicity. Replacement of the nitro group with an acetyl group and addition of a methyl on the aryl ring afforded loviride, which had further improved potency and low cytotoxicity. Although the initial discovery was based on inhibition of viral replication,

Figure 11.39 Early leads in the development of rilpivirine: from APA lead to loviride. The APA lead was identified by screening for inhibition of HIV-1 replication. Aryl substitutions led to the nitro analog R18893, with improved potency and reduced cytotoxicity. Further substitutions led to the acetyl derivative loviride, which progressed to clinical trials (changes to structure shown in red).

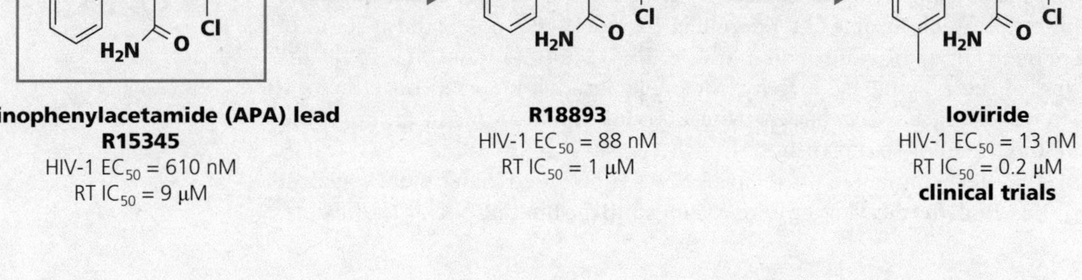

α-aminophenylacetamide (APA) lead R15345
HIV-1 EC_{50} = 610 nM
RT IC_{50} = 9 μM

R18893
HIV-1 EC_{50} = 88 nM
RT IC_{50} = 1 μM

loviride
HIV-1 EC_{50} = 13 nM
RT IC_{50} = 0.2 μM
clinical trials

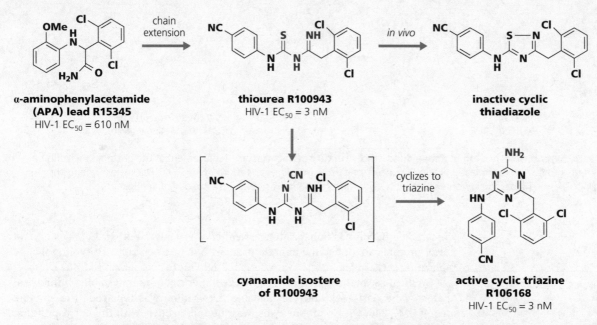

Figure 11.40 Early leads in the development of rilpivirine: from APA lead to cyclic triazine. Chain extension of the APA lead afforded a potent thiourea; however, it cyclized *in vivo* to an inactive thiadiazole metabolite. Incorporation of the *N*-cyano bioisostere gave the cyanamide, which spontaneously cyclized to an active triazine. This compound was highly potent. Changes in structure shown in red.

the specific mechanism was investigated and found to be inhibition of RT, with IC_{50} values of 9 μM for the APA lead and 0.2 μM for loviride.

On the basis of potency as well as pharmacokinetic profile, loviride progressed to clinical trials. Although active, loviride had no advantage over other NNRTIs such as delavirdine that were already on the market.

In addition to the aryl modifications that afforded loviride, lead modification also included chain extension of the aryl linker of R15345, and although most analogs lost activity, a thiourea analog showed increased potency. This finding led to the synthesis of thiourea R100943, a second clinical candidate (**Figure 11.40**). Unfortunately, its activity was limited by rapid metabolism to an inactive metabolite, a thiadiazole, which resulted from cyclization of the thiourea moiety. In an attempt to avoid formation of the metabolite, the cyanamide isostere was synthesized. However, this compound was not isolated, as it also cyclized as soon as it was formed to the triazine R106168. Unlike the cyclic thiadiazole, the triazine had excellent potency.

Replacement of one of the triazine ring nitrogens by a carbon to generate a diarylpyrimidine was based on molecular modeling studies, and after further optimization led to the diarylpyrimidine R147681 (dapivirine) (**Figure 11.41**), as well as the bis(nitrile) R165335 (etravirine).

One of the most promising aspects of dapivirine was its activity against strains of the virus that were resistant to other NNRTIs. In a further medicinal chemistry optimization effort, extensive SAR studies were carried out, based on further improving potency against resistant strains. Modeling into the binding pocket of RT shows adoption of a butterfly-like conformation where one wing interacts with tyrosines Y181 and Y188, as well as tryptophan W229, and the NH bonds to the backbone amide of lysine K101, as seen in NNRTIs such as efavirenz. The allosteric NNRTI binding pocket is flexible and lipophilic. The pocket is small in the absence of a ligand but opens upon binding of an inhibitor. This conformational change results in inhibition of the polymerase activity. Molecular modeling based on etravirine indicated that inserting a spacer between one aryl ring and the *p*-nitrile group would improve binding, leading to rilpivirine.

Goals in the development of these novel NNRTIs included high potency against resistant strains. Both the diarylpyrimidine analogs and the binding pocket are flexible,

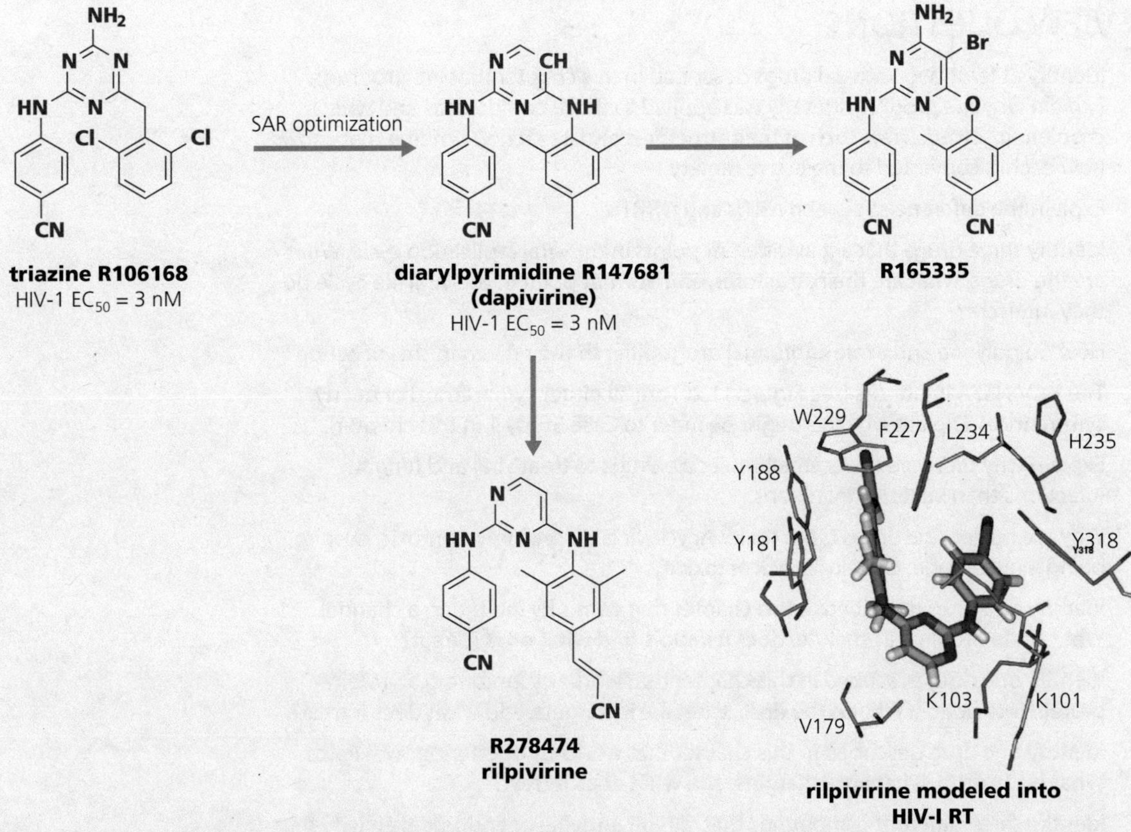

Figure 11.41 Development of rilpivirine: from triazines to diaminopyrazines. SAR optimization of the triazine R106168 led to the diarylpyrimidines. Both R147681 (dapivirine) and R165335 (etravirine) advanced to clinical trials. Molecular modeling based on R165335 indicated that inserting a spacer between one aryl ring and the nitrile would improve binding, leading to rilpivirine. Rilpivirine is seen modeled into HIV-1 RT, showing binding between the nitrile and W229, as well as hydrophobic interactions with Y181 and Y188. (From Janssen PAJ, Lewi PJ, Arnold E et al. [2005] *J Med Chem* 48:1901–1909. With permission from American Chemical Society.)

which may contribute to activity against resistant strains. Other goals included a long half-life and high oral bioavailability to allow once-daily dosing, minimal side effects, and ease of synthesis and formulation. Rilpivirine fulfilled all of these criteria, with high potency, a half-life of up to 39 h (in dogs), and oral availability of approximately 35%. Rilpivirine also exhibited no side effects in multiple animal models and is synthetically accessible in a six-step sequence.

REVIEW QUESTIONS

1. Identify at least two antiviral drugs described in this chapter that are prodrugs. Explain why the prodrug strategy was applied to these compounds and what problem it solved. Draw each of their structures and a reaction scheme that shows how each is converted to the active moiety.

2. Explain the difference between NRTIs and NNRTIs.

3. Identify three drugs that act at different points in the viral replication cycle. What are the drugs, what are their structures, and at what point in the viral life cycle do they interfere?

4. How do polyene and azole antifungal drugs differ in their mechanisms of action?

5. The HCV NS5A inhibitors (see Figure 11.20) are all either symmetrical or nearly symmetrical. Explain why this might be (refer to Case Study 1 in this chapter).

6. Explain why there are fewer small-molecule drugs to treat viral and fungal infections than bacterial infections.

7. Why are nucleoside drugs often toxic? Acyclovir is surprisingly nontoxic, despite being a nucleoside. Explain its lack of toxicity.

8. Identify one drug described in this chapter that works by inhibiting a channel. What is the drug, what channel does it inhibit, and what does it treat?

9. Identify one drug described in this chapter that works by inhibiting a protein–protein interaction. What is the drug, what are its targets, and what does it treat?

10. Identify one drug described in this chapter that works by interfering with lipids. What is the drug, what are its targets, and what does it treat?

11. Identify three different compounds that exhibit antiviral or antifungal activity that are natural products.

APPLICATION QUESTIONS

1. HCV NS3 is a serine protease described in Section 11.6, and its inhibitors boceprevir and telaprevir (see Figure 11.17) contain a warhead like those described in Chapter 7.

    (a) Draw the general structure of the tetrahedral intermediate formed by reaction of one of these inhibitors with HCV NS3.

    (b) Design two new inhibitors based on the structure of boceprevir or telaprevir by incorporating different warheads into the inhibitor scaffold.

2. Using the structures of the neuraminidase inhibitors in Figure 11.25, apply Lipinski's rules to each of them. What are the parameters for each compound? Do these drugs comply with Lipinski rules?

3. Viruses are examples of a type of agent causing a disease that can be eradicated or cured. Name one example of a virus that has been eradicated or nearly eradicated. Research the history of its eradication.

4. Compare the structures of penciclovir and ganciclovir to the natural substrate they mimic. How does each differ from guanosine? What is the mechanism of action of ganciclovir? Draw the structures of the intermediate products.

guanosine
(natural ligand)

ganciclovir

penciclovir

5.   For three different enzymes, identify one representative antiviral or antifungal drug that works through its inhibition. Applying the concepts in Chapter 7, describe the enzyme, what reaction the enzyme catalyzes, and how the inhibitor works.

6.   From the examples in this chapter, find five different examples of molecules containing a privileged structure. Draw the structures and highlight the privileged structures.

7.   Many of the HIV protease inhibitors in Figure 11.15 contain a hydroxyethylene transition-state mimetic. Based on information from Chapter 4, design three other possible inhibitors based on the structure of saquinavir by incorporating alternative transition-state mimetics.

8.   AZT was the first compound approved to treat HIV. Research its history. Who synthesized it, when, and why? Draw the initial synthesis. Research a more recent synthesis and compare the two.

9.   A number of individuals were awarded Nobel prizes for their work on HIV over several years. Name four of them, with the years of their awards, and describe their contributions.

10.   Ebola is a life-threatening virus. Research the small-molecule approaches that are being taken to identify drugs to fight it. Draw the structures of two and describe their mechanisms of action.

FURTHER READING

HIV/HCV

Thematic issue on HCV therapy. (2014) *J Med Chem* 57:1625–2166.

De Clercq E (2007) The design of drugs for HIV and HCV. *Nat Rev Drug Discovery* 6:1001–1018.

De Corte BL (2005) From 4,5,6,7-Tetrahydro-5-methylimidazo[4,5,1-*jk*] (1,4)benzodiazepin-2(1*H*)-one (TIBO) to etravirine (TMC125): Fifteen years of research on non-nucleoside inhibitors of HIV-1 reverse transcriptase. *J Med Chem* 48:1689–1696.

Huryn DM & Okabe M (1992) AIDS-driven nucleoside chemistry. *Chem Rev* 92:1745–1768.

Gordon CP & Keller PA (2005) Control of hepatitis C: a medicinal chemistry perspective. *J Med Chem* 48:1–20.

Ghosh AK, Chapsal BD, Weber IT & Mitsuya H (2008) Design of HIV protease inhibitors targeting protein backbone: an effective strategy for combating drug resistance. *Acc Chem Res* 41:78–86.

Pommier Y, Johnson AA & Marchand C (2005) Integrase inhibitors to treat HIV/AIDS. *Nat Rev Drug Discovery* 4:236–248.

Acyclic nucleosides and phosphonates

Fyfe JA, Keller PM, Furman PA et al. (1978) Thymidine kinase from herpes simplex virus phosphorylates the new antiviral compound, 9-(2-hydroxyethoxymethyl)guanine. *J Biol Chem* 253:8721–8727.

Freeman S & Gardiner JM (1996) Acyclic nucleosides as antiviral compounds. *Mol Biotechnol* 5:125–137.

De Clerq E & Holy A (2005) Acyclic nucleoside phosphonates: a key class of antiviral drugs. *Nat Rev Drug Discovery* 4:928–940.

Neuraminidase inhibitors

von Itzstein M (2007) The war against influenza: discovery and development of sialidase inhibitors. *Nat Rev Drug Discovery* 6:967–974.

Varghese JN, McKimm-Breschkin JL, Caldwell JB et al. (1992) The structure of the complex between influenza virus neuraminidase and sialic acid, the viral receptor. *Proteins: Struct Funct Genet* 14:327–332.

von Itzstein M, Wu W-Y, Kik GB et al. (1993) Rational design of potent sialidase-based inhibitors of influenza virus replication. *Nature* 363:418–423.

Antifungal agents

Odds FC, Brown AJP & Gow NAR (2003) Antifungal agents: mechanisms of action. *Trends Microbiol* 11:272–279.

Denning DW (1997) Echinocandins and pneumocandins: a new antifungal class with a novel mode of action. *Antimicrob Agents Chemother* 40:611–614.

Petranyi G, Meingassner JG & Mieth H (1987) Activity of terbinafine in experimental fungal infections of laboratory animals. *Antimicrob Agents Chemother* 31:1558–1561.

Richardson K, Cooper K, Marriott MS et al. (1990) Discovery of fluconazole, a novel antifungal agent. *Clin Infect Dis* 12(Suppl 3):S267–S271.

Georgopapadakou N (1998) Antifungals: mechanism of action and resistance, novel and established drugs. *Curr Opin Microbiol* 1:547–557.

Nussbaumer P, Petranyi G & Stutz A (1991) Synthesis and structure–activity relationships of benzo[*b*]thienylallylamine antimycotics. *J Med Chem* 34:65–73.

Antibacterial and antiparasitic drugs

12

LEARNING OBJECTIVES

- Learn the historical background of the discovery and development of antibacterial and antiparasitic drugs.
- Describe different mechanisms of action of antibacterial agents.
- Identify different classes of antibacterial drugs acting by each mechanism.
- Explain antibacterial drug resistance mechanisms.
- Understand the structure–activity relationships of several classes of antibacterial drugs.
- Become familiar with drugs used to treat parasitic infections and their mechanism of action.

Infections caused by bacteria and parasites have historically been, and continue to be, a significant worldwide cause of mortality. It has been estimated that almost half of the world's population is at risk of malaria, a disease that has been known for over 4000 years and is the result of infection by *Plasmodium* parasites. Prior to the early 1900s, bacterial infections, such as tuberculosis, typhoid fever, syphilis, bubonic plague, leprosy, and sepsis from infected wounds, were a leading cause of death. The antibiotic age brought about new treatment for bacterial infections, and the increase in life expectancy in the 20th century has been attributed, in part, to the introduction of antibiotics such as penicillin. Similar advances have been made in the area of antiparasitic drugs.

Today, these infections continue to be a source of morbidity and mortality but with less of an impact than they once had. Efforts to purify water sources, minimize exposure to infectious agents, and eliminate vectors of parasites have significantly reduced the incidence of certain bacterial and parasitic infections. Several bacterial infections are also preventable by vaccination, with a few examples being diphtheria, pertussis, meningococcal disease, and typhoid, as well as *Haemophilus influenzae* and *Streptococcus pneumoniae* infections.

Despite the large variety of bacteria and parasites, the same drug is often effective against multiple species, thereby broadening the utility and number of drugs available to treat these infections. In some cases, however, the complex life cycle of certain parasites makes drug discovery particularly challenging, and there are fewer drugs to treat infections caused by parasites than by bacteria. For both bacteria and parasites, resistance to current drugs is a serious problem, and drug discovery efforts are focusing on addressing this issue.

ANTIBACTERIAL AGENTS: BACTERIAL STRUCTURE, POINTS OF DRUG INTERACTION, AND IMPACT

Bacteria are prokaryotic microorganisms, and unlike eukaryotes, they do not have a nucleus and typically do not have organelles. Their DNA and ribosomes are surrounded by a cell wall in addition to a cell membrane. Each of these are drug targets. Bacteria display pili and flagella on their surface that are responsible for adhesion and locomotion, respectively. They are broadly divided into two classes, Gram-positive and Gram-negative, on the basis of their ability to take up the crystal violet of the Gram stain. Gram-positive bacteria have a high percentage (50–70%) of peptidoglycan content in the bacterial cell wall, whereas the cell walls of Gram-negative bacteria are only about 10% peptidoglycan but contain an additional outer membrane that contains pore proteins (porins) and displays lipopolysaccharide (LPS) on the cell surface. LPS is a macromolecule composed of a hydrophobic lipid portion (lipid A), linked to a polysaccharide core, which is linked to O-antigenic oligosaccharides. Gram-positive bacteria contain different molecules on their surface, including lipoteichoic acid and wall teichoic acid. Both contain integral membrane and peripheral membrane proteins, as well as wall-associated proteins such as those involved in peptidoglycan synthesis. A representation of a bacterial cell is shown in **Figure 12.1A**, with key structural

A: STRUCTURE OF A BACTERIUM

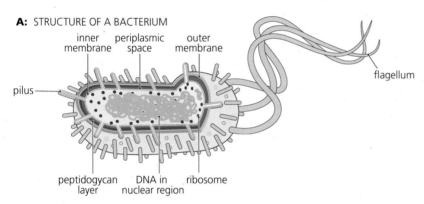

B: DIFFERENCES IN CELL WALL OF GRAM-POSITIVE AND GRAM-NEGATIVE BACTERIA

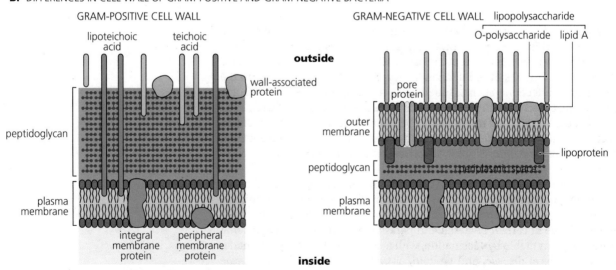

Figure 12.1 Bacterial structure and cell-wall details. A: General structure of a bacterium consisting of pilus (for adhesion) and flagella (for motility), as well as drug targets such as the cell wall, cell membrane, ribosomes, and DNA. B: Differences in the bacterial cell wall between Gram-positive and Gram-negative bacteria. Gram-positive bacteria have a thick peptidoglycan layer in the cell wall with teichoic and lipoteichoic acid displayed on the surface. Gram-negative bacteria have a thin peptidoglycan layer but have an outer membrane that contains pore proteins (porins) and displays lipopolysaccharides (made up of a lipid A linked to a polysaccharide core). Various proteins (wall-associated, peripheral membrane, and integral membrane) are found in each. (A, adapted from Strelkauskas A, Edwards E, Fahnert B et al. [2015] Microbiology: A Clinical Approach, 2nd ed. Garland Science. B, adapted from Alberts B, Johnson A, Lewis J et al. [2014] Molecular Biology of the Cell, 6th ed. Garland Science.)

elements highlighted as well as points for drug intervention. **Figure 12.1B** illustrates the differences in the cell wall between Gram-positive and Gram-negative bacteria.

The process of infection by bacteria involves entering the host, adhering to cells, and then multiplying and spreading. Bacteria tend to colonize tissues that are in contact with the external environment, like wounds or the respiratory tract. Adhesion takes place either by nonspecific interactions between the host cell and the bacterium or by specific interaction between the pili on the bacterial cell surface and host cell-surface receptors.

Unlike viruses, most bacteria multiply outside of cells, forming microcolonies that can spread either to multiple tissues or into the lymph and bloodstream (bacteremia). Bacteria may or may not be pathogenic and can be classified as primary pathogens, which always cause disease; opportunistic pathogens, which usually cause disease only in immunocompromised patients, and nonpathogens, which are part of the normal flora in a human body and do not cause disease.

The pathogenicity of a specific organism, or **virulence**, is the result of numerous factors including the effectiveness and specific nature of the host's own immune response, the route of entry into the body, and specific virulence factors of the bacterium. Symptoms of a bacterial infection are the result of not only the bacteria themselves and often their toxic secretions but also the host defense mechanisms. In the latter case, immune cells release toxic factors in an effort to eliminate the infection, but at the same time these factors can destroy surrounding tissue.

Since bacteria are rapidly evolving systems, the emergence of resistant organisms is a constant problem, and its impact on health is growing. The inappropriate use of antibiotics contributes to the development of resistant organisms. Bacteria can pass on their resistance genes either in a linear fashion, to their progeny, or horizontally through plasmids to other nonresistant bacteria, exacerbating the problem. The most common causes of resistance are mutations in the bacteria that result in the following:

- production of drug-inactivating enzymes

- evolution of altered drug targets with reduced drug affinity

- decreased permeability of the bacterium to drugs

- production of drug efflux systems

In 2016, the US Centers for Disease Control (CDC) estimated that, each year in the United States, 2 million people are infected with resistant organisms and 23,000 die from those infections. Even more alarming are estimates that, if resistance continues unchecked, the number of deaths per year worldwide will grow to 10 million. While there are currently many antibacterial drugs, there is clearly a need for new agents due to this escalation in resistant organisms.

ANTIBACTERIAL DRUG DISCOVERY

In this day and age, it is difficult to appreciate the importance of the discovery of antibacterial drugs. Treatment of bacterial infections with highly toxic metals, such as mercuric chloride and arsenic, was common from the Middle Ages until the early 1900s. At that time, Ehrlich began a systematic investigation of agents to treat syphilis, a significant public health problem. On the basis of the recent identification of the causative agent, *Treponema pallidum*, and his interest in the use of organic dyes to stain bacteria, he and his colleagues embarked on a study of organoarsenic compounds. Number 606, Salvarsan or arsphenamine (**Figure 12.2**), was introduced in 1910. It was effective against *T. pallidum*, as well as the parasite that causes sleeping sickness, but did not target a wide range of bacteria. For many years the structure of Salvarsan was believed to be analogous to that of azo dyes, containing an As=As double bond; however, the correct structure was determined in 2005 by Brian Nicholson to be a mixture of cyclic species (see Figure 12.2).

Other early drugs used as antiseptics to inhibit the growth of microorganisms were aminoflavins such as proflavine (see Figure 12.2), introduced in the early 1900s to treat topical infections. The first broadly effective and safe antibacterial agents were

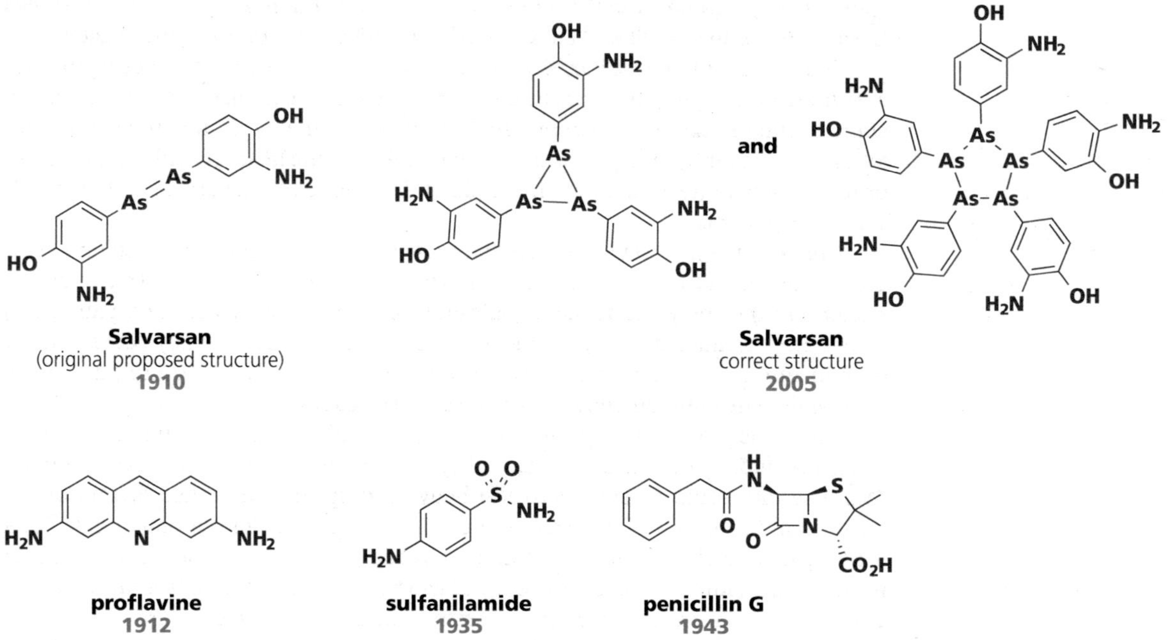

Salvarsan
(original proposed structure)
1910

Salvarsan
correct structure
2005

proflavine
1912

sulfanilamide
1935

penicillin G
1943

the sulfonamides (commonly called sulfa drugs), such as the prototype sulfanilamide, that was launched in 1935. Soon after, in the early 1940s, the penicillin fungal metabolites represented by penicillin G became widely used. They were bactericidal rather than bacteriostatic like the sulfa drugs, and they had a lower incidence of side effects. Since then, there have been hundreds of antibacterial drugs introduced that led to successful treatment of most bacterial infections. Despite these advances, there is a continual need for new antibacterial agents, primarily due to the development of drug resistance.

A particular problem is that of nosocomial or hospital-acquired infections, which result in approximately 100,000 deaths per year. Many of these infections are due to drug-resistant organisms. The increased severity of this problem is evidenced by the fact that in 1975 only 2% of strains of *Staphylococcus aureus* (SA) were penicillin-resistant, but by 1988 that number had increased to 80%. Of those, 40% were also resistant to another drug, methicillin; and a significant portion of methicillin-resistant *Staphylococcus aureus* (MRSA) strains (78%) have developed cross-resistance to other classes of antibacterial drugs. Even organisms that were nearly eradicated have made a comeback: between 1980 and 1992, deaths from *Mycobacterium tuberculosis* increased by 58%. Some of the most problematic organisms have been labeled as ESKAPE pathogens, since they cause most hospital infections and escape the action of antibacterial drugs. These include *S. aureus*, *Klebsiella pneumoniae*, *Acinetobacter baumannii*, *Pseudomonas aeruginosa*, and *Enterobacter* species. Despite this increase in resistant organisms and lack of efficacy of current drug classes towards them, from 2000 to 2016, of the approximately 25 new antibacterial drugs that were introduced, only two are from novel structural classes (cyclic lipopeptides and oxazolidinones).

Over the last several years, increasing attention has been focused on the very real possibility of a return to the pre-antibacterial era. In the United States, promising new developments include recent passage of the Generating Antibiotics Incentive Now Act (GAIN), which gives an extra 5–7 years of patent life for antibacterial drugs. In the European Union, the establishment of the Innovative Medicines Initiative New Drugs for Bad Bugs (IMI ND4BB) is a $280 million fund that supports clinical development of new antibacterial drugs, as well as basic research. These initiatives have spurred renewed interest in developing new antibacterial drugs, and some compounds that languished for years due to regulatory issues have recently been approved. One example is dalbavancin, which was discovered in 1996 but did not receive FDA approval until 2014.

Figure 12.2 Early antibacterial drugs and years introduced. Structures of Salvarsan (purported and actual), proflavine (an aminoflavin), sulfanilamide (from the sulfonamide, or sulfa, drug class), and penicillin G are shown.

Although the terms are often used interchangeably, the term **antibiotic** refers to products such as penicillin that are derived from microorganisms and inhibit bacterial growth. An **antibacterial agent** is any compound, natural or synthetic, that inhibits bacterial growth. Some drugs are **bactericidal**, killing the bacteria, while others are **bacteriostatic** and inhibit replication but do not kill existing bacteria. **Antiseptics** include a number of common compounds, such as phenols and alcohols, that do not have a defined mechanism but are used topically on skin and tissue to inhibit growth of microorganisms. Some common pathogenic bacteria include the Gram-positive bacteria *S. aureus*, *Streptococcus pyogenes*, and *S. pneumoniae*. One important group of pathogenic Gram-positive bacteria is mycobacteria, with *M. tuberculosis* causing about 2 million deaths per year worldwide. Mycobacteria have an outer waxy cell wall that is difficult for drugs to penetrate. Examples of Gram-negative bacteria that cause disease include *Escherichia coli*, *Neisseria gonorrhoeae*, *Salmonella* species, and *P. aeruginosa*. **Table 12.1** highlights some disease-causing bacteria and classes of drugs that are effective against them.

Some of the components of bacteria targeted by drugs include the cell wall, plasma membrane, ribosomes, and DNA function (see Figure 12.1A). The four major categories of antibacterial drugs, based on mechanism of action, include cell-wall synthesis inhibitors, protein synthesis inhibitors, nucleic acid synthesis inhibitors, and drugs that affect membrane permeability. Ideal antibacterial drugs work against multiple strains of both Gram-positive and Gram-negative bacteria and are orally active with low toxicity.

Table 12.1 **Examples of common pathogenic bacteria, associated diseases and conditions, and drugs or drug classes used to treat each.**

Bacterium	Disease or condition	Drugs
Gram-positive bacteria		
Streptococcus pneumoniae	pneumonia, meningitis	β-lactams, tetracyclines, macrolides
Streptococcus pyogenes	strep throat, skin infections, rheumatic fever	β-lactams, macrolides
Staphylococcus aureus	pneumonia, blood infections, skin infections	β-lactams, tetracyclines, (resistant: vancomycin, daptomycin, sulfa)
Clostridium difficile	diarrhea	vancomycin, metronidazole
Mycobacterium tuberculosis	tuberculosis	isoniazid, rifampicin, ethambutol, pyrazinamide, quinolones, aminoglycosides
Gram–negative bacteria		
Escherichia coli	food poisoning, gastroenteritis	β-lactams, aminoglycosides, quinolones, sulfonamides
Salmonella species	food poisoning, typhoid	β-lactams, quinolones, sulfonamides
Neisseria gonorrhoeae	gonorrhea	β-lactams, macrolides
Shigella species	food poisoning, dysentery	β-lactams, quinolones
Pseudomonas aeruginosa	pneumonia, sepsis	β-lactams, aminoglycosides, quinolones
Helicobacter pylori	gastritis, ulcers	β-lactams, metronidazole, macrolides
Legionella pneumophila	Legionnaire's disease	macrolides, quinolones, tetracyclines
Haemophilus influenzae	pneumonia, meningitis	β-lactams, quinolones, macrolides
Borrelia burgdorferi	Lyme disease	tetracyclines, β-lactams
Treponema pallidum	syphilis	β-lactams, tetracyclines
Klebsiella pneumoniae	pneumonia, sepsis	β-lactams, aminoglycosides, quinolones

BACTERIAL CELL-WALL SYNTHESIS INHIBITORS

The bacterial cell-wall structure depends on the cross-linking of **peptidoglycan** strands. The strands are composed of *N*-acetylmuramic acid (NAM) and *N*-acetylglucosamine (NAG) polysaccharides, with peptide strands linked to the NAM strand, containing diaminopimelic acid (DAP) and terminating in D-Ala-D-Ala residues. Cross-linkage is catalyzed by peptidoglycan transpeptidase, a serine protease, also known as **penicillin-binding protein** (PBP), of which there are multiple isoforms. These enzymes react at the amide between the D-Ala-D-Ala residues to generate an acyl-enzyme intermediate, and then the amine of DAP on a second peptidoglycan strand displaces the enzyme. The basic process for the cross-linking step is outlined in **Figure 12.3** (see Chapter 7 for the specific mechanism of serine proteases).

Cell-wall synthesis inhibitors comprise about 44% of all antibacterial drugs on the market and include the β-lactam antibacterial compounds, as well as vancomycin and its analogs. The discovery of penicillin led the way to the discovery and development of numerous analogs of β-lactams, including the penicillins, cephalosporins, carbapenems, penems, and monobactams.

β-Lactam antibacterial compounds are irreversible inhibitors of the bacterial serine protease, with the active-site serine adding to the β-lactam's reactive carbonyl, acylating the enzyme (mechanism outlined in Figure 7.26). Vancomycin and its analogs also inhibit cell-wall synthesis, but instead of acting as enzyme inhibitors, they bind to the D-Ala-D-Ala portion of the enzyme substrate.

12.1 β-Lactam antibacterial compounds are the largest class of cell-wall synthesis inhibitors

The discovery of penicillin in 1928 by Alexander Fleming is one of the most important chapters in medicinal chemistry. A bacteriologist, Fleming had previously isolated the enzyme lysozyme and was studying the lysis, or cell breakdown, of bacteria.

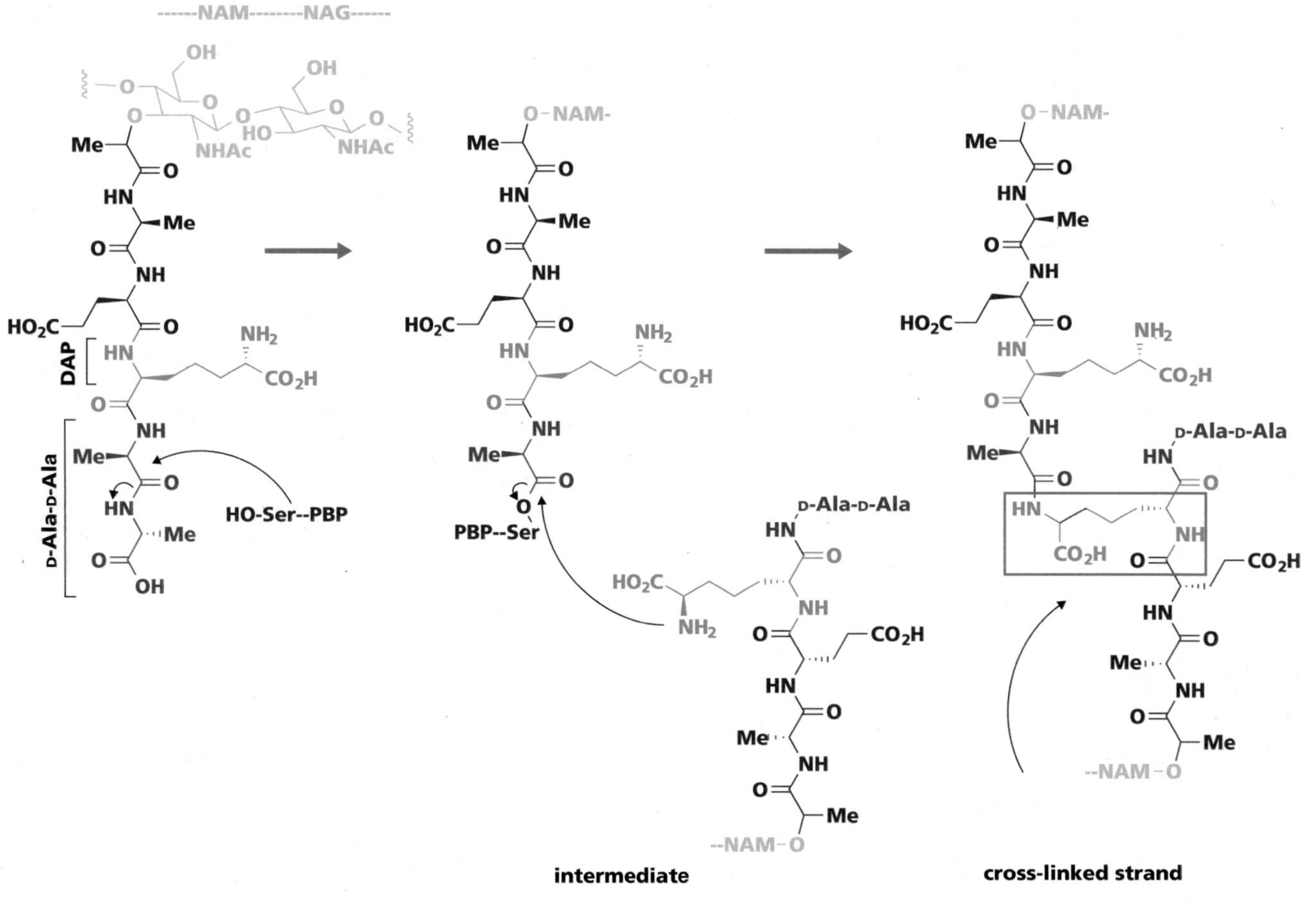

Figure 12.3 Formation of bacterial cell-wall cross-links catalyzed by penicillin-binding protein. Cell walls are composed of *N*-acetylmuramic acid (NAM) and *N*-acetylglucosamine (NAG) polysaccharides (green), with peptide strands linked to the NAM strand, containing diaminopimelic acid (DAP, blue) and terminating in D-Ala-D-Ala residues (red). The serine hydroxyl group in PBP attacks the amide bond between the two terminal D-alanine residues of a peptidoglycan strand; addition of the amino group of DAP from a second peptidoglycan strand to the acyl-enzyme intermediate forms a cross-link (boxed) and releases the enzyme.

intermediate   **cross-linked strand**

thiazolidine oxazolone

β-lactam structure

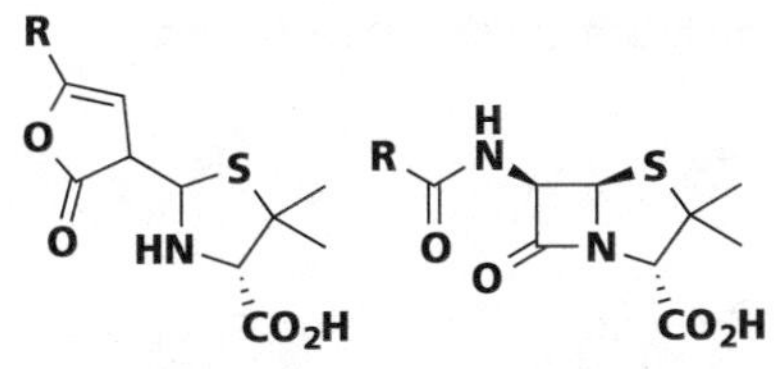

Figure 12.4 Proposed penicillin structures. The incorrect thiazolidine oxazolone and the correct β-lactam structure, confirmed by X-ray crystallography (R = benzyl), are shown.

Upon returning from several weeks of vacation, he observed that an uncovered plate of the bacterium *S. aureus* had been contaminated with a mold, and lysis had occurred where the bacterial colonies were in contact with the mold. He identified the mold as *Penicillium rubrum* (later corrected to *Penicillium notatum*), cultured the broth, and found it to be an effective antibacterial agent against a number of Gram-positive organisms, as well as the Gram-negative *N. gonorrhoeae*. He also injected the mold into rabbits and mice and noted its lack of toxicity. However, he was unable to isolate the active component, and his isolation attempts were abandoned in 1932. Three years later saw the introduction of the synthetic sulfonamide antibacterial drugs, and then in 1938 Ernst Chain and Howard Florey carried out a systematic study of all reported antibacterial compounds. Believing the active ingredient in Fleming's mold to be an enzyme, Chain was able to isolate penicillin in 1938 by using milder techniques than conventional isolations that used acid and base extractions (see Chapter 1.1). With the advent of World War II in Europe, the need for antibacterial agents became urgent, and the scale-up and production of penicillin through isolation was primarily done in the United States, at Merck, Squibb, and Pfizer pharmaceutical companies. Until 1944, penicillin was in short supply and availability was restricted mainly to the military. The structure of penicillin was not fully clarified until Dorothy Hodgkin elucidated it by use of X-ray crystallography. Until then, the two most common structures proposed were a thiazolidine oxazolone, supported by Sir Robert Robinson, and a β-lactam, proposed by Robert B. Woodward and supported by Ernst Chain (**Figure 12.4**). The X-ray structure unequivocally confirmed the bicyclic β-lactam structure.

Penicillins are bicyclic β-lactam antibacterial compounds, with the lactam ring fused to a five-membered thiazolidine ring (**Figure 12.5**). As found by Fleming and later confirmed by Chain and Florey, penicillins exhibit good activity against Gram-positive bacteria.

The original fermentation products were penicillin G (benzylpenicillin) and penicillin V (phenoxymethylpenicillin), which are still in clinical use. Only one enantiomer is active, and requirements for activity include the β-lactam thiazolidine bicyclic core, a free carboxylic acid at C3, and an amide side chain at C6 (see Figure 12.5). The amide substituent can be varied, as long as it contains an aryl group. Many active amide substituents also contain an amine or carboxylic acid at the position α to the carbonyl. The specific amide substituent can have a profound influence on the activity of the compound. In some cases, its steric bulk protects the lactam ring from deactivation by β-lactamases, and in others it can afford improved permeability. Substitution of either oxygen or carbon for the sulfur atom in the thiazolidine ring maintains activity, but no compounds based on these scaffolds are used clinically. Substitution on one of the C2 methyls with a heterocycle maintains potency. Due to the mechanism of action (reaction with the serine protease), reactivity of the β-lactam carbonyl is essential.

There are approximately 20 penicillin derivatives marketed, with the majority being semisynthetic C6 amide derivatives. Variations in the side-chain amide are prepared by selective amide hydrolysis of the readily available natural products penicillin V or G (**Figure 12.6A**) to give 6-aminopenicillanic acid (6-APA), followed by coupling to a wide variety of acids or acid chlorides, as seen in **Figure 12.6B**.

Numerous semisynthetic analogs have been prepared, and penicillins are still some of the most widely used antibacterial drugs. Methicillin (1959) is an example of an early analog that has some activity against resistant organisms (see Figure 12.6A). All penicillins are susceptible to acid degradation in the stomach, with some having better oral availability than others. Resistance to penicillins has been a problem

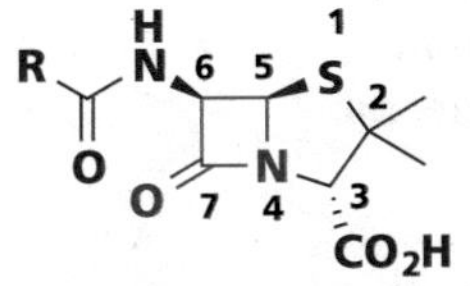

Figure 12.5 Structure–activity relationships of penicillins. All active penicillins contain the bicyclic core, with the stereochemistry shown. An amide at C6 is required, as is the C3 acid. The sulfur may be replaced with either oxygen or carbon, and one of the C2 methyl groups may be substituted with a heterocycle.

penicillin structure (β-lactam in red)

STRUCTURE–ACTIVITY RELATIONSHIPS

position 1 = usually sulfur; oxygen or carbon also active
postion 2 = usually dimethyl; substitution on methyl with heterocycle tolerated
position 3 = carboxylic acid required
position 4, 7 = β-lactam moiety required
position 6 = amide; R group variable aryl
stereochemistry: as shown

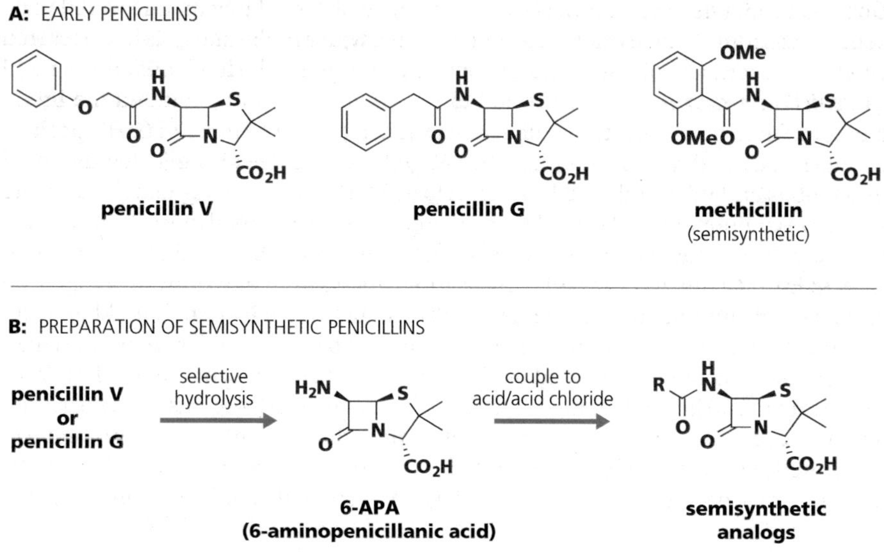

A: EARLY PENICILLINS

penicillin V   penicillin G   **methicillin**
                                            (semisynthetic)

B: PREPARATION OF SEMISYNTHETIC PENICILLINS

penicillin V   selective   **6-APA**   couple to   **semisynthetic**
or   hydrolysis   (6-aminopenicillanic acid) acid/acid chloride   **analogs**
penicillin G

Figure 12.6 Structures of early penicillins and preparation of semisynthetic analogs. A: Early penicillins include natural products penicillin V and G and semisynthetic analog methicillin. B: Synthesis of semisynthetic analogs. Hydrolysis of the natural products penicillin V or G affords 6-APA which is used to prepare various amide semisynthetic derivatives.

almost since their introduction, in part due to bacterial production of the penicillin-inactivating enzyme β-lactamase. Some penicillins that have activity against β-lactamase-producing strains include dicloxacillin, oxacillin, and nafcillin. These are active against Gram-positive bacteria exclusively (**Figure 12.7**).

Amine analogs of penicillin G (aminopenicillins), such as amoxicillin and ampicillin, show improved acid stability as well as activity against some Gram-negative bacteria such as *E. coli* and *H. influenzae.* Of the two, amoxicillin has better oral activity than ampicillin, which is used as its prodrug, pivampicillin. The prodrug contains a pivaloyloxymethyl ester at C3 that is hydrolyzed *in vivo* to give ampicillin. The ester, although inactive until hydrolyzed, provides greater oral bioavailability. The carboxypenicillins and ureidopenicillins have a broader spectrum of activity than the earlier penicillins and can be used to treat Gram-negative infections. The carboxypenicillins, examples of which are ticarcillin and carbenicillin (used for veterinary medicine), contain a carboxylic acid group as part of the C6 amide side chain. The ureidopenicillins, such as mezlocillin, azlocillin, and piperacillin, were introduced in the 1980s and can be considered analogs of the aminopenicillins. They have improved activity against *P. aeruginosa* as well as some anaerobic bacteria. Of these, piperacillin is still used clinically.

As mentioned above, a major antibiotic resistance mechanism is the production of β-lactamase, an enzyme that evolved from PBP and hydrolyzes the β-lactam ring in penicillins and other β-lactam antibacterial compounds. It has no function in cell-wall biosynthesis and serves only to inactivate the β-lactams. Successful strategies to mitigate this resistance mechanism include identifying drugs with low susceptibility to β-lactamase and identifying inhibitors of it that can be co-administered with β-lactam antibacterial drugs. The most commonly used β-lactamase inhibitor is clavulanic acid, a natural product isolated from *Streptomyces clavuligerus* in the 1970s (**Figure 12.8**). Although this oxapenem possesses a bicyclic β-lactam, it has no amide at C6 and has only minimal antibacterial activity. However, it is a potent inhibitor of the β-lactamase enzyme and is an example of a suicide inhibitor, or mechanism-based inactivator (see Figure 7.27).

To increase its effectiveness, amoxicillin is widely prescribed in combination with the β-lactamase inhibitor clavulanate and the carboxypenicillin ticarcillin is used almost exclusively in combination with clavulanate. Other β-lactamase inhibitors used in combination with penicillins include the penicillin sulfones tazobactam and sulbactam (see Figure 12.8).

Another resistance mechanism used by bacteria is the production of PBPs that can still catalyze cell-wall biosynthesis but have reduced affinity for penicillins. This type of resistance is seen in MRSA, an organism that carries the *mecA* gene, which encodes a mutant PBP. This modified enzyme does not bind the drug methicillin but β-LACTAMASE-RESISTANT

dicloxacillin

oxacillin

nafcillin

AMINOPENICILLINS

amoxicillin

ampicillin

pivampicillin
(pro-drug)

CARBOXYPENICILLINS

ticarcillin

carbenicillin

UREIDOPENICILLINS

mezlocillin

azlocillin

piperacillin

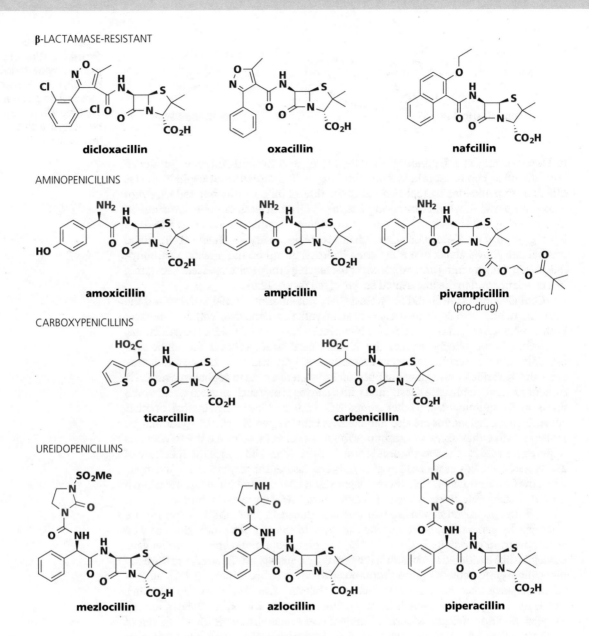

Figure 12.7 **Structures of semisynthetic penicillins.** Families include β-lactamase-resistant penicillins; aminopenicillins, characterized by the presence of a primary amine; carboxypenicillins, which all contain a carboxylic acid in the amide side chain; and ureidopenicillins, typified by a cyclic urea in the amide side chain. Common structural features within each family are shown in red.

still catalyzes cell-wall biosynthesis. Other resistant bacteria with altered PBPs include *S. pneumoniae* and *N. gonorrhoeae*.

Cephalosporins were the second family of β-lactam antibiotics to be isolated. Cephalosporin C was found in a fungus by Giuseppe Brotzu in Sardinia in the early 1940s. This discovery was prompted by efforts to reduce the incidence of typhoid fever (caused by *Salmonella typhi*) in Sardinia. The *S. typhi* organism was found in the sewers but not in nearby seawater, so Brotzu cultured the seawater and identified a fungus (*Cephalosporium acremonium*) responsible for the antibacterial activity. He isolated an active component that he named mycetin and used it to treat patients with typhoid as well as other bacterial infections. During World War II, he was unable to pursue further development, but after the war, a sample of the fungus was sent

clavulanic acid

tazobactam

sulbactam

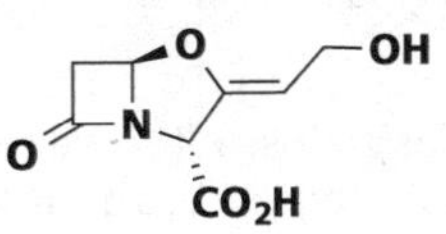

Figure 12.8 **Structures of β-lactamase inhibitors.** The natural product clavulanic acid and the semisynthetic analogs tazobactam and sulbactam, which are used in combination with penicillins, are shown.

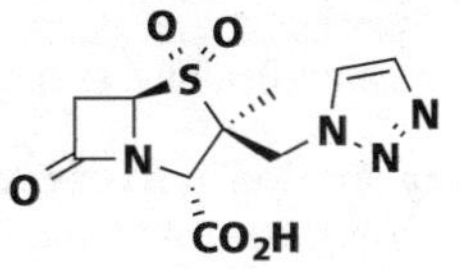

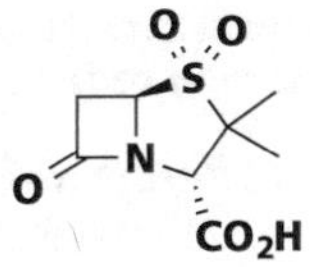

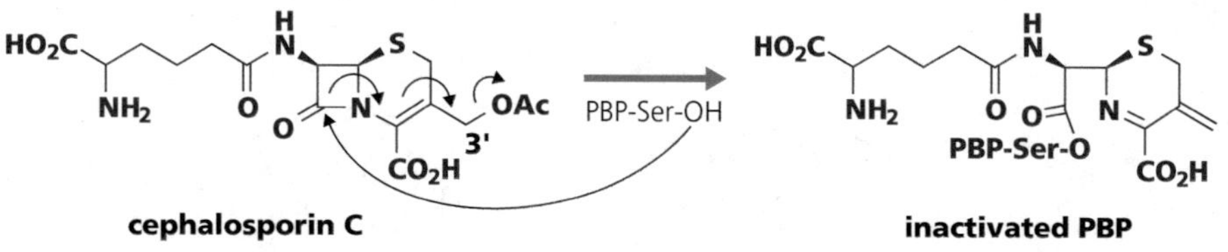

Figure 12.9 Abbreviated mechanism for inactivation of penicillin-binding protein by cephalosporin C. A serine hydroxyl of PBP attacks the β-lactam carbonyl, and a leaving group at C3′ is expelled when the β-lactam ring opens, resulting in a covalently modified, inactivated PBP.

to Florey in England. Ultimately, in 1962, Florey and Edward Abraham produced and identified cephalosporin C from the fungus. The structure of cephalosporins differs from penicillins by replacement of the thiazolidine five-membered ring with a six-membered dihydrothiazine ring (**Figure 12.9**), but both contain the strained β-lactam ring that is essential for activity. In addition, cephalosporins may contain a leaving group at the 3′-position, although this is not necessary for activity. A simplified mechanism shows attack of a PBP serine hydroxyl group on the β-lactam carbonyl, followed by ring opening and expulsion of the leaving group (when present), resulting in a covalent bond to the inactivated enzyme (see Figure 12.9).

Cephalosporin C itself did not possess very potent antibacterial activity, and the most frequently used cephalosporins are semisynthetic derivatives with variations at both the side-chain amide and the 3- or 3′-position (**Figure 12.10**). Like the penicillins, requirements for activity include the bicyclic core structure with the embedded β-lactam with the stereochemistry as drawn, a carboxylic acid at C4 and an amide side chain at C7. Various substitutions at position 3 are tolerated. As in cephalosporin C, C3 sometimes has a methylene substituted with a leaving group such as acetoxy. However, this is not a requirement, and other groups at C3 such as chloro, vinyl, methyl, or other substituted methyl groups are also tolerated. As with the penicillins, the sulfur may be replaced with either oxygen or carbon without loss of activity. While the β-lactam is required for activity, the specific amide and C3 substituents influence the spectrum of antibacterial activity, as well as physical and pharmaceutical properties. For example, when the C3 substituent is CH_2OAc, analogs exhibit Gram-positive activity, but when it is a CH_2-heterocycle, the derivatives have an improved Gram-negative profile.

The first approved cephalosporin was introduced in 1964. Cephalosporins are classified by generation, corresponding roughly to the era of introduction, as well as by spectrum of activity (**Figure 12.11**). The first-generation cephalosporins have penicillin-like amide side chains, and they exhibit an activity profile similar to the early penicillins: good activity against Gram-positive bacteria but limited activity against Gram-negative bacteria. Examples include cefalotin (also known as cephalothin), which requires parenteral administration, due in part to acetoxy hydrolysis, as well as cefazolin and cefalexin. Most have limited oral availability, with the exception of cefalexin. In the late 1970s and 1980s, medicinal chemistry efforts focused on variation of the C7 amide and the 3-position, leading to second-generation cephalosporins such as cefuroxime, cefoxitin, and cefaclor. These are all characterized by improved Gram-negative potency but reduced Gram-positive potency. The oxime in the amide side chain of cefuroxime provides improved stability toward β-lactamase. Cefoxitin is an example of a cephamycin, a semisynthetic derivative of a naturally occurring cephem that possesses an α-methoxy group at C7.

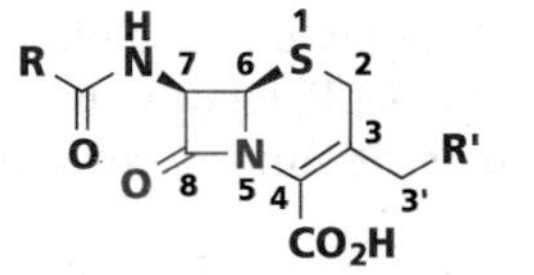

**cephalosporin structure
(β-lactam in red)**

STRUCTURE–ACTIVITY RELATIONSHIPS

position 1 = usually sulfur; oxygen or carbon also active
position 3 = Cl, vinyl, propenyl, methyl, CH_2R (R = OAc, heterocycle)
postion 3′ (R′) = acetate (Gram-positive), heterocycle (improved Gram-negative)
position 4 = carboxylic acid
position 5, 8 = β-lactam moiety required
position 7 = amide; many R groups tolerated
stereochemistry: as shown

Figure 12.10 Structure–activity relationships of cephalosporins. All active cephalosporins contain a β-lactam embedded within a bicyclic core, with stereochemistry as drawn. An amide at C7 is required, as is the C4 acid. The sulfur atom may be replaced with either oxygen or carbon. The C3-position may be substituted with a small lipophilic group or methylene group containing a leaving group or heterocycle.

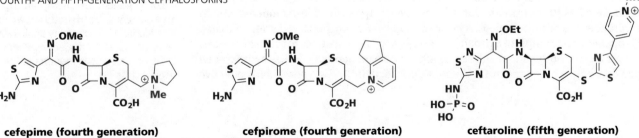

Figure 12.11 First- through fifth-generation cephalosporin structures. Generations correspond roughly to era of introduction as well as spectrum of activity. First-generation drugs (1964–1970s) contain penicillin-like side chains and have activity against Gram-positive organisms; second-generation cephalosporins such as cefuroxime and cefaclor, introduced in the late 1970s, have improved activity toward Gram-negative bacteria, with cephamycins such as cefoxitin (methoxy group shown in red) adding anaerobic activity against organisms typically found in the GI tract. Third-generation cephalosporins (1980s) have improved activity against Gram-negative bacteria; many contain a common aminothiazole oxime, shown in red. Fourth-generation compounds (1990s) have an extended spectrum of activity against Gram-negative organisms and some resistant organisms and are characterized by a cationic C3′-substituent (shown in red). The fifth-generation cephalosporin ceftaroline is a broad-spectrum antibacterial agent, with Gram-positive and Gram-negative activity, as well as activity against resistant organisms such as MRSA due to the 1,3-thiazole ring (shown in red) at C3′.

Further discovery efforts in cephalosporins were driven by a focus on achieving a broader spectrum of activity, including activity against resistant organisms, and enhancements in pharmacokinetics. Major improvements in Gram-negative activity were seen with the third-generation cephalosporins developed in the 1980s. The major structural change involved adding an aminothiazole ring to the oxime amide side chain that had proved successful in the second-generation analog cefuroxime. This combination is found in all third-generation cephalosporins. These changes both broaden the spectrum of activity and improve β-lactamase stability. Examples include cefotaxime, ceftriaxone (which has a long half-life and can be dosed once a day), ceftazidime (which has improved activity against *P. aeruginosa*) and cefixime. Many of these drugs are not orally available, with the exception of cefixime.

The newest cephalosporins are considered members of the fourth and fifth generations. Those in the fourth generation have a broad spectrum of activity, as well as activity against problem organisms such as the ESKAPE pathogens *P. aeruginosa* and *K. pneumoniae*. These compounds retain the aminothiazole oxime-containing amide side chains, and most, such as cefepime and cefpirome, are zwitterions with improved penetration into Gram-negative organisms. The most recent, ceftaroline, is a fifth-generation cephalosporin. It has a broad spectrum of activity, including activity against MRSA, due to the 1,3-thiazole at the C3′-position.

Resistance to cephalosporins occurs through the production of β-lactamase and altered PBPs, as for penicillins. A third prominent mechanism in Gram-negative organisms is the production of mutant porins, which reduces the ability of cephalosporins to penetrate the bacterial cell wall. Porins are transmembrane channels in the outer membrane of Gram-negative bacteria, through which antibacterial compounds, including β-lactams, enter the cell. Mutations in the genes that encode porins produce modified channels that restrict the entry of antibacterial drugs.

The **penems and carbapenems** are a much smaller family of bicyclic β-lactam antibacterial drugs than the penicillins and cephalosporins (**Figure 12.12**). While the penems are synthetic, the carbapenems constitute both natural and semisynthetic products. Both contain a β-lactam fused to an unsaturated five-membered ring. The penem structure was originally proposed as a hybrid of penicillin (4,5 ring system) and cephalosporin (unsaturated sulfur-containing ring) by Woodward, and analogs with and without an amide side chain were prepared but were found to be unstable. Carbapenems are the corresponding analogs in which the sulfur atom is replaced with a carbon. Discovery of the naturally occurring carbapenem thienamycin in 1976, which had the unusual hydroxyethyl side chain, inspired the synthesis of the more stable and less toxic amidine analog imipenem. Both penems and carbapenems are susceptible to hydrolysis by the kidney enzyme renal dehydropeptidase (DHP); therefore, one strategy is to co-administer a DHP inhibitor such as cilastatin (see Figure 12.12). The combination of imipenem and cilastatin is highly effective and is marketed as Primaxin. Addition of a methyl group on the five-membered ring in a carbapenem affords analogs such as meropenem with improved DHP stability. Faropenem, an example of a penem, is the only approved member of the penem class.

As a class, both natural and semisynthetic carbapenems, as well as hydroxyethyl penems, have a broad spectrum of antibacterial activity and are particularly effective

Figure 12.12 Penem and carbapenem structures. Thienamycin, a carbapenem natural product, provided insight into how to generate less toxic and more stable synthetic analogs such as imipenem and meropenem. The combination of imipenem and cilastatin, an inhibitor of renal dehydropeptidase (DHP), sold as Primaxin, extends the half-life of imipenem. The methyl analog meropenem (methyl group shown in red) has improved stability against DHP. Faropenem, an example of a penem, is the only approved member of the penem class.

thienamycin
1976
(carbapenem)

imipenem
1985
(carbapenem)

cilastatin
(DHP inhibitor)

meropenem
1995
(carbapenem)

faropenem
1997
(penem)

Primaxin combination

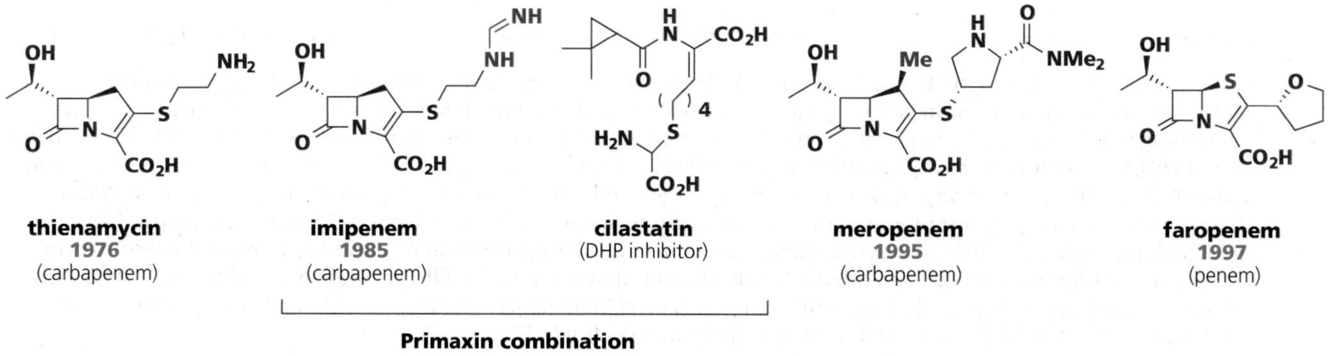

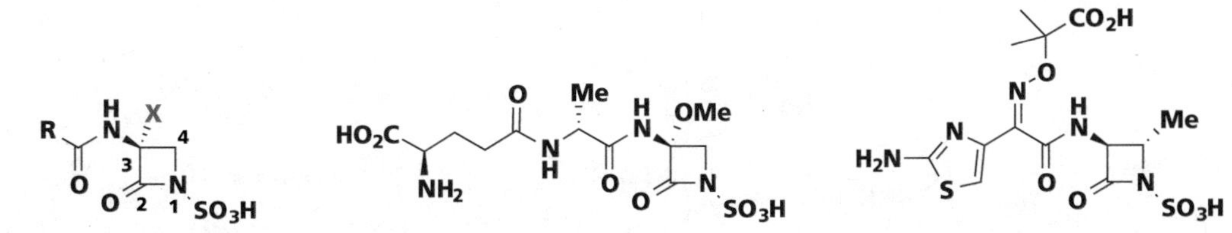

Figure 12.13 Monobactam structures. All monobactams have the general structure on the left with either a proton or methoxy at the 3-position. In addition to the amide, SQ 26,445 was one of the first monobactams reported. The semisynthetic aztreonam, containing a 3rd generation cephalosporin-like aminothiazole oxime, has improved activity compared to the natural product as well as β-lactamase stability.

against many types of anaerobic bacteria. They have also recently been found to be active against *M. tuberculosis*, unlike other β-lactam antibacterial drugs.

Monobactams are monocyclic β-lactams, and aztreonam is the one example on the market. As a class, they are particularly potent against Gram-negative bacteria. The monobactams, represented by the simplified β-lactam ring (**Figure 12.13**), were discovered at Squibb Institute for Medical Research in the late 1970s. Scientists used a strain of *Bacillus licheniformis* that was genetically engineered to be overly sensitive to β-lactams in an effort to identify novel β-lactams. The first monobactams were identified in 1979, with one of the earliest reported being SQ 26,445 (see Figure 12.13). Most of the naturally occurring monobactams contain a sulfonate at position 1, and many possess a methoxy substituent at C3, along with simple amide side chains.

Although the early monobactams typically had only modest antibacterial activity, many synthetic analogs bearing both penicillin- and cephalosporin-like side chains were investigated. The N-sulfonate was found to be necessary for activity; however, the C3 α-methoxy group could be eliminated. A substituent at C4 improved both potency and resistance to β-lactamase, as did incorporation of the aminothiazole oxime amide side chain found in third-generation cephalosporins. A 2-methyl-2-propionic acid moiety on the oxime imparts improved potency against *Pseudomonas*. All of these SAR features are evident in aztreonam (see Figure 12.13), a monobactam introduced in 1984 and still used today to treat severe blood infections.

12.2 Glycopeptide antibacterial agents inhibit cell-wall synthesis by a different mechanism than β-lactams

Vancomycin and teicoplanin are dalbaheptide glycopeptide antibacterial agents; the term dalbaheptide was derived from D-Ala-binding antibiotics having a heptapeptide structure. Vancomycin was isolated in 1953 from a soil bacterium found in Borneo, as a result of a search by Eli Lilly for antibacterial agents with activity against penicillin-resistant *Staphylococcus*. Although vancomycin was approved in 1958, toxicity attributed to impurities in early preparations, as well as the introduction of methicillin in the same year, led to infrequent use of this intravenous drug. In the 1980s, vancomycin began to be used much more frequently to treat postoperative colitis, usually caused by *S. aureus* or *Clostridium difficile*, as well as infections caused by MRSA. Teicoplanin was isolated from a soil bacterium in 1984 and has the same dalbaheptide core as vancomycin (**Figure 12.14**). It contains an additional diphenyl ether bridge, as well as two glycosides (D-mannose and *N*-Ac-glucosamine) and an amide group in place of the L-vancosaminyl unit found in vancomycin. This amide substituent is typically a C8 or C9 chain in place of the L-vancosaminyl carbohydrate of vancomycin. Dalbavancin is very similar in structure to teicoplanin, but has one less carbohydrate unit (*N*-Ac-glucosamine) and converts the acid to an amide, as well as other minor variations.

Like the β-lactam antibacterial drugs, vancomycin, teicoplanin, and dalbavancin inhibit synthesis of the peptidoglycan component of the bacterial cell wall. However, they are not enzyme inhibitors but bind to the peptidoglycan substrate through a series of hydrogen bonds, thus preventing the enzyme from binding.

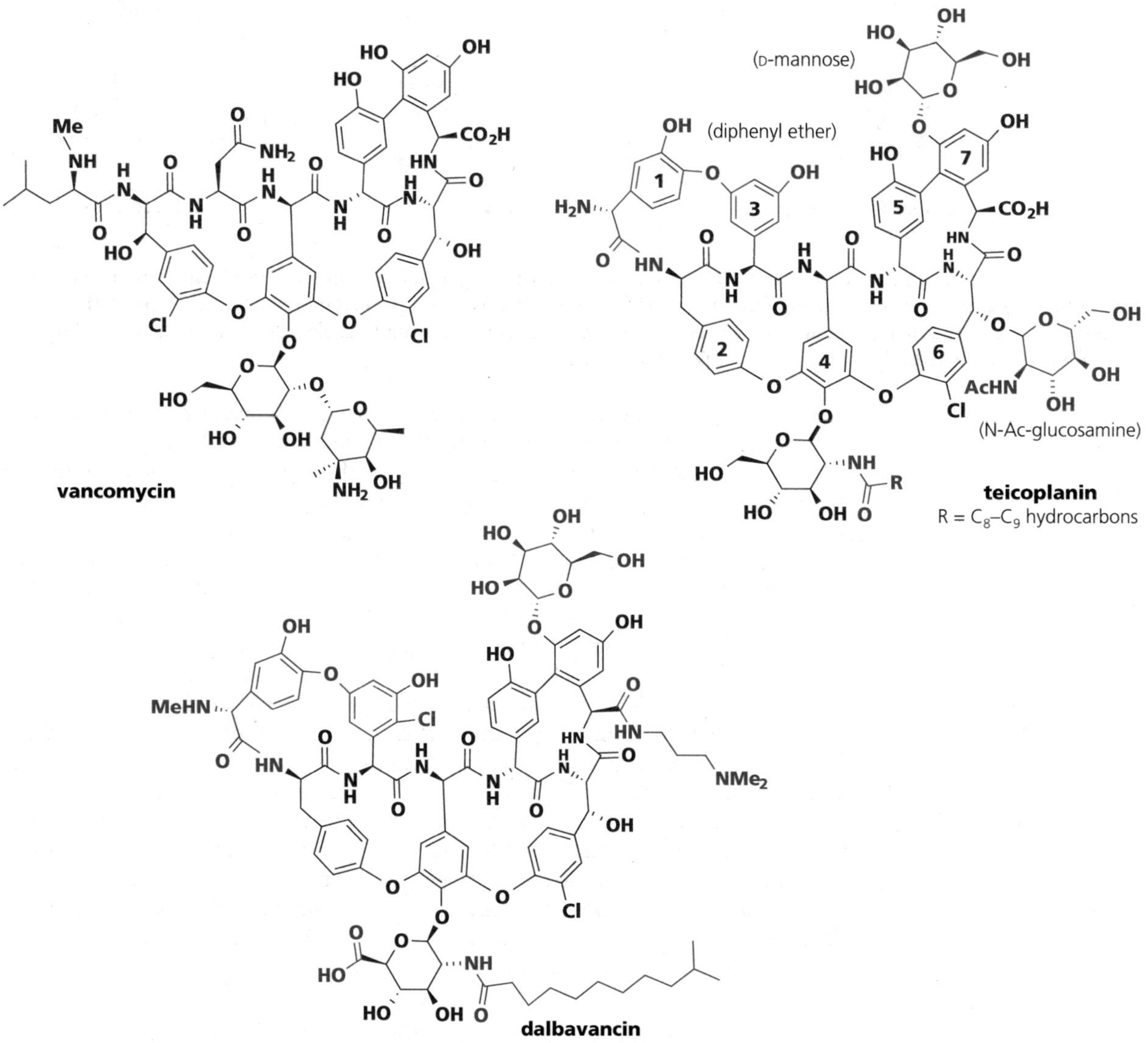

vancomycin

teicoplanin
R = C_8–C_9 hydrocarbons

dalbavancin

An X-ray structure of vancomycin bound to L-Lys-D-Ala-D-Ala is shown in **Figure 12.15**. This mode of binding includes five hydrogen bonds to the carboxylate and backbone of the D-Ala-D-Ala fragment and can be considered an example of a drug interrupting a protein–protein interaction, such as those described in Chapter 8.

Vancomycin resistance is conferred by mutations that change the target D-Ala-D-Ala terminus of the peptidoglycan strand to D-Ala-D-lactate, replacing the peptide bond with an ester or D-Ala-D-Ser, sterically extending the methyl group. These simple changes result in reduced affinity of the target for the drug by 1000-fold. Most mutations that result in resistance to vancomycin do not confer resistance to teicoplanin.

Figure 12.14 Glycopeptide antibiotics. Structures of vancomycin, teicoplanin, and dalbavancin are presented (the aryl amino acid numbering system is shown for teicoplanin). Structural changes compared to vancomycin are shown in red, with the cores in teicoplanin and dalbavancin that are common to vancomycin in black.

BACTERIAL PROTEIN SYNTHESIS INHIBITORS

While many antibacterial agents target the structure of the organism, another class affects the ability to replicate and survive by inhibiting bacterial protein synthesis. There are four major families of drugs in this class: aminoglycosides, tetracyclines, macrolides, and oxazolidinones. All but the oxazolidinones are natural or semisynthetic products, and all act by a similar mechanism, binding to bacterial ribosomes. This binding leads to the synthesis of faulty bacterial proteins, so that eventually protein synthesis is arrested and bacterial cell death occurs.

The process of protein synthesis is outlined in **Figure 12.16**, showing messenger RNA (mRNA) binding to each incoming aminoacyl-transfer RNA (tRNA) in the ribosome. As each tRNA enters the ribosomal machinery, carrying an individual

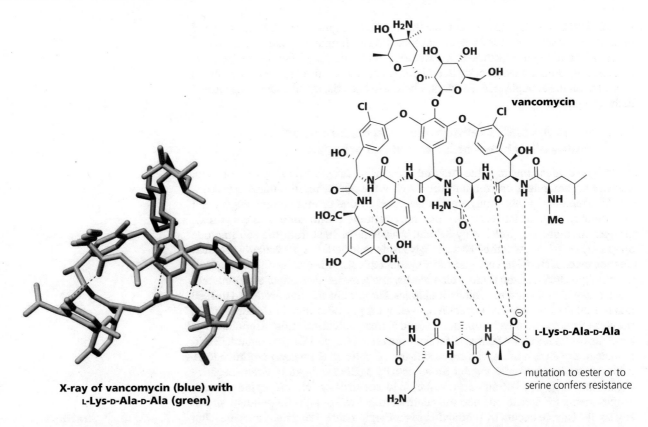

X-ray of vancomycin (blue) with
L-Lys-D-Ala-D-Ala (green)

Figure 12.15 X-ray structure of vancomycin and details of binding interactions. (Left: Vancomycin (blue) hydrogen-bonded to L-Lys-D-Ala-D-Ala (green). Right: Schematic of the five hydrogen bonds (shown as dotted lines) between four amide N-H groups and one carbonyl to the L-Lys-D-Ala-D-Ala substrate. Resistant organisms produce mutant D-Ala-D-Ala-lactate with an ester linkage, resulting in loss of a hydrogen bond and reduced affinity, or a change to serine. (Photo by M. Stone/Wikimedia Commons, CC BY-SA 3.0.)

amino acid, it binds to the aminoacyl (A) site. Here, proofreading occurs to ensure the correct amino acid is matched to the corresponding codon. The tRNA then moves to the peptidyl (P) site, where its amino acid is transferred to the growing peptide chain. Finally, the tRNA shifts to the exit (E) site, where it leaves the ribosome.

Ribosomes are complexes of ribosomal RNA (rRNA) and proteins and are characterized in terms of Svedberg units (S). Bacteria contain 70S ribosomes, consisting of a 30S and 50S subunit. The function of the 30S subunit, which consists of protein

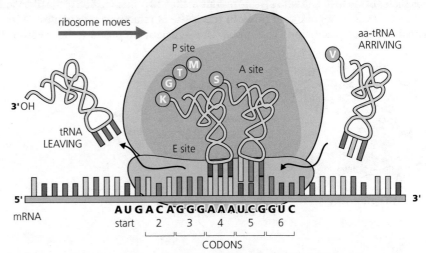

Figure 12.16 Process of protein synthesis on the ribosome. The ribosome, where protein synthesis occurs, consists of multiple proteins and several ribosomal RNA molecules. A template mRNA guides protein synthesis; the two subunits of the bacterial ribosome are shaded pink: the lower part is the 30S subunit, and the upper part is the 50S subunit. On the ribosome, charged aminoacyl-tRNA enters the A site carrying an amino acid; the amino acid is transferred to the growing peptide strand in the P site, and then the tRNA moves to the E site, where uncharged tRNA exits. (Adapted from Kuriyan J, Konforti B &Wemmer D [2012] The Molecules of Life: Physical and Chemical Principles. Garland Science.)

and 16S rRNA, is to decode the incoming tRNA so that the growing peptide is translated properly. Drug selectivity for bacterial ribosomes versus human ribosomes is conferred by both location and structure. Eukaryotic ribosomes are larger (80S) than bacterial ribosomes and have a different rRNA and protein composition. They are located in the cytosol or on the endoplasmic reticulum, whereas in bacteria, the ribosomes are located in the cytoplasm.

12.3 Aminoglycosides, tetracyclines, and erythromycins are protein synthesis inhibitors based on natural products

Aminoglycosides include the natural products streptomycin, paromomycin, neomycin, gentamicin, and tobramycin as well as the semisynthetic amikacin (**Figure 12.17**). Members of this family are characterized by one or more amino sugars and an aminocyclitol, which is a cyclohexane substituted with amino and hydroxyl groups. Streptomycin, isolated by Selman Waksman in 1943 from the soil microbe *Streptomyces griseus*, was the first aminoglycoside reported. It is particularly useful in treating mycobacterial infections, primarily tuberculosis. This was the first example of a natural product isolated from a soil microbe, and it initiated an era of exploration of these organisms as sources of other antibiotics. Paromomycin was introduced in 1960 and is used to treat intestinal infections as well as the parasitic infection leishmaniasis; the closely related neomycin is primarily used to treat topical infections. Gentamicin is a mixture of three closely related natural products (C1, C2, and C1a). Gentamicin and amikacin, as well as tobramycin, are used to treat *E. coli* and *K. pneumoniae* infections. Although aminoglycosides exhibit broad activity against a range of Gram-negative organisms, their use is limited by kidney and ear toxicity (ototoxicity). Structural requirements for activity include the central aminocyclitol and the pendant amino sugars. Resistance occurs by production of aminoglycoside transferase enzymes that modify the amine and alcohol substituents of the drug. Both tobramycin and the semisynthetic amide amikacin have activity against resistant organisms.

The aminoglycosides bind to ribosomal RNA and associated proteins, specifically the A site of the 16S rRNA portion of the 30S subunit of bacterial ribosomes, resulting in inaccurate translational reading. Insight into the mechanism of aminoglycosides comes from an X-ray co-structure with the 30S subunit. **Figure 12.18** shows hydrogen-bonding and ionic interactions between streptomycin and specific residues in the A site. Hydroxyl, aldehyde, amino, and guanidine groups of streptomycin make interactions with phosphates of the RNA and with a lysine residue in the S12 protein region of the ribosome.

Accuracy in recognition of tRNA in the A site is related to two conformations, termed accuracy-prone and error-prone. One segment proposed to be involved in

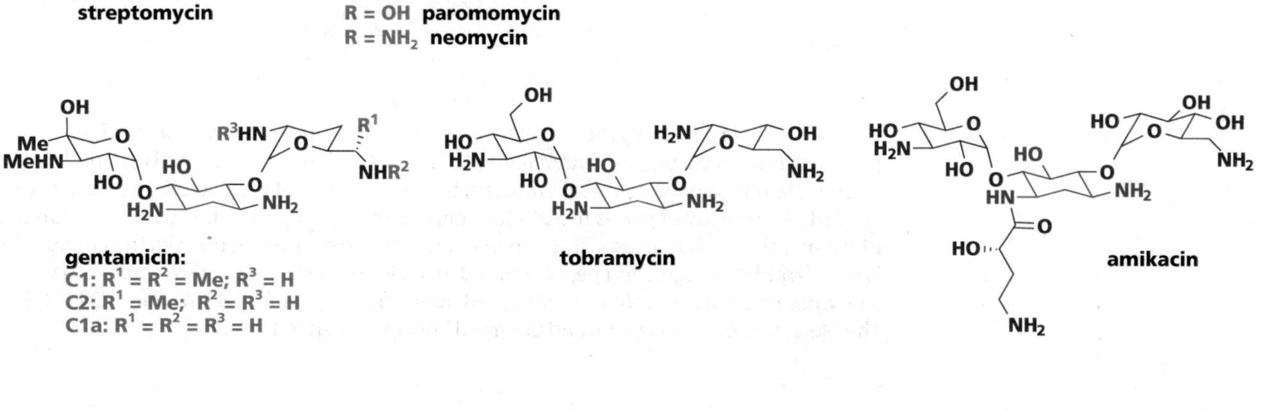

Figure 12.17 Structures of aminoglycoside antibiotics. Common structural features include an aminocyclitol unit called 2-deoxystreptamine (shown in red; note that streptomycin is hydroxylated at position 2) and amino sugars. Streptomycin, paromomycin, and neomycin contain a furanose and a pyranose unit; gentamicin, tobramycin, and the semisynthetic amikacin (from kanamycin) are substituted with pyranose units only.

streptomycin

R = OH **paromomycin**
R = NH$_2$ **neomycin**

gentamicin:
C1: R^1 = R^2 = Me; R^3 = H
C2: R^1 = Me; R^2 = R^3 = H
C1a: R^1 = R^2 = R^3 = H

tobramycin

amikacin

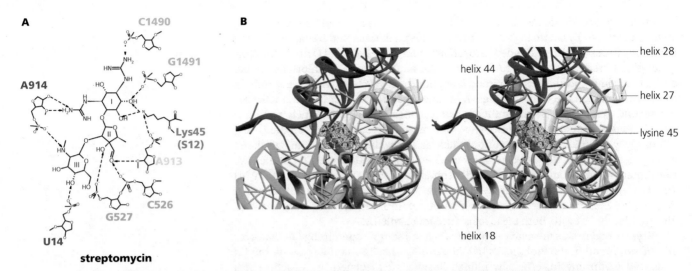

Figure 12.18 X-ray structure of streptomycin in the 30S ribosome subunit. A: Schematic of specific binding interactions, including ionic interactions and hydrogen bonds, between streptomycin and the 30S ribosomal subunit, which is composed of protein and 16S rRNA. Lys45 of ribosomal protein S12 (brown) forms an ionic interaction with the phosphate of A913 (adenine 913) on helix 27 of rRNA (yellow), and also hydrogen-bonds to hydroxyl groups of the aminocyclitol ring of streptomycin, stabilizing the error prone form. A913 interacts with the aldehyde carbonyl group of streptomycin; this aldehyde group also binds to a phosphate between C526 and G527. Other nucleotides that participate in binding include C1490 and G1491 of helix 44 (blue), A914 of helix 28 (purple), and G527 and C526 of helix 18 in rRNA (teal). B: Stereoview of streptomycin bound in the ribosome, showing helix 27, known as the accuracy helix (depicted in yellow) and the S12 ribosomal protein component (depicted in brown); other helices colored as described in A. (From Carter AP, Clemons WM, Brodersen DE et al. [2000] *Nature* 407:340–348. With permission from Macmillan Publishers Limited.)

the conformational change between the two is helix 27 (yellow in Figure 12.18B), sometimes called the accuracy helix, which adopts different conformations in each state. When tRNA binds to the error-prone conformation, it leads to faulty protein translation, while binding to the other conformation leads to accurate translation. Streptomycin binds to and stabilizes the error-prone form, leading to mistakes in the translation of proteins, arrest of protein synthesis, and bacterial growth inhibition.

Tetracyclines, characterized by four fused six-membered rings, were discovered in 1948 when chlortetracycline was isolated from the soil bacteria *Streptomyces aureofaciens* (**Figure 12.19**). They are exemplified by oral activity as well as a broad spectrum of activity against Gram-positive, Gram-negative, and some parasitic infections. As such, they are used to treat sinusitis, bronchitis, and urinary tract infections (UTIs) caused by *H. influenzae*, pneumococci, and *E. coli*, as well as gonococci and *Chlamydia*. This class is particularly useful as a treatment for *Borrelia burgdorferi*, the causative agent of Lyme disease. Tetracyclines are most likely complexed to magnesium ions and then transported into cells through porins. They bind to the 16S RNA of the 30S subunit of the bacterial ribosome and prevent tRNA from binding at the A site.

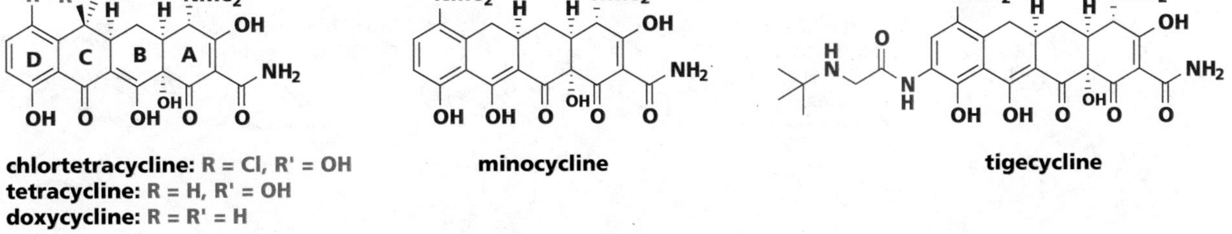

chlortetracycline: R = Cl, R' = OH
tetracycline: R = H, R' = OH
doxycycline: R = R' = H

minocycline

tigecycline

Figure 12.19 Structures of tetracyclines. First-generation analogs are represented by chlortetracycline, tetracycline, and doxycycline, and differ in the substituents on the C and D rings. Minocycline is a second-generation derivative, and semi-synthetic tigecycline is a third-generation derivative. The glycylcycline substituent of tigecycline is shown in red, and may contribute to its activity against resistant organisms.

Structural requirements for activity include the linear fused tetracyclic ring system; the naturally occurring stereochemistry found in the A and B rings, including the *cis* ring fusion; and the extended keto–enol system of the B, C, and D rings. The first-generation tetracyclines (1962–1973) include the natural products chlortetracycline and tetracycline and the semisynthetic compound doxycycline, which vary only in the substituents on the C and D rings. A broader spectrum of activity characterizes the second-generation (semi-synthetic) tetracyclines (1973–1990), such as minocycline. With the emergence of resistance to tetracyclines, substitution on the D ring led to glycylcyclines (third-generation) such as tigecycline, also a semi-synthetic analog (see Figure 12.19). The two major mechanisms for tetracycline resistance are ribosomal protection and drug efflux. Ribosomal protection proteins such as Tet(M) and Tet(O) act by dislodging tetracyclines from the ribosome, and the drug efflux systems are membrane-associated proteins that pump tetracyclines from the cell. The glycylcyclines evade both these resistance mechanisms.

Erythromycin was the active ingredient in a soil sample containing *Streptomyces erythraeus*, found in the Philippines by Abelardo Aguilar. The sample was sent to Eli Lilly, and erythromycin, originally named ilosone, was isolated, its structure was elucidated, and the drug was approved and marketed in 1952. The complex macrolide is polyhydroxylated, with a desosamine sugar at C5 and a cladinose sugar unit at C3. It has potent activity against Gram-positive and some Gram-negative bacteria and is used to treat respiratory, skin, and soft tissue infections, as well as infections caused by *Mycoplasma* and *Legionella*. One liability is its instability in the acidic environment of the stomach. Under those conditions, a significant fraction of the equilibrium mixture is present as the inactive anhydroerythromycin shown in **Figure 12.20**. Formation is initiated when the C12 hydroxyl attacks the C9 ketone to form a 9,12-hemiacetal. This reversible, acid-catalyzed process leads to formation of the 6,9-acetal anhydroerythromycin, limiting the bioavailability of active erythromycin.

One solution to this problem was the development of the C6 methoxy analog clarithromycin, which cannot undergo the ketalization reaction (**Figure 12.21**). Another semisynthetic analog, roxithromycin, contains the C6 methoxy group as well as an oxime (both shown in red) at the original C9 ketone. This modification maintains the activity of the parent but has enhanced stability. Azithromycin, also lacking the C9 ketone, was prepared from erythromycin by a Beckmann rearrangement of a C9 oxime at Pliva Pharmaceuticals in Croatia and was subsequently licensed to Pfizer. This analog replaces the ketone with an amine and expands the ring size of the macrocycle from 14 to 15. Azithromycin has improved potency, acid stability, and spectrum of activity over erythromycin, with a low incidence of side effects.

With increased use of erythromycin, roxithromycin, and azithromycin has come a corresponding increase in emergence of resistant organisms. For example, these drugs are frequently prescribed to treat common infections such as strep throat and upper respiratory infections; however, there are now many *Streptococcus* strains that are resistant to azithromycin.

Macrolides bind to 23S ribosomal RNA of the 50S subunit of ribosomes and prevent translocation of tRNA from the A site to the P site. One mechanism of

Figure 12.20 Erythromycin and its conversion to hemiacetal and acetal forms. Erythromycin is in equilibrium with its 9,12-hemiacetal; loss of H_2O occurs with formation of the 6,9-acetal to generate anhydroerythromycin, which is inactive.

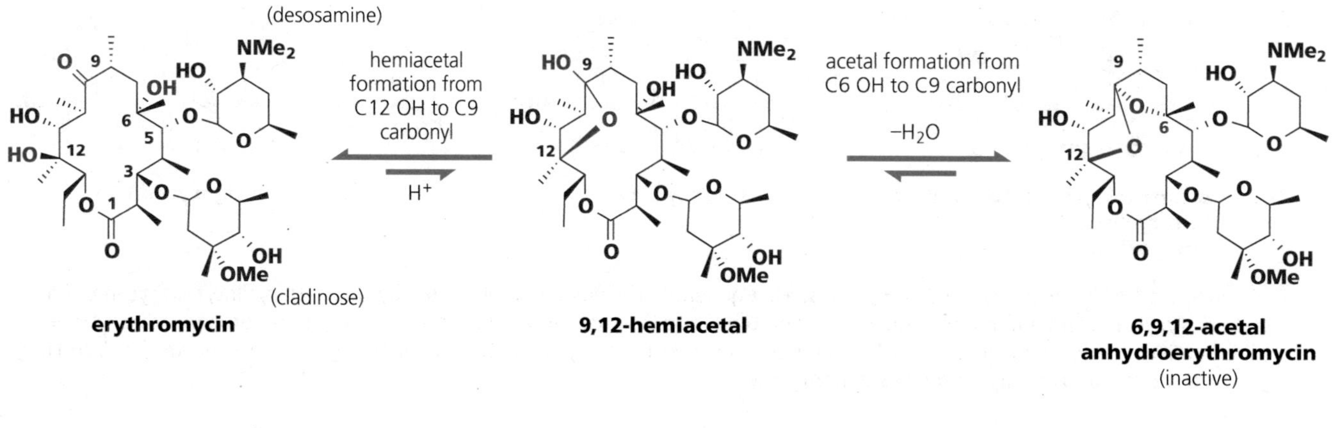

erythromycin   9,12-hemiacetal   6,9,12-acetal anhydroerythromycin (inactive)

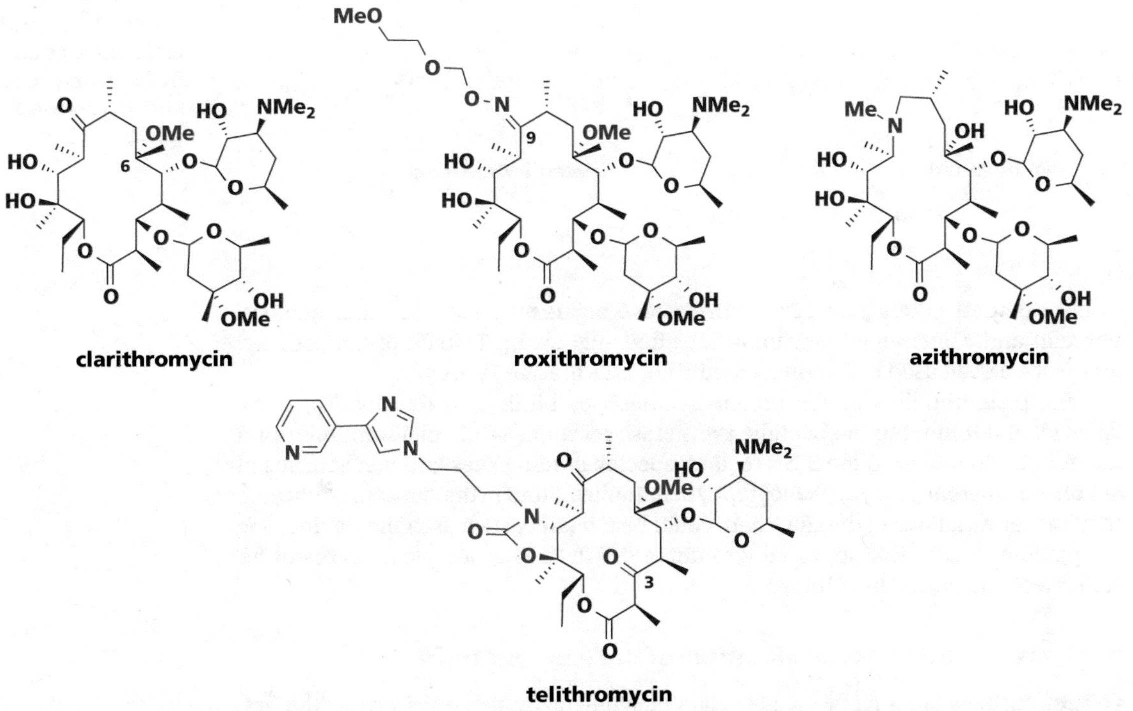

Figure 12.21 Structures of semisynthetic macrolide antibacterial drugs. Clarithromycin, roxithromycin, azithromycin, and telithromycin are shown, with key structural features that are modified compared to erythromycin highlighted in red. These structural changes result in improved stability, and in some cases activity against erythromycin-resistant organisms.

resistance is modification of the ribosome via mono- or dimethylation of an adenine on the 23S ribosomal RNA component of the 50S subunit, which decreases binding to the cladinose of erythromycins. The enzymes carrying out this methylation are known as erythromycin ribosome methylation (Erm) enzymes and are found in resistant organisms. One approach to address this type of resistance is the use of Erm inhibitors, several of which have been identified, although none are used clinically. Another resistance mechanism that has been identified is the production of macrolide efflux proteins, which effectively reduces the amount of macrolide that is absorbed by the bacteria. Further medicinal chemistry optimization of this scaffold found that addition of a cyclic carbamate improved activity against resistant organisms, and replacement of the C3 cladinose ring with a ketone improved activity against efflux-mediated resistance. These modifications led to the ketolide telithromycin.

The **pleuromutilins** (**Figure 12.22**) are antimicrobial compounds from *Pleurotus mutilus*, an edible mushroom. They were initially discovered in 1950 and were found

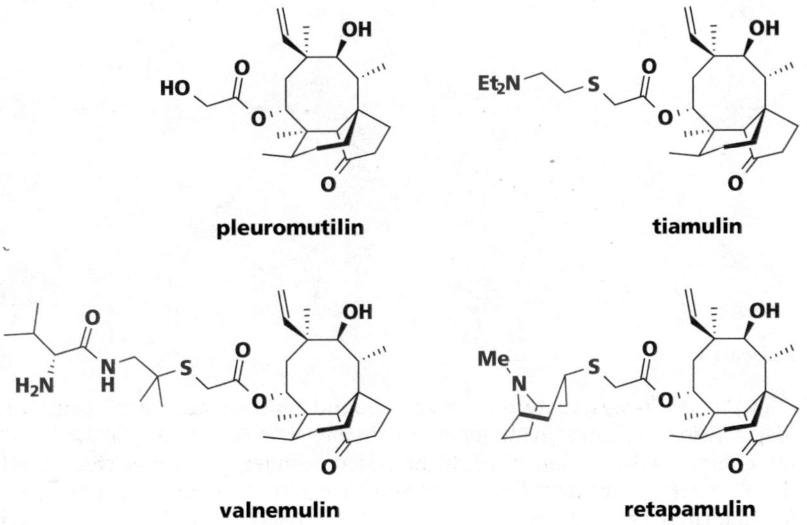

Figure 12.22 Structures of pleuromutilin and thioether analogs. Pleuromutilin is a natural product with modest antibacterial activity. Thioether modifications (shown in red) generated the drugs tiamulin, valnemulin, and retapamulin. Tiamulin and valnemulin are used in veterinary medicine, and retapamulin is approved for use in humans. All inhibit protein synthesis by inhibiting the peptidyl transferase reaction.

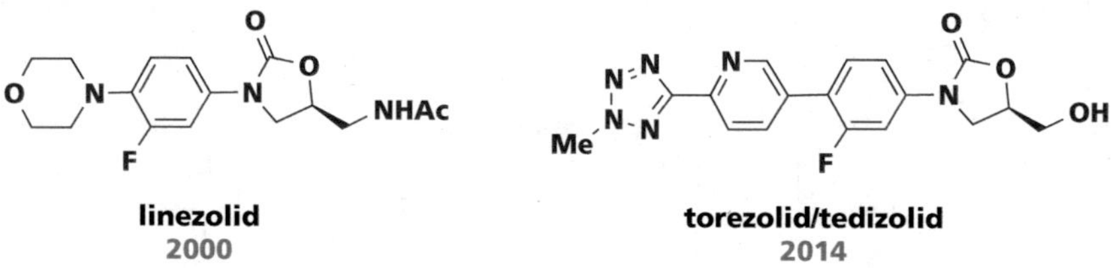

Figure 12.23 Structures of oxazolidinone antibacterial drugs. Linezolid and tedizolid (formerly known as torezolid) are shown.

linezolid
2000

torezolid/tedizolid
2014

to have modest potency against Gram-positive organisms. Two thioether analogs, tiamulin and valnemulin, containing extended side chains instead of the hydroxyl group, have been used in veterinary medicine since the late 1990s.

The pleuromutilins inhibit protein synthesis by binding to nucleotides in the 23S site, and inhibiting the peptidyl transferase reaction. While pleuromutilins and macrolides both bind to the 23S site, their specific binding sites and mechanisms of action are different. X-ray crystallography of tiamulin bound in the ribosome indicated that further variations of the side chain could be tolerated, such as in the rigid analog retapamulin, which was approved for human use in 2006 as a topical treatment for skin infections caused by MRSA.

12.4 Oxazolidinones are inhibitors of protein synthesis

Oxazolidinones are a relatively new class of synthetic antibacterial drugs. The first member of the family, linezolid, was approved in 2000. As of 2017 only one additional oxazolidinone, tedizolid (formerly known as torezolid), is marketed (**Figure 12.23**). This class exhibits potent activity against Gram-positive organisms, particularly against MRSA and vancomycin-resistant enterococci (VRE), as well as activity against *M. tuberculosis*.

On the basis of an X-ray crystal co-structure (**Figure 12.24**), linezolid was shown to bind to the A site of the 50S subunit, and is proposed to prevent tRNA from entering the site.

Hydrophobic interactions are observed between linezolid's aromatic ring and the bases of C2452 and A2451 in 23S ribosomal RNA. Although, as a new class of drugs, resistance has been slow to develop, there were reports of linezolid-resistant organisms within 4 years of its introduction. The resistance mechanism appears to be mainly conferred by mutations to the 23S RNA.

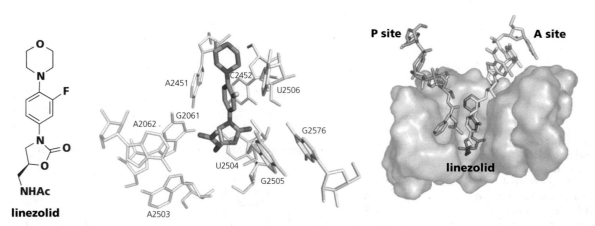

Figure 12.24 X-ray structure of linezolid bound in ribosome. Left: Structure of linezolid. Center, representation of linezolid (depicted in pink) bound in ribosome. Specific interactions include hydrophobic interactions between the aromatic ring of linezolid and nucleobases of the ribosomal RNA. Right: Surface features of ribosome with bound linezolid (depicted in pink). The A and P sites are defined by tRNA substrates shown in blue and tan, respectively. Linezolid occupies the same site as incoming tRNA, blocking its entry. (Adapted from Leach KL, Swaney SM, Colca JR et al. [2007] *Mol Cell* 26:393–402. With permission from Elsevier.)

DRUGS TARGETING BACTERIAL DNA REPLICATION

Two main categories of drugs, DNA gyrase inhibitors (quinolones) and dihydropteroate synthase inhibitors (sulfonamides), specifically prevent bacterial DNA replication and ultimately the ability of bacteria to reproduce and proliferate. Both classes inhibit bacterial enzymes that have human homologs. DNA gyrase is a topoisomerase, involved in supercoiling and uncoiling of DNA during the bacterial replication process. The mechanism of topoisomerases was discussed in Chapter 10, and inhibitors of human topoisomerase are effective anti-cancer agents. Dihydropteroate synthase is an enzyme in the bacterial folic acid biosynthesis pathway. Folic acid is required for DNA synthesis, specifically as the source of the methyl group in thymidine, as was also described in Chapter 10. While humans do not efficiently synthesize folic acid, inhibitors of the related human dihydrofolate reductase, required for biosynthesis of purines and pyrimidines in the DNA replication process, are also used as anti-cancer agents.

12.5 Quinolone antibacterial agents inhibit DNA gyrase

Quinolone antibacterial agents, characterized by the scaffold in **Figure 12.25**, are synthetic compounds that were discovered in 1962. Nalidixic acid is a naphthyridone that was identified by George Lesher at Sterling Pharmaceuticals. This by-product, formed during the synthesis of the antimalarial drug chloroquine, was found to have potent activity against Gram-negative organisms and was the starting point for development of the more useful class of fluoroquinolones. Since the original discovery of nalidixic acid, thousands of quinolones have been reported in the literature, and over 20 are used clinically. Requirements for activity include the quinolone or naphthyridone core, a carboxylic acid or equivalent at position 3, and an aliphatic or aromatic substituent on the N-1 nitrogen. Early calculations indicated that either an ethyl group or the constrained cyclopropyl moiety was the optimal size for the N-substituent, although it was later found that aryl substituents are also tolerated. Addition of a nitrogen heterocycle at C7 results in increased potency against Gram-positive bacteria and improves the compound's half-life. A fluorine atom at the C6-position, which characterizes the fluoroquinolines, improves potency toward DNA gyrase inhibition as well as cell penetration. More recent quinolones include those containing a substituent at C8 (chlorine, fluorine, or methoxy), which improves the overall spectrum of activity. A summary of the quinolone structure–activity relationships is shown in Figure 12.25.

Quinolones are categorized by generation, based primarily on the spectrum of activity. Nalidixic acid, oxolinic acid, and cinoxacin are examples of first-generation compounds, with activity against Gram-positive bacteria (**Figure 12.26**). The 1980s saw the advent of the fluoroquinolones (second generation), which typically contain a cyclic amine at C7. Examples include ciprofloxacin, ofloxacin, levofloxacin, and norfloxacin. These analogs maintain Gram-positive activity and add activity against Gram-negative bacteria. The third-generation agents, closely related in structure to the second-generation fluoroquinolones, have an expanded spectrum of activity against Gram-positive bacteria, especially pneumococci. Examples include sparfloxacin and temafloxacin. The most recent drugs, the fourth generation, have additional activity against anaerobic bacteria and pneumococci. This generation includes compounds such as moxifloxacin, gemifloxacin, and trovafloxacin. The addition of larger, more structurally complex substituents at C7 both decreases susceptibility to efflux and increases activity against certain bacteria. The importance of this class of antibacterial drugs is evidenced by the fact that eight of the nine synthetic antibacterial agents introduced between 2000 and 2009 were fluoroquinolones.

Figure 12.25 Structure of nalidixic acid and structure–activity relationships of quinolone antibacterials. Nalidixic acid was an early example of a DNA gyrase inhibitor and served as the basis for the class of quinolone antibiotics. Active compounds contain a quinolone or naphthyridone core and an acid at C3. Small alkyl or aryl substituents are preferred at N1. A variety of substitutions at C6 are possible, but F is preferred (fluoroquinolones). Cyclic amines at C7 improve potency and duration. C8 may be substituted with halogen or methoxy, which improves the spectrum of activity.

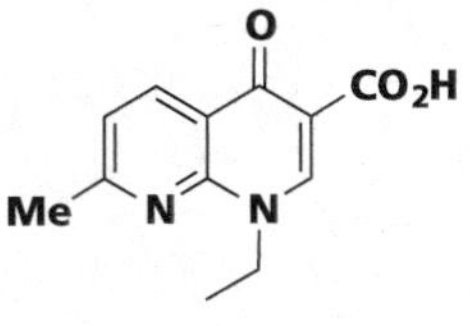

nalidixic acid

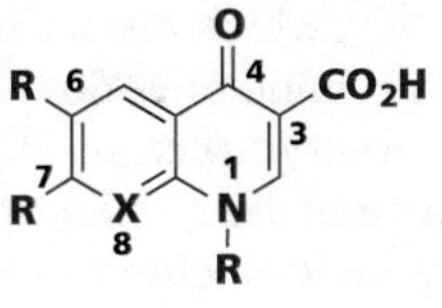

STRUCTURE–ACTIVITY RELATIONSHIPS
position 1 = nitrogen with small alkyl or aryl
position 3 = carboxylic acid or equivalent required
position 4 = carbonyl
position 6 = multiple possibilities; F preferred for potency/permeability
position 7 = H, cyclic amines improve potency and $t_{1/2}$
position 8 = N, C-R; R = halogen or OMe

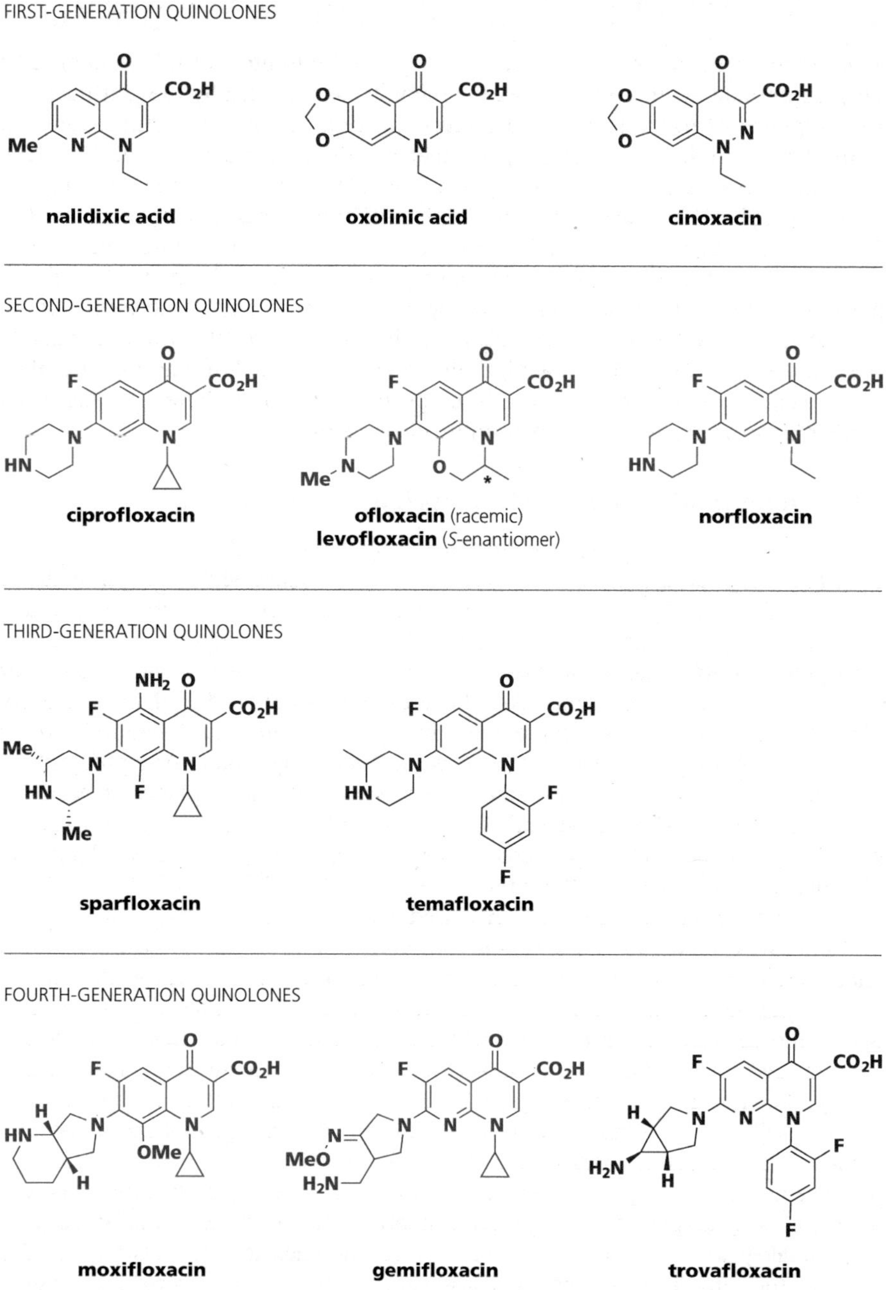

FIRST-GENERATION QUINOLONES

nalidixic acid

oxolinic acid

cinoxacin

SECOND-GENERATION QUINOLONES

ciprofloxacin

ofloxacin (racemic)
levofloxacin (S-enantiomer)

norfloxacin

THIRD-GENERATION QUINOLONES

sparfloxacin

temafloxacin

FOURTH-GENERATION QUINOLONES

moxifloxacin

gemifloxacin

trovafloxacin

Figure 12.26 Examples of quinolone antibacterial drugs according to generation. First-generation quinolones include nalidixic acid (technically a naphthyridone) as well as oxolinic acid and cinoxacin, none of which are still used. Second-generation drugs are all fluoroquinolones, with a fluorine atom at C6 and cyclic amine at C7, which imparts improved potency and permeability. Ciprofloxacin, ofloxacin, levofloxacin, and norfloxacin are still used clinically. Third-generation compounds have branching on the C7 heterocycles and have improved Gram-positive activity; examples include sparfloxacin and temafloxacin, although both have been withdrawn. Examples of fourth-generation compounds include moxifloxacin, gemifloxacin and trovafloxcin (withdrawn). These have bicyclic or complex C7 heterocycles and are active against anaerobes. Those remaining on the market in the United States as of 2017 are shown in red.

However, this class is also plagued by safety issues due to musculoskeletal, cardiovascular, and CNS side effects, leading to removal of several of them from the market.

The quinolone antibacterial drugs are inhibitors of the bacterial enzyme DNA gyrase, or bacterial topoisomerase II. In Gram-positive bacteria, topoisomerase IV is also a target, and it is the primary target of fourth-generation quinolones. DNA gyrase and topoiosmerase IV catalyze the cleavage of double-stranded DNA and introduce negative superhelical turns. The enzyme is a tetrameric (A_2B_2) 400 kDa protein. Subunit A is responsible for cleavage and resealing of the phosphate backbone, and Tyr124 of this subunit makes a covalent bond to DNA. The ATPase activity, which resides in the B subunit, hydrolyzes ATP to produce energy for supercoiling. Quinolones do not bind directly to DNA but to the DNA–gyrase complex to form a ternary structure. The mechanism is similar to that described for human topoisomerases and their inhibitors found in Chapter 10 (see Figure 10.6). Two molecules of the quinolone bind to the DNA–enzyme complex by intercalation into DNA, increasing the concentration of the ternary cleavage complexes and acting as poisons.

Figure 12.27 Representation of quinolone binding to topoisomerase IV. Left: Representation of Mg²⁺ complex with a quinolone, with binding interactions to serine (Ser) and the side chain of an acidic residue (Glu or Asp) mediated through water molecules. Right: X-ray structure of two molecules of moxifloxacin (red) bound to DNA (yellow)–topoisomerase IV (green/blue) complex. Two views are shown. (Adapted from Aldred KJ, Kerns RJ & Osheroff N [2014] *Biochemistry* 53:1565–1574. With permission from American Chemical Society.)

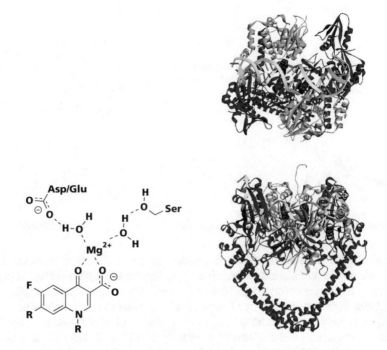

Recent X-ray crystallography has provided detailed insight into the binding and mechanism of action of the quinolones. For example, it had long been proposed that there was a role for Mg²⁺ in quinolone binding, and this was confirmed in 2010. The carbonyl at C4 and the acid at C3 form a complex with a magnesium ion, which forms a bridge to serine and acidic (Asp, Glu) residues on the enzyme, mediated by water molecules (**Figure 12.27**). These residues are absent in human topoisomerase, providing some explanation for the selectivity of quinolones for bacterial DNA gyrase and topoisomerase IV. The planar aromatic quinolone also intercalates into DNA, distorting the helix. An X-ray structure of bound moxifloxacin shows two molecules intercalating into the DNA–enzyme complex, four base pairs apart (see Figure 12.27).

Mechanisms of resistance to quinolones include modification of the target, particularly mutations of the serine and acidic residues that bind to the magnesium complex. Resistance can also be conferred through plasmids, encoding both efflux pumps and proteins that metabolize or acetylate heterocyclic amines present at C7 in second and beyond generation drugs, thereby reducing its activity. Porin mutations in Gram-negative bacteria are also an important resistance mechanism, resulting in both lower expression and decreased ability of quinolones to permeate bacteria.

12.6 Sulfonamide antibacterial compounds inhibit folic acid biosynthesis

The sulfonamides were the first nontoxic synthetic antibacterial drugs. The prototype, the prodrug prontosil, a red dye, was marketed in 1936. Gerhard Domagk and Josef Klarer, at Bayer in Germany, investigated a series of dyes as potential magic bullets that might target bacteria, since they were known to specifically dye bacteria. After a lack of toxicity was demonstrated in mice infected with *Streptococcus*, trials in humans showed both efficacy and safety. Most famously, in 1936, while still a little-known drug, prontosil was used to treat and cure Franklin Roosevelt's son, who was seriously ill from complications of strep throat. The resulting publicity helped to market the drug. Although prontosil is active *in vivo*, it is inactive *in vitro* and is converted by the enzyme azoreductase to sulfanilamide, the active form (**Figure 12.28**).

Since the active component, sulfanilamide, was a known compound used in dye synthesis, numerous preparations were made and sold. Due to lack of regulations and oversight at the time, one of these preparations, in sweet-tasting ethylene glycol, led to the deaths of over 100 patients (see Chapter 5). This tragedy resulted in the passage of the Federal Food, Drug, and Cosmetic Act in 1938, and prontosil is no longer used.

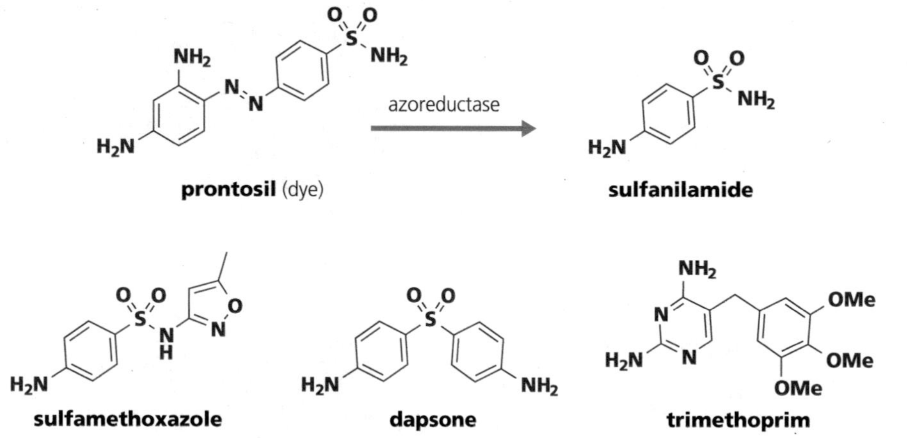

Figure 12.28 Inhibitors of folate biosynthesis. Prontosil is a prodrug that generates sulfanilamide *in vivo*, which inhibits dihydropteroate synthase. Sulfamethoxazole, the only sulfonamide antibacterial drug still in use, and dapsone also inhibit dihydropteroate synthase. Trimethoprim inhibits a different enzyme in the folic acid biosynthesis pathway, dihydrofolate reductase.

The basic structure of all antibacterial sulfonamides includes a *p*-aminosulfonamide moiety, where the sulfonamide nitrogen may be substituted with a variety of groups. Allergic reactions were common, and the sulfa drugs were widely replaced by penicillins in the 1940s. Sulfamethoxazole (see Figure 12.28) is the one example still in use.

The sulfonamide antibacterial drugs are inhibitors of dihydropteroate synthase, an enzyme required for the synthesis of tetrahydrofolic acid, which is a coenzyme required for DNA synthesis in bacteria. In a reaction catalyzed by dihydropteroate synthase, *p*-aminobenzoic acid (PABA) reacts with dihydropteroate diphosphate in a displacement reaction to give dihydropteroic acid. This product is the substrate for a series of additional steps that includes installation of the amide bond (shown in red) found in tetrahydrofolic acid, as shown in **Figure 12.29A**. The sulfonamide

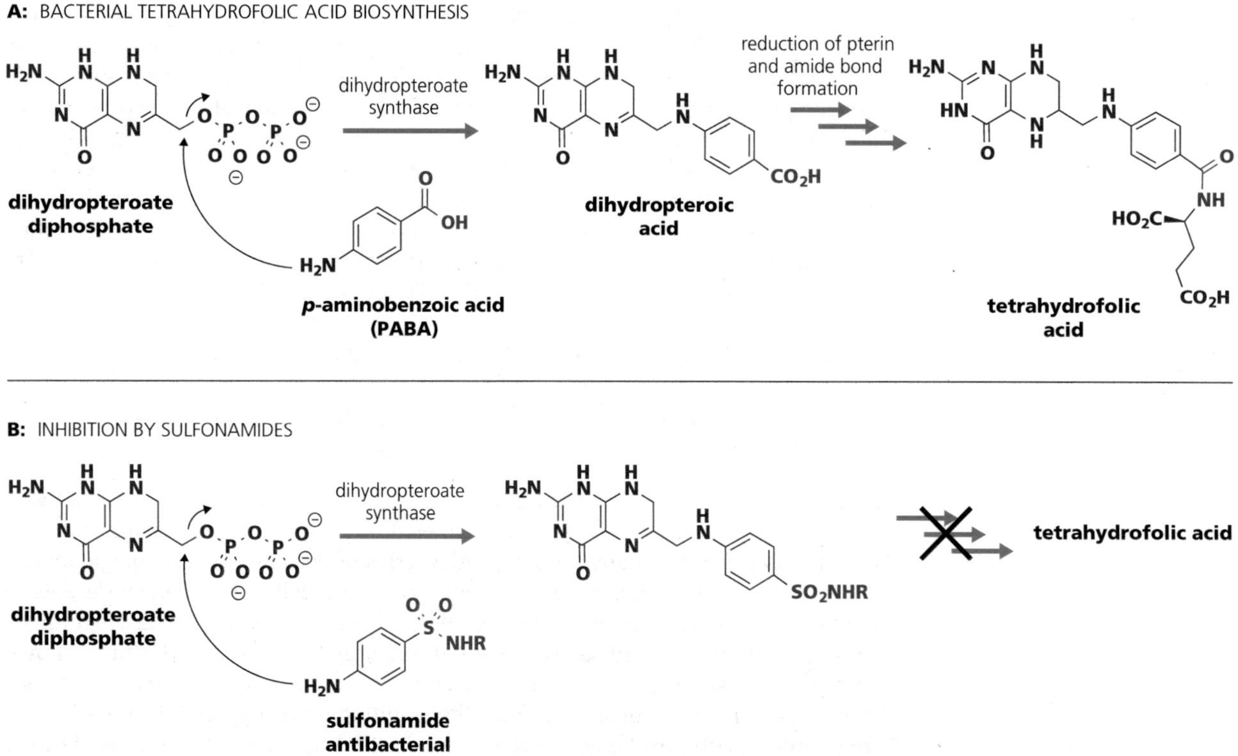

A: BACTERIAL TETRAHYDROFOLIC ACID BIOSYNTHESIS

B: INHIBITION BY SULFONAMIDES

Figure 12.29 Mechanism of action of sulfonamide antibacterial drugs. A: Generalized biosynthesis of tetrahydrofolic acid, an intermediate in the biosynthesis of folic acid. The amine of *p*-aminobenzoic acid displaces the diphosphate of dihydropteroate diphosphate, leading to dihydropteroic acid; subsequent reactions include conversion of the acid (shown in red) to the amide in tetrahydrofolic acid. Tetrahydrofolic acid eventually is converted to folic acid. B: Mechanism of inhibition of sulfonamide. In an analogous reaction, the amine of a sulfonamide adds to dihydropteroate diphosphate, but the sulfonamide product cannot participate in the subsequent reactions for the final conversion to tetrahydrofolic acid, leading to inhibition of folic acid synthesis.

antibacterial drugs are substrates for dihydropteroate synthase and compete with the natural substrate, displacing the diphosphate to form the sulfonamide analog of dihydropteroic acid; however, no further reactions proceed since the requisite acid moiety is not present (**Figure 12.29B**).

Dapsone (See Figure 12.28) although not a sulfonamide, is a sulfone that also acts as an inhibitor of dihydropteroate synthase by competing with PABA. This drug is particularly effective against mycobacterial infections and is used to treat both tuberculosis (*M. tuberculosis*) and leprosy (*M. leprae*). Another antibacterial that inhibits this pathway is trimethoprim, which inhibits the bacterial enzyme dihydrofolate reductase, blocking conversion of dihydrofolic acid to tetrahydrofolic acid. It is used most frequently to treat UTIs as a formulation in combination with sulfamethoxazole.

DRUGS AFFECTING BACTERIAL CELL-MEMBRANE PERMEABILITY

Drugs that affect bacterial cell-membrane permeability include the polymyxins and daptomycin (**Figure 12.30**). Polyethers such as monensin and lasalocid also affect cell membrane permeability and are used as supplements in animal feed; they affect the flora and aid digestion. Polymyxins are cationic cyclic peptides with a long hydrophobic tail that binds to the lipopolysaccharide of Gram-negative bacteria. They are relatively toxic and were not widely used until recently, even though they have been available for years. With the increase in multi-drug-resistant bacteria such as

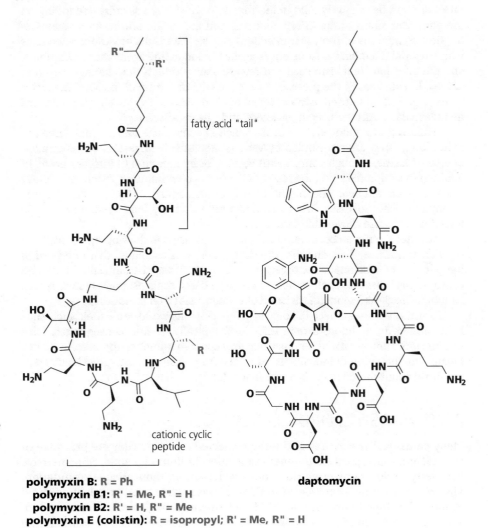

Figure 12.30 Structures of polymyxins and daptomycin. Both are cyclic peptides with lipophilic tails that disrupt bacterial cell membranes; points of variation in the polymyxins are shown in red. Polymyxin B is a mixture of polymyxins B1 and B2, differing in the substitution pattern on the fatty acid side chain. Polymyxin E (colistin) has the same fatty acid side chain as polymyxin B1 but substitutes D-Leu for D-Phe.

fatty acid "tail"

cationic cyclic peptide

polymyxin B: R = Ph
polymyxin B1: R' = Me, R" = H
polymyxin B2: R' = H, R" = Me
polymyxin E (colistin): R = isopropyl; R' = Me, R" = H

daptomycin

P. aeruginosa, A. baumannii, and carbapenem-resistant Enterobacteriaceae, there has been renewed interest in polymyxins. Several polymyxins (labelled A–E) were isolated in the 1940s from the soil bacterium *Paenibacillus polymyxa*; both polymyxins B and E (also known as colistin) are used clinically. Polymyxin B is a mixture (of B1 and B2) that varies in the composition of the fatty acid side chain. Polymyxin E varies from polymyxin B1 by substitution of D-Leu for D-Phe (see Figure 12.30).

The cationic cyclic peptide displaces Ca^{2+} and Mg^{2+} from the membrane, destabilizing it. The fatty acid tail then interacts with LPS, inserting into the membrane and allowing leakage of cellular components. Due to toxicity, primarily in the kidney, their use was very limited until recently, when they have become a drug of last resort to treat patients infected with multi-drug-resistant Gram-negative bacteria. This mechanism is similar to that proposed for daptomycin (described in detail in Section 8.4), which also interacts with the lipid bilayer of the cell membrane.

ANTIPARASITIC DRUGS: COMMON PARASITE FEATURES, INFECTIOUS PROCESS, AND IMPACT

A number of infectious diseases are caused not by bacteria but by parasitic organisms. These include both unicellular organisms, formerly called protozoa, and more complex worms (helminths). Protozoan parasites are microscopic, unicellular, eukaryotic organisms that are transmitted to humans through vectors, usually blood-feeding insects such as mosquitoes. They proceed through several life stages in the infected host cell; some have capabilities for movement or propulsion. Protozoal infections can be relatively mild to life-threatening, with the severity depending on the particular strain of the infectious agent and the health and immune status of the host. Symptoms of protozoal infections can be the results of various effects. As with bacterial infections, host defenses against the infecting agent cause symptoms, and the infectious organism itself can release toxic products that damage cells and tissues. In some cases, the presence of the parasite in the small intestine interferes with absorption of nutrients. Examples of diseases caused by unicellular organisms include malaria, African sleeping sickness, and Chagas' disease.

Helminths are multicellular worms, which in some cases can be quite large (>1 meter long). They are transmitted by various methods: by ingestion or penetration of eggs or larvae, through contact with vectors, or by ingestion of infected hosts. In addition to symptoms being the result of the host's own immune system, pathology can also be caused by the helminths' activity or metabolism or by physical blockage of physiological processes. Many helminths are extremely long-lived, and chronic infection can cause irreversible damage.

Parasites are the most common infectious organisms in developing countries in sub-Saharan Africa, Asia, and the Americas, where it is estimated that one-third of the population is infected. The organisms often infect the gastrointestinal tract and cause tropical diseases such as hookworm, ascariasis, schistosomiasis (snail fever), lymphatic filariasis (elephantiasis), and onchocerciasis (river blindness).

Parasitic diseases affect billions of people in the world, and their incidence is increasing. In addition, certain infections, typically of little consequence, have become more prevalent and serious when they occur in immunosuppressed patients. Finally, the migration of individuals infected with parasites to low-prevalence areas has further contributed to the increase in incidence.

ANTIPARASITIC DRUG DISCOVERY

Many parasitic diseases are considered neglected diseases. They are prevalent in tropical and subtropical environments and affect billions of people, who often live in poverty, in close contact with infectious vectors and without adequate sanitation. They are termed neglected because these diseases have been largely eradicated in more developed parts of the world. Treatment strategies rely on prevention, such as elimination of vectors and safe food and water sources. In addition, drug therapy needs to consider the specific patients affected and their environment. As such, low cost, short treatment regimens, and ease of administration are primary criteria.

Many older drugs were developed on the basis of known activity against other organisms, relying on phenotypic screens. In fact, a number of antibacterial drugs are also used to treat parasitic diseases. However, the number of drugs that specifically target parasites is far fewer than the number that target bacteria. Challenges include the highly complex life cycle of some parasites and development of resistance. While there were few drugs approved from the 1970s to the 1990s, there has been an increase in activity in the development of new antiparasitic agents in the 21st century. Advances in sequencing the genomes of these organisms and formation of private–public partnerships to support drug discovery for neglected tropical diseases are partly responsible for this change. **Table 12.2** highlights examples of antiparasitic agents.

Table 12.2 Examples of pathogenic parasites, associated diseases and conditions, drugs or drug classes used to treat each and their mechanism of action.

Organism	Disease or condition	Drug	Mechanism
Protozoal parasites			
Plasmodium falciparum and other *Plasmodium* species	malaria	quinine	inhibition of hemozoin crystallization
		artemisinin	ROS generation
		mefloquine, chloroquine (prevention)	inhibition of hemozoin crystallization
		doxycycline (prevention)	protein synthesis inhibition
Leishmania	leishmaniasis	pentamidine	not clarified; interferes with nuclear metabolism
		amphotericin B	cell-wall disruption
Trypanosoma brucei gambiense	African trypanosomiasis (sleeping sickness)	suramin	inhibition of glycolytic enzymes
		pentamidine	not clarified; interferes with nuclear metabolism
Trypanosoma cruzi	Chagas' disease	nifurtimox	ROS generation
		benznidazole	ROS generation
Helminths			
Onchocerca volvulus	onchocerciasis (river blindness)	ivermectin	increased permeability of invertebrate nerve/muscle cells
Schistosoma mansoni	schistosomiasis (snail fever)	praziquantel	muscle paralysis due to Ca^{2+} influx
Necator americanus	hookworm	albendazole, mebendazole	inhibition of microtubule polymerization
Ascaris lumbricoides	roundworms (ascariasis)	albendazole, mebendazole	inhibition of microtubule polymerization
Strongyloides stercoralis	strongyloidiasis	mebendazole	inhibition of microtubule polymerization
Wuchereria bancrofti	elephantiasis (lymphatic filariasis)	ivermectin	increased permeability of invertebrate nerve/muscle cells

12.7   Current drugs used to treat malaria are derivatives of natural products

Malaria is a mosquito-borne disease that affects approximately 3 billion people worldwide, resulting in roughly 1 million deaths per year. The disease is caused by various organisms of the *Plasmodium* genus, which have become increasingly resistant to treatment. Humans are infected with the parasite in its sporozoite form by the mosquito vector. The sporozoite then travels to the liver and matures to a schizont, containing merozoites, which then infect other blood cells and produce more merozoites in the blood (erythrocytic) stage. There the parasites degrade hemoglobin, releasing iron-bound heme. However, heme is toxic to the parasite, so the parasites then convert the toxic heme to nontoxic hemozoin crystals (also called "malaria pigment") (**Figure 12.31**).

Despite renewed efforts to develop antimalarial drugs, there are only two classes in use. Both inhibit hemozoin formation, albeit via different mechanisms. The earliest drug used to treat malaria was quinine, an alkaloid isolated from the bark of the *Cinchona* tree and introduced into Western medicine in the 17th century. More recent analogs of quinine include chloroquine, introduced in the 1950s, and

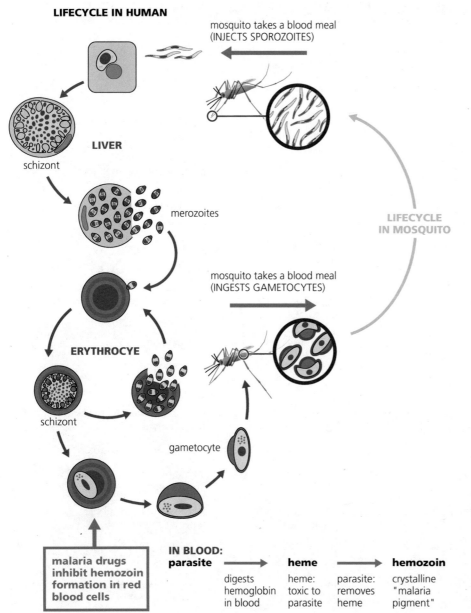

Figure 12.31 Life cycle of malaria parasite. The infected *Anopheles* mosquito injects the parasite as a sporozoite into the blood; the sporozoite enters the liver and matures to a schizont, which contains thousands of merozoites. Release of merozoites into the blood leads to destruction of blood cells. In this blood stage, the parasite digests hemoglobin, forming heme, which is toxic to the parasite; the parasite then removes heme, forming hemozoin. Malaria drugs inhibit hemozoin formation, leading to toxic buildup of heme.

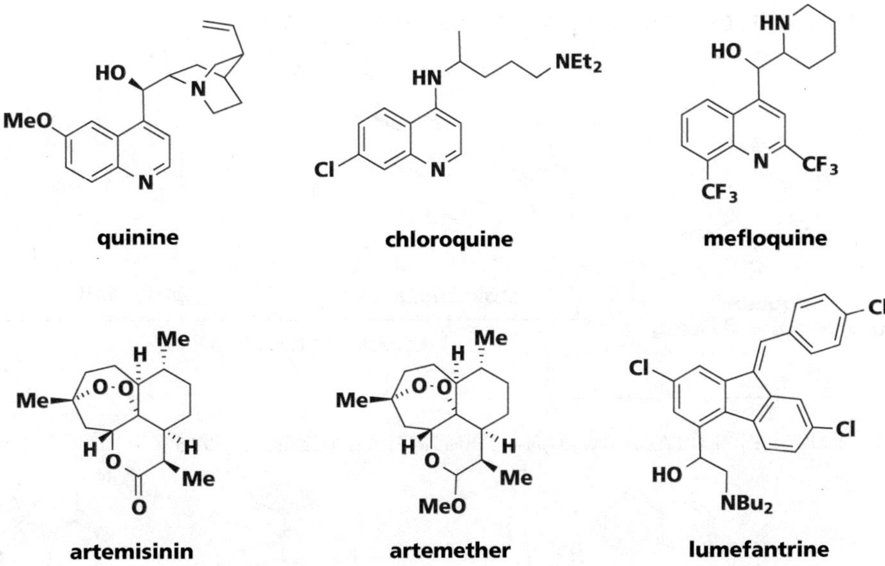

**Figure 12.32 Structures of quinine-
and artemisinin-based antimalarial
drugs.** The natural product quinine
has been in use since the 17th
century to treat malaria. More recent
synthetic analogs include chloroquine
and mefloquine, both of which are
administered as racemic mixtures.
The natural product artemisinin
was discovered in the 1970s, and its
semisynthetic analog artemether
is widely used, in combination with
lumefantrine.

**Figure 12.32 Structures of quinine-
and artemisinin-based antimalarial
drugs.** The natural product quinine
has been in use since the 17th
century to treat malaria. More recent
synthetic analogs include chloroquine
and mefloquine, both of which are
administered as racemic mixtures.
The natural product artemisinin
was discovered in the 1970s, and its
semisynthetic analog artemether
is widely used, in combination with
lumefantrine.

mefloquine, developed in the 1970s (**Figure 12.32**). The mechanism of the quinine-based antimalarial drugs involves inhibition of hemozoin crystallization, resulting in buildup of heme, which then kills the parasites.

Although the early quinine-based antimalarial drugs have been effective, multi-drug-resistant organisms are a serious threat. To combat this issue, in 2006, the WHO advocated the use of artemisinin-based therapies, which are now used in many countries. Artemisinin was discovered in the 1970s, as a result of Project 523, an effort by the Chinese government to find new antimalarial drugs during the Vietnam War (see Case Study 1 in Chapter 1). It contains an unusual peroxide moiety and has poor solubility. The reduced semisynthetic analog artemether is most widely used. Unlike the quinine derivatives, which act in the blood stage, artemisinin and artemether are active at all stages of the parasite life cycle. The mechanism of action is still not fully defined but involves bioactivation by heme iron to generate reactive oxygen species (ROS). The free radicals inhibit hemozoin formation and also damage cellular targets in the parasite. Artemether has a short half-life and is usually given in combination with a longer-acting drug such as lumefantrine. Lumefantrine was also discovered in China, as part of Project 523, and interferes with the conversion of heme to hemozoin. The Nobel Prize in Physiology or Medicine 2015 was awarded to Youyou Tu for her work on the isolation of artemisinin.

In addition to treatment of malaria, several drugs are used prophylactically, so that they will be present in the body if a person is infected with the parasite by an insect bite. One commonly used prophylactic drug is Malarone, a combination of atovaquone and proguanil (**Figure 12.33A**). As part of the Malaria Research Committee, hundreds of hydroxynaphthoquinones, structurally related to atovaquone, were synthesized in the 1940s in an effort to find quinine alternatives due to shortages of it during World War II. Although many of these compounds were found to inhibit respiration of the organism, they were not metabolically stable and therefore not an effective quinine alternative.

These hydroxynaphthoquinones were re-investigated years later when, in the late 1960s, it was found that malarial ubiquinones (coenzymes present in eukaryotes) differed from their mammalian counterparts at the polyprenyl chain. The ubiquinones (see Figure 12.33A) are involved in electron transfer reactions required for cell respiration, and therefore it was suggested that ubiquinone analogs might selectively inhibit electron transfer in the malaria parasite and be an effective therapeutic. In the 1990s, investigation of atovaquone showed that it irreversibly blocks ubiquinol–ubiquinone redox cycling.

The ubiquinol–ubiquinone process is involved in pyrimidine biosynthesis, and blockage leads to death of the organism. Although as a single agent atovaquone had a 70% cure rate in infected patients, it was found to act synergistically with another drug,

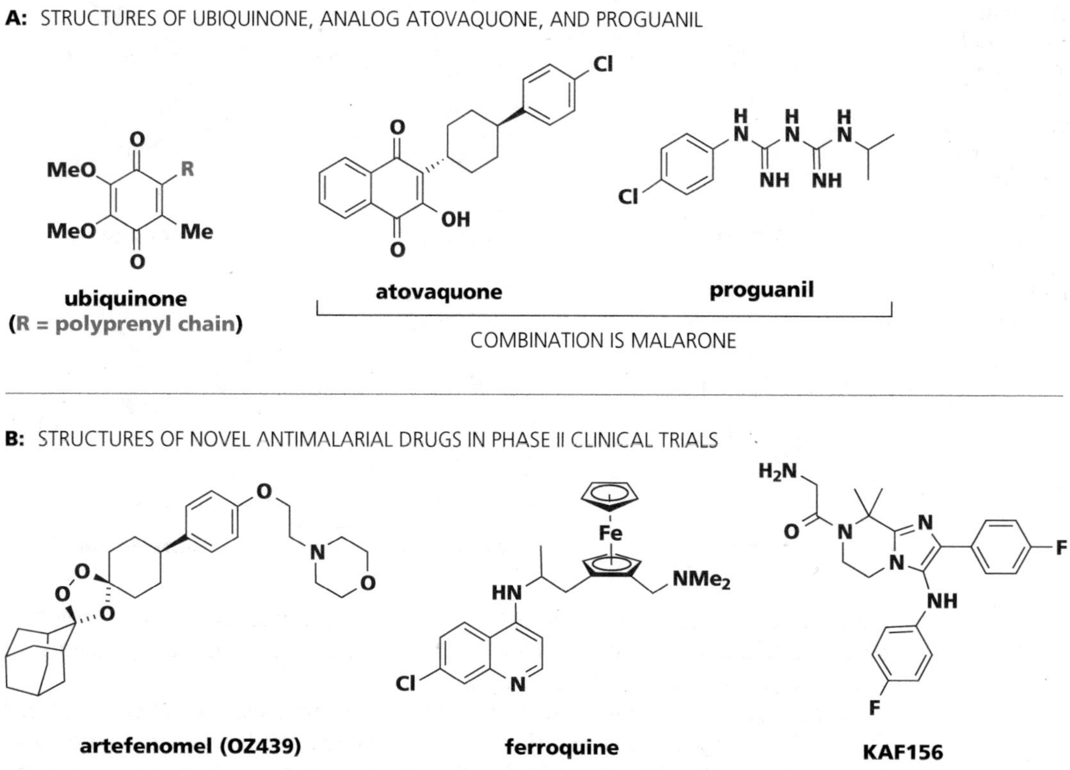

A: STRUCTURES OF UBIQUINONE, ANALOG ATOVAQUONE, AND PROGUANIL

ubiquinone
(R = polyprenyl chain)   **atovaquone**   **proguanil**

COMBINATION IS MALARONE

B: STRUCTURES OF NOVEL ANTIMALARIAL DRUGS IN PHASE II CLINICAL TRIALS

artefenomel (OZ439)   **ferroquine**   **KAF156**

proguanil, which had been discovered in the 1940s; when used in combination, cure rates are nearly 95%. Proguanil is a dihydrofolate reductase (DHFR) inhibitor, with selectivity for the parasite form of the enzyme.

In 1999, the Medicines for Malaria Venture (MMV), a public–private foundation, was launched to develop novel medicines to treat malaria. As of 2017, several compounds from this initiative have progressed to phase II clinical trials, including the synthetic ozonide artefenomel, a peroxide that works by the same mechanism as artemesinin, and the quinine-based organometallic drug ferroquine (**Figure 12.33B**). In addition, Novartis has developed KAF156, a novel imidazolopiperazine that was optimized from a hit identified from a high-throughput screening campaign of 2 million compounds to detect compounds that inhibited proliferation of *Plasmodium falciparum* (see Journal Club 1 in Chapter 4).

Figure 12.33 Structures of quinone-based antimalarial prophylactic drugs and novel drugs in clinical trials. A: The malaria parasite relies on a unique ubiquinone for respiration. The prophylatic antimalarial drug atovaquone is an analog of ubiquinone and is used in combination with the DHFR inhibitor proguanil as Malarone. B: Structures of several novel anti-malarial drugs that have advanced to clinical trials, that work through various mechanisms.

12.8 There are few effective treatments for trypanosomal diseases

Trypanosomes are a type of protozoal parasite transmitted by insect vectors, in a similar fashion to malaria. *Trypanosoma brucei gambiense* is transmitted by the tsetse fly and is seen mainly in sub-Saharan Africa, where it causes African sleeping sickness, or human African trypanosomiasis (HAT). A similar organism, *Trypanosoma cruzi*, causes American trypanosomiasis, or Chagas' disease, and is transmitted by the kissing bug. The disease is found throughout South America and Central America and in the southern United States.

In response to an epidemic of HAT in the Congo and Kenya in the late 1800s, a cure was sought by colonial governments. Ehrlich investigated a number of dyes, which led to the identification of a series of compounds such as trypan blue, which was effective in mice but not other mammals, and the closely related trypan red, which was effective in humans but dyed the skin red. Inclusion of a urea linking the structural elements eventually led to the dimeric compound suramin, which did not have trypan red's pigmenting side effects. Suramin was developed at Bayer in Germany in 1916, where it was originally named Germanin. Its value was so high that it was actually offered to the British in return for some German colonies that had been lost in World War I, without disclosing the structure. The British declined, and the structure was determined independently by the French pharmacist Ernest Fourneau. Suramin is still used to treat the early stages of HAT (**Figure 12.34A**).

Another class of compounds investigated during the early 1900s was the arsenicals. Although toxic, particularly to the optic nerve, tryparsamide was used until the 1960s when it was replaced by the less toxic analog melarsoprol, which is still used

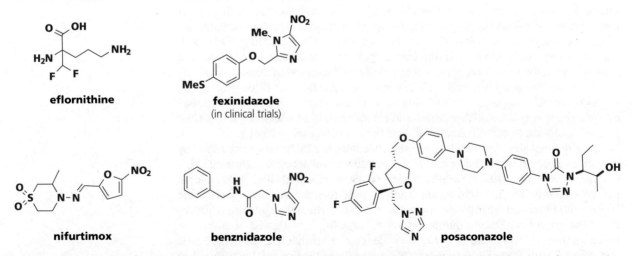

A: EARLY ANTI-TRYPANOSOMAL DRUGS

trypan red

suramin

tryparsamide

melarsoprol

pentamidine

B: ANTI-TRYPANOSOMAL DRUGS DEVELOPED IN THE LATE 1900s AND 2000s

eflornithine

fexinidazole
(in clinical trials)

nifurtimox

benznidazole

posaconazole

Figure 12.34 Structures of anti-trypanosomal drugs. A: Early anti-trypanosomal drugs. The structure and activity of trypan red served as the basis for suramin, which is used to treat HAT. Other early drugs include the arsenicals tryparsamide and melarsoprol (still used to treat later stages of HAT), as well as pentamidine. B: Later anti-trypanosomal drugs. Eflornithine inhibits ornithine decarboxylase and is used to treat HAT. Fexinidazole, an analog of benznidazole is in advanced clinical trials to treat the late stages of HAT. The nitrofuran nifurtimox and the nitroimidazole benznidazole likely work through ROS generation, and are effective in Chagas' disease. Posconazole, an anti-fungal agent, inhibits Cyp51 and is effective in animal models as a treatment for Chagas' disease.

to treat the later stages of HAT. Pentamidine, invented in 1940, is an analog of the early anti-diabetic drug synthalin, or decane-1,10-bis(guanidine), and was found to have anti-trypanosomal activity, and has been used to treat HAT and Chagas' disease. Its mechanism is has not been clarified, but involves interfering with nuclear metabolism (see Figure 12.34A).

The connection between anti-diabetics and drugs to treat trypanosome infection came from the observation that trypanosomes need glucose to reproduce. Synthalin, discovered in the 1920s, was based on a folk remedy, the French lilac *Galega officinalis*, used in medieval Europe for the diabetic condition. This plant contains both guanidine and *N*-isoprenylguanidine), and alkyl analogs such as synthalin were investigated in the 1920s for diabetes.

The most recent drug approved to treat HAT is eflornithine (**Figure 12.34B**), which was investigated as an anti-cancer compound in the 1970s. It was designed as a suicide inhibitor of ornithine decarboxylase, where inhibition leads to reduced cell proliferation. It was ineffective as an anti-tumor agent, but testing in the 1980s showed it to be an effective inhibitor of the proliferation of *T. brucei gambiense*. It was approved in 1990 to treat African sleeping sickness. One promising compound for the treatment of HAT is fexinidazole, which is in clinical trials as of 2017. It was first synthesized in the 1980s and is closely related to benznidazole. It was rediscovered due to the efforts of DNDi, and it is the first new drug to treat late-stage HAT that has entered clinical trials in the last 30 years.

Like the MMV for malaria drugs, the public–private Drugs for Neglected Diseases Initiative (DNDi) was launched in 2003, with the goal of identifying novel accessible treatments for HAT, leishmaniasis, Chagas' disease, pediatric HIV, and helminth infections.

Drugs used to treat Chagas' disease include nifurtimox and benznidazole. The mechanism of these aromatic nitro compounds is believed to involve reduction of the nitro group to afford reactive oxygen species (ROS), which then cause cell damage. Increased interest in addressing neglected diseases has led to several compounds that have entered clinical trials. Antifungal compounds such as posaconazole (Figure 12.34B) and others from this class are effective in models of Chagas' disease; they act by CYP51 (sterol 14α-demethylase) inhibition. Since *T. cruzi* requires ergosterol, it is susceptible to these inhibitors, more commonly used as antifungal drugs (see Chapter 11).

12.9 Drugs that treat helminthic diseases are used in both veterinary and human medicine

Although diseases caused by helminths (worms) have existed for thousands of years and affect many millions of people, there are very few drugs to treat these conditions. Like protozoal parasites, helminths have complex life cycles and can grow in both mammals and invertebrates. Only four new drugs were introduced between 1975 and 2004; however, their effectiveness has nearly eradicated some conditions.

The azole drugs such as mebendazole and albendazole were discovered in the 1970s. These carbamates are less toxic analogs of thiabendazole, first reported in 1961 as a veterinary medicine. Mebendazole and albendazole bind selectively to parasitic β-tubulin, blocking microtubule formation in the parasite (**Figure 12.35**).

Praziquantel and oxamniquine, introduced in the early 1980s, were discovered by the collaborative efforts of Bayer and Merck to find treatments for schistosomiasis, a disease caused by parasitic flatworms that infects 250 million and kills 200,000 people per year worldwide. The schistosomes infect both mammalian and invertebrate (river snail) hosts and are found in contaminated water, where they penetrate human skin. The parent pyrazinoisoquinolines were originally investigated at Merck as potential tranquilizers in the early 1970s. While inactive for that use, the compounds were shared with Bayer for veterinary screening, where praziquantel was found to be effective against a number of parasitic helminths. Testing in humans indicated high effectiveness against schistosomes (parasitic flatworms) in a single-dose oral formulation and with low toxicity. Its mechanism involves increasing the parasite's membrane permeability toward Ca^{2+}, leading to death of the organisms. Oxamniquine is effective against only one species, *Schistosoma mansoni*.

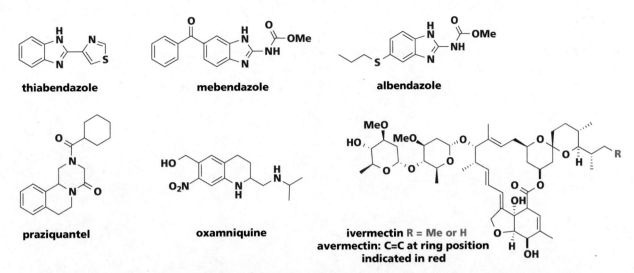

Figure 12.35 Structures of drugs used to treat helminthic diseases. The veterinary medicine thiabendazole was the basis of less toxic analogs mebendazole and albendazole, used for human disease. The synthetic quinolines praziquantel and oxamniquine are effective against schistosomiasis. Avermectin, a natural product isolated from soil bacteria, and ivermectin, a semisynthetic analog, are used to treat river blindness.

Ivermectin is a semisynthetic derivative of avermectin and differs only by reduction of a carbon–carbon double bond in the spiroketal ring (shown in red in Figure 12.35). Avermectin was discovered by Satoshi Ōmura in the soil bacterium *Streptomyces avermitilis*. It was purified and identified by William Campbell at Merck Pharmaceuticals, who had also discovered thiabendazole. Ivermectin acts against many parasitic helminths at low doses and with low toxicity. The mechanism involves modulation of parasite-specific chloride ion channels, leading to death of the organism. It has become one of the most widely used drugs and is an important part of a program to eradicate river blindness and elephantiasis. Ōmura and Campbell were awarded the Nobel Prize in Physiology or Medicine 2015 for the discovery of avermectin.

SUMMARY

Antibacterial and antiparasitic drugs are some of the oldest drugs that have been developed, starting with suramin and Salvarsan in the early 1900s and the sulfonamides in the 1930s. The introduction of antibacterial drugs has had a profound effect on life span, and penicillin is considered a wonder drug. While there are relatively few antiparasitic drugs, there are hundreds of antibacterial drugs. Unlike viruses (see Chapter 11), bacteria have a number of unique targets, and these are acted on by different classes of antibacterial drugs. These targets are primarily involved in DNA replication and the integrity of the cell wall. Discovery of antibacterial drugs has most often come about by screening of both natural products and synthetic compounds, rather than *a priori* drug design, although a vast majority of modern antibacterial drugs are derived from medicinal chemistry optimization of natural products. Resistance toward antibiotics is a continual issue, and newer drugs are those that are not prone to those mechanisms. In addition, strategies to avoid common resistance mechanisms constitute an emerging approach. The development of antiparasitic drugs lags behind that of antibacterial drugs. Despite the fact that malaria affects over 3 billion people, only a few effective therapies are available, and resistance toward those is becoming a concern. Older drugs were discovered on the basis of phenotypic screening, and many drugs that are used for other infections (fungal or bacterial) have found use as antiparasitic agents. Drug discovery efforts for neglected diseases, however, have increased due to the significant need, and novel therapeutics from these initiatives are currently in development.

CASE STUDY 1   DISCOVERY OF LINEZOLID

Linezolid was discovered at Upjohn Pharmaceuticals (now part of Pfizer) and, when introduced in 2000, it was the first entirely new class of antibacterial drug introduced in 30 years. It was based on a series of oxazolidinone-containing compounds, represented as DuP 105 and DuP 721, first reported by chemists from DuPont Merck in 1987 (Figure 12.36).

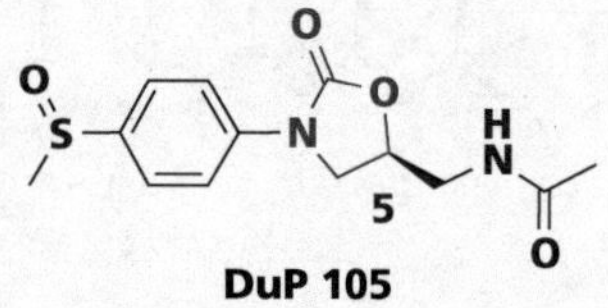

DuP 105

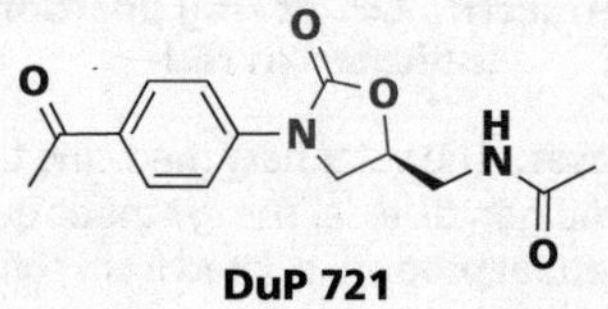

DuP 721

Figure 12.36 Initial oxazolidinone leads for linezolid. Two oxazolidinone antibacterial lead compounds, DuP 105 and DuP 721, were reported by DuPont Merck Pharmaceuticals in 1987. The oxazolidinone group is shown in red.

Promising characteristics of these leads included good *in vitro* and oral activity versus MRSA and *M. tuberculosis* as well as good pharmacokinetics in rats. In addition, there was no induction of resistance observed in *in vitro* studies. Structure–activity relationships reported included an aryl substituent containing a para electron-withdrawing substituent on the oxazolidinone nitrogen, and a C5 (*S*)-acetamidomethyl group being important for potency. However, efforts in this series were suspended due to toxicity issues.

On the basis of these reports, chemists at Upjohn initiated a program to identify novel oxazolidinones. One strategy was to use conformational constraints to improve activity as well as to impart novelty. Compound **1** is a bicyclic analog of DuP 721 and exhibited potent MRSA *in vitro* and *in vivo* activity (in mice) as well as favorable pharmacokinetics (Figure 12.37). Surprisingly, although DuP 721 causes bone marrow toxicity, **1** had no such effects; since it was covered in the DuPont patent, further structure elaboration was pursued. A second series, in which the ketone was replaced with an acylated amine, provided the novel and patentable 5′-indolinyloxazolidinones **2** and **3**, which also exhibited potent activity and low toxicity.

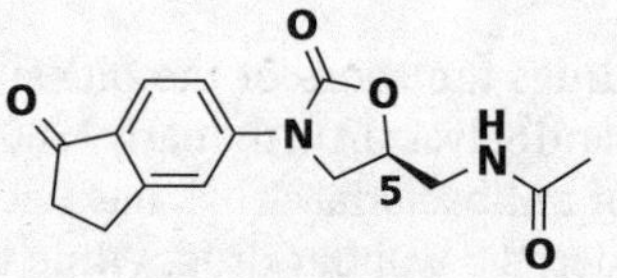

compound 1

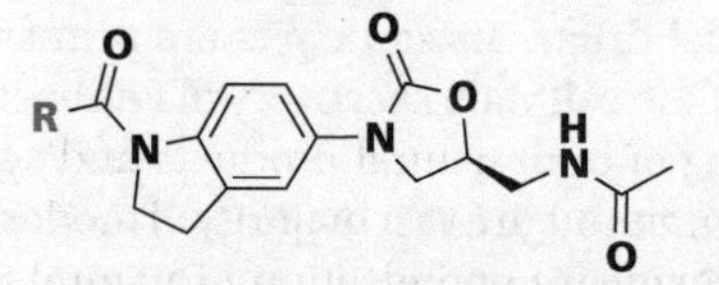

compound 2: R = CH₂OH
compound 3: R = 2-thiophene

Figure 12.37 Structures of constrained analogs of oxazolidinones. Chemists at Upjohn investigated the oxazolidinones further, giving compound **1**, a bicyclic analog of DuP 721. Compounds **2** and **3** replace the ketone of **1** with acylated amines, and both were potent and had low toxicity.

The project goal was to further optimize the compounds to develop two clinical candidates, each with a vancomycin-like profile, that were effective both intravenously and orally. Three teams of chemists were assigned, and they developed three series of compounds: tropinone, indolinyl, and piperazinyl (Figure 12.38).

In the tropinone series, fluorination on the aryl group improved potency, but the compounds had poor solubility and were difficult to synthesize. The indolinyl compounds had a good safety profile, but were less potent than the original series.

The optimal series proved to be the piperazinyl compounds, which displayed good pharmacokinetics, solubility, potency, and toxicity profiles.

Figure 12.38 Three series of oxazolidinone antibacterial leads. Three series of leads were developed: the tropinone, indolinyl and piperazinyl structures; the piperazinyl series had the optimal combination of properties.

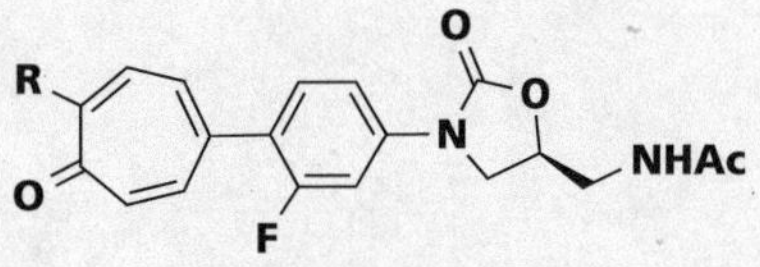

tropinone series

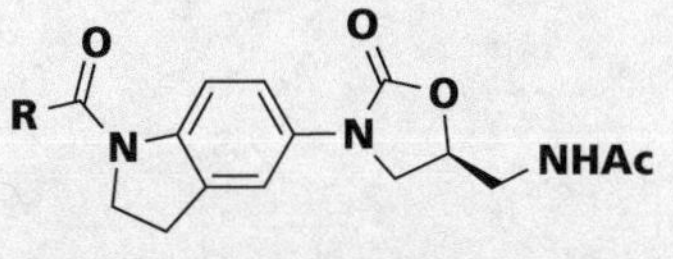

indolinyl series

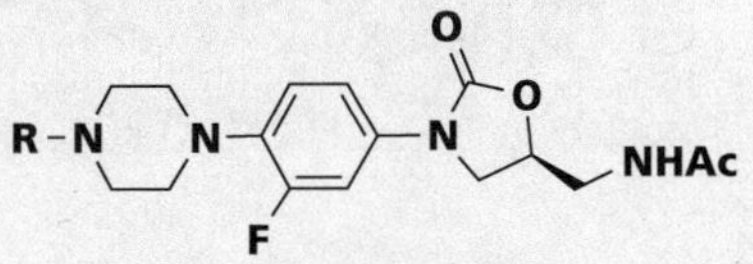

piperazinyl series

Focus on this series led to eperezolid, which entered into phase I trials in 1994 (**Figure 12.39**). The compound had high solubility and was well tolerated up to 2000 mg/kg when dosed orally. The fluorine substituent on the aryl ring doubled potency *in vitro* as compared to the unsubstituted analog, and while addition of a second fluorine atom to the aromatic ring increased potency, that derivative had lower solubility.

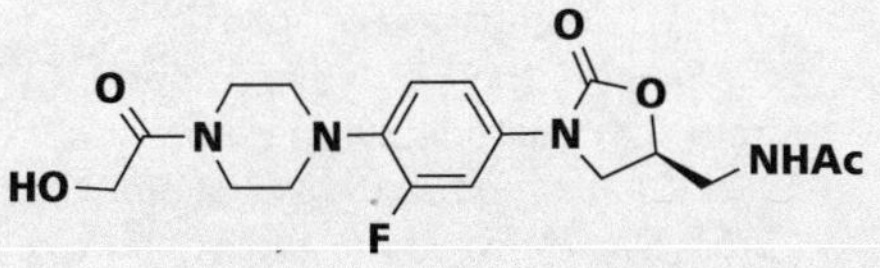

eperezolid
(early clinical candidate)

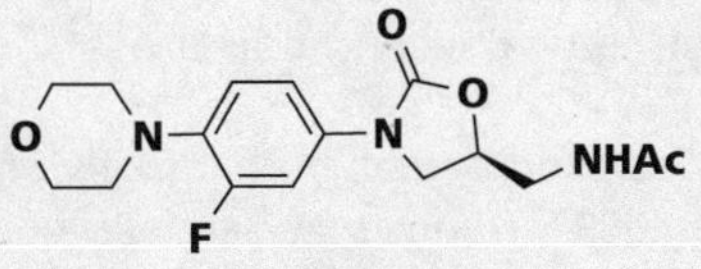

linezolid
2000

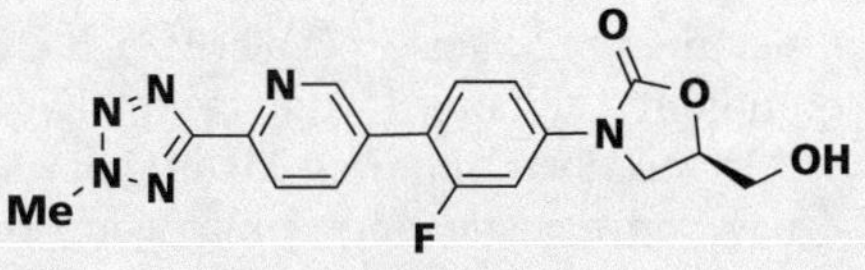

torezolid/tedizolid
2014

Figure 12.39 Structures of oxazolidinone antibacterial drugs. Eperezolid and linezolid both advanced to phase I clinical trials; with linezolid having better pharmacokinetic properties and advancing to an approved drug. Torezolid (tedizolid) is the only other approved oxazolidinone antibacterial drug.

Linezolid, the morpholine analog, has a similar profile to eperezolid and entered phase I trials at the same time. Although very similar in potency, linezolid progressed further due to a superior PK profile in humans. It had 100% oral bioavailability with rapid absorption and minimal metabolism. Minimal toxicity was also seen in clinical trials, and very slow development of resistance to linezolid was observed. Linezolid is bacteriostatic for enterococci and staphylococci and bactericidal for streptococci.

While a number of other oxazolidinones have entered clinical trials, as of 2017, only one other has received FDA approval. Torezolid (now called tedizolid) is a biaryltetrazole that has some improvements over linezolid and received approval in 2014.

CASE STUDY 2 SQ109 FOR MULTI-DRUG-RESISTANT TUBERCULOSIS

Tuberculosis is the world's leading cause of death from a single microorganism and kills over 3 million people per year. The infectious agent is *Mycobacterium tuberculosis* (Mtb), and many of the common antibacterial drugs are ineffective against it.

Mycobacteria are Gram-positive bacteria which are also acid-fast bacteria; they possess small amounts of peptidoglycan but have a waxy outer layer of glycolipids composed of mycolic acid and arabinogalactan (**Figure 12.40**).

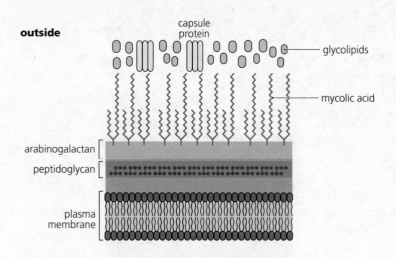

Figure 12.40 Structure of the cell wall of mycobacteria. These bacteria possess an outer capsule (blue/green) of proteins and glycolipids, a waxy layer of of mycolic acid (orange), arabinogalactan (orange), and peptidoglycan (purple).

The standard drug treatment for tuberculosis includes a combination of isoniazid (INH), rifampicin (RIF), pyrazinamide (PZA), and ethambutol (EMB), all of which have been used for over 40 years. The combination must be given for 2 months, followed by just INH and RIF for 4–6 months. This lengthy regimen, along with the toxicity of the drugs, results in poor compliance. Noncompliance has led to multi-drug-resistant tuberculosis (MDR-TB), which is resistant to both drugs, as well as extensive-drug-resistant tuberculosis (XDR-TB), which is resistant to second-line drugs such as quinolones, kanamycin, and capreomycin.

In the 1990s, renewed TB drug discovery efforts focused on both identifying new drugs and investigating repurposed drugs. In 1999, scientists at Sequella began a combinatorial chemistry approach to synthesizing analogs of EMB (**Figure 12.41**). Ethambutol had been discovered in the 1950s, and no extensive SAR was reported. Although it is part of the standard regimen, the drug causes toxicity to the eye, which limits the dose that can be administered.

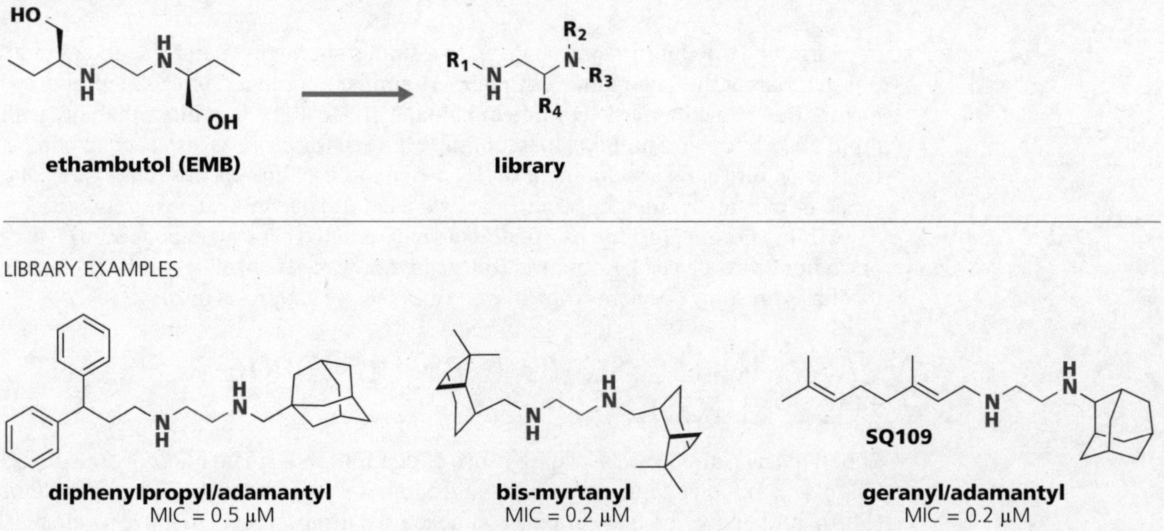

Figure 12.41 Ethambutol scaffold and library design. Ethambutol was the basis for combinatorial synthesis of 63,238 compounds (top). Three examples of the 170 active compounds from combinatorial synthesis are shown and include representatives of diphenyl propyl, myrtanyl amine and isoprenoid scaffolds. The geranyl/adamantyl analog SQ109 advanced to clinical trials. The common ethylene diamine core in each is shown in red.

ethambutol (EMB) → **library**

LIBRARY EXAMPLES

diphenylpropyl/adamantyl
MIC = 0.5 μM

bis-myrtanyl
MIC = 0.2 μM

SQ109
geranyl/adamantyl
MIC = 0.2 μM

By use of split-pool combinatorial chemistry techniques (see Section 2.8), a library of 63,238 compounds was created, based on the ethylenediamine core (see Figure 12.41). Compounds were synthesized in groups of 10 and evaluated as mixtures in a broth microdilution assay to determine the minimum inhibitory concentration (MIC) versus Mtb as well as in a bioluminescence assay for inhibition of Mtb cell-wall formation. Components of active 10-compound pools were resynthesized individually to identify active compounds, and the SAR was evaluated. They identified 2796 10-compound mixtures as active, and deconvolution generated 170 individual compounds that had MICs in the <0.6 μM range in both screens.

Most of the active compounds were lipophilic, with examples being extensively α-branched aliphatic, diphenylethyl, and diphenylpropyl fragments; tricyclic skeletons from adamantanes, myrtanylamine, and isopinocamphylamine; and isoprenoids (select examples shown in Figure 12.41).

The top 27 compounds, based on potency, were evaluated more extensively in cytotoxicity assays in HepG2 cells to determine a selectivity index (SI). SQ109 had the lowest MIC and highest SI in this group. The top 13, based on potency and high SI, were also tested in secondary assays for effects in Mtb-infected macrophages. The top 11, based on potency and efficacy in that intracellular assay, proceeded to *in vivo* trials in mice. The three most promising were investigated in further *in vivo* studies (mice) to determine their maximum tolerated dose (MTD) and evaluate pharmacokinetic (PK) parameters. Overall, SQ109 exhibited the most potent activity, lowest toxicity, and best MTD/PK profile, and it had activity against MDR strains. It was also found to be effective in a chronic model of TB in mice at 10 mg/kg, and it became the lead candidate for clinical trials after PK and toxicity studies in rats, dogs, and primates.

The ADMET profile in preclinical trials showed the highest concentrations of the drug in the liver but also significant levels in the lung and spleen, which are TB target organs. Metabolism was primarily by cytochrome P-450 enzymes from oxidation, epoxidation, and N-dealkylation. No significant toxicity was observed at doses well above the effective dose. SQ109 received Fast Track designation by the FDA in 2007 as well as Orphan Drug Status. Safety testing in phase I clinical trials showed no adverse effects; however, in phase II clinical trials, it has shown little efficacy.

SQ109 works by inhibition of MmpL3, which is different from the mechanism by which EMB works. EMB inhibits synthesis of the arabinogalactan of the cell wall and is bacteriostatic. In contrast, with SQ109 treatment, there is a decrease not in synthesis of cell-wall components but in incorporation of mycolic acids into the cell wall, specifically, trehalose dimycolate and arabinogalactan mycolates. There is evidence that SQ109 targets transport of mycolates, which is supported by the fact that mutants resistant to SQ109 had a mutant TMM transporter, called MmpL3. This transporter is found only in mycobacteria.

REVIEW QUESTIONS

1. Outline three mechanisms of action of antibacterial drugs.

2. Both quinolones and sulfonamides target bacterial DNA synthesis. Explain how their mechanisms are different.

3. Describe three classes of cell-wall synthesis inhibitors that act by covalent binding.

4. Describe two different mechanisms that are utilized by bacteria to resist penicillins.

5. Describe the main difference between Gram-positive and Gram-negative bacteria and why drugs might be effective against one and not the other.

6. What are neglected tropical diseases, and what specific requirements should be considered for drug discovery and development programs for these diseases?

7. What are the two classes of drugs used to treat malaria, and what are their mechanisms?

8. What drug discovery projects have contributed to increased numbers of drugs to treat parasitic disease?

9. Identify three antiparasitic drugs that are either natural products or derived from natural products, and for each, briefly describe what the drug is used for and its mechanism of action.

10. Explain why some drug discovery targets for antibacterial agents are similar to those used in anti-cancer drug discovery.

APPLICATION QUESTIONS

1. Draw the products of the reaction of PBP (particularly the active-site serine OH) with cefuroxime.

2. Using the examples in the chapter, identify two different compounds that are conformationally constrained.

3. Using the examples in the chapter, identify a compound that uses a prodrug strategy, and research the advantage of using the prodrug.

4. Using the examples in the chapter, identify three different compounds that incorporate isosteric replacements.

5. The Nobel Prize in Physiology or Medicine 2015 was awarded for the discovery of medicines for infectious diseases. Research the awardees and the medicines to which they contributed.

6. PBP is a serine protease. On the basis of your knowledge of serine protease inhibitors from Chapter 7, list other functional groups that could be used in place of the β-lactam in compounds such as penicillin.

7. Review the structures in this chapter and identify at least two that do not obey Lipinski's rule. For these two, calculate their Lipinski parameters. Use public data (such as PubChem) or other programs (such as ChemDraw) to approximate log P. Investigate whether they are orally active.

8. Research the structure and activity of anthracycline anti-cancer agents. Compare them to the tetracyclines described in this chapter. What are the similarities and differences in structure and activities?

9. Vancomycin resistance can occur when the D-Ala-D-Ala terminus of the substrate is mutated to D-Ala-D-lactate (substitution of oxygen for N-H). Design an analog of vancomycin that would be effective against the D-Ala-D-lactate mutant.

10. Many third- and fourth-generation quinolones contain a fluorine atom at several different positions. Given what you have learned about the properties of fluorine (see Chapter 4), speculate on how introduction of that atom changes and improves the properties of these drugs.

FURTHER READING

Butler MS, Blaskovich MA & Cooper MA (2013) Antibiotics in the clinical pipeline in 2013. *J Antibiot* 66:571–591.

Kohanski MA, Dwyer DJ & Collins JJ (2010) How antibiotics kill bacteria: from targets to networks. *Nat Rev Drug Discovery* 8:423–435.

Neu H (1992) The crisis in antibiotic resistance. *Science* 257:1064–1073.

Cell-wall synthesis inhibitors

Llarrull LI, Testero SA, Fisher JF & Mobashery S (2010) The future of β-lactams. *Curr Opin Microbiol* 13:551–557.

Papp-Wallace KM, Endimiani A, Taracila MA & Bonomo RA (2011) Carbapenems: past, present, and future. *Antimicrob Agents Chemother* 55:4943–4960.

Fleming A (1929) On the antibacterial action of cultures of a *Penicillium*, with special reference to their use in the isolation of *B. influenzae*. *Br J Exp Pathol* 10:226–236.

Levine DP (2006) Vancomycin: a history. *Clin Infect Dis* 42 (Suppl 1): S5–S12.

Knox JR & Pratt RF (1990) Different modes of vancomycin and D-alanyl-D-alanine peptidase binding to cell wall peptide and a possible role for the vancomycin resistance protein. *Antimicrob Agents Chemother* 34:1342–1347.

Protein synthesis inhibitors

Kotra LP, Haddad J & Mobashery S (2000) Aminoglycosides: perspectives on mechanisms of action and resistance and strategies to counter resistance. *Antimicrob Agents Chemother* 44:3249–3256.

Carter AP, Clemons WM, Brodersen DE et al. (2000) Functional insights from the structure of the 30S ribosomal subunit and its interactions with antibiotics. *Nature* 407:340–348.

Recht MI, Douthwaite S & Puglisi JD (1999) Basis for prokaryotic specificity of action of aminoglycoside antibiotics. *EMBO J* 18:3133–3138.

Beringer M & Rodnina MV (2007) The ribosomal peptidyl transferase. *Mol Cell* 26:311–321.

Brodersen DE, Clemons WM, Carter AP et al. (2000) The structure basis for the action of the antibiotics tetracycline, pactamycin, and hygromycin B on the 30S ribosomal subunit. *Cell* 103:1143–1154.

Connell SR, Tracz DM, Nierhaus KH & Taylor DE (2003) Ribosomal protection proteins and their mechanism of tetracycline resistance. *Antimicrob Agents Chemother* 47:3675–3681.

Chopra I & Roberts M (2001) Tetracycline antibiotics: mode of action, applications, molecular biology, and epidemiology of bacterial resistance. *Microbiol Mol Biol Rev* 65:232–260.

Pal S (2006) A journey across the sequential development of macrolides and ketolides related to erythromycin. *Tetrahedron* 62:3171–3200.

Zuckerman JM (2004) Macrolides and ketolides: azithromycin, clarithromycin, telithromycin. *Infect Dis Clin N Am* 18:621–649.

Rafie S, MacDougall C & James CL (2010) Cethromycin: a promising new ketolide antibiotic for respiratory infections. *Pharmacotherapy* 30:290–303.

DNA synthesis inhibitors

Aldred KJ, Kerns RJ & Osheroff N (2014) Mechanism of quinolone action and resistance. *Biochemistry* 53:1565–1574.

Andriole VT (2005) Quinolones: past, present, and future. *Clin Infect Dis* 41:S113–119.

Wohlkonig A, Chan PF, Fosberry AP et al. (2010) Structural basis of quinolone inhibition of type II topoisomerases and target-mediated resistance. *Nat Struct Mol Biol* 17:1152–1153.

Chu CT & Fernandes PB (1980) Structure activity relationships of the fluoroquinolones. *Antimicrob Agents Chemother* 33:131–135.

Gleckman R, Blagg N & Joubert DW (1981) Trimethoprim: mechanisms of action, antimicrobial activity, bacterial resistance, pharmacokinetics, adverse reactions, and therapeutic indication. *Pharmacotherapy* 1:14–19.

Antiparasitic drugs

Andrews KT, Fisher G & Skinner-Adams TS (2014) Drug repurposing and human parasitic protozoan diseases. *Int J Parasitol: Drugs Drug Resist* 4:95–111.

Hotez PJ, Brindley PJ, Bethony JM et al. (2008) Helminth infections: the great neglected tropical disease. *J Clin Invest* 118:1311–1321.

Pink R, Hudson A, Mouries M-A & Bendig M (2005) Opportunities and challenges in antiparasitic drug discovery. *Nat Rev Drug Discovery* 4:727–740.

Chabala JC, Mrozik H, Tolman RL et al. (1980) Ivermectin, a new broad-spectrum antiparasitic agent. *J Med Chem* 23:1134–1136.

Headrick DR (2014) Sleeping sickness epidemics and colonial responses in east and central Africa, 1900–1940. *PLoS Neglected Trop Dis* 8:e2772.

SQ 109

Lee RE, Protopova M, Crooks E et al. (2003) Combinatorial lead optimization of [1,2]-diamines based on ethambutol as potential antituberculosis preclinical candidates. *J Comb Chem* 5:172–187.

Tahlan K, Wilson R, Kastrinsky DB et al. (2012) SQ109 targets MmpL3, a membrane transporter of trehalose monomycolate involved in mycolic acid donation to the cell wall core of *Mycobacterium tuberculosis*. *Antimicrob Agents Chemother* 56:1797–1809.

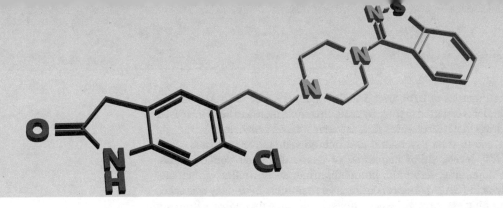

Drugs acting on the central nervous system

13

LEARNING OBJECTIVES

- Learn the history of treatment for psychiatric and neurodegenerative conditions.
- Become familiar with CNS-acting drugs and how they were developed.
- Identify mechanisms of drugs used to treat psychiatric disorders.
- Describe targets and approaches to treat neurodegenerative diseases.
- Develop an appreciation for the challenges of CNS drug discovery.
- Learn some novel approaches to future CNS drugs.

Disorders of the central nervous system (CNS) affect many millions of people worldwide and, according to the World Health Organization, account for over 11% of total deaths. They are typically divided into neuropsychiatric (or mental health) disorders and neurodegenerative diseases. Examples of mental health disorders include anxiety, depression, bipolar disorder, and schizophrenia. Neurodegenerative diseases such as Parkinson's and Alzheimer's diseases, whose incidence increases with age, affect about 7 million people in the United States, and this number is expected to increase as baby boomers age. In addition, pain is also considered a CNS disorder; whether chronic or more transient, it can be debilitating and affects roughly 17% of the population in the United States alone.

Some of the oldest medicines known were used to treat CNS disorders: plant preparations from the opium poppy or willow bark were used to alleviate pain. However, other CNS conditions, particularly neuropsychiatric disorders such as psychoses and depression, which have been known for thousands of years, were not treatable until the 20th century when psychotherapy and drug therapy were introduced. Even today, while there are many drugs available to treat these diseases, patients find varying levels of success with them. Some are effective, but only in a subset of the patient population, and/or are accompanied by significant side effects that impact compliance. Others improve some symptoms but not all. Finally, some work for a limited time, after which patients become refractory. It is generally believed that there is still considerable room for improvement in drugs that treat most psychiatric disorders.

Similarly, while symptoms of certain neurodegenerative diseases were reported in ancient times, there are few drugs that effectively treat them. While some neurodegenerative disorders are the result of injury or genetic factors, a majority are associated with advanced age. With an increase in the number of people reaching their eighties, nineties, and even 100 years old, the numbers of patients who suffer from neurodegenerative diseases is expected to increase dramatically. In fact, in the United States, it has been estimated that, as of 2016, over 5 million people suffer from Alzheimer's disease, and that number is expected to triple by 2050. Therefore, there has been increased urgency to identify drugs that treat diseases such as Parkinson's and Alzheimer's.

Many drugs in use to treat psychiatric and neurodegenerative disorders affect neurotransmitter (NT) levels, either increasing or decreasing their concentration. These NTs include dopamine, serotonin, norepinephrine, acetylcholine, glutamate, and γ-aminobutyric acid (GABA). The role of neurotransmitters is to relay messages along their corresponding neurons; this is accomplished through their release from the presynaptic neuron into the synapse and interaction with receptors on the postsynaptic neuron. This release affects transmission of ions, such as Na^+, Ca^{2+}, K^+, and Cl^-, and changes the electron potential. The resting potential of a neuron is –70 mV; **excitatory neurotransmitters** (NTs) increase the concentration of cations, causing depolarization and relay of an electrical signal along the axon (action potential). **Inhibitory neurotransmitters** increase the concentration of anions, causing hyperpolarization and decreasing the relay. Important drug targets are the GPCR neurotransmitter receptors, ion channels, and neurotransmitter transporters (see Chapter 6) involved in reuptake. The pre- and postsynaptic neurons and associated receptors, channels, and transporters of these neurotransmitters are illustrated in **Figure 13.1**.

Synaptic vesicles containing neurotransmitters release them when their membranes fuse with the outer cell membrane of the neuron. Once released, some neurotransmitter molecules cross the synaptic cleft and bind to receptors, including ligand-gated ion channels (LGICs) and G protein-coupled receptors (GPCRs) on the postsynaptic neuron. Binding to these receptors results in changes in ion concentration, either directly for LGICs or indirectly through GPCRs.

When concentrations of NTs in the synaptic cleft reach certain levels, NT transporters remove them in a process called reuptake as one mechanism to regulate the concentration of NTs and their signaling. Once removed from the cleft, the NTs are repackaged in vesicles.

The release and reuptake of various NTs is controlled by multiple factors, and there is interplay between individual NTs. Neurological diseases are sometimes caused by an imbalance in NT levels, with NT roles in the disease state depending on their location in the brain. Structures of some small-molecule neurotransmitters are shown in **Figure 13.2**, and an overview of the role of specific neurotransmitters involved in CNS disorders is given here. While all are amines, serotonin, dopamine, and norepinephrine are commonly referred to as **monoamine neurotransmitters**.

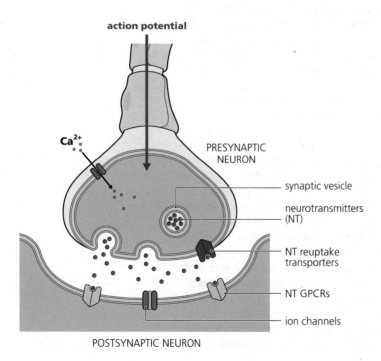

action potential

Ca^{2+}

PRESYNAPTIC NEURON

synaptic vesicle

neurotransmitters (NT)

NT reuptake transporters

NT GPCRs

ion channels

POSTSYNAPTIC NEURON

Figure 13.1 Schematic drawing of two neurons (presynaptic and postsynaptic) and the synapse between them. The action potential travels along the axon, ultimately effecting release of neurotransmitters (NTs, shown as pink circles) from the synaptic vesicles. NTs bind to receptors, such as GPCRs (green) on the postsynaptic neuron, and to NT reuptake transporters (purple) on the presynaptic neuron. They also affect voltage- and ligand-gated ion channels (orange) on either neuron causing ions such as Ca^{2+} to enter (shown) or be released.

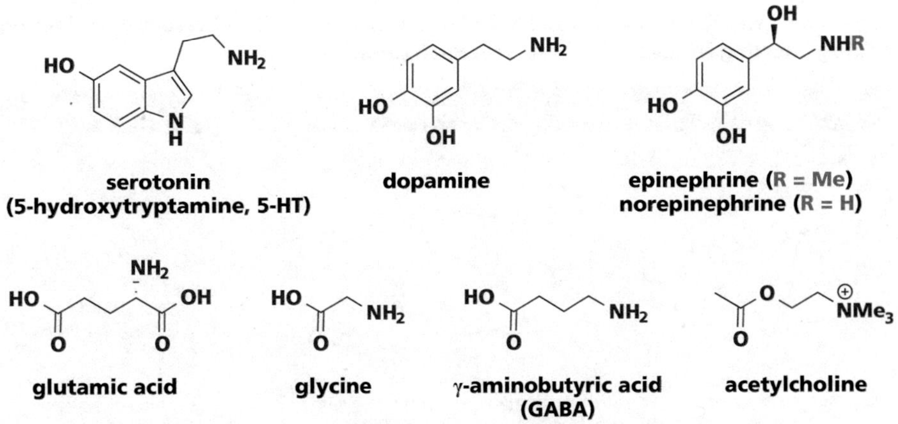

Figure 13.2 Structures of neurotransmitters involved in CNS disorders. Small molecules that interact with GPCRs, reuptake transporters, and ion channels to regulate synaptic transmission include serotonin, dopamine, norepinephrine, epinephrine, glutamic acid, glycine, γ-amino butyric acid and acetylcholine.

serotonin
(5-hydroxytryptamine, 5-HT)

dopamine

epinephrine (R = Me)
norepinephrine (R = H)

glutamic acid

glycine

γ-aminobutyric acid
(GABA)

acetylcholine

Serotonin, or **5-hydroxytryptamine** (5-HT), is an inhibitory neurotransmitter that regulates mood as well as sleep, appetite, memory, body temperature, and sexual function. Low levels of serotonin are associated with both anxiety and depression, and its dysregulation is also thought to have a role in schizophrenia, as well as bipolar disorder. **Dopamine** is both inhibitory and excitatory and plays roles in motor behavior, motivation, and emotion. Two conditions that are caused by an imbalance in dopamine levels, although in opposite directions, are Parkinson's disease and schizophrenia. Low levels of dopamine and loss of dopaminergic neurons (neurons primarily releasing dopamine) are implicated in Parkinson's disease, while increased dopamine levels and dopaminergic neuron activity are thought to contribute to the psychoses experienced by schizophrenics. Dopamine levels are regulated in part by other neurotransmitters, and nearly all drugs of abuse raise dopamine levels either directly or indirectly. This relationship is the basis for the **dopamine reward system**, also known as the mesolimbic dopamine system in the brain. This circuit connects the ventral tegmental area (VTA) and the nucleus accumbens (NAc), and activation controls responses to rewards such as food and sex.

Epinephrine and **norepinephrine** (also known as noradrenaline and adrenaline) are excitatory neurotransmitters. They are involved in the regulation of sleep and alertness in the CNS, and in the periphery they also have roles in controlling heart rate and bronchodilation. In the CNS, high levels of these NTs cause anxiety and can induce paranoid psychosis. **Glutamic acid** is also an excitatory neurotransmitter with roles in synaptic plasticity, which refers to changes in the connections between neurons. Hyperfunction of its receptors causes excitotoxicity that may lead to seizures. **Glycine** is an inhibitory neurotransmitter and plays a role in movement. In fact, several movement disorders are associated with mutations in the glycine receptor. Glycine is also a co-agonist at the *N*-methyl-D-aspartate (NMDA) subtype of glutamate receptors, and in that role it is excitatory. **γ-Aminobutyric acid** (GABA) is an inhibitory neurotransmitter, which balances the excitatory NTs. Low levels can lead to anxiety, depression, and convulsions. **Acetylcholine** affects muscle contraction and has a role in memory. **Table 13.1** summarizes these neurotransmitters and their roles in psychiatric and neurodegenerative disorders.

The brain's architecture relies on a unique barrier, the **blood–brain barrier** (BBB), to protect it. Paul Ehrlich demonstrated the existence of the BBB in the late 1880s when he injected a dye into the bloodstream of mice and saw that all the organs become stained except the brain. In a related experiment almost 30 years later, injection of the same dye into mouse brains only stained the brains, and no other organs, proving the existence of a barrier between the brain and the bloodstream. The BBB is made up of tightly packed endothelial cells that are denser than other membrane structures. This architecture protects the brain from toxins and infectious agents but also provides an additional barrier for drugs to penetrate. A number of studies have attempted to characterize the physical properties of drugs that are active in the CNS, and therefore must cross the BBB, and compare them to properties of drugs that affect other organ systems. In general, CNS-active agents are of lower molecular weight, higher

Table 13.1   Neurotransmitters and drug targets that modulate NT levels, disorders implicated in NT imbalance, and examples of drug affecting NT levels (*indicates research probe).

Neurotransmitter	Drug target or mechanism	Disorder	Drug examples
serotonin (5-HT)	5-HT transporter and receptors	depression	fluoxetine, citalopram
		migraine	sumatriptan
		schizophrenia	aripirazole, quetiapine
		social anxiety	paroxetine, citalopram
		obesity	lorcaserin
dopamine	dopamine receptors and transporter; biosynthesis	Parkinson's disease	L-dopa
		schizophrenia	Thorazine, clozapine
GABA	GABA receptor	anesthesia	phenobarbital, lorazepam, alprazolam
		anxiety	lorazepam, alprazolam
		epilepsy	phenobarbital
		insomnia	zolpidem
norepinephrine	norepinephrine receptors and transporter	anxiety	duloxetine
		depression	reboxetine
		ADHD	methylphenidate
acetylcholine	acetylcholine receptors, biosynthesis	Alzheimer's disease	tacrine, donepezil
glutamate	glutamate receptors	Alzheimer's disease	memantine
		schizophrenia	pomaglumetad*
glycine	glycine transporters and NMDA receptors	schizophrenia	bitopertin*
		OCD	bitopertin

lipophilicity (log P), contain fewer H-bond donors and acceptors, and have smaller polar surface areas compared to drugs that act in the periphery. Of these, lipophilicity is considered the most important determinant. In addition to the tightly packed cells that prevent diffusion across the BBB, the brain also expresses high levels of the P-glycoprotein transporter (also called MDR1), which expels molecules that have diffused into the brain. There are assays available with cells that express MDR1, which can be used to predict brain penetration of a drug candidate.

Many drugs targeting neuropsychiatric disorders are based on neurotransmitters and are either agonists or antagonists at their receptors. Ligand-based drug design and the use of pharmacophore models have been widely used in the development of most of these agents. There are far fewer drugs approved to treat neurodegenerative diseases, and while some affect neurotransmitter levels, others are in development that inhibit enzymes involved in these diseases. The challenges in understanding the basis for many CNS disorders make drug discovery particularly challenging.

DRUGS TARGETING ANXIETY AND DEPRESSION

Anxiety disorders are the most common mental health disorder, affecting about 25 million Americans. Depression is a little less common but still affects approximately 7% of the U.S. population. These are related conditions, with about half of those being diagnosed with depression also suffering from anxiety disorders, and both are challenging to treat. Some patients may respond to drug treatment while others are refractory, and drug trials are complicated by a large placebo effect. In addition, some drugs have a multiweek lag time before they take effect, resulting in lower patient compliance.

Neurotransmitters involved in anxiety disorders include GABA, serotonin, and norepinephrine. GABA binds at the $GABA_A$, $GABA_B$, and $GABA_C$ receptors: the A and C receptor subtypes are chloride ion channels, and the B subtype is a GPCR. Of these, $GABA_A$ is the most important target in terms of treating anxiety and depression, where increased GABA activity reduces anxiety. Low levels of serotonin and norepinephrine are both implicated in depression, and many drugs used to treat depression raise levels of these NTs. A prominent mechanism for raising levels is inhibition of the NT transporters, which raises levels by blocking reuptake of the NTs.

13.1 Positive allosteric modulators at the $GABA_A$ receptor are sedatives and anticonvulsants

The $GABA_A$ receptor is a ligand-gated chloride ion channel, and positive allosteric modulators (PAMs) act as sedatives as well as anticonvulsants. Binding of either GABA or PAMs increases intracellular chloride ion concentration, resulting in membrane hyperpolarization and reduced transmission of the action potential.

The basic structure of the $GABA_A$ receptor is a hetero-oligomer, with different combinations of various subunits resulting in a variety of subtypes (**Figure 13.3**). However, the majority of $GABA_A$ receptors identified in the brain are composed of two α, two β, and one γ subunit. The natural ligand, GABA, binds at two extracellular sites on the α/β interface. Different classes of drugs acting at the GABA receptor bind at different allosteric sites on the receptor.

Barbiturates, as a class, act as sedatives and hypnotics. The first approved member of this class, barbital, was marketed in 1904 (**Figure 13.4**). It is a derivative of barbituric acid, synthesized in the 1860s as a condensation product of urea and malonic acid. Although barbituric acid is not pharmacologically active, it is the parent for the barbiturates. In Germany, chemists Josef von Mering and Emil Fischer made barbital, the diethyl analog of barbituric acid, in part on the basis of the observation that the bis(diethylsulfone), sulfonal, had activity as a hypnotic. Prior to that time, the most widely used sedative was the salt potassium bromide, which was introduced in 1857 as a sedative and anticonvulsant. Barbital was used to treat insomnia, sedate psychotic patients, and induce anesthesia. Its use to treat epileptic seizures was also described in 1912. Many

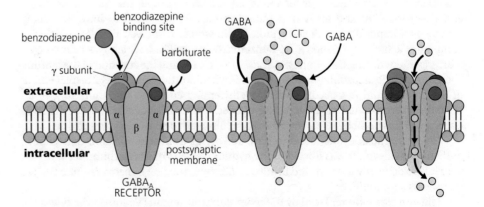

Figure 13.3 Simplified structure and binding sites of small molecules on the $GABA_A$ receptor chloride ion channel. Left: The $GABA_A$ receptor, located on the postsynaptic neuron, is a ligand-gated channel for chloride ions (shown as yellow circles). It consists of two α subunits (orange), two β subunits (green), and one γ subunit (blue). Center: Two molecules of GABA (red circles) bind between the α and β subunits, resulting in channel opening. Right: Benzodiazepines (blue circles) bind at the α/γ interface, resulting in increased binding of GABA and increases in channel opening, and barbiturates (gray circles) are thought to bind on the α subunit.

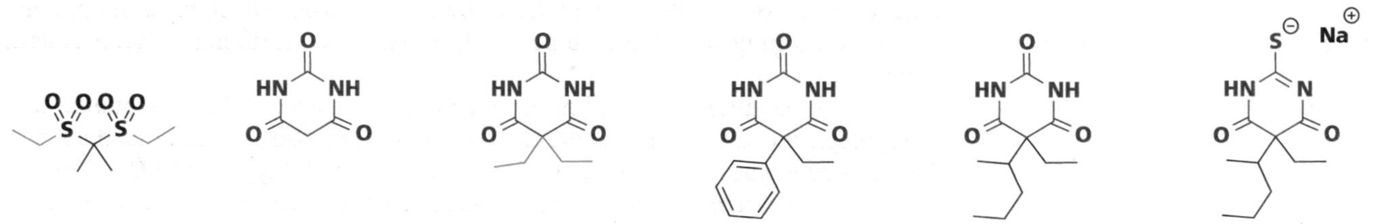

| sulfonal | barbituric acid | barbital | phenobarbital | pentobarbital | sodium thiopental |

analogs of the barbiturates were made in industrial and academic laboratories. The barbital scaffold is the basis of a number of drugs that are used for various indications.

The derivative phenobarbital is one of the most widely used agents to treat seizure disorders, and pentobarbital is primarily used as a sedative and in anesthesia. Sodium thiopental, a sulfur analog, is used as a rapid onset, short-acting anesthetic. It is also one of a cocktail of drugs used for lethal injection and has been used as a truth serum, although the lowered inhibitions may lead to false as well as true statements.

With the wide use of barbiturates, it became obvious that their frequent use could result in dependence. In fact, by 1960 there were an estimated 250,000 barbiturate addicts in the United States. In addition, these drugs have a low therapeutic index, sometimes resulting in fatal overdose. While their use to treat anxiety has been supplanted with much safer drugs, the barbiturates are still used as anticonvulsants and in anesthesia. They are thought to bind near the GABA binding sites on the α subunit (see Figure 13.3). The mechanism of barbiturates was not fully understood until the late 1970s, when they were shown to potentiate inhibitory effects on neurotransmission of GABA.

The **benzodiazepines** (BZs) were discovered in the 1950s in Leo Sternbach's lab at Hoffmann-La Roche. As with other synthetic drugs discovered in this era, the program was driven by ease of synthesis and *in vivo* activity rather than a specific target; the GABA receptor activity was identified much later. Although sometimes erroneously classified in popular literature as accidental, the discovery was driven by a rational search for tranquilizers. Sternbach synthesized many compounds that were derivatives of structures originally assigned in the 1850s as benzheptoxdiazines (**Figure 13.5A**). During the course of his work, these structures were reassigned as quinazoline-3-oxides. None of the compounds synthesized was active in mouse models of sedation, and after several years the project was abandoned. At the time of the work, purification methods were limited, and only compounds that could be recrystallized (as a method for purification) were subjected to testing. During a cleanup of the lab, Sternbach's associate Earl Reeder found an untested sample that had crystallized, and upon isolation and assay in a mouse model, it was found to have promising activity as a tranquilizer. Reinvestigation of the structure showed that this particular compound actually contained a 1,4-benzodiazepine scaffold, which was formed by a rearrangement during the synthesis (**Figure 13.5B**). During the reaction of the starting α-chloromethylquinazoline-3-oxide with methylamine, the expected S_N2 displacement of the chloride did not occur. Instead, methylamine added to the imine to give an unstable intermediate that led to a ring-opened oxime. Displacement of the chloride occurred at this point by reaction of the oxime nitrogen to give chlordiazepoxide.

Chlordiazepoxide was found to have activity as a muscle relaxant, tranquilizer, and anticonvulsant. It was devoid of the hypnotic effects of the barbiturates and had very low toxicity. It was marketed in 1960 as Librium, the first benzodiazepine (BZ) to be used as a tranquilizer.

Librium was soon replaced by the more stable diazepam (Valium), which was the top-selling drug between 1968 and 1982 (**Figure 13.6**). While their low toxicity and profile of muscle relaxation without sedation meant that benzodiazepines rapidly replaced barbiturates, their mechanism of action remained unknown until 1977, when they were found to interact with specific receptors in the brain. These were cloned and identified as the $GABA_A$ receptors in 1987. Benzodiazepines bind between the α and γ subunits of the receptor and modulate binding of GABA (see Figure 13.3). Positive allosteric modulators (PAMs) such as diazepam enhance GABA activity and are used to treat anxiety and convulsive disorders such as epilepsy. As of 2017, lorazepam and

Figure 13.4 Structural basis and examples of barbiturate drugs, in order of increasing complexity. Sulfonal was an early hypnotic, and combining some of its structural features (ethyl moieties) with inactive barbituric acid formed the basis for the barbiturate analog barbital. Drugs used today include phenobarbital, pentobarbital, and sodium thiopental. The ethyl groups of sulfonal and barbital are shown in blue, and the barbituric acid core is shown in red.

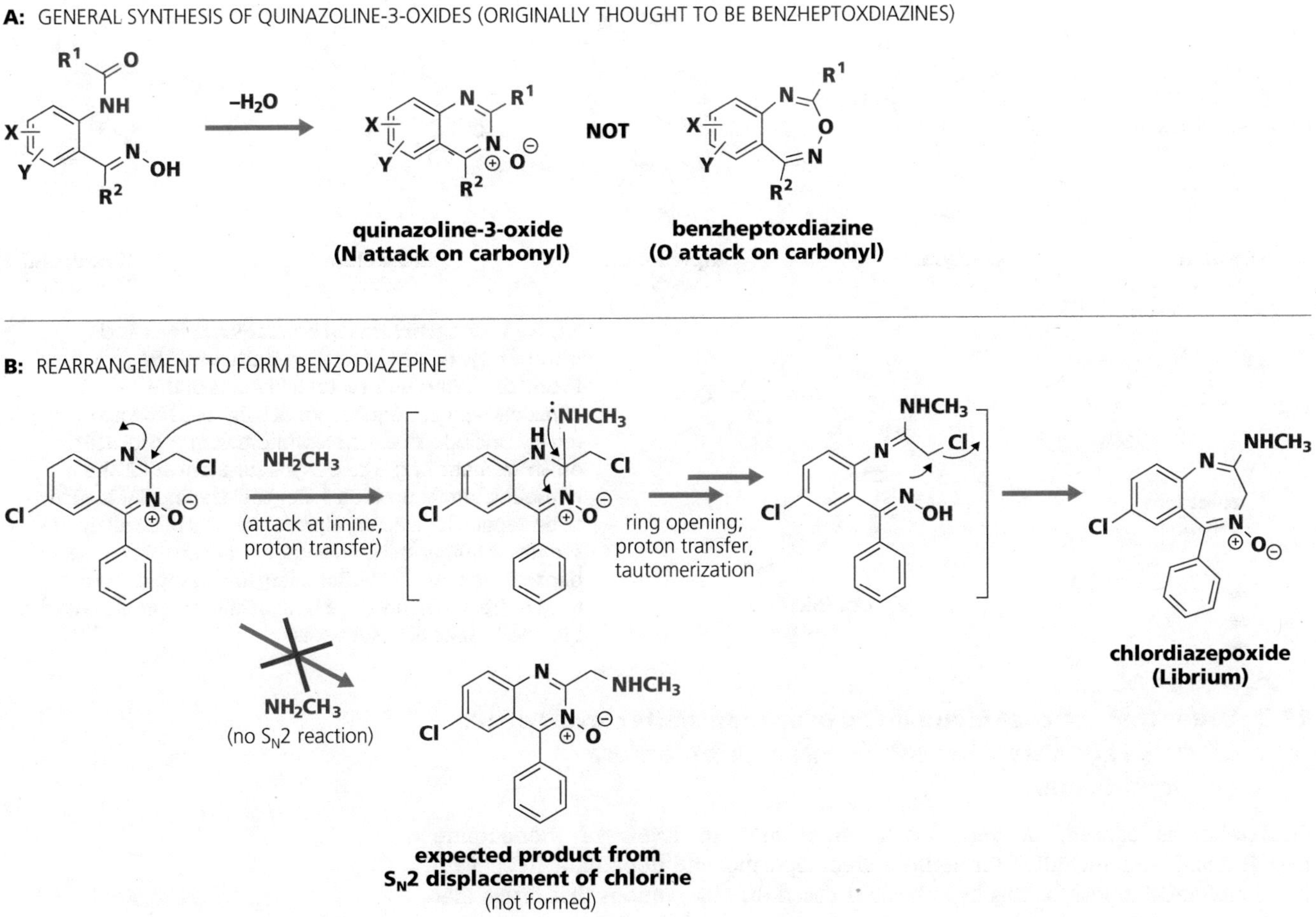

A: GENERAL SYNTHESIS OF QUINAZOLINE-3-OXIDES (ORIGINALLY THOUGHT TO BE BENZHEPTOXDIAZINES)

quinazoline-3-oxide
(N attack on carbonyl)

NOT

benzheptoxdiazine
(O attack on carbonyl)

B: REARRANGEMENT TO FORM BENZODIAZEPINE

(attack at imine, proton transfer)

ring opening;
proton transfer,
tautomerization

**chlordiazepoxide
(Librium)**

NH₂CH₃
(no S_N2 reaction)

**expected product from
S_N2 displacement of chlorine**
(not formed)

Figure 13.5 History of chlordiazepoxide synthesis. A: General synthesis of quinazoline-3-oxides. Compounds with various aryl substituents (X, Y) and varying the amide substituent R^1 (amide shown in red) were prepared. Attack of the hydroxylamine nitrogen at the amide carbonyl gives the quinazoline-3-oxide. The structure was originally assigned as the benzheptoxdiazine that would result from attack by the oxime oxygen on the amide. B: Rearrangement of a specific quinazoline-3-oxide (X = 6-chloro, Y = H, R^1 = CH₂Cl, R^2 = Ph) to benzodiazepine scaffold. Reaction of 6-chloro-2-chloromethyl-quinazoline-3-oxide with an amine was expected to generate the simple displacement product via S_N2 reaction. In the case of methylamine, addition to the imine occurred instead of the expected S_N2 displacement. Ring opening, proton transfer, and ring closure produced chlordiazepoxide (abbreviated mechanism shown).

alprazolam are the most widely prescribed benzodiazepines for anxiety and panic disorders. The short-acting drug midazolam is commonly used for the induction of anesthesia. Antagonists of benzodiazepine binding, such as flumazenil, can be used to treat benzodiazepine overdose. Although benzodiazepines were originally believed to be nonaddictive, and therefore much safer than barbiturates, dependence is indeed seen with their long-term use. The structure–activity relationships (SAR) for benzodiazepines PAMs include an aromatic A-ring with an electron-withdrawing group at C7, a carbonyl or equivalent unsaturation at C2, and a nitrogen at position 1. Pharmacophore models for the benzodiazepines have been developed and used in virtual screening programs to identify new ligands for the GABA BZ binding site (see Section 3.5).

In addition to the benzodiazepines, zolpidem and eszopiclone also have been found to bind at the benzodiazepine site on the GABA_A receptor. These drugs have hypnotic effects at a low dose, resulting in less impact on cognition and psychomotor reflexes than benzodiazepines, and they are primarily used to treat insomnia. Unlike BZs which bind to multiple subtypes of the α subunit, zolpidem binds at the BZ site only on certain α subunits, specifically the α_1 subtype; it is believed this selectivity results in its hypnotic effects and differentiates it from the BZs that bind to the α_1, α_3, and α_4 subtypes, a characteristic of drugs that have anti-anxiety and anticonvulsant effects.

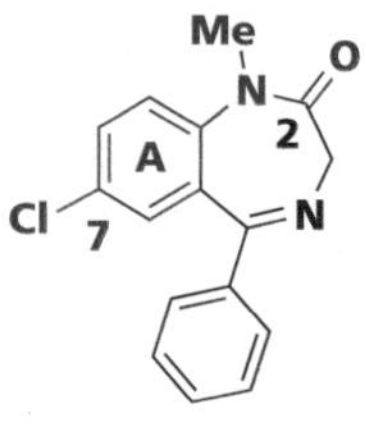

diazepam
Valium

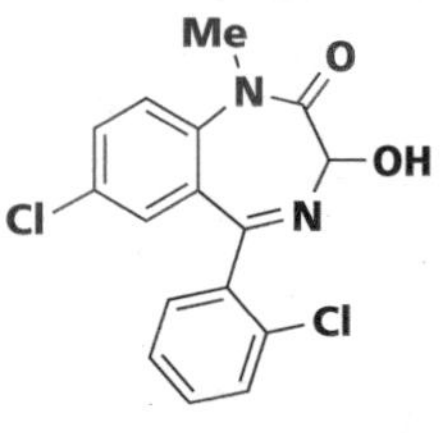

lorazepam
Ativan

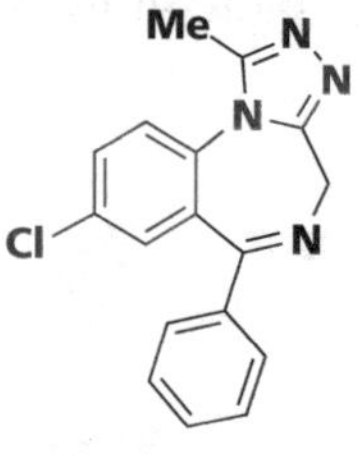

alprazolam
Xanax

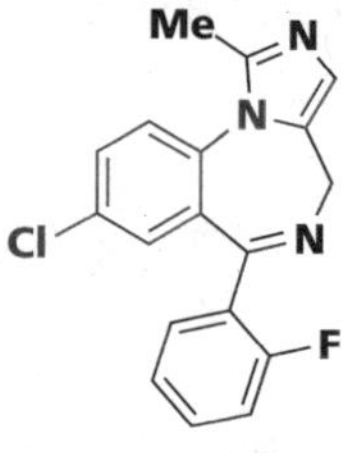

midazolam
Versed

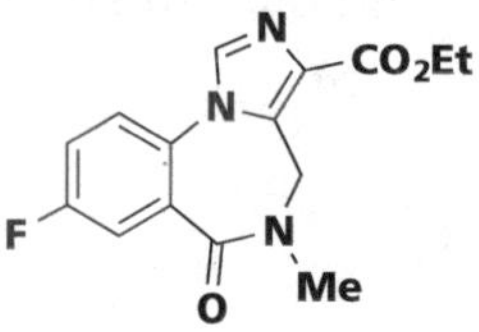

flumazenil
BZ antagonist

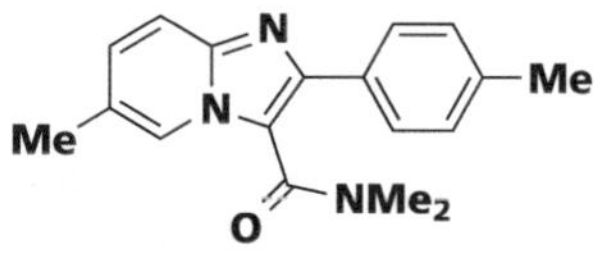

zolpidem
Ambien

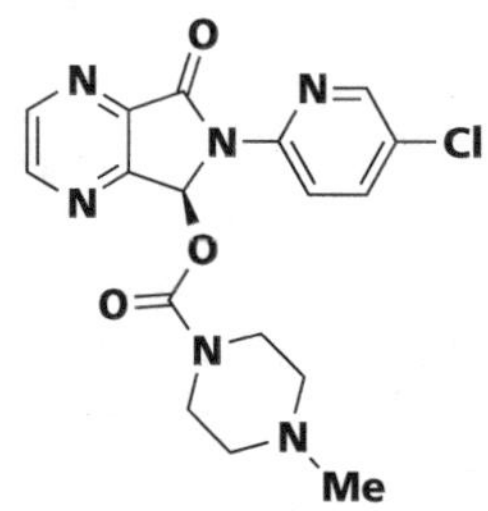

eszopiclone
Lunesta

Figure 13.6 Structures of benzodiazepines and other drugs that bind at the BZ site of GABA$_A$ receptor. Common structural features of the benzodiazepines, required for activity, are shown in red and include an electron-withdrawing substituent on an aromatic ring, a carbonyl equivalent at C2 and a nitrogen atom at position 1. Benzodiazepine PAMs such as diazepam, lorazepam, alprazolam, and midazolam are sedatives; flumazenil is an antagonist used for reversal of benzodiazepine effects. Zolpidem and ezsopiclone are used to treat insomnia and have a different profile based on binding to specific α subtypes.

13.2 Drugs that increase monoamine neurotransmitter levels or act as partial agonists at neurotransmitter receptors are antidepressants

Depression is caused, in part, by an imbalance in levels of monoamine neurotransmitters, including serotonin, norepinephrine, and dopamine, in specific brain regions. Support for this hypothesis is based on observations that drugs that are effective in humans modulate brain concentration of these monoamines in animal models. The mechanisms of these drugs include monoamine oxidase (MAO) inhibition, inhibition of monoamine reuptake, and mimicking the action of these neurotransmitters. Because monoamine oxidases are also involved in the metabolism of many drugs, MAO inhibitors are not widely used due to their potential to cause drug–drug interactions. Currently, the most common treatment for depression relies on increasing levels of serotonin or mimicking its effects. This may be accomplished by use of partial agonists or, more often, reuptake inhibitors. Since there are multiple subtypes of serotonin (5-HT) receptors (see Chapter 6), with effects on mood, appetite, energy, sexual function, vasodilation, and locomotion, selectivity for specific subtypes is desirable. Partial agonism at the 5-HT$_{1A}$ receptor subtype is particularly effective in treating depression.

Selective serotonin reuptake inhibitors (SSRIs) are currently the most widely used drugs to treat depression. In the transmission of messages by nerve cells, neurotransmitters such as serotonin are released into the synaptic cleft and bind to receptors on the postsynaptic cell. As neurotransmitters are released from the receptors, they are taken up by monoamine transporters (see Section 6.11) back into the presynaptic cell in a process known as **reuptake** (refer to Figure 13.1). Reuptake inhibitors maintain concentrations of monoamine neurotransmitters in the synapse for a longer period of time. Early drugs in this category were the tricyclic antidepressants, and newer examples include the selective serotonin reuptake inhibitors (SSRIs).

The earliest **tricyclic antidepressant** approved was imipramine, developed in the 1950s at Geigy. Imipramine was synthesized as an analog of the antipsychotic drug chlorpromazine but was found to be effective as an antidepressant. The carbon analog amitriptyline and its metabolite, nortriptyline, were introduced by Merck in the early 1960s (**Figure 13.7A**). The tricyclic antidepressants all act as serotonin reuptake inhibitors, although they are not selective and also act as norepinephrine reuptake inhibitors. In fact, their antidepressant effects were originally thought to be due to their effects on norepinephrine. They also block adrenergic, muscarinic acetylcholine, and

A: TRICYCLIC ANTIDEPRESSANTS (YEAR APPROVED)

B: BROMPHENIRAMINE LEAD AND FIRST SSRI ZIMELIDINE

C: SELECTIVE SEROTONIN REUPTAKE INHIBITORS

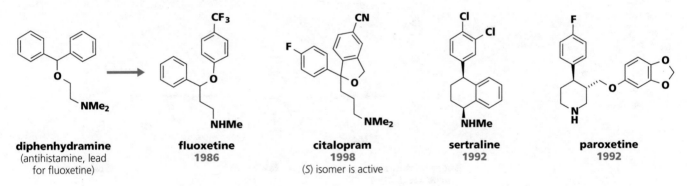

Figure 13.7 Examples of drugs used to treat depression that work through serotonin reuptake inhibition. A: Tricyclic antidepressants. These include drugs such as imipramine, amytriptyline and nortriptyline, which are serotonin reuptake inhibitors but are not selective, and exhibit significant side effects. B: Brompheniramine lead and first SSRI zimelidine. Pheniramine and brompheniramine were the basis for the first SSRI introduced (in Europe), zimelidine. C: Selective serotonin reuptake inhibitors. Drugs such as fluoxetine, citalopram, sertraline, and paroxetine are relatively safe and are the most widely prescribed class of antidepressants. The antihistamine diphenhydramine served as the structural basis for fluoxetine.

histamine receptors, leading to undesirable cardiac and sedative effects, and therefore they have a narrow therapeutic index.

The concept of developing SSRIs was based on ideas that the mode of action of tricyclic antidepressants involved blocking reuptake of serotonin. Arvid Carlsson and co-workers identified antihistamines, which also had serotonin and norepinephrine reuptake inhibition (termed SRI and NRI, respectively) properties, and began to optimize for serotonin reuptake inhibition activity. Among a group of pheniramine antihistamines, brompheniramine was identified as having a promising profile based on some selectivity for serotonin reuptake inhibition (**Figure 13.7B**). Modification of the nitrogen heterocycle and conformational constraint by introduction of a rigid alkene led to zimelidine. Zimelidine is considered the first SSRI to be approved (1982, Europe) but was quickly withdrawn due to its association with Guillain–Barré syndrome.

The first SSRI to be introduced in the United States was fluoxetine (**Figure 13.7C**), and it has a considerably improved safety profile compared to zimelidine. The starting point for fluoxetine was diphenhydramine, a potent histamine antagonist with a similar structure to pheniramine that also had activity as a monoamine reuptake inhibitor. The success of fluoxetine led to the development of additional members of this class of drugs that have selectivity for the serotonin transporter compared to other transporters and receptors (see also Case Study 1 in Chapter 5). Fluoxetine was first reported in 1974, approved in 1986, and marketed as Prozac. It became the most widely prescribed antidepressant, and within 10 years of its introduction, its sales reached $2.5 billion per year. As of 2017, there are nine SSRIs approved for the treatment of depression. Examples shown in Figure 13.7C include citalopram, sertraline, and paroxetine.

Citalopram's structure was based on an older antidepressant called talopram that worked through selective norepinephrine reuptake inhibition (SNRI), rather than as an SSRI. Talopram entered clinical trials, but development was stopped due to side effects such as increased psychomotor activity. Like the benzodiazepines, talopram was the result of a synthesis that did not yield the expected product (**Figure 13.8**). In 1965, Klaus Bøgesø at Lundbeck was trying to synthesize an analog of tricyclic

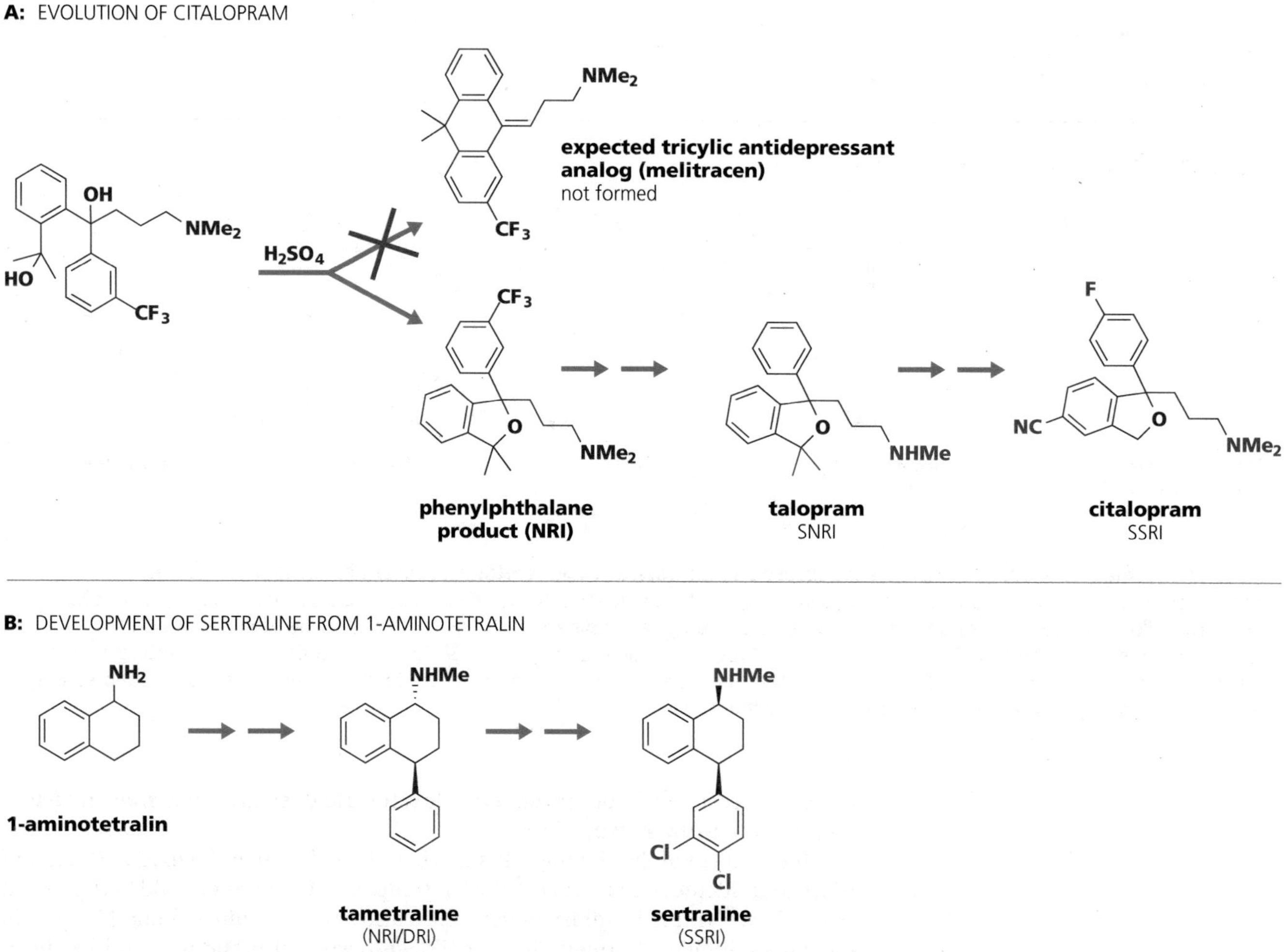

A: EVOLUTION OF CITALOPRAM

B: DEVELOPMENT OF SERTRALINE FROM 1-AMINOTETRALIN

Figure 13.8 Development of citalopram and sertraline. A: Evolution of citalopram. An attempt to synthesize melitracen, an analog of tricyclic antidepressants, via electrophilic aromatic substitution of the diol, resulted instead in formation of the phenylphthalane cyclic ether. This scaffold also had antidepressant activity, and modifications (shown in red) led to the SNRI talopram and then to the SSRI citalopram. B: Development of sertraline from 1-aminotetralin. Aminotetralins were found to have anti-anxiety effects. The parent 1-aminotetralin was modified to give the phenyl analog tametraline, the lead for sertraline. Changes included inversion of stereochemistry and incorporation of aryl substituents (shown in red).

antidepressants, called melitracen, but the reaction followed an alternate pathway, and a phenylphthalane was produced instead. Unexpectedly, the alternate structure was also effective as an antidepressant and was a potent NRI. Modification of the structure led to talopram, which was a highly selective inhibitor of norepinephrine reuptake (SNRI). Converting the secondary amine to a tertiary amine, removing the geminal di-methyl groups from the bicyclic structure, and introducing aryl substituents led to citalopram and changed the reuptake inhibition selectivity from norepinephrine to serotonin. While it was originally marketed as the racemate, the S-enantiomer of citalopram (escitalopram) is the active stereoisomer and is also approved.

Sertraline, initially reported in 1973, was synthesized by William Welch at Pfizer as part of a program to develop antipsychotics. A series of 1-aminotetralins based on the antipsychotic chlorpromazine was investigated, and while they were not active as antipsychotics, they did exhibit anti-anxiety effects. This observation led to synthesis of a number of analogs, including the *trans*-aryl-substituted tametraline, which exhibited activity as both a norepinephrine and dopamine reuptake inhibitor (DRI). Interest in pursuing SSRIs in the early 1980s led Kenneth Koe at Pfizer to reinvestigate this series. Changing the ring substituent stereochemistry to the *cis* orientation and introducing aryl substituents ultimately led to sertraline.

Based on the importance of SSRIs as antidepressants, there have been studies to identify the required pharmacophore for binding. The target, the human serotonin transporter (hSERT), is a sodium neurotransmitter symporter (see Section 6.11). Prior to solution of the X-ray structure of (S)-citalopram bound to hSERT in 2016, homology models based on an X-ray structure of a related transporter, bacterial LeuT, were used to dock SSRIs and develop binding hypotheses. For example, one model of (S)-citalopram bound to hSERT based on the LeuT model is shown in **Figure 13.9**, along with an X-ray structure of (S)-citalopram bound to hSERT.

In this docking model, interactions in the binding pocket include a salt bridge between the amine on the drug to Asp98, π–π interactions of aryl rings with Phe335 and Tyr176, and hydrophobic interactions with Ala411, Tyr95, Ala173, and Ile172 (see Figure 13.9A). A pharmacophore model based on this binding pose includes a cationic site (P1) corresponding to the amine found in all SSRIs, as well as two aryl sites (R1, R2) and a hydrophobic area (H1). While the SSRIs in use were developed by use of traditional SAR to identify modifications providing selectivity, pharmacophore models may be used in virtual screening programs to identify novel SSRIs. A recent X-ray structure confirms that (S)-citalopram binds in the central cavity of SERT (see Figure 13.9B), with a slightly different orientation than the model in Figure 13.9A. Important interactions include nitrogen to Asp98 (as predicted), fluorophenyl to Tyr176, and bicyclic aryl to Phe335. The orientation of the aryl groups is opposite to what was predicted. In addition, the crystal structure shows a second molecule of citalopram binds at a nearby allosteric site, preventing the molecule in the central cavity from dissociating.

Reuptake inhibitors that target other neurotransmitters also have important clinical uses. Duloxetine and venlafaxine both have activity as combined serotonin and norepinephrine reuptake inhibitors, although they are more potent inhibitors of the serotonin transporter than the norepinephrine transporter. Both are used to treat both depression and anxiety. Reboxetine is a selective norepinephrine reuptake inhibitor (SNRI) developed in the 1990s and is used in Europe to treat depression. SNRIs such as atomoxetine and dopamine reuptake inhibitors (DRI) such as methylphenidate (Ritalin) can be used to treat attention-deficit hyperactivity disorder (ADHD), although methylphenidate is not a selective inhibitor and has additional activity at the adrenergic receptor (**Figure 13.10A**).

Positive clinical results for use of SSRIs in combination with dopamine agonists have led to the idea of developing triple reuptake inhibitors (TRIs) that affect levels of serotonin, norepinephrine, and dopamine. Amitifadine, which progressed to phase III clinical trials, is an example of a TRI. Others include ansofaxine, which is in phase II trials as of 2017 and liafensine, which advanced to phase II trials (**Figure 13.10B**). While amitifadine and liafensine did not progress further due to lack of superiority over marketed drugs, this approach is still under investigation.

A: MODEL OF hSERT WITH (*S*)-CITALOPRAM AND PHARMACOPHORE MODEL

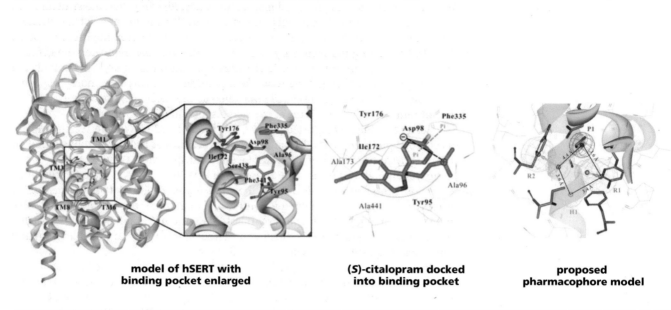

**model of hSERT with
binding pocket enlarged**

**(*S*)-citalopram docked
into binding pocket**

**proposed
pharmacophore model**

B: X-RAY CRYSTAL STRUCTURE OF (*S*)-CITALOPRAM BOUND TO hSERT

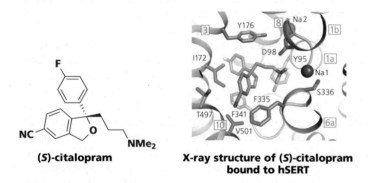

(*S*)-citalopram

**X-ray structure of (*S*)-citalopram
bound to hSERT**

Figure 13.9 Homology and pharmacophore model of the human serotonin transporter and X-ray co-structure.
A: Models of hSERT with (S)-citalopram, and phamacophore model. Left: homology model of hSERT with binding site enlarged to show key side chains. Middle: (S)-citalopram docked to the homology model shows proposed interactions including ion–ion interaction between the amine and Asp98 (black dotted line), π-stacking of the aryl ring with Phe335 (gold dotted line), and a hydrophobic region (Ile172, Ala441, Tyr95, and Ala173, light blue lines) where the bicyclic portion binds. Right: The pharmacophore model is based on the binding model where R1, R2 = aryl; H1 = hydrophobic; and P1 = cationic (model defined by distances between dots that are centered in pharmacophore grid points). B: Solved X-ray structure of (S)-citalopram (green) bound to hSERT (red). Several proposed binding interactions are confirmed including specific binding site and ionic interaction between citalopram nitrogen to Asp98. The aryl groups sit in a slightly different orientation than the model; important interactions observed include fluorophenyl to Tyr176, and bicyclic aryl to Phe335. Red balls = sodium ions. A second molecule of (S)-citalopram bound at an allosteric site is not shown. (A, adapted from Zhou Z-L, Liu H-L, Wu JW et al. [2013] *Chem Biol Drug Des* 82:705–717. B, from Coleman JA, Green EM & Gouaux E [2016] *Nature* 532:334–339. With permission from Macmillan Publishers Limited.)

In addition to the neurotransmitter reuptake inhibitors, partial agonists at the 5-HT$_{1A}$ receptor are also effective as antidepressants and anti-anxiety agents. **Buspirone** (**Figure 13.11**), an azapirone, is one such example. The 5-HT$_{1A}$ receptor subtype is located in the hippocampus and frontal cortex, which are areas of the brain involved in anxiety modulation. Buspirone is as effective as benzodiazepines but with no addiction potential. Since buspirone does not target the GABA receptor, it is lacking in the sedative and anticonvulsant effects of benzodiazepines. It was originally prepared in 1969 during a search for tranquilizers devoid of the sedation side effects that characterized earlier drugs.

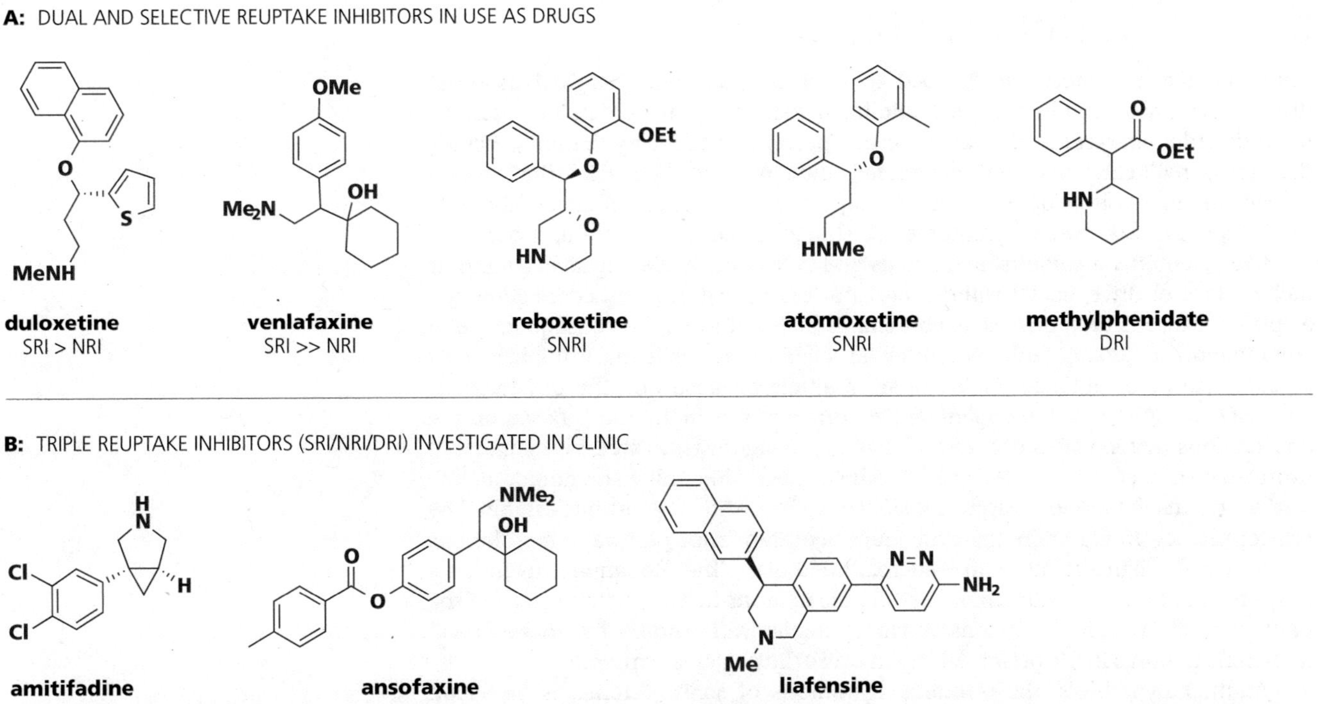

A: DUAL AND SELECTIVE REUPTAKE INHIBITORS IN USE AS DRUGS

duloxetine
SRI > NRI

venlafaxine
SRI >> NRI

reboxetine
SNRI

atomoxetine
SNRI

methylphenidate
DRI

B: TRIPLE REUPTAKE INHIBITORS (SRI/NRI/DRI) INVESTIGATED IN CLINIC

amitifadine

ansofaxine

liafensine

Figure 13.10 Structures of reuptake inhibitors targeting multiple neurotransmitters. A: Dual and selective reuptake inhibitors in use as drugs. Duloxetine and venlafaxine are dual SRI/NRIs (predominant target indicated) used to treat depression and anxiety. Reboxetine (for depression) and atomoxetine (for ADHD) are selective NRIs. Methylphenidate, a dopamine reuptake inhibitor, is used to treat ADHD. B: Triple reuptake inhibitors investigated in clinic. Several triple reuptake inhibitors (SRI/NRI/DRI) have entered clinical trials to treat depression, including amitifadine, ansofaxine, and liafensine.

One shortcoming of SSRIs is a delay in onset of effectiveness, which may take 3–4 weeks. It has been suggested that this delay is because the increase in concentration in 5-HT in the synapse, resulting from inhibition of the transporter, leads to feedback inhibition of 5-HT$_{1A}$ receptors, resulting in a decrease in release of 5-HT. After a few weeks of treatment, however, the 5-HT$_{1A}$ receptors are desensitized, restoring release of serotonin. A recent approach has been the development of compounds with dual activity as 5-HT$_{1A}$ partial agonists and serotonin reuptake inhibitors. This approach should circumvent the receptor sensitization that is believed to cause the delay in response. The first compound approved in this class is vilazodone (see Figure 13.11), which may have a shorter onset than other SSRIs and exhibits fewer side effects, such as sexual dysfunction (see Case Study 1 in this chapter).

As seen in these examples, a focus on neurotransmitter reuptake has provided many drugs that are effective in treating anxiety and depression. These have progressed from early nonselective drugs like the tricyclic antidepressants to SSRIs and SNRIs, as well as TRIs, which affect levels of serotonin, norepinephrine, and dopamine concurrently. Other indications for reuptake inhibitors include ADHD and insomnia. As these drugs have been used more widely, additional indications have also been approved, including use in sleep disorders, treatment of neuropathic pain, and smoking cessation.

Figure 13.11 Serotonin partial agonists. Buspirone is a 5-HT$_{1A}$ partial agonist, while vilazodone is both an SSRI and a 5-HT$_{1A}$ partial agonist.

buspirone
5-HT$_{1A}$ partial agonist

vilazodone
SSRI/5-HT$_{1A}$ partial agonist

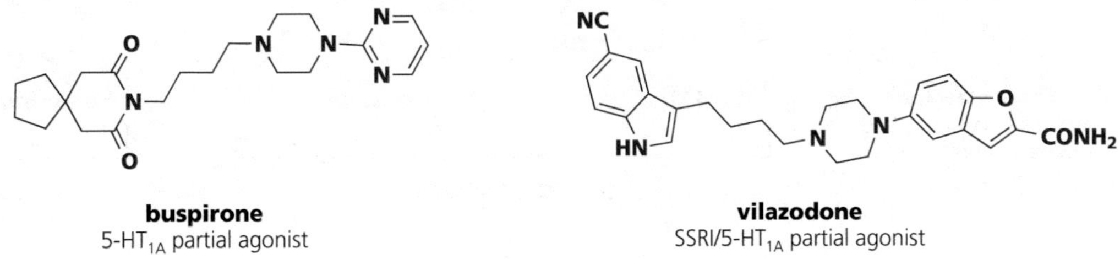

DRUGS TARGETING PSYCHOSIS

Antipsychotics are most widely used to treat schizophrenia, as well as other disorders characterized by delusions and hallucinations. Schizophrenia is a serious brain disorder characterized by an abnormal perception of reality that may include delusions, hallucinations, and disordered thinking and behavior. The disease typically manifests in people between the ages of 15 and 45, and it affects about 24 million people worldwide. Symptoms are characterized as positive and negative; positive symptoms include hallucinations and delusions, while negative symptoms include loss of drive, social withdrawal, and loss of cognitive function. Although a specific cause is unknown, schizophrenia is believed to be the consequence of a combination of genetic and environmental factors that result in an imbalance in certain neurotransmitter levels. There are multiple proposals on the physiological basis of schizophrenia. The dopamine hypothesis of schizophrenia is based on the observations that effective drugs are dopamine antagonists, as well as the fact that overuse of amphetamine (**Figure 13.12**), which causes dopamine and noradrenaline release, results in paranoid psychosis, similar to the positive symptoms exhibited by schizophrenics. In the brain, there are four major dopamine pathways: mesolimbic, mesocortical, nigrostriatal, and tuberoinfundibular. The dopamine hypothesis purports that overactive dopamine mesolimbic neurons in the striatal regions of the brain cause the positive symptoms of schizophrenia, while underactive mesocortical dopamine neurons in the prefrontal region cause the negative symptoms.

Another hypothesis, the serotonin hypothesis of schizophrenia, is based on evidence that serotonin agonists such as lysergic acid diethylamide (LSD) and mescaline produce hallucinations. Although these compounds are nonselective, agonism at the 5-HT$_{2A}$ receptor is thought to be responsible for their hallucinogenic effects. The glutamate hypothesis proposes that insufficient glutamate levels contribute to disease symptoms. It has its basis in the observation of reduced levels of glutamate in the cerebrospinal fluid of patients, as well as higher levels of NMDA receptors in the brain of patients compared to unaffected individuals. In addition, the NMDA antagonists ketamine and phencyclidine (PCP), a drug of abuse, cause schizophrenia-like psychosis (see Figure 13.12). It has been suggested that neurodevelopmental abnormalities result in dysfunctional NMDA receptors and predispose those affected to the development of schizophrenia. NMDA receptors are involved in the regulation of dopaminergic neurons, providing an explanation for the observed changes in these neurons and a link to the dopamine hypothesis.

Treatment of schizophrenia prior to the 1950s involved convulsive therapy, partial lobotomy, and treatment with the plant alkaloid reserpine. Convulsive therapy included medical and electroconvulsive treatment as well as insulin injections to induce coma. Reserpine, from the Indian snakeroot plant, has been used in India for centuries to treat psychoses. However, it has serious side effects, including lowering blood pressure and decreasing heart rate. Beginning in the 1950s, several safer drugs were introduced to treat schizophrenia, and some have found use as treatments for other conditions, such as bipolar disorder.

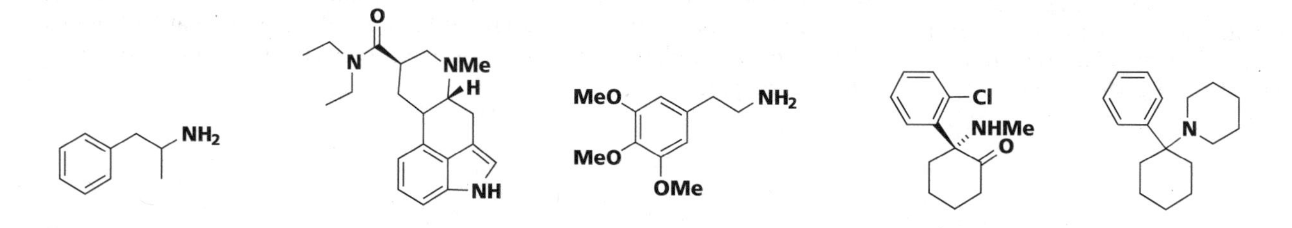

Figure 13.12 Compounds that can cause schizophrenia-like symptoms. Compounds with effects on dopamine, serotonin, and glutamate levels are known to cause schizophrenia-like symptoms. Amphetamine increases dopamine and norepinephrine levels and overuse causes paranoid psychoses; LSD and mescaline are serotonin agonists and produce hallucinations; ketamine and PCP are NMDA antagonists, which antagonize glutamate effects, and cause schizophrenia-like psychoses.

amphetamine
increases dopamine and
norepinephrine levels

LSD   **mescaline**

SEROTONIN AGONISTS

ketamine   **PCP (phencyclidine)**

NMDA ANTAGONISTS,
antagonizes glutamate effects

13.3 Typical antipsychotics act as dopamine receptor antagonists

Early drugs used to treat schizophrenia are termed **typical antipsychotics**; they act as antagonists at dopamine receptors. The five subtypes of dopamine receptors are all GPCRs and are divided into either the D_1-like family (including the D_1 and D_5 subtypes) or the D_2-like family (including D_2, D_3, and D_4 subtypes). Binding of dopamine at the D_1-like family of receptors activates inhibitory G proteins, while binding at the D_2-like subtypes activates stimulatory G proteins. Within the D_2-like receptor family, binding of dopamine at the D_2 receptor activates psychomotor pathways, and binding at the D_3 and D_4 receptors regulates emotion and cognition.

The first drugs used in treating psychosis associated with schizophrenia were the **phenothiazines**, characterized by the tricyclic ring system (red, in **Figure 13.13**). The prototype, chlorpromazine, was first synthesized in 1951 at Rhone-Poulenc in France. Its discovery can be traced to the benzodioxane antihistamines and the phenothiazine compound promethazine. Phenothiazine itself (not shown), first synthesized in 1883, was used as an anti-helminthic drug but had no antipsychotic activity. However its derivative, promethazine, had activity as both a sedative and antihistamine. Lengthening the alkyl chain, along with adding a chlorine atom to the aryl ring, led to chlorpromazine, which is both a D_2 and D_3 antagonist. Chlorpromazine was originally introduced early in 1952 to potentiate the effects of anesthesia, but due to its sedating effect, it was approved by the end of that year to control psychosis. As early as 1955, it was noted that its sedating effects were related to anti-serotonin effects, which are weak. However, in the 1960s, Arvid Carlsson demonstrated its anti-dopamine effects as the primary antipsychotic mechanism. He later won the Nobel Prize in Physiology or Medicine 2000 for this discovery. The importance of dopamine effects led to searches for dopamine antagonists as new anti-schizophrenic agents. Chlorpromazine is effective on the positive symptoms of schizophrenia but not the negative symptoms. Currently there are several phenothiazines, with variations in the nitrogen and aryl substituents, that are used clinically, including fluphenazine and perphenazine (see Figure 13.13).

Although phenothiazines were the first effective antipsychotics to be approved, they are limited by their side effects. These include extrapyramidal symptoms (EPS) such as tremors and muscle rigidity that are similar to symptoms of Parkinson's disease. Other side effects include sedation and weight gain. These side effects are so debilitating that they often limit patient compliance.

Haloperidol, approved in 1958 in Europe and 1967 in the United States, is an example of the **butyrophenone** class of antipsychotics (**Figure 13.14A**). It was first synthesized at Janssen Pharmaceuticals in the 1950s as a derivative of the opiate meperidine (pethidine), as part of a program to identify analgesics (**Figure 13.14B**). Replacement of the N-methyl group of meperidine with a propiophenone moiety led to R-951, which exhibited improved analgesic activity. However, patent issues with the propiophenones led to synthesis of the butyrophenone homologs. Surprisingly, the homolog R-1187 was only a short-acting analgesic, but it had activity as a tranquilizer and cataleptic agent (causing rigidity), with an activity profile like chlorpromazine. Over 400 analogs of R-1187 were synthesized, including haloperidol.

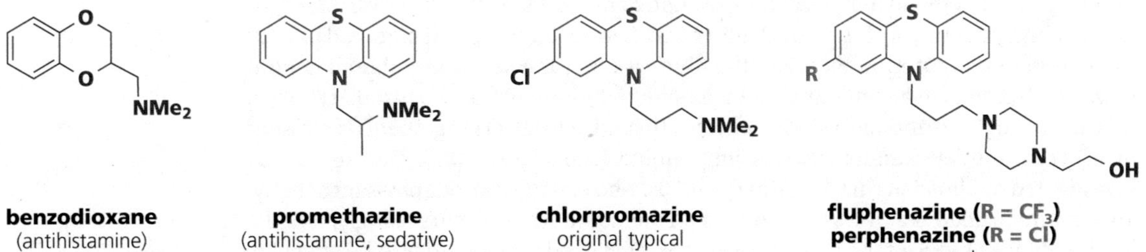

Figure 13.13 Structures of phenothiazines. Phenothiazines were synthesized as analogs of benzodioxane and promethazine, both antihistamines. The phenothiazine core is shown in red. Chlorpromazine is considered a typical antipsychotic; fluphenazine and perphenazine are more recent analogs. All three are used to treat positive symptoms of schizophrenia.

benzodioxane
(antihistamine)
structural basis for
chlorpromazine

promethazine
(antihistamine, sedative)
structural basis for
chlorpromazine

chlorpromazine
original typical
antipsychotic

fluphenazine (R = CF$_3$)
perphenazine (R = Cl)
more modern
typical antipsychotics

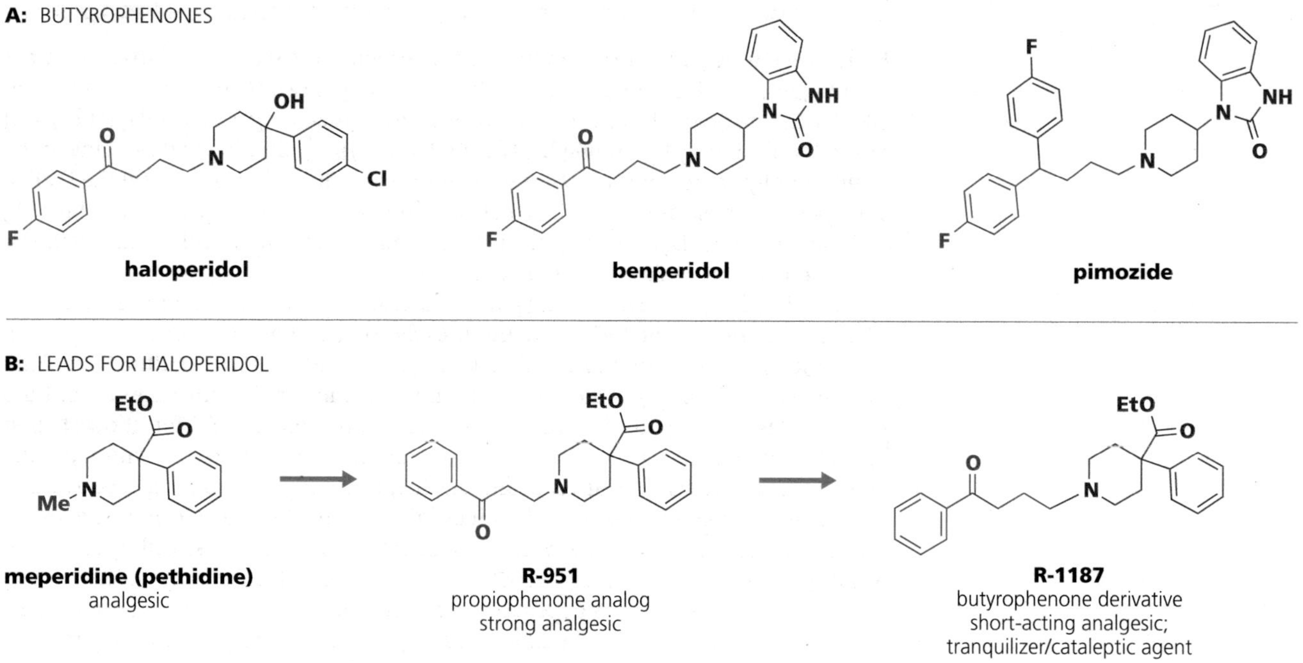

A: BUTYROPHENONES

haloperidol

benperidol

pimozide

B: LEADS FOR HALOPERIDOL

meperidine (pethidine)
analgesic

R-951
propiophenone analog
strong analgesic

R-1187
butyrophenone derivative
short-acting analgesic;
tranquilizer/cataleptic agent

Figure 13.14 Development of the antipsychotic butyrophenones. A: Butyrophenones. Members of the class of butyrophenones include haloperidol, benperidol, and pimozide (butyrophenone substructure/derivative in red). B: Leads for haloperidol. The propiophenone R-951 was synthesized as an analog of meperidine (substitution shown in red). The butyrophenone homolog R-1187 was prepared to circumvent patent issues and was a tranquilizer and cataleptic agent and had a chlorpromazine-like profile, rather than strong analgesic activity.

Although haloperidol is less sedating than chlorpromazine, patients still experience a high incidence of EPS. Despite this effect, several butyrophenones are used clinically, including haloperidol and benperidol. They act primarily as D_2 antagonists, with some activity at the 5-HT$_2$ receptor. Some other analogs, such as pimozide, have a fluorophenyl group in place of the carbonyl group. This compound, in addition to being used as an antipsychotic, is also used to treat severe symptoms of Tourette's syndrome. The typical antipsychotics have largely been replaced as first-line therapy by the atypical antipsychotics, most of which were developed in the 1990s.

13.4 The mechanism of atypical antipsychotics involves dopamine receptor antagonism combined with serotonin receptor antagonism

The **atypical antipsychotics** are characterized by a binding profile that includes stronger antagonism at D_4 than D_2 receptors, as well as 5-HT$_{2A}$ antagonism. They are more effective than earlier antipsychotics against the negative symptoms of schizophrenia, as well as positive symptoms, and have a lower incidence of EPS.

Clozapine, a member of the class termed **dibenzodiazepines** developed at Sandoz in the 1990s, was the first atypical antipsychotic approved, in 1990 (**Figure 13.15**). It had originally been synthesized by Wander AG Pharmaceuticals, and patented in 1960 as an antidepressant. One theory at the time was that the seven-membered central ring, which results in a bent rather than planar orientation of the two fused aryl rings, was necessary for antidepressant activity. This structural arrangement is present in tricyclic antidepressants such as imipramine (see Figure 13.7). Clozapine was investigated by clinicians in Europe in the 1960s, who expected antidepressant activity. They found instead that it was effective as an antipsychotic and, surprisingly, it had a low incidence of EPS. At the time, in 1966, it was believed that, in order to be effective,

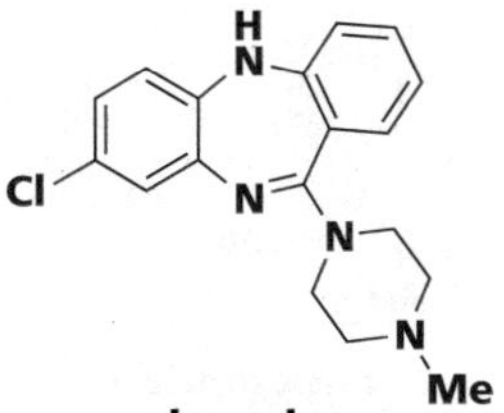

clozapine

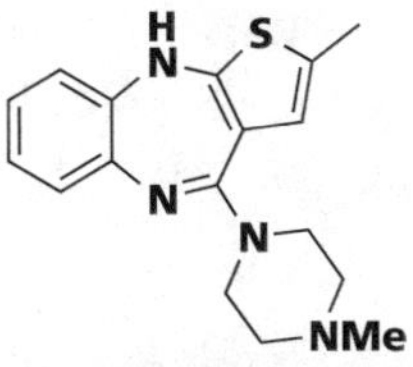

olanzapine

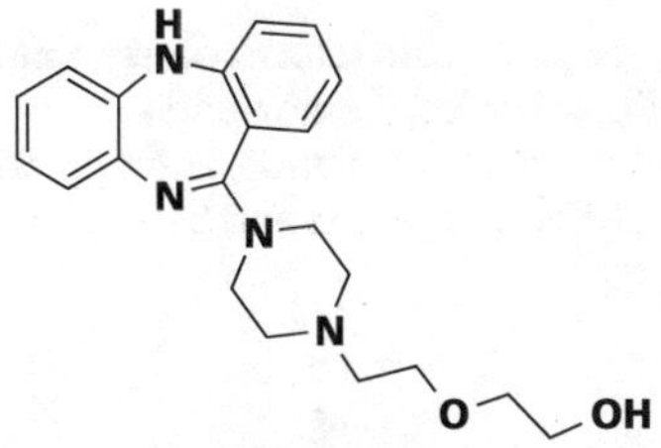

quetiapine

Figure 13.15 **Structures of dibenzodiazepine atypical antipsychotics.**
Clozapine, olanzapine, and quetiapine are examples of atypical antipsychotics which exhibit a lower incidence of EPS.

an antipsychotic needed to cause EPS, so interest in clozapine was low. In spite of this belief, clozapine entered clinical trials as an antipsychotic in the 1970s, and its efficacy was confirmed, but it was withdrawn due to serious side effects. Agranulocytosis was seen in about 1% of patients taking clozapine, and roughly half those patients died. It was reinvestigated and finally approved in 1990, but weekly monitoring of white blood cell count is required with its use. Later analogs such as olanzapine (1996) and quetiapine (1997) do not exhibit the same side-effect profile.

The binding profile of drugs related to clozapine, compared to the typical antipsychotics, is one explanation for the differences in their profiles. For example, clozapine binds more strongly to the D_4 receptor than to D_2, with $K_i = 74$ nM at the D_4 receptor and 254 nM at the D_2 receptor, whereas haloperidol has roughly equivalent binding at both (D_4, $K_i = 7.3$ nM; D_2, $K_i = 4.8$ nM). The atypical antipsychotics such as clozapine are also antagonists at the 5-HT_{2A} receptor.

Like the dibenzodiazepines, the **benzisoxazoles** are antagonists at both the D_2 and 5-HT_{2A} receptors (**Figure 13.16**). Risperidone was first synthesized at Janssen Pharmaceuticals in 1984 and was approved to treat both schizophrenia (in 1993) and bipolar disorder (in 2003). Its metabolite, paliperidone, is also used as an antipsychotic. Ziprasidone and lurasidone are in the same family; they contain a sulfur bioisostere in place of the oxygen of the benzisoxazole ring, as well as different bicyclic heterocycles.

Today, aripiprazole and brexpiprazole are among the drugs most frequently used to treat schizophrenia. These phenylpiperidines are also considered atypical antipsychotics on the basis of their side-effect profile, but they are D_2 and 5-HT_{1A} partial agonists as well as antagonists at the 5-HT_{2A} receptor.

As with the antidepressants that target neurotransmitter levels, antipsychotic drugs that have been developed to treat schizophrenia have also found other uses. For example, aripiprazole is used in combination with other drugs, to treat depression, and many antipsychotics are useful in treating bipolar disorder. Aripiprazole is also used to treat autism, where it reduces some symptoms such as stereotypy.

Benzamides, such as remoxipride, act as D_2/D_3 antagonists and have a relatively low incidence of EPS due to some selectivity for the D_2 receptor. However, remoxipride

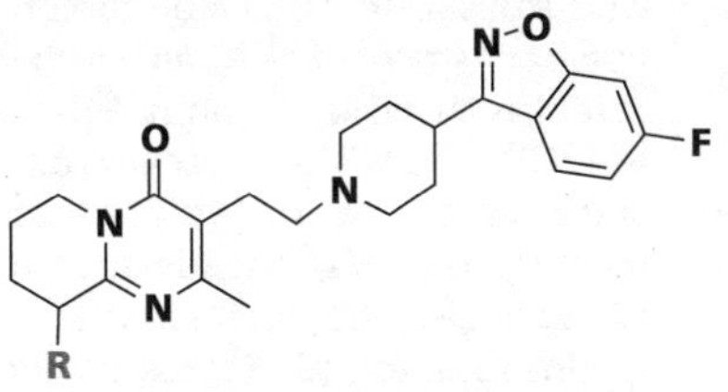

risperidone (R = H)
paliperidone (R = OH)

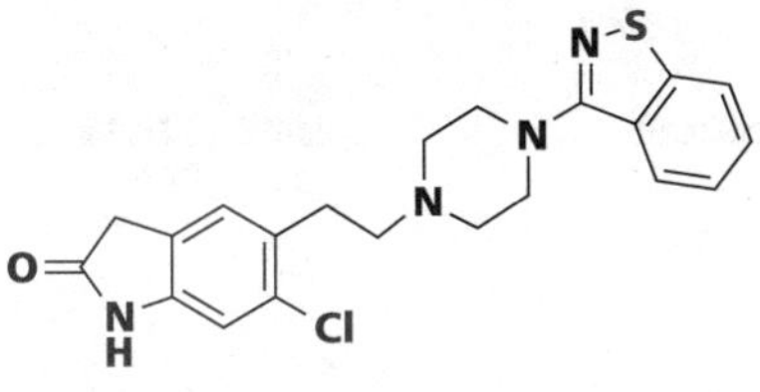

ziprasidone

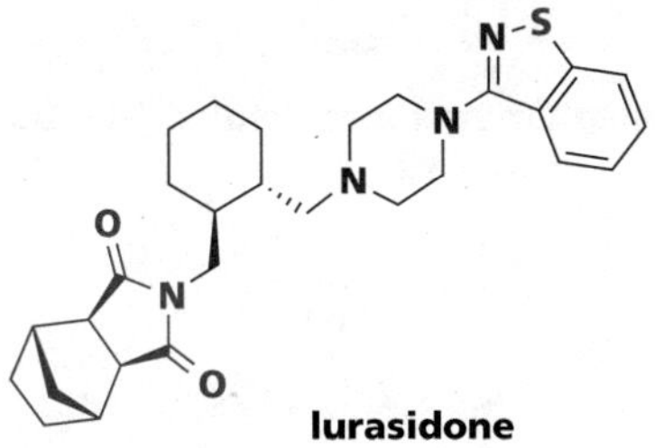

lurasidone

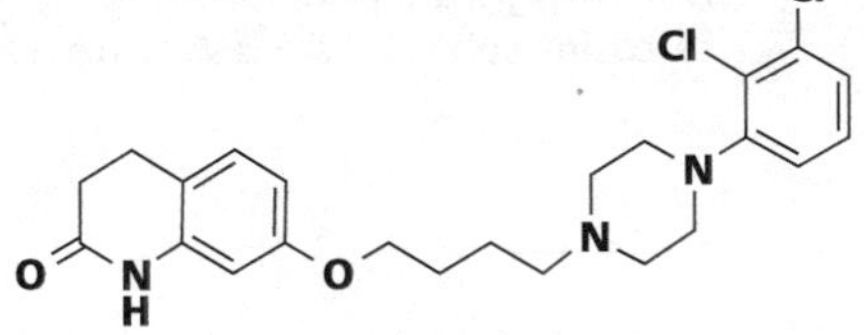

aripiprazole

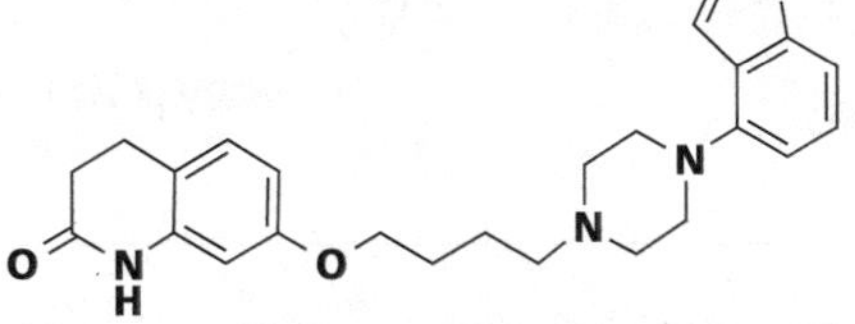

brexpiprazole

Figure 13.16 **Benzisoxazole and phenylpiperidine atypical antipsychotics.** The benzisoxazoles risperidone and its metabolite paliperidone, as well as analogs ziprasidone and lurasidone, are characterized by D_2 and 5-HT_{2A} receptor antagonism (red indicates bioisosteres and modified heterocycles of ziprasidone and lurasidone). The phenylpiperidines aripiprazole and brexpiprazole are D_2 and 5-HT_{1A} partial agonists as well as antagonists at the 5-HT_{2A} receptor.

was withdrawn several years after its introduction in 1990 due to occurrences of aplastic anemia (**Figure 13.17**). Other approved analogs include amisulpride and sulpiride.

13.5 Drugs targeting glutamate and phosphodiesterase 10A have potential as antipsychotics

As mentioned previously, the molecular basis of schizophrenia is not completely understood, and there are multiple hypotheses that attempt to link dysregulation of levels of specific NTs to disease state. Current drugs affect serotonin and dopamine receptors; however, other hypotheses are also being pursued. The glutamate hypothesis is based on the idea that hypofunction in NMDA receptor-mediated neurotransmission is involved in schizophrenia. The NMDA receptor is a ligand-gated ion channel (see Section 6.6), with binding sites for both glutamate and glycine, both of which are required for opening of the channel. Glutamate also binds to the AMPA receptor, another ionotropic receptor. Several approaches have been investigated to increase glutamate levels with the goal of treating schizophrenia, as well as other afflictions such as obsessive–compulsive disorder (OCD). One approach has been to develop modulators of the metabotropic glutamate receptors (mGluR). These GPCRs are either postsynaptic (mGlu$_1$ and mGlu$_5$) and increase NMDA receptor activity or presynaptic (mGlu$_2$ and mGlu$_3$) and decrease NMDA receptor activity (mGlu$_{4,6,7,8}$ receptors have not been as widely targeted). **Figure 13.18A** shows several examples

remoxipride

amisulpride (R = NH$_2$)
sulpiride (R = H)

Figure 13.17 Structures of benzamide antipsychotics. Remoxipride (withdrawn), amisulpride, and sulpiride are D$_2$/D$_3$ antagonists and approved drugs.

A: EXPERIMENTAL COMPOUNDS AFFECTING METABOTROPIC GLUTAMATE (mGlu) RECEPTORS

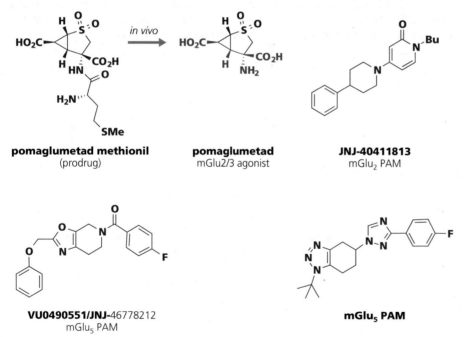

pomaglumetad methionil
(prodrug)

pomaglumetad
mGlu2/3 agonist

JNJ-40411813
mGlu$_2$ PAM

VU0490551/JNJ-46778212
mGlu$_5$ PAM

mGlu$_5$ PAM

Figure 13.18 Examples of experimental compounds based on the glutamate hypothesis of schizophrenia. A: Experimental compounds affecting the metabotropic glutamate (mGlu) receptors. Several compounds that act at mGlu receptors have advanced to clinical trials. Pomaglumetad, adminstered as a prodrug, whose design was based on conformational constraint of glutamate (shown in red), is an mGlu$_{2/3}$ agonist. JNJ-40411813, VU0400551/JNJ-46778212 and a benztriazole are positive allosteric modulators (PAMs) that advanced to clinical trials. B: Compounds affecting glycine receptors (GlyT1). Experimental drugs that affect glycine levels by inhibiting the GlyT1 transporter include bitopertin and compounds such as AMG747 and Org25935, containing an N-methylglycine (sarcosine) moiety (the sarcosine substructure is shown in red).

B: EXPERIMENTAL COMPOUNDS AFFECTING GLYCINE TRANSPORTERS (GlyT1)

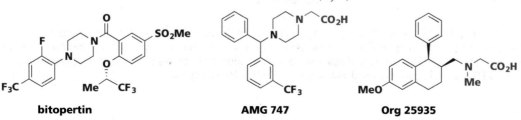

bitopertin

AMG 747

Org 25935

of modulators of mGlu receptors that have advanced to clinical trials, including the mGlu$_{2/3}$ agonist pomaglumetad, based on the idea of developing a conformationally constrained analog of glutamate (see Section 4.13). An amide prodrug, pomaglumetad methionil, developed at Eli Lilly, advanced to phase II trials but was ineffective against the negative symptoms of schizophrenia. Another example is the mGlu$_2$ positive allosteric modulator JNJ-40411813, which was based on a hit discovered through an HTS program and advanced to phase II clinical trials. Several mGlu$_5$ modulators have also advanced to phase I clinical trials, including the PAM VU0490551/JNJ-46778212 and a benztriazole mGlu$_5$ PAM developed at Eisai (see Figure 13.18A). It is proposed that compounds targeting mGluRs would avoid the EPS seen with the marketed drugs that affect dopamine levels.

Another approach based on the glutamate hypothesis has led to the development of inhibitors of the glycine transporter GlyT1. This sodium transporter regulates glycine levels, which binds to and activates the NMDA receptor. One known competitive inhibitor of GlyT1 is *N*-methylglycine (sarcosine). Design based on this compound and high-throughput screening hits have led to several compounds that advanced to clinical trials. One example is bitopertin, which progressed to phase III trials for both schizophrenia and OCD (see Figure 13.18B). While it was not sufficiently effective against the negative symptoms of schizophrenia for further advancement, as of 2017 it remained in trials for OCD. Other examples include the sarcosine analogs AMG 747 and Org25935, which also progressed to phase II trials but were discontinued due to safety concerns.

One novel strategy for treating schizophrenia that is distinct from directly affecting NT receptors is based on inhibiting phosphodiesterases. There are multiple forms of these enzymes, all of which hydrolyze phosphodiester bonds (see Chapter 7). Phosphodiesterase 10A (PDE10A) is primarily found in the striatal region of the brain, and abnormalities in this region are seen in patients with schizophrenia. PDE10A regulates cAMP/PKC signaling and affects both glutamate and dopamine pathways. Since its discovery in 1999, many groups have been investigating selective inhibitors of PDE10A as a potential treatment for schizophrenia, as well as other disorders such as Huntington's disease. Several have advanced to clinical trials, including OMS824, AMG 579, and PF-2545920 (Figure 13.19).

The quinoline PF-2545920 was developed at Pfizer and was the first PDE10A inhibitor to enter clinical trials (see Figure 13.19). It was based on a hit from library screening that binds in a selectivity pocket of PDE10A. All phosphodiesterases have a conserved glutamine at the active site, which in most cases forms a hydrogen bond

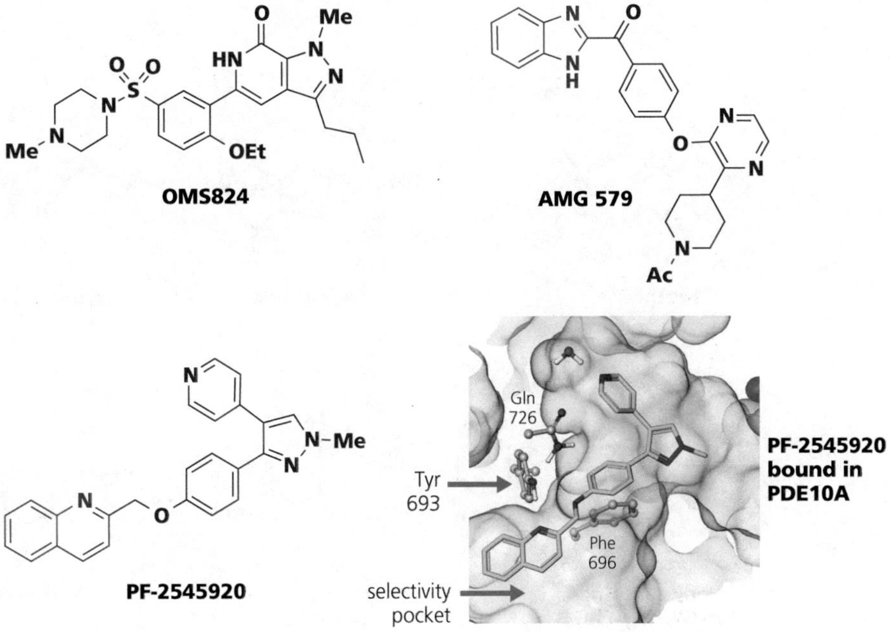

Figure 13.19 Targeting phosphodiesterase 10A to treat schizophrenia.
Structures of PDE10A inhibitors OMS824, AMG 579 and PF-2545920 that have advanced to clinical trials are shown, along with an X-ray structure of PF-2545920 (depicted in green) bound to PDE10, showing an H-bond between the quinoline nitrogen and Tyr693 in the selectivity pocket. Selectivity over other PDEs can be conferred by a substituent that binds in the selectivity pocket of the enzyme (red heterocycles in PF 2545920 (quinoline) and AMG 579 (benzimidazole) indicates moiety occupying selectivity pocket and making H-bond to Tyr683). (From Verhoest PR, Chapin DS, Corman M et al. [2009] *J Med Chem* 52:5188–5196. With permission from American Chemical Society.)

with known inhibitors. In PDE10A, the adjacent residue is a glycine, and its small size opens a selectivity pocket found only in PDE10A. Inhibitors with moieties that occupy this selectivity pocket form a hydrogen bond to Tyr693. Rather than an H-bond to Gln726, these selective inhibitors bind to Gln726 by a cation-π interaction. In the case of PF-2545920, the quinoline binds in the selectivity pocket, and its nitrogen acts as an H-bond acceptor. Other interactions include π-stacking between Phe residues with the aryl rings (see Figure 13.19), and an H-bond between the pyridyl nitrogen and a water molecule that bridges to the PDE10A backbone. Both OMS824 and AMG 579 were also based on hits found through library screening for selective compounds; in AMG 579, the benzimidazole occupies the selectivity pocket and makes an H-bond to Tyr683.

In summary, numerous advances in the treatment of schizophrenia have been made since the first drugs were introduced in the 1950s. The earliest drugs, the typical antipsychotics, are still in use but have mostly given way to the atypical antipsychotics, which have fewer side effects. These approved drugs all modulate levels of dopamine as well as serotonin. Newer approaches are focused in two areas and include experimental drugs to affect glutamate receptors as well as PDE10A inhibitors, which would indirectly affect levels of both glutamate and dopamine.

DRUGS TARGETING PAIN

Various forms of pain affect 20% of the world population and lead to health care and lost worktime costs of approximately $600 billion per year in the United States alone. Pain can be categorized as either **nociceptive**, resulting from injury to muscle or bone tissue, or **neuropathic**, resulting from injury to nerves. Nociceptive pain is typically acute and of shorter duration, whereas neuropathic pain is long-lasting and more resistant to treatment. Conditions that may cause neuropathic pain include osteoarthritis, fibromyalgia, diabetes, stroke, and certain chemotherapy drugs.

13.6 Drugs used to treat pain include opiates and nonsteroidal anti-inflammatory drugs as well as antidepressants

The oldest treatments for pain are the opiates, such as morphine (see Section 1.3), which have been used for thousands of years. While effective against nociceptive pain, opiates are not as effective against neuropathic pain and exhibit dangerous side effects, including respiratory depression and addiction potential. Morphine and its semisynthetic analogs (differing mainly in oxidation states), such as oxycodone and hydrocodone, are agonists at the opiate receptors, which are GPCRs (**Figure 13.20**).

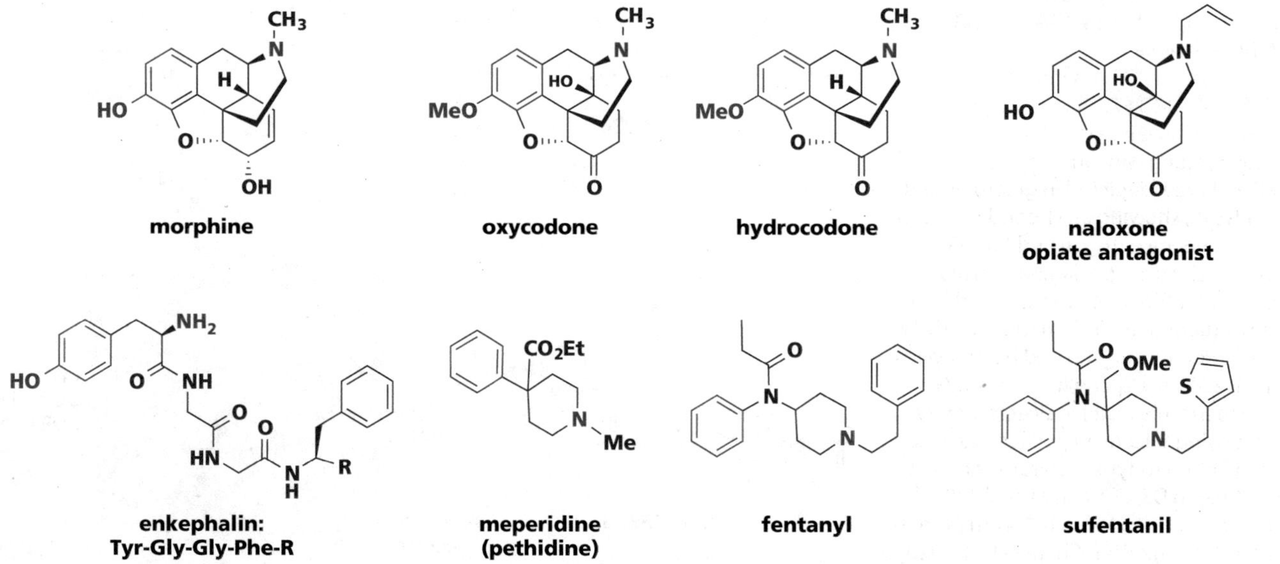

Figure 13.20 Structures of compounds that bind to opioid receptors.
Morphine and the semisynthetic analogs oxycodone and hydrocodone are agonists at opiate receptors; the related analog, naloxone, is an antagonist used to treat opiate overdose. The Tyr-Gly-Gly-Phe fragment of the natural ligand enkephalin (R = Met or Leu) displays key pharmacophoric elements for activating the opioid receptor. Synthetic agents used to treat pain include meperidine, fentanyl, and sufentanil. The shared pharmacophore elements for agonists are shown in red.

morphine

oxycodone

hydrocodone

naloxone
opiate antagonist

enkephalin:
Tyr-Gly-Gly-Phe-R

meperidine
(pethidine)

fentanyl

sufentanil

Increasing steric bulk on the amine substituent leads to antagonists, such as naloxone, which is used to treat opiate overdose.

There are three different subtypes of the opioid receptor, μ, δ, and κ, with agonism at the μ receptor primarily responsible for reducing pain. It is believed that activity at the δ receptor mediates the addictive characteristics of opioids, and numerous efforts have been made to develop subtype-selective drugs. In the 1980s, the natural ligands for the opiate receptors were identified as the enkephalin peptides (see Figure 13.20). The structural feature essential for activating the receptor is the N-terminal Tyr-Gly-Gly-Phe sequence. Some of these can be mapped onto the opiates: Tyr1 corresponds to the aryl and amine moieties found in the opioids, as seen in red in Figure 13.20. Other analgesics that bind at the opiate receptors include the synthetic drug meperidine (or pethidine), synthesized in the late 1930s as an anti-cholinergic agent and later found to have analgesic activity. Fentanyl, synthesized by Paul Janssen in 1960 as an analog of meperidine, is 100× more potent than morphine, as is its analog sufentanil. These analogs all maintain the aryl and nitrogen elements of the opioid pharmacophore.

Acetaminophen and the nonsteroidal anti-inflammatory drugs (NSAIDs), as well as muscle relaxants are also used to treat nociceptive pain. The NSAIDs are inhibitors of cyclooxygenase and are discussed in Section 7.9. These include aspirin as well as the selective COX-2 inhibitors such as celecoxib, which primarily act on COX-2 to reduce inflammation; these compounds work in the periphery rather than the brain.

One pain medication with a unique mechanism of action is ziconotide, which selectively targets the N-type calcium channel Ca_v2.2 and must be administered intrathecally (injected into spinal fluid). This 25-amino-acid peptide (ω-conotoxin) is produced by cone snails as one of a cocktail of peptides that are used to immobilize fish so that the snail can eat them. Investigation of these peptides by Baldomero Olivera at the University of Utah led to the discovery of the utility of ω-conotoxin, which is 1000× more potent than morphine as an analgesic. The neuronal N-type calcium channel is a voltage-gated ion channel found on presynaptic terminals, and ziconotide blocks the entry of this channel. One model, shown in **Figure 13.21**, shows a molecule of ω-conotoxin (green) bound in the ion channel through an ionic interaction between an aspartate (D178) on the channel and a lysine (K2, blue) on the peptide toxin located just above the selectivity filter. An additional interaction between the N-terminal cysteine (C1, blue) and subunit IV glutamate (E177, red) is also evident. The large molecular weight and peptidic nature of this agent require it to be delivered intrathecally.

Neuropathic pain has been more difficult to treat than nociceptive pain. Drugs that have some utility include tricyclic antidepressants such as amitriptyline (see Figure 13.7); monoamine reuptake inhibitors such as duloxetine and venlafaxine (see Figure 13.10); and anticonvulsants such as carbamazepine, lamotrigine, and phenytoin (**Figure 13.22**).

These anticonvulsants inhibit pain by varying mechanisms. Both carbamazepine and lamotrigine act primarily by blockage of voltage-gated sodium channels, while phenytoin is a barbiturate, acting as a PAM at the GABA_A chloride ion channel.

13.7 Novel approaches to pain treatment include selective ion channel blockers

While pain accounts for 20% of all doctor visits and 10% of all drug sales, there have been few new pain medications in the last 20 years. This is despite the limitations

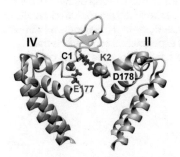

Figure 13.21 Model of ω-conotoxin (green and blue) blocking entry to the Ca_v2.2 ion channel (gray). The salt bridge between peptide lysine (blue, K2) and subunit II aspartate (teal, D178) is shown. An additional interaction between the N-terminal cysteine (C1) and subunit IV glutamate (E177, red) is also shown. (From Chen R & Chung S-H [2013] *Biochemistry* 52:3765–3772. With permission from American Chemical Society.)

Figure 13.22 Structures of anticonvulsants that are also used to treat neuropathic pain. Carbamazepine and lamotrigine act primarily by blockage of voltage-gated sodium channels. Phenytoin is a barbiturate, acting as a PAM at the GABA_A chloride ion channel. Both pregabalin and gabapentin block the formation of functional voltage-gated calcium channels.

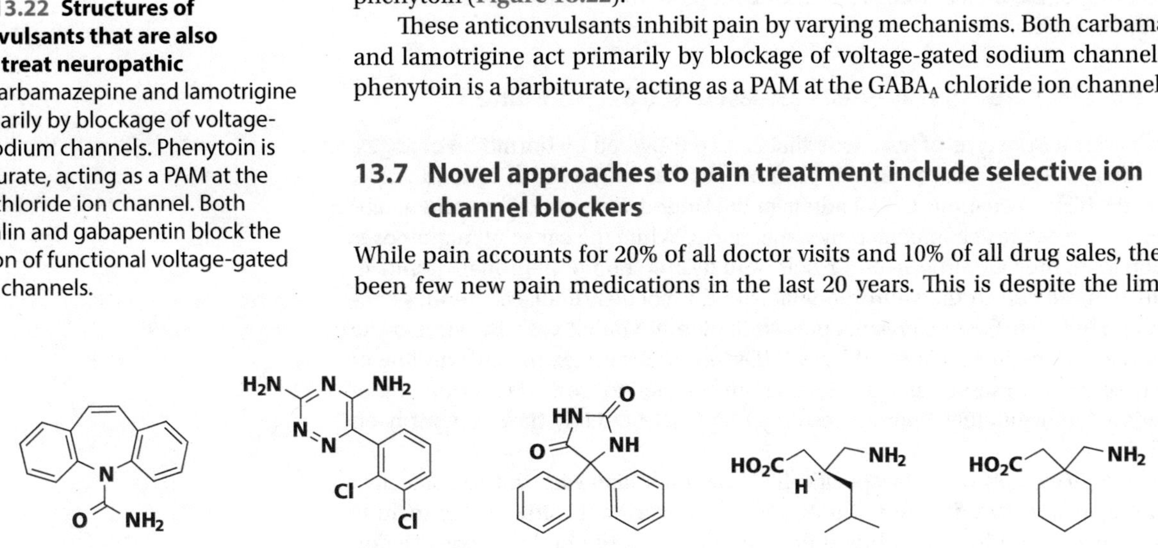

carbamazepine   **lamotrigine**   **phenytoin**   **pregabalin**   **gabapentin**

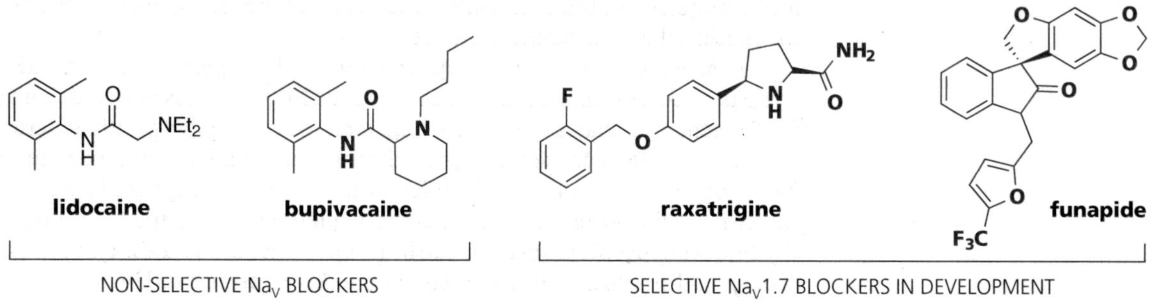

NON-SELECTIVE Na$_V$ BLOCKERS   SELECTIVE Na$_V$1.7 BLOCKERS IN DEVELOPMENT

Figure 13.23 Structures of nonselective and selective Na$_V$ inhibitors used to treat pain. Lidocaine and bupivacaine bind indiscriminately to sodium channels. Raxatrigine and funapide are examples of experimental compounds that selectively block the Na$_V$1.7 channel.

of current drugs, including the abuse potential of the opioids and the relative lack of efficacy of drugs to treat neuropathic pain. Some newer areas of research have advanced compounds to clinical trials, but few novel compounds have received approval since 2004.

Pregabalin and gabapentin, both approved as anticonvulsants (see Figure 13.22), were originally developed as analogs of GABA but actually target the $\alpha_2\delta$ subunit of voltage-gated calcium channels, which are up-regulated in models of neuropathic pain. They bind to the Ca$_V$ channel, which reduces Ca^{2+} influx into presynaptic terminals and thus indirectly blocks release of the excitatory NT glutamate as well as other NTs.

The voltage-gated sodium channels (Na$_V$) are the targets of the caine anesthetics such as lidocaine and bupivacaine (**Figure 13.23**, see also Section 6.9). These are nonselective ligands that bind at a conserved local anesthetic binding site. There are nine subtypes of the Na$_V$ channels, with Na$_V$1.7 located primarily in the peripheral nervous system. Interest in subtype Na$_V$1.7 as a target for pain is based on the observation that individuals with no functional Na$_V$1.7 channel are insensitive to pain, while those with gain-of-function mutations in these channels suffer from severe chronic pain syndromes. There are several compounds in clinical trials for neuropathic pain that are selective Na$_V$1.7 blockers, including raxatrigine and funapide (see Figure 13.23). Drug discovery for this target has relied on screening and design based on known modulators.

Treatments for pain have been available for thousands of years, with two major classes of drugs, opiates and NSAIDS, originally derived from natural sources. However, there are limitations to these drugs based on side effects and abuse potential; therefore, there is a continued effort to identify novel drugs, especially those to treat neuropathic pain and those acting through new mechanisms. Most of the older drugs have been discovered on the basis of effects found through *in vivo* assays. New approaches are based on genetic data that have identified new targets. With an understanding of the mechanisms responsible for pain, more selective and effective drugs may be developed.

13.8 Selective serotonin agonists are used to treat migraine

Migraines are a severe type of headache that can be triggered by hormonal changes, certain foods, stress, or environmental prompts such as bright lights or loud noise. These headaches affect about 13% of adults in the United States, mostly women, and about 25% of cases are accompanied by visual auras. While the cause of migraines is not understood, they are proposed to result from dysfunction of neuronal circuits in the brainstem, related to the neuromodulator and vasoconstrictor calcitonin gene-related peptide (CGRP), which results in vasodilation in cranial vessels. While these headaches are sometimes alleviated by NSAIDs and other drugs, the current line of therapy uses selective serotonin agonists that are believed to work via modulation of vasodilation. Unfortunately, approaches targeting CGRP directly have not yet been successful.

The first drug approved to specifically treat migraine was the nonselective serotonin agonist ergotamine (a natural product); however, its side effects include vomiting, nausea, and increased blood pressure due to peripheral vasoconstriction (**Figure 13.24A**).

A: SEROTONIN AGONISTS USED TO TREAT MIGRAINES

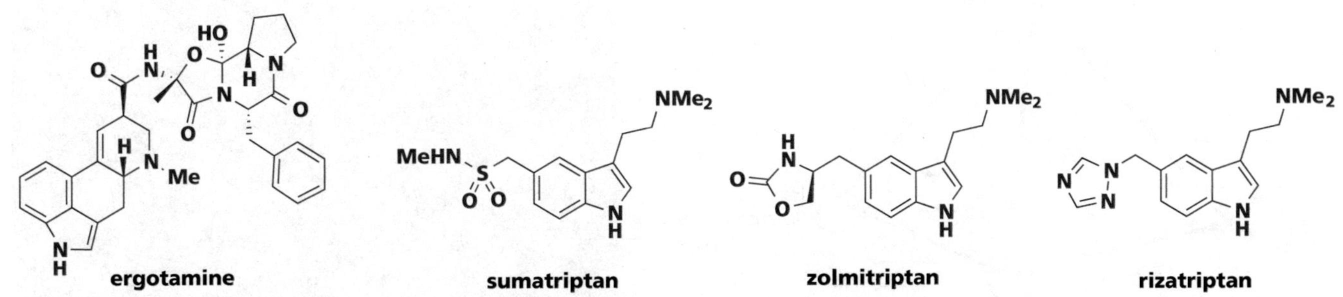

ergotamine

sumatriptan

zolmitriptan

rizatriptan

B: NEUROSTABILIZERS THAT ACT THROUGH SEVERAL MECHANISMS

topiramate

sodium valproate

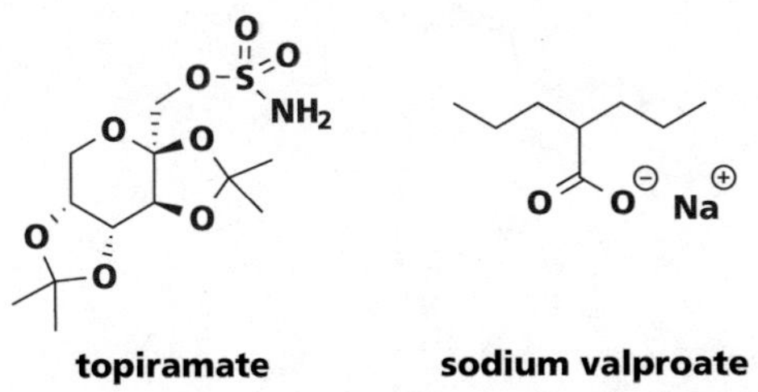

Figure 13.24 Structures of drugs used to treat migraines.
A: Serotonin agonists used to treat migraines. Ergotamine is a natural product that is nonselective. Sumatriptan is a selective $5\text{-HT}_{1B}/5\text{-HT}_{1D}$ agonist, as are zolmitriptan and rizatriptan. B: Neurostabilizers that act through several mechanisms. Topiramate and valproate are considered neurostabilizers, lowering the excitability of neuronal pathways through multiple mechanisms.

Sumatriptan is a selective $5\text{-HT}_{1B}/5\text{-HT}_{1D}$ agonist and acts by constricting blood vessels in the brain. While it had been known that migraines were associated with decreased levels of serotonin, the 5-HT_{1B} receptor subtype was not identified until the 1970s. This subtype is a GPCR located in the cranial vessels, and selective constriction of those vessels increases the rate of blood flow in the brain, providing migraine relief. Later analogs such as zolmitriptan and rizatriptan are more lipophilic and may have better BBB penetration.

Zolmitriptan was developed from a 5-HT_{1D} agonist pharmacophore model that was derived by the active analog approach (**Figure 13.25**). This model was based on data from a series of serotonin analogs that were evaluated for agonism at both 5-HT_{1D} (desired) and 5-HT_{2A} (undesired) receptors in order to generate a model that would predict binding to both subtypes. This pharmacophore exercise identified optimal regions for a protonated amine, an H-bond acceptor, an H-bond donor or acceptor and an aryl group. In addition, a hydrophobic region was identified between the H-bonding regions. Overlaying both selective and nonselective compounds identified a selectivity pocket in the hydrophobic region that was occupied by compounds with selectivity for 5-HT_{1D} subtype over the 5-HT_{2A} subtype. How zolmitriptan adheres to this pharmacophore is illustrated in Figure 13.25.

Several drugs that were originally marketed as anticonvulsants have been approved to prevent migraines. These include topiramate and valproate (see **Figure 13.24B**). Topiramate was originally synthesized in 1979 by Bruce Maryanoff at Johnson & Johnson as a chemical intermediate and became part of their chemical library. Testing in a mouse model showed potent anticonvulsant activity, and the compound entered preclinical testing in 1983. After it was approved as an anticonvulsant in 1996, subsequent clinical testing for other symptoms led to its additional approval to treat migraines. Topiramate has been found to operate through multiple mechanisms, including blockage of the Na_v channel and acting as a PAM of the GABA_A receptor at a site that is neither the benzodiazepine nor the barbiturate binding site, as well as several other mechanisms. Overall, it is considered a neurostabilizer, lowering excitability of several neuronal pathways. Another drug considered a neurostabilizer is valproate. Originally synthesized in 1881, it was marketed as an anticonvulsant in 1962 and is also effective in migraine prevention. Valproate has multiple mechanisms, effecting increased GABA synthesis as well as inhibiting glutamate function.

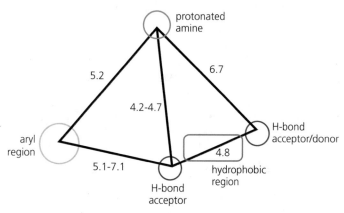

5–HT$_{1D}$ pharmacophore model
(numbers are distances in angstroms)

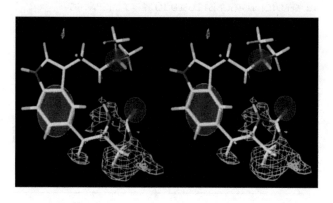

stereodiagram of zolmitriptan superimposed on model

zolmitriptan

Figure 13.25 Pharmacophore model for antagonists of the 5-HT$_{1D}$ receptor. The pharmacophore model on the left was generated from a series of serotonin analogs based on affinity at 5-HT$_{1D}$ (desired) and 5-HT$_{2A}$ (undesired) receptors. Specific elements with distance constraints are shown, and include a protonated amine (blue), an aromatic region (green), H-bond do-nor/ acceptor (red) and hydrophobic region (gray). Modeling of both selective and nonselective compounds onto the pharmaco-phore model identified the volume of a hydrophobic selectivity pocket that must be occupied for selectivity at 5-HT$_{1D}$ (orange, figure on right). This model was used to develop zolmitriptan, shown in a stereodiagram on the right, superimposed on part of the model. The amine (blue) fits the protonated amine region, the indole (green) fits the aryl region, and the carbonyl (red) fits the H-bond acceptor/donor region. The ring CH$_2$ fits into the selectivity pocket (yellow grid) in the hydrophobic region (gray in pharmacophore model). (From Glen R, Martin GR, Hill AP et al. [1995] *J Med Chem* 38:3566–3580. With permission from American Chemical Society.)

DRUGS TARGETING NEURODEGENERATION

Neurodegenerative diseases are considered those resulting from the degeneration and death or loss of neurons. Many neurodegenerative diseases, such as Parkinson's and Alzheimer's diseases, are associated with aging. For example, 11% of Americans over 65 have been diagnosed with Alzheimer's disease, but that number rises to 45% for people over the age of 85. Other neurodegenerative diseases, like Huntington's disease, are due to congenital conditions or to autoimmune attack on the CNS, such as occurs in patients with multiple sclerosis (MS). These varied conditions, unfortunately, have few effective treatments.

13.9   Approved drugs to treat Alzheimer's disease affect acetylcholine or glutamate levels

Alzheimer's disease (AD) was first described by Alois Alzheimer in 1907 and is characterized by loss of memory and cognitive function, behavioral changes, and dementia. Loss of cholinergic neurons as well as the presence of amyloid plaques (aggregated β-amyloid protein) and neurofibrillary tangles (composed of phosphorylated τ protein in the brain) constitute a modern definition of the disease. A diagnosis of AD is based on a constellation of symptoms; however, the ultimate diagnosis cannot be made until autopsy. Further complicating disease treatment is the fact that there are many forms of dementia, but not all forms result from AD.

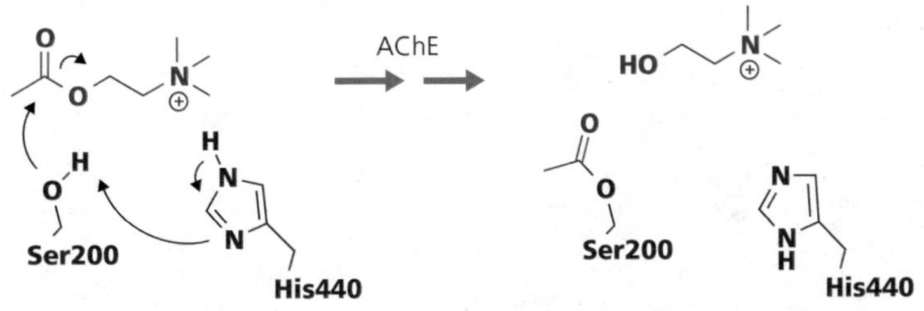

Figure 13.26 Abbreviated mechanism for hydrolysis of acetylcholine, catalyzed by acetylcholinesterase (AChE). Acid–base catalysis in the active site results in deprotonation of Ser200, which then reacts with the acetate carbonyl; cleavage of the ester bond generates choline and acetylated enzyme. For a more complete mechanism, see Figure 7.2.

acetylcholine in enzyme   choline and acetylated enzyme

While there is neither a cure nor a preventative for Alzheimer's disease, nor even drugs to change the course of the disease, there are some drugs that improve cognition and perhaps slow the progression in AD patients. Acetylcholinesterase inhibitors are one such class of approved drugs. The **cholinergic hypothesis** proposes that low levels of the neurotransmitter acetylcholine in AD patients contribute to cognitive decline. Levels of acetylcholine are regulated by its hydrolysis to choline, a reaction catalyzed by the enzyme acetylcholinesterase (AChE) (**Figure 13.26**). In this reaction, the catalytic Ser200, located at the bottom of a hydrophobic pocket termed the aromatic gorge, reacts with the ester of acetylcholine to generate choline and the acylated enzyme. By inhibition of AChE, the concentration of acetylcholine is maintained, and cognitive function should improve.

The first drug approved to treat Alzheimer's disease was the AChE inhibitor tacrine (**Figure 13.27**). Adrian Albert originally discovered this aminoacridine in the 1940s during a search for antibacterial drugs. While tacrine was only weakly antibacterial, it was observed that it reversed anesthetic sleep and exhibited activity as an AChE inhibitor. It was used as an antidote for anti-cholinergic drug overdose from the 1950s through the 1970s but was not considered as a potential Alzheimer's disease treatment until 1981. A report by William K. Summers on its intravenous use in Alzheimer's

Figure 13.27 Structures of drugs used to treat Alzheimer's disease. The AChE inhibitors include the synthetic drugs tacrine and donepezil (noncompetitive), as well as the natural product galantamine and natural-product-derived rivastigmine, both competitive inhibitors. Memantine acts by a different mechanism, as an NMDA antagonist.

ACETYLCHOLINESTERASE INHIBITORS

tacrine   donepezil   galantamine

physostigmine   rivastigmine
(toxic alkaloid)

NMDA ANTAGONIST

memantine

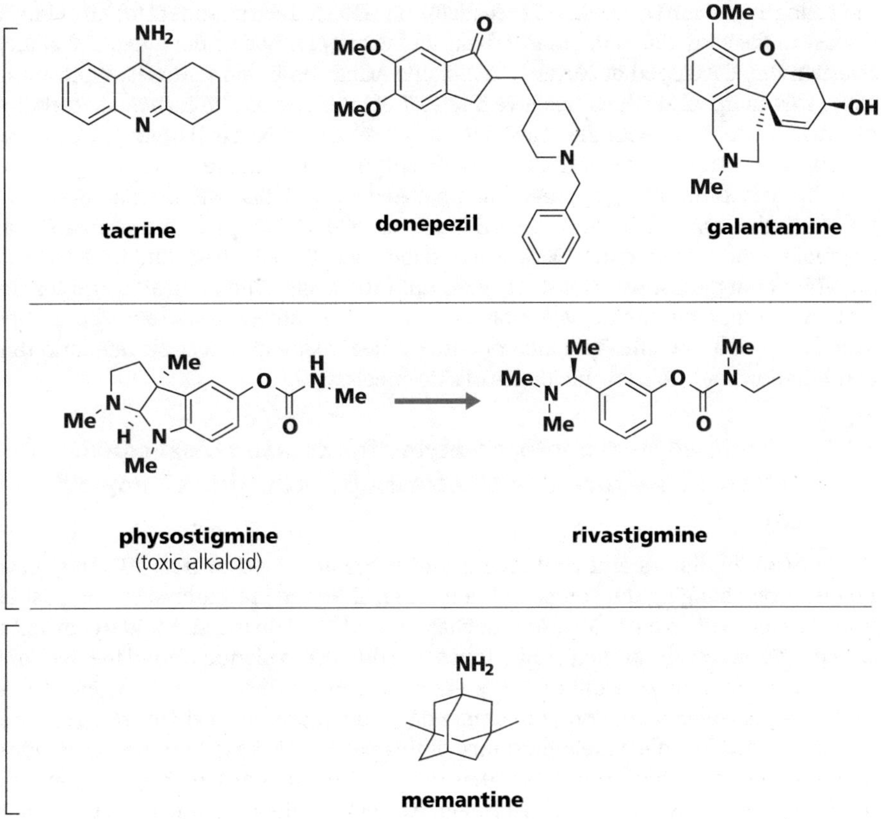

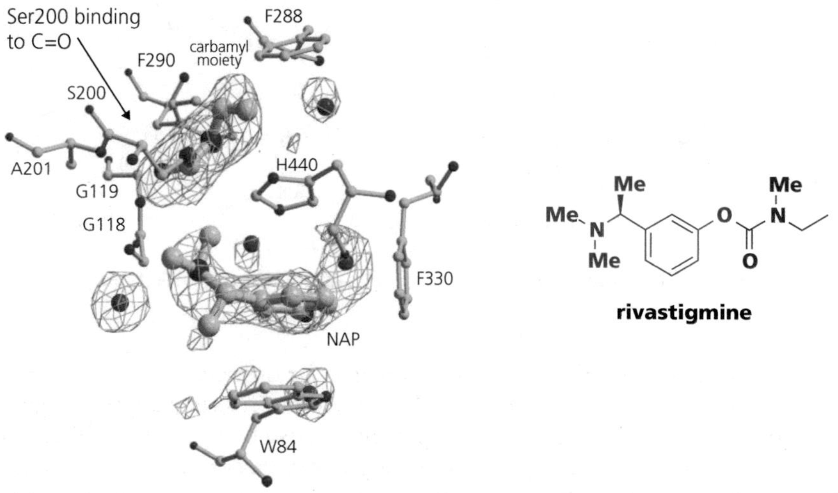

Figure 13.28 X-ray co-structure of AChE inhibitor rivastigmine bound to the enzyme AChE. Rivastigmine fragments are shown in yellow and enzyme in green. The carbamate carbonyl of rivastigmine reacts with the active-site Ser200, forming a covalent bond to the carbamyl moiety and releasing the dimethylamino-ethylphenol (NAP). The NAP residue shows π-stacking with W84 and F330 (NAP portion colored red in rivastigmine structure on the right). (From Bar-On P, Millard CB, Harel M et al. [2002] *Biochemistry* 41:3555–3564. With permission from American Chemical Society.)

patients described brief reversal of mild cognitive impairment. This observation ultimately led to its approval as an oral medication in 1993.

Tacrine is a noncompetitive reversible inhibitor of AChE. Due to limited oral availability and liver toxicity, it is no longer used; it has been replaced by donepezil, another noncompetitive reversible inhibitor. Donepezil was discovered by researchers at Eisai in the early 1980s while searching for an alternative to tacrine that had reduced toxicity. High-throughput screening identified an *N*-benzylpiperazine that exhibited *in vivo* activity and had AChE inhibitory activity in the rat brain. After synthesis of ~700 derivatives, donepezil emerged as the clinical candidate and received approval in 1997 (see Case Study 2 in this chapter).

The two other approved AChE inhibitors, galantamine and rivastigmine, are based on natural products and are competitive inhibitors of AChE. The lead for rivastigmine was physostigmine, an alkaloid found in the Calabar bean from western Africa. Ingestion of this poisonous plant was used by indigenous tribes as a test for witchcraft, with death indicating the person was a witch. Physostigmine was tested as a treatment for Alzheimer's disease in the early 1980s, but its instability and toxicity limited its potential. The analog rivastigmine, developed at Novartis, maintains AChE inhibition and was approved in 1997. This compound is a competitive inhibitor of the enzyme. The carbamate carbonyl of rivastigmine reacts with the active-site Ser200 releasing dimethylamino-ethylphenol (NAP). **Figure 13.28** shows NAP and acylated enzyme bound in the active site.

The only other drug approved to treat Alzheimer's disease, memantine, does not work through inhibition of AChE but is an NMDA receptor antagonist. It was originally synthesized in the 1960s as a possible anti-diabetic drug, and its activity as an NMDA antagonist was not discovered until the 1980s. The natural ligand for the NMDA receptor, glutamate, is excitatory, and excess activity leads to neurotoxicity. Memantine is a low-affinity noncompetitive antagonist with a fast off-rate, and that combination leads to a low incidence of side effects.

13.10 Recent approaches to modifying the course of Alzheimer's disease have focused on decreasing production of amyloid plaques

While AChE inhibitors and NMDA antagonists are approved to treat AD, they have no effect on changing the course of the disease. Therefore, research over the past 20 years has focused on alternative approaches. One is based on the **amyloid hypothesis**, which suggests that inhibiting production of the β-amyloid plaques found in the brains of Alzheimer's patients would modify the course of the disease. It is believed that these plaques precede the onset of dementia, and either they or their precursors are neurotoxic. Evidence for the importance of this pathway is based on the observation that some forms of early-onset AD occur in people with mutations in the genes that code for the protein (amyloid precursor protein, APP) that ultimately generates β-amyloid

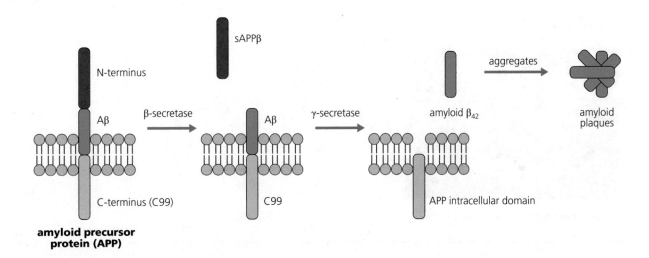

Figure 13.29 Sequential enzymatic cleavage of APP to provide amyloid β. The membrane-spanning amyloid precursor protein (APP) is cleaved on the extracellular N-terminal side by the enzyme β-secretase to release a soluble APPβ fragment (sAPPβ) (shown in red). Cleavage of the remaining C-terminal fragment (C99) by γ-secretase generates free amyloid β (blue), of 39-49 amino acid lengths, and the APP intracellular domain (green). The 42-amino acid amyloid β_{42} goes on to aggregate and form amyloid plaques.

plaques. The plaques are formed by aggregation of amyloid β_{42} protein (**Figure 13.29**), which is produced by proteolytic cleavage of APP by sequential enzyme processing.

APP is a membrane-bound substrate whose normal function is not well understood. The membrane-associated aspartyl protease β-secretase 1 (BACE1) cleaves the extracellular N-terminal portion of APP in the rate-limiting step to generate a soluble fragment (sAPPβ) and a membrane-bound fragment, C99. BACE1 was isolated in 1999 and is primarily found in neurons (another isoform, BACE2, is found in the periphery). The BACE1-catalyzed reaction is followed by cleavage of the intracellular portion catalyzed by a second protease, γ-secretase. This reaction generates small amyloid β peptides from 39 to 49 amino acids, including amyloid β_{42}, which is highly prone to aggregation and forms amyloid plaques. Approaches have targeted both γ-secretase and BACE inhibition.

γ-Secretase, also a membrane-bound protease, consists of a multidomain protein that was difficult to isolate. Most approaches utilized high-throughput screening with phenotypic assays for hit identification and optimization. While a number of compounds advanced into clinical trials, most fell out for a variety of reasons, including lack of efficacy, toxicity, or poor pharmacokinetics (**Figure 13.30**). Semagacestat was a γ-secretase inhibitor developed at Eli Lilly that advanced to phase III clinical trials based on reduction in plasma Aβ levels, however in patients, symptoms of the disease actually worsened and trials were halted. Trials of other inhibitors, including begacestat and avagacestat have also been halted. γ-Secretase is also involved in processing other substrates, including the Notch receptor that plays an essential role in a number of biological processes. Interference with the Notch signaling pathway produced side effects such as an increase in skin cancer and decreased lymphocyte levels, however some of these drugs are finding potential use as anti-cancer agents.

In addition to enzyme inhibitors, several γ-secretase modulators were identified, including *R*-tarenflurbil. This compound resulted from an epidemiological study showing that there was a lower incidence of Alzheimer's disease in patients taking NSAIDS. Investigation of these drugs showed that they decreased levels of $A\beta_{42}$ while increasing levels of the non-plaque-generating $A\beta_{38}$. (*R*)-Tarenflurbil is an enantiomer of

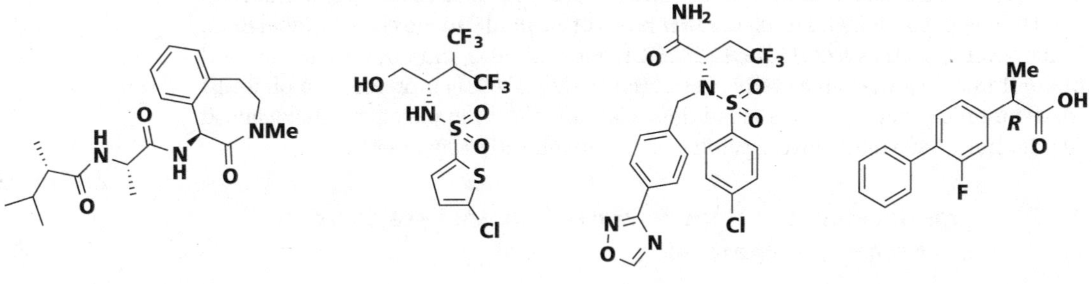

Figure 13.30 Select examples of γ-secretase inhibitors and modulators that advanced to clinical trials for Alzheimer's disease. Semagacestat, begacestat, and avagacestat are all enzyme inhibitors that advanced to clinical trials, but were ineffective. (*R*)-Tarenflurbil is a γ-secretase modulator (GSM). Unfortunately none have proved successful as treatments for the disease.

semagacestat   begacestat   avagacestat   (*R*)-tarenflurbil (GSM)

A: PEPTIDOMIMETIC BACE INHIBITOR

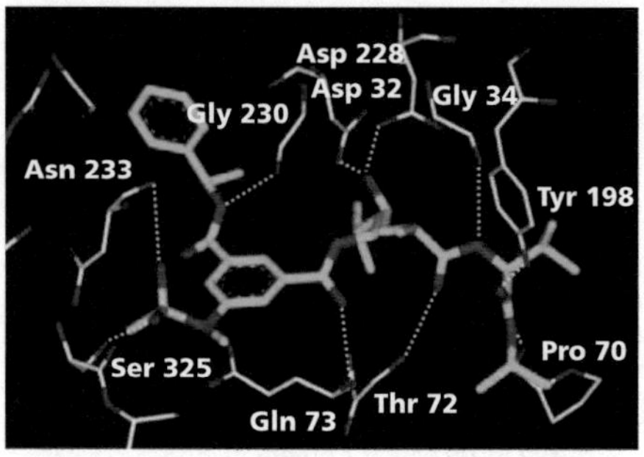

CTS-21166 bound in BACE active site

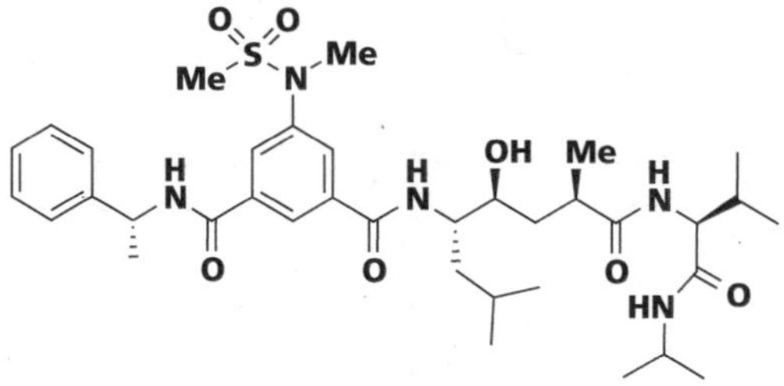

CTS-21166

B: BACE INHIBITORS DEVELOPED FROM SCREENING HITS

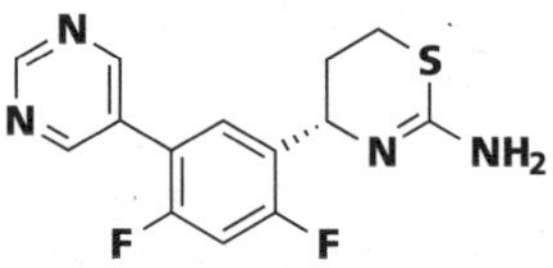

LY2811376

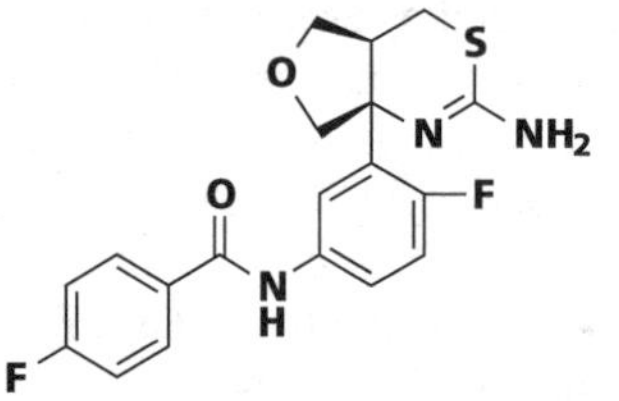

LY2886721

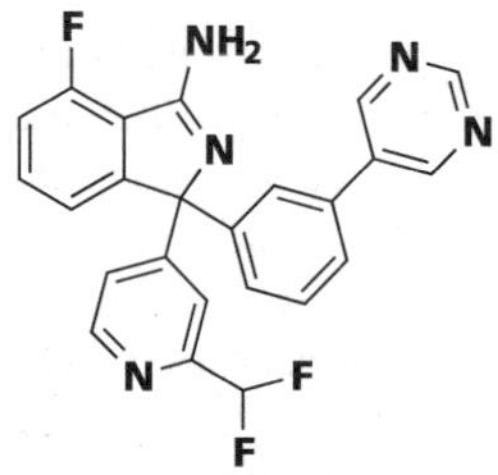

AZD3839

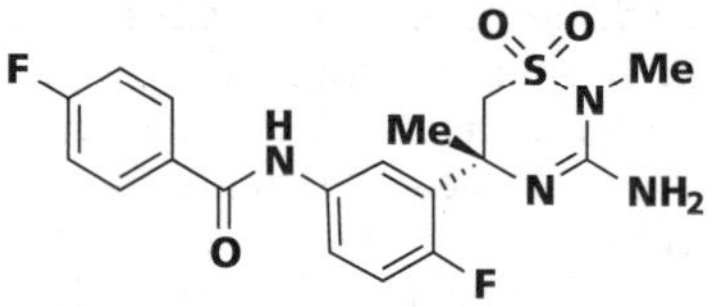

verubecestat

an anti-inflammatory drug, which has no activity as a COX inhibitor, but modulates the Aβ levels so that much less of the Aβ$_{42}$ is produced. Although this drug was not successful in clinical trials, many other modulators of γ-secretase have also been investigated.

Targeting BACE was facilitated by the vast knowledge acquired while developing other aspartyl protease inhibitors, most notably the HIV protease inhibitors used to treat AIDS. Several design approaches have been pursued in the development of BACE inhibitors, with a number of compounds progressing to clinical trials. However, while levels of amyloid β$_{42}$ were lowered in some cases, clinical improvement in Alzheimer's symptoms has not yet been realized.

Most early examples that advanced to clinical trials were peptidomimetics, such as CTS-21166 (**Figure 13.31A**), that were optimized by structure-based drug design. This compound, developed by Arun Ghosh, at Purdue University, inhibits BACE by binding at the active site, making key interactions with Asp32 and Asp228 (see Figure 13.31A). However, in clinical trials, while levels of amyloid β were reduced in plasma and the compound was safe, there was little efficacy based on cognition and daily function. In addition, the peptidomimetics had poor brain penetration due to their high surface area, flexibility, and polarity and they were removed by efflux via P-glycoprotein (P-gp).

The sources of other BACE inhibitors were discovered through high-throughput and fragment-based screening programs and optimized by structure-based design. Examples that have advanced to clinical trials are shown in **Figure 13.31B**. These compounds have good brain penetration and result in lower levels of amyloid β in the cerebrospinal fluid. While several, such as LY2811376, LY2886721, and AZD3839, did not progress beyond phase II trials, a few, such as verubecestat (formerly MK-8931) progressed to phase III trials but unfortunately were dropped due to lack of efficacy in patients with advanced AD. Several are still under investigation in patients with early stages of AD.

Figure 13.31 Structures of BACE inhibitors investigated to treat Alzheimer's disease. A: Peptidomimetic BACE inhibitor. X-ray co-structure of an early peptidomimetic, CTS-21166, bound in the BACE active site. Binding interactions include H-bonding to the active-site aspartates and additional H-bonds to the backbone. (Courtesy of Ghosh laboratories.) B: BACE inhibitors developed from screening hits. Other BACE inhibitors, such as LY2811376, LY2886721, AZD3839 and verubecestat originated from screening programs and were optimized by structure-based design. Several advanced to phase II and III clinical trials.

13.11 Drugs developed to treat Parkinson's disease are based on increasing dopamine levels

Parkinson's disease (PD) is characterized by loss of dopaminergic neurons and reduced dopamine levels in the part of the brain called the substantia nigra. This damage

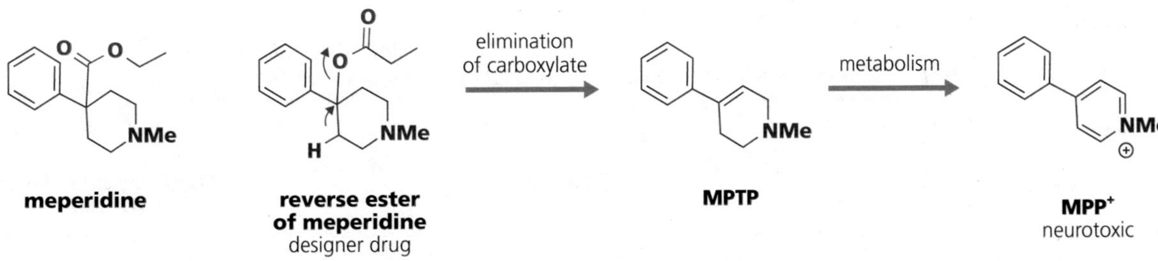

Figure 13.32 Elimination and metabolism of meperidine analog to give MPP⁺ neurotoxin. The reverse ester of meperidine, MPPP, was made as a designer drug (change in red). This change makes the ester susceptible to elimination, and the product, MPTP, an impurity in the designer drug preparation, is metabolized to generate the neurotoxic MPP⁺.

results in movement disorders including tremors and rigidity. An additional marker for Parkinson's disease, observed upon autopsy, is the presence of structures called Lewy bodies in the brain, which are composed of aggregates of the protein α-synuclein. While the cause of PD is unknown, it is believed to be due in small part to a genetic predisposition, possibly combined with prolonged exposure to environmental toxins and aging. Some support for the idea that external exposure can cause Parkinsonism came in the 1980s, with reports of young drug users being hospitalized with Parkinson-like symptoms. Investigation found that these patients had been taking a designer drug based on meperidine. Reversing the ester linkage of meperidine gave MPPP, a compound that had some of the analgesic effects of meperidine but was never marketed. The reverse ester readily underwent elimination to afford an alkene (MPTP), which was an impurity in the drug preparations (**Figure 13.32**). Metabolism of MPTP gives MPP⁺, which is neurotoxic and destroys dopaminergic neurons in the substantia nigra. Prior to this discovery, there were no animal models for Parkinson's disease, and MPP⁺ is now used to induce Parkinsonism in animal models for PD drug discovery.

While no drugs are currently available to cure Parkinson's disease, the few that are on the market alleviate symptoms by restoring levels and activity of dopamine. Since dopamine does not cross the blood–brain barrier, treatment with it would not be effective. Instead, the precursor L-dopa is administered and is taken up by amino acid transporters and delivered to the brain. Once in the brain, it is then converted to dopamine by the enzyme DOPA decarboxylase, as shown in **Figures 13.33A** and **C**.

The bioavailability of L-dopa is low due to first-pass metabolism, and about 95% of the drug is decarboxylated to dopamine before it can cross the BBB. Hence, it is given in combination with the DOPA decarboxylase inhibitor carbidopa (see **Figure 13.33B**) to improve safety and bioavailability. Another strategy for increasing dopamine levels is the use of deprenyl, a monoamine oxidase B (MAO-B) inhibitor that slows the degradation of dopamine to inactive 3,4-dihydroxyphenylacetic acid (DOPAC), see Figure 13.33A. Figure 13.33C illustrates the interactions and effects of these various drugs.

Instead of increasing dopamine levels, another approach uses dopamine agonists to mimic the effects of dopamine. Several drugs have been developed by this approach. The earliest drug approved that works through this mechanism, apomorphine, is formed upon acid degradation of morphine (**Figure 13.34**).

Apomorphine occurs naturally in the water lily and was used in both Mayan and Egyptian cultures as a hallucinogen and aphrodisiac. It is a nonselective D_2–D_5 agonist but lacks the opiate activity of morphine. Apomorphine was first investigated by Erick Harnack in the late 1880s for its emetic effects and effects on stereotypy (repetitive behaviors) in farm animals. While its use to treat PD was postulated in 1884, this was not put into practice until the 1970s.

Other dopamine agonists were developed on the basis of their structural similarity to apomorphine. These include pramipexole, ropinirole, and rotigotine. The common key structural element is based on the 2-aminotetralin core of apomorphine (shown in red in Figure 13.34) that is mimicked in the synthetic analogs by various isosteric aryl groups and an appropriately positioned substituted amine. The dopamine agonist pergolide is based on the ergot alkaloid structure. This compound was used briefly but was withdrawn due to cardiac side effects.

Neurodegenerative diseases have proven to be some of the most difficult to treat, as seen by the two examples discussed here. While Alzheimer's and Parkinson's diseases are primarily diseases related to aging, there are a number of others that are

A: BIOSYNTHESIS AND METABOLISM OF DOPAMINE

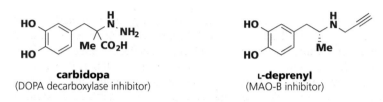

L-dopa → (DOPA decarboxylase) → dopamine → (MAO-B and MAO-A (monoamine oxidases)) → 3,4-dihydroxyphenylacetic acid (DOPAC)

B: DRUGS USED TO RAISE DOPAMINE LEVELS IN THE BRAIN

carbidopa
(DOPA decarboxylase inhibitor)

L-deprenyl
(MAO-B inhibitor)

C: PATHWAYS FOR L-DOPA AND DOPAMINE ACTION

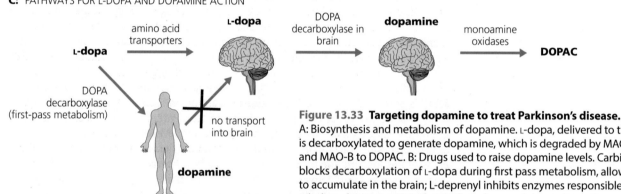

Figure 13.33 Targeting dopamine to treat Parkinson's disease.
A: Biosynthesis and metabolism of dopamine. L-dopa, delivered to the brain, is decarboxylated to generate dopamine, which is degraded by MAO-A and MAO-B to DOPAC. B: Drugs used to raise dopamine levels. Carbidopa blocks decarboxylation of L-dopa during first pass metabolism, allowing it to accumulate in the brain; L-deprenyl inhibits enzymes responsible for metabolism dopamine. C: Pathways for L-dopa and dopamine action; L-dopa is taken into the brain by amino acid transporters, while dopamine is not. First-pass metabolism by DOPA decarboxylase lowers L-dopa levels, converting it into dopamine. Metabolism of L-dopa in the brain increases dopamine levels; these are lowered by subsequent metabolism by monoamine oxidases.

related to genetic factors. Older drugs to treat AD and PD relied on increasing levels of NT levels in an effort to modify symptoms. Newer approaches are based on disease-modifying agents and include perhaps the first examples of structure-based drug design applied to CNS diseases. However, none of these newer approaches has yet successfully translated to drugs.

apomorphine
(D₂–D₅ agonist)

pramipexole

ropinirole

rotigotine

pergolide

Figure 13.34 Structures of dopamine agonists used to treat Parkinson's disease. Apomorphine, a natural product, was the earliest dopamine agonist used to treat PD. Pramipexole, ropinirole and rotigotine are based on the apomorphine scaffold, with all compounds containing an aromatic group and amine (similarities to apomorphine are shown in red). Pergolide was developed on the basis of the structure and activity of ergot alkaloids but is no longer prescribed.

DRUGS OF ABUSE

Unfortunately, a number of the drugs mentioned in this chapter that have valid medicinal uses are also misused. Drug abuse and addiction are related to the self-reward system, which is initiated by dopamine release from dopaminergic neurons in certain parts of the brain. Any drug that increases dopamine transmission in the mesolimbic dopamine system (self-reward system), either directly or indirectly, potentiates self-reward and has a potential for abuse. Drug addiction is characterized by physical and/or psychological dependence. With drugs that cause physical dependence, a tolerance to the drug causes a need for larger doses of drug to achieve the desired effect. Physical withdrawal symptoms include nausea, sweating, difficulty breathing, tremors, and heart palpitations. Drugs that cause psychological dependence lead to uncontrolled compulsive use of the drug, and withdrawal symptoms include anxiety, depression, insomnia, and irritability.

13.12 Stimulants include both legal and illegal drugs

Stimulants cause improvement in both mental and physical function, increasing alertness and endurance. They also can increase heart rate and blood pressure and may decrease food intake and act as appetite suppressants. Caffeine, the most widely used legal stimulant, is isolated from the beans of the *Coffea* plant but is also found in other plant sources (**Figure 13.35**). Its structure resembles the purine base of adenosine, and it acts as a competitive antagonist at adenosine A_{2A} receptors, which are involved in the sleep–wake cycle. Caffeine is nonselective and is also an agonist at the β-adrenergic receptors in the heart, increasing heart rate. Nicotine, found in the tobacco plant, is another widely used legal stimulant. This plant alkaloid acts as an agonist at the nicotinic acetylcholine receptor (see Section 6.6). Its action on receptors in the adrenal medulla indirectly increases levels of dopamine as well as adrenaline, raising both heart rate and blood pressure.

Other stimulants include the phenethylamine amphetamines, both legal and illegal, as well as cocaine. Amphetamines are derived from ephedrine and act as norepinephrine and dopamine reuptake inhibitors, causing increases in synaptic concentrations of both neurotransmitters. Ephedrine, found in *Ephedra sinica*, has been used for thousands of years as a stimulant and asthma treatment (see Section 1.1). Although still legal as a treatment for asthma and colds, its use as a dietary supplement (as a stimulant and for weight loss) was banned in the U.S. in 2004. Two similar compounds, cathinone and cathine, are found in the plant *Catha edulis*. The plant is found in East Africa and its leaves, known as khat or qat, are chewed for stimulant and euphoric effects. Both are controlled substances in the U.S.

While legal and beneficial drugs, such as methylphenidate, used for the treatment of ADHD, have been developed from amphetamines, a number of drugs of abuse

Figure 13.35 Naturally occurring plant-based stimulants and their sources. Caffeine and nicotine are legal stimulants, while ephedrine has been banned as a dietary supplement. The closely related stimulants cathinone and cathine are controlled substances in the U.S. (Coffee photo by Jean-Marie Hullot/Wikimedia Commons, CC BY-SA 3.0. *Nicotiana tabacum* photo by Joachim Mullerchen/Wikimedia Commons, CC BY-2.5. *Ephedra* photo by Lazare Gagnidze/Wikimedia Commons, CC BY-SA 4.0.)

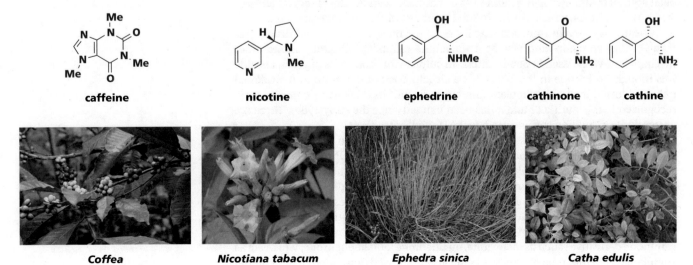

caffeine   nicotine   ephedrine   cathinone   cathine

Coffea   *Nicotiana tabacum*   *Ephedra sinica*   *Catha edulis*

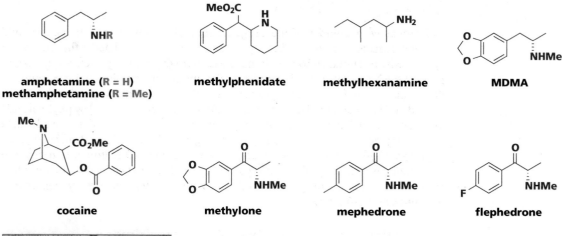

amphetamine (R = H)
methamphetamine (R = Me)

methylphenidate

methylhexanamine

MDMA

cocaine

methylone

mephedrone

flephedrone

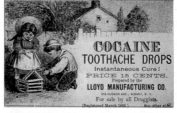

Figure 13.36 Structures of psychostimulants. Amphetamine and methamphetamine were originally used to treat asthma, and as stimulants. Methylphenidate, prescribed to treat ADHD, is a derivative of amphetamine, as is methylhexanamine. Cocaine is a natural product originally used as a local anesthetic. MDMA, methylone, mephedrone, and flephedrone are all stimulants and empathogens.

also come from this family (**Figure 13.36**). Amphetamine was originally synthesized in the 1880s, and methamphetamine was synthesized from ephedrine in 1919. In the 1930s, amphetamine was marketed as Benzedrine, a treatment for asthma as well as for bronchial congestion. Its stimulant and anorectic effects led to it being prescribed to treat narcolepsy and as diet pills. Methamphetamine was widely used by soldiers in World War II and afterward as a stimulant.

By the 1960s methamphetamine was becoming widely abused, with extended use causing amphetamine psychosis. It was made illegal in 1970, and as of 2017, methamphetamine is the most widely abused illegal drug in the United States, with some states reporting that 1% of their population is addicted. Amphetamine is still a legal drug; it is marketed as Adderall to treat ADHD. Methylhexanamine is commonly known as DMAA (1,3-dimethylamylamine) and was originally marketed in the 1960s as a nasal decongestant. Later, in 2006, it was marketed as a natural dietary supplement, in products such as OxyElite Pro and Jack3d, and used as a stimulant. Although DMAA has been touted as being found in geraniums, the FDA found no evidence that this is true and issued warnings in 2012 for its removal. This drug has been abused by athletes and is banned as a stimulant, with deaths of several athletes attributed to DMAA, which causes elevated heart rate and high blood pressure.

Cocaine is a psychostimulant that is one of the most widely abused drugs. This highly addictive compound acts as a dopamine reuptake inhibitor, among other mechanisms. While used in South American cultures for thousands of years, cocaine was brought to Europe in the 1800s. It was legally used at that time to treat dental pain and introduced as a stimulant and euphoric, but its addictive properties were recognized in the late 1800s and it has been banned since the early 1900s. There are currently over 1 million cocaine users in the United States alone.

Other phenylethylamines include MDMA, or ecstasy, which is an empathogen, increasing feelings of empathy and social connection. MDMA was originally synthesized in 1912 as a stimulant but was not marketed. Its psychotropic effects were noted in the 1970s, and it became a schedule I drug in 1985. In addition to acting at the dopamine and norepinephrine transporters, MDMA also increases levels of serotonin. It has weak agonist activity at the 5-HT$_1$ and 5-HT$_2$ receptors, resulting in an increase of oxytocin levels and its activity as an empathogen. A more recent trend is the use of cathinone derivatives such as methylone, mephedrone, and flephedrone, which act as stimulants and empathogens. These chemicals are sprayed onto dried plant material

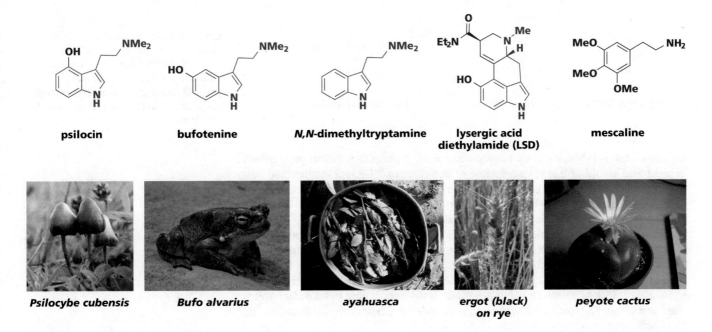

psilocin bufotenine *N,N*-dimethyltryptamine lysergic acid diethylamide (LSD) mescaline

Psilocybe cubensis *Bufo alvarius* ayahuasca ergot (black) on rye peyote cactus

Figure 13.37 Structures of naturally occurring and derived hallucinogens and their sources. These include the indole alkylamines psilocin, bufotenine, *N,N*-dimethyltryptamine, and LSD and the phenylalkylamine mescaline. Most contain a common indole alkylamine substructure (shown in red). The natural sources of each compound or precursor are also shown. (*Psilocybe* photo by the Mushroom Observer/Wikimedia Commons, CC BY-SA 3.0. Ayahuasca photo by Awkipuma/Wikimedia Commons, CC BY-SA 3.0. Ergot photo by JoJan/Wikimedia Commons, CC BY-SA 2.5.)

and sold under names such as plant food and bath salts in convenience stores, labeled not for human consumption.

13.13 Hallucinogens include serotonin receptor agonists and *N*-methyl-D-aspartate antagonists

The classical hallucinogens have the general structure Ar-C-C-N and are structurally related to serotonin. They bind at the 5-HT$_{2A}$ receptor, acting as agonists, although serotonin itself is not hallucinogenic. The indole alkylamines, natural products or derivatives thereof that are found in a variety of sources, are one category. Psilocin is a hallucinogenic serotonin analog that is found in *Psilocybe* mushrooms (**Figure 13.37**). Bufotenine, the *N,N*-dimethyl analog of serotonin, is secreted by psychoactive toads such as *Bufo alvarius* that are found in the American southwest. It has also been isolated from some mushrooms. The closely related *N,N*-dimethyltryptamine has been used in the Amazonian Indian cultures as a spiritual medicine and is found in the ayahuasca brew made of several plant preparations. A more complex structure in this family is LSD, lysergic acid diethylamide. It is a semisynthetic derivative of an ergot alkaloid found in the fungus ergot, which infects grasses. Ingestion of these fungus-infected plants led to a condition called St. Anthony's fire, with symptoms including hallucinations. Historically, these symptoms are believed to have led to accusations of witchcraft. While studying the ergot compounds, Albert Hofmann, at Sandoz Pharmaceuticals, synthesized the *N,N*-diethylamide LSD in 1938. Although his goal was to make a circulatory stimulant, accidental ingestion of a small amount of this compound resulted in hallucinations and an altered state of consciousness. The drug was used in psychiatry in the 1950s and was popularized in the 1960s as a recreational drug, most notably by Timothy Leary, a Harvard psychologist.

Currently, LSD is still widely used, with estimates of about 200,000 teens per year using it in the United States, and reports in the popular press of microdoses being useful to treat certain neuropsychiatric disorders. Ayahuasca is legal in most South American countries and is actually promoted in healing tours to Peru. There are anecdotal reports of its use to treat posttraumatic stress disorder (PTSD) as well as drug addiction. Another category of hallucinogens is the phenylalkylamines, such as mescaline, found in peyote cactus. Like the indole alkaloids, mescaline is a serotonin agonist. Mescaline has been used by Native American tribes in the southwest United States for thousands of years and gained popular attention in Aldous Huxley's book *The Doors of Perception*.

Phencyclidine (PCP), ketamine, and dextromethorphan act as noncompetitive NMDA receptor antagonists and, as such, have the indirect effect of increasing

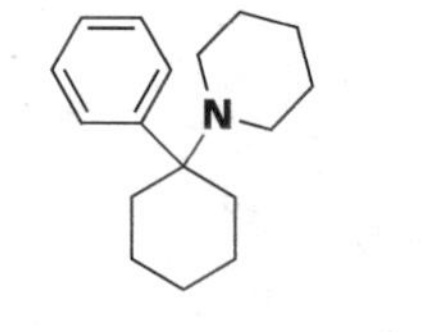

phencylidine (PCP) 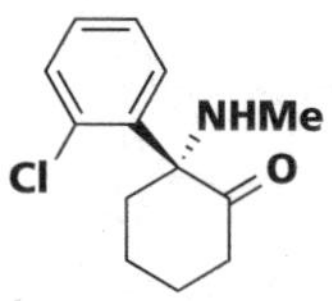   **ketamine** 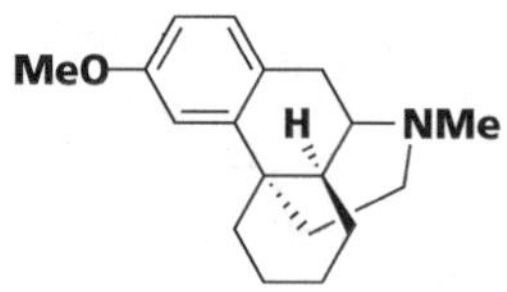   **dextromethorphan**

Figure 13.38 Structures of NMDA antagonists drugs of abuse. Both phencyclidine and ketamine were originally developed as anesthetics, with ketamine still used for that purpose. Dextromethorphan is a cough suppressant, but is also a weak NMDA antagonist.

dopamine levels (**Figure 13.38**). They are dissociative drugs that distort perceptions of sight and sound and lead to a feeling of detachment. PCP was synthesized and used as an anesthetic in the 1950s and was originally believed to be relatively safe since it caused no cardiac or respiratory suppression. However, it was found to induce schizophrenia-like psychosis and was withdrawn from use in 1965.

PCP binds at an allosteric site inside the NMDA receptor, which is an ion channel (Na^+ and Ca^{2+}). Binding of N-methyl-D-aspartate and glycine opens the channel, and PCP prevents this and inhibits depolarization. Both ketamine and dextromorphan bind at the same site, blocking the channel. Ketamine is used legally as an anesthetic but is also a drug of abuse. Dextromethorphan is the enantiomer of an opiate and is used as a cough suppressant. However, in high doses, it can cause hallucinations due to its activity as an NMDA antagonist.

13.14 Cannabinoids have potential medical uses

The cannabinoids are found in the *Cannabis sativa* plant, which has been used for medicinal purposes since about 6000 BC. Their effects include euphoria and enhanced sensory perception as well as alleviation of pain; less desirable effects consist of difficulty in concentration and memory impairment. The component primarily responsible for the psychoactive effects among various related analogs is Δ^9-THC (tetrahydrocannabinol) (**Figure 13.39**). In the 1990s, the receptors at which THC acts were discovered: CB_1 in the brain and CB_2 in the periphery. Both are GPCRs; the CB_1 receptor is responsible for the euphoric and anticonvulsant effects of cannabinoids, while the CB_2 receptor may be involved in immune effects. As a class, cannabinoids indirectly increase activity of dopaminergic neurons.

Anandamide was identified as the CB receptors' natural ligand in the early 1990s (see Figure 13.39). It is hydrolyzed by the enzyme fatty acid amide hydrolase (FAAH), and inhibitors of this enzyme have been investigated as potential antidepressants. There are few actual clinical trials of THC, due to the listing of marijuana as a schedule I drug, which requires DEA approval for studies. In spite of this, synthetic Δ^9-THC was approved by the FDA in the 1990s to treat nausea associated with cancer chemotherapy.

CB_1 agonists have the potential to be anti-nausea agents and appetite stimulants, and hundreds of synthetic cannabinoids have been investigated in academic and industrial laboratories. Agonists at the CB_2 receptor have been investigated to treat neuropathic pain, inflammation, and seizures. Antagonists have been investigated as appetite suppressants and memory enhancers. One CB_1 antagonist, rimonabant (**Figure 13.40**), was approved in Europe in 2006 to treat obesity but was later withdrawn due to psychiatric side effects, including severe depression.

Some of these synthetic analogs, such as JWH-018 and CP 47,497, have been used as designer drugs or synthetic cannabis (see Figure 13.40) and have become dangerous drugs of abuse. Spice and K2 are preparations of cheap herbs and a mixture of synthetic cannabinoids sprayed onto the plant material. Since the components were, in most cases, never tested on humans, serious side effects are common. These range from seizures, psychosis, and agitation, to death from heart attack, sometimes even after one dose. Although JWH-018 and other N-alkyl analogs, as well as CP 47,497, are now illegal in many countries, there are many analogs being sold that are still not classified as illegal.

Many drugs of abuse are based on natural products that have been known for centuries and exert dangerous psychotropic effects. However, the study of these agents and their mechanism of action has served to help the development of legitimate and

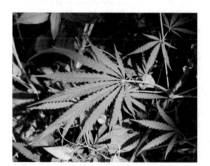

Cannabis sativa

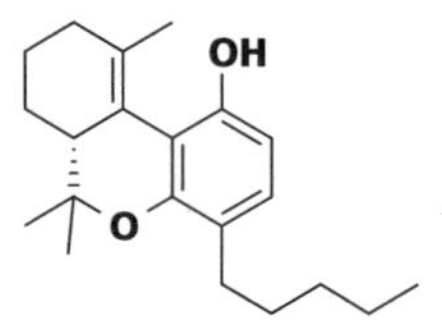

Δ^9-THC (tetrahydrocannabinol)

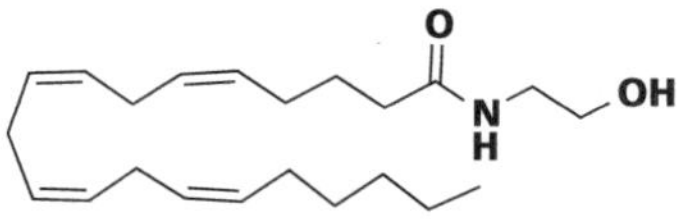

anandamide

Figure 13.39 Structures of natural cannabinoid Δ^9-THC, found in *Cannabis sativa*, and anandamide, the cannabinoid receptor's natural ligand. Δ^9-Tetrahydrocannabinol is the main psychoactive ingredient in *Cannabis sativa*. Anandamide, the ethanolamine amide of arachidonic acid, is an endogenous ligand of CB receptors.

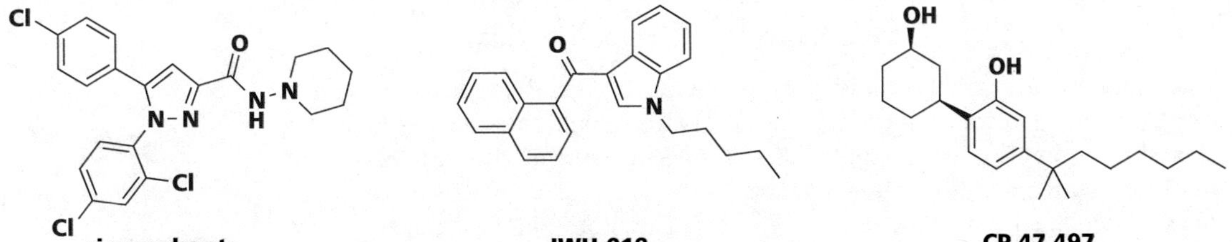

rimonabant:
CB₁ antagonist

JWH-018

CP 47,497

EXAMPLES OF CANNABINOID AGONISTS FOUND IN "SPICE" AND "K2"

Figure 13.40 Examples of synthetic cannabinoids. Rimonabant, a CB₁ antagonist, was approved to treat obesity but was later withdrawn. JWH-018 and CB 47,497 are CB agonists and have been found in illegal drug substances.

potentially valuable drugs. For example, study of cannabis led to identification of the cannabinoid receptors and potential new drug targets CB_1 and CB_2.

SUMMARY

For thousands of years, people have used plant preparations that have effects on the CNS for relief of pain, as stimulants, and for euphoric effects. However, until the 20th century there were no known medications for mental health conditions such as schizophrenia, anxiety, and depression. Likewise, there were no treatments for neurodegenerative diseases. There are now many useful drugs that alleviate neuropsychiatric conditions, and some promising approaches are being tested to treat neurodegenerative diseases such as Alzheimer's disease. Many of the drugs available originated in the mid-20th century and were based on clinical observations, with knowledge of their molecular target not found until later. However, newer treatments are target-driven and based on modern understanding of how neurotransmitters are regulated. The complexity of pathways in the brain and maintaining a balance of neurotransmitters makes drug discovery in this area very challenging. Furthermore, patients may respond differently, or not at all, even when given the same drug.

Neurodegenerative diseases are particularly challenging, and with an aging population there is a more urgent need for effective drugs. With a better understanding of the causes of diseases such as Alzheimer's and Parkinson's, there have been numerous efforts put into developing drugs. While a number have advanced to clinical trials, as yet there are no drugs that affect the course of these diseases.

CASE STUDY 1 DEVELOPMENT OF VILAZODONE

Vilazodone was added to the arsenal of antidepressants in 2011; it exhibits combined SSRI activity and partial agonism at the 5-HT$_{1A}$ receptor. This combination helps to avoid the typical slow onset of antidepressant effects of the SSRIs and also exemplifies the complexity of targeting neurotransmission. The slow onset of SSRIs is believed to be due to a negative feedback loop: SSRIs increase levels of serotonin in the synapse, which leads to activation of presynaptic 5-HT$_{1A}$ autoreceptors and inhibition of firing of serotonergic neurons; this feedback loop limits the rise in extracellular serotonin that SSRIs cause. Chronic use of SSRIs over a period of weeks desensitizes the 5-HT$_{1A}$ autoreceptors, allowing neurons to resume normal firing. The observation, made in the mid-1990s, that coadministration of the 5-HT$_{1A}$ antagonist pindolol and SSRIs led to faster onset of antidepressant effects in humans was the basis of the idea of finding a dual SSRI/5-HT$_{1A}$ antagonist. However, antagonism of postsynaptic 5-HT receptors would be undesirable since the overall goal is to increase serotonin activity. Alternatively, use of a 5-HT$_{1A}$ agonist (rather than antagonist) along with an SSRI could speed up the desensitization, also leading to a faster overall increase in extracellular serotonin.

The discovery of vilazodone began in the 1990s with Merck's investigation of the indole alkylamine roxindole as a potential antipsychotic. Roxindole is similar in structure to the butyrophenone antipsychotics such as haloperidol, but it lacks the ketone moiety. While roxindole had high affinity for dopamine receptors D$_2$ and D$_3$, in functional assays it is an agonist, and in animal models it was found to have activity predictive of anxiolytic and antidepressant action. In addition to its dopamine activity, it is also a potent, selective serotonin agonist, with selectivity for the presynaptic 5-HT$_{1A}$ receptor subtype, and it inhibits the serotonin transporter (**Figure 13.41**).

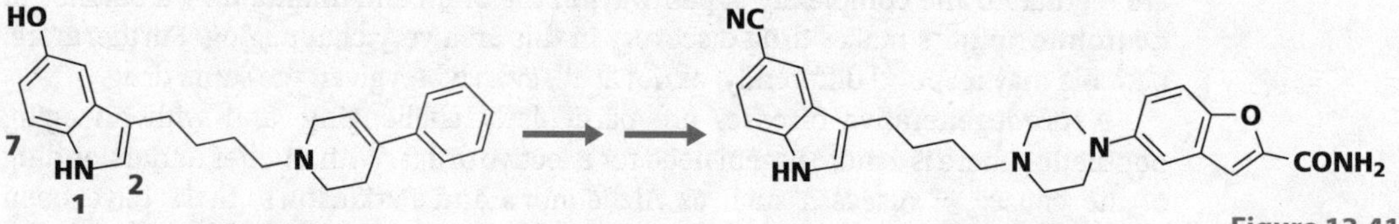

roxindole

IC_{50} $\begin{cases} D_2 = 5.6\ nM \\ 5\text{-}HT_{1A} = 0.8\ nM \\ SRI = 1.4\ nM \end{cases}$

vilazodone

IC_{50} $\begin{cases} D_2 = 666\ nM \\ 5\text{-}HT_{1A} = 0.2\ nM \\ SRI = 0.5\ nM \end{cases}$

Figure 13.41 Structures of roxindole and vilazodone. The lead, roxindole, is a mixed agonist (requirements for D$_2$ agonism are shown in red). The final drug, vilazodone, is a selective 5HT$_{1A}$ agonist and SSRI.

During the course of studies to differentiate dopamine agonist activity from 5-HT$_{1A}$ receptor binding, SAR for each activity emerged. For binding to dopamine (D$_2$) receptors, requirements are the unsubstituted phenyl ring appended to the 4-phenyltetrahydropyridine; unsaturation in the heterocyclic piperidine ring; a saturated butyl linker between the indole and basic nitrogen; and an indole with no substituents at positions 1, 2, or 7. Addition of substituents on the phenyl ring (in particular, hydroxyls and ethers) of roxindole led to selective 5-HT$_{1A}$ agonists and most eliminated dopamine binding while maintaining serotonin reuptake inhibition, as seen in **Figure 13.42**.

While the 5-hydroxyindole piperidine analog exhibited the desired binding profile, the alkoxy analogs were preferred due to greater metabolic stability. Changes to the unsaturated piperidine system were made by replacement with saturated piperidines as well as piperazines. In particular, the piperazines (see Figure 13.42) were investigated further.

In this series, substitution of an electron-withdrawing group at the 5-position on the indole maintained serotonin reuptake inhibition (SRI), and the 5-F and 5-CN analogs were chosen for further study. Although the SRI and 5-HT$_{1A}$ binding profile was optimal, the 5-cyano derivative still had substantial binding to the D$_2$ receptor. A series of compounds was prepared in which the benzo[1,4]dioxane was replaced

ANALOGS WITH SUBSTITUTED PHENYL RING

PIPERAZINE ANALOGS WITH BENZO-[1,4]DIOXANE RING

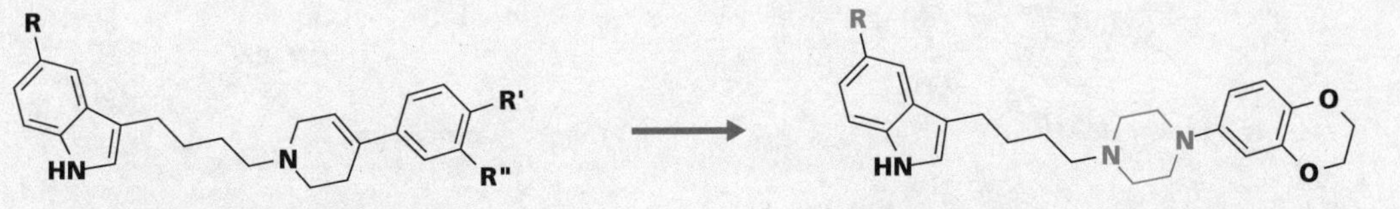

analogs with reduced D_2 affinity

analogs with combined 5-HT$_{1A}$/SRI affinity

R	R'	R''	5-HT$_{1A}$	D$_2$
OH	OH	H	0.4 nM	~100 nM
OCH$_3$	OCH$_3$	H	0.6 nM	>100 nM
OCH$_3$	OCH$_2$ — CH$_2$O		0.4 nM	>100 nM

R	5-HT$_{1A}$	SRI	D$_2$
OCH$_3$	0.4 nM	100 nM	>100 nM
F	5 nM	1 nM	>100 nM
CO$_2$CH$_3$	0.6 nM	50 nM	>100 nM
CN	1 nM	0.4 nM	5.6 nM

Figure 13.42 Examples of series investigated to optimize 5-HT$_{1A}$ and serotonin transporter binding profile and eliminate dopamine effects. Introduction of substitution on the phenyl ring of roxindole with hydroxyl and ether groups eliminated D$_2$ affinity. Substitution of piperazine (blue) for the unsaturated piperidine and incorporation of a substituent on the indole ring at position 5 (blue) decreased dopamine activity but maintained 5-HT$_{1A}$ potency. The benzo[1,4]dioxane series had the desired 5-HT$_{1A}$/SRI profile with either fluoro or cyano substituents on the indole ring, although the cyano analog (red in table) had undesirable D$_2$ affinity.

with other heterocycles such as benzofuran while the 5-fluoro and 5-cyano indole substituents were maintained. Of these, the carboxamide-substituted benzofuran known as vilazodone exhibited the optimal binding profile, maintaining transporter and 5-HT$_{1A}$ binding but decreasing D$_2$ binding from 5.6 to 666 nM.

In addition to binding assays, compounds were tested *in vivo* (in rats) in assays for ultrasonic vocalization as well as elevation of core temperature, which are reflections of activation of presynaptic 5-HT$_{1A}$ autoreceptors. Inhibition of apomorphine-induced climbing in mice was used as a measure of D$_2$ antagonism. In these animal models, vilazodone showed an *in vivo* profile of 5-HT$_{1A}$ agonism with no evidence of D$_2$ antagonism.

Vilazodone entered clinical trials in the early 2000s and showed efficacy against major depressive disorder, with side effects primarily being diarrhea and nausea. Advantages include decreased sexual dysfunction as compared to other SSRIs, as well as anti-anxiety activity. Although there has not been a direct comparison in time of onset, one clinical trial showed improvement in symptoms after 1 week, while other SSRIs typically take 3–4 weeks to be effective. Vilazodone was licensed to Forest Pharmaceuticals and received FDA approval in 2011.

CASE STUDY 2 DISCOVERY OF DONEPEZIL

The first drug approved to treat Alzheimer's dementia was tacrine, in 1993. Although there was some improvement in the memory of treated patients, shortly after its introduction, concerns developed over hepatic toxicity. At Eisai in Japan, library screening for acetylcholinesterase inhibitors identified N-benzylpiperazine **1**, which had originally been synthesized as a potential treatment for arterial sclerosis (**Figure 13.43**). Compound **1** had an IC$_{50}$ of 12,600 nM against rat brain AChE, and a program was initiated to improve its potency. A large number of analogs were prepared, including substitutions on and for the heterocyclic ring, which led to N-benzylpiperidine **2** with binding of 340 nM. Replacement of the ether linkage with an amide further improved potency. Investigation of aryl substituents led to a promising candidate, sulfonate **4**, with 21,000× better binding to AChE than the lead compound **1**. However, while novel and selective, **4** had a short duration of action.

One of the goals of the program was to develop inhibitors that were selective for acetylcholinesterase (AChE) over butyrylcholinesterase (BuChE). Both enzymes hydrolyze esters of choline. However, AChE is found primarily in the brain while BuChE exists primarily in the periphery, specifically in the heart and intestines. It was

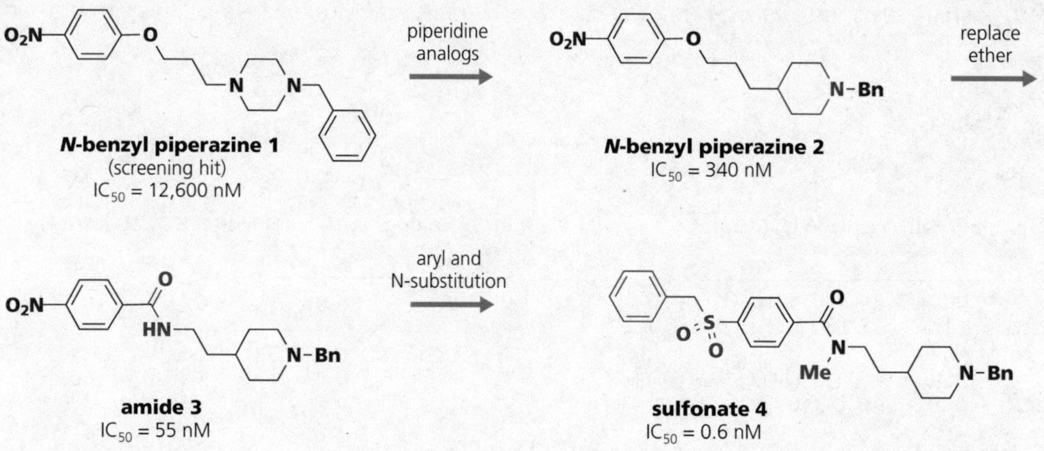

Figure 13.43 Evolution of a screening hit during development of donepezil. The screening hit, *N*-benzylpiperazine **1**, was modified to give the more potent *N*-benzylpiperidine **2**. Replacement of the ether linkage led to the amide **3**, and then N-methylation and substitution for the nitro gave sulfonate **4**, which exhibited potent AChE activity but poor pharmaceutical properties.

thought that selectivity would help to prevent some of the toxicity of tacrine, which inhibits both enzymes equally. The sulfonate **4**, while not ideal, showed 18,000-fold selectivity for AChE over BuChE and was a reversible inhibitor.

The next advances in structure modification came through cyclization of the amide to the aryl ring (**5**) and then replacement of the labile amide with a ketone moiety (**6**). The constrained analog **5** was twice as potent as its parent acyclic *N*-methylamide, and the ketone (indanone) **6** maintained selective enzyme inhibition and had a longer duration of action (**Figure 13.44**). Further optimization of linker length and indanone substitution led to donepezil, a reversible noncompetitive inhibitor of AChE with high enzyme affinity and 1100× selectivity for AChE over BuChE.

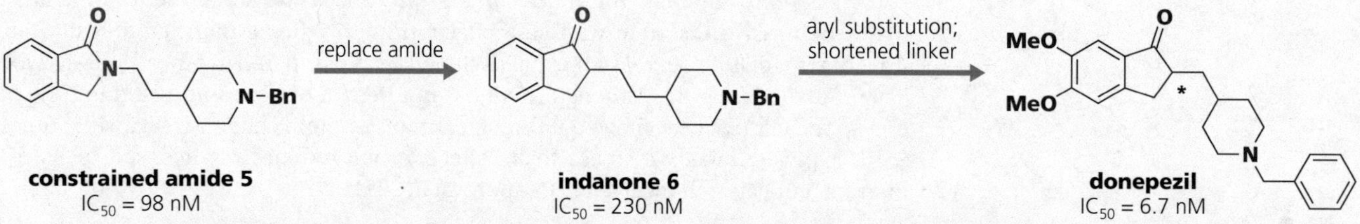

Figure 13.44 Late lead development of donepezil. The constrained amide **5** was modified to the indanone **6**, which exhibited a longer half-life. Substitution on the aryl ring and shortening of the linker led to donepezil.

Prior to solution of the X-ray structure of acetylcholinesterase, donepezil was proposed to bind as shown in **Figure 13.45**: with both aryl groups binding in hydrophobic pockets, the required nitrogen of the piperidine binding to an anionic site, and the ketone accepting a hydrogen bond from a serine OH. Some of these interactions are seen in the actual X-ray structure of donepezil co-crystallized with acetylcholinesterase, which also gives some understanding of its selectivity over BChE.

The active site of acetylcholinesterase sits at the base of a long cleft called the aromatic gorge. While tacrine binds near the active site, the solved X-ray structure showed that donepezil extends through the gorge. Key interactions include binding of the benzyl group through π–π interactions to Trp84 near the active site, binding of the nitrogen to Phe330 through a cation–π interaction, and binding of the aromatic ring of the indanone to Trp279 at the opposite end of the gorge through a π–π interaction. Although there is no H-bond between the serine OH and the indanone carbonyl observed (as proposed), a bridging bond to the backbone through a water molecule is

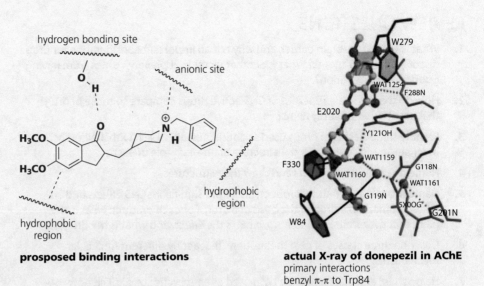

prosposed binding interactions

actual X-ray of donepezil in AChE
primary interactions
benzyl π-π to Trp84
nitrogen cation-π to Phe330
indanone π-π to Trp279

Figure 13.45 Proposed and observed binding of donepezil (E2020) in AChE. Left: the originally proposed binding had both aryl groups in hydrophobic pockets, the piperidine nitrogen in an anionic site and the ketone as an H-bond acceptor. Right: X-ray co-crystal structure shows donepezil (green) with π–π interactions of the benzyl to Trp84 and indanone to Trp279; the piperidine nitrogen has a cation-pi interaction to Phe330. (From Kryger G, Silman I & Sussman JL [1999] *Structure* 7:297–307. With permission from Elsevier.)

evident. Since BChE does not have the Phe330 and Trp279 residues, the X-ray provides an explanation for selectivity.

In animal models, donepezil exhibited inhibition of AChE in rats at an oral dose of 2.6 mg/kg, as compared to 9.5 mg/kg for tacrine. It also showed good brain permeability, and selectivity was evidenced by 14× better inhibition of brain AChE than plasma AChE. Donepezil was shown to increase ACh levels in rat brain and to be effective in several learning and memory models in rats and monkeys. Donepezil entered clinical trials in 1989, and while early trials did not show promising efficacy, phase III trials showed improvement in memory for patients with mild to moderate Alzheimer's disease and only mild side effects. Donepezil was approved by the FDA in 1996, with once-daily oral dosing. While not a cure or a disease-modifying agent for Alzheimer's disease, it can slow progression of memory loss.

REVIEW QUESTIONS

1. What is the blood–brain barrier, and why is it an important consideration for drug discovery for CNS agents? What is another factor that prevents drugs from having good brain penetration?

2. How do the physical properties of CNS-active drugs compare to those of drugs that act at other organ systems?

3. Identify three classes of drugs used as antidepressants, each with a different mechanism of action. Draw the structure of one example of each.

4. Name five neurotransmitters and draw their structures.

5. Name five different natural products that have significant CNS effects and are either themselves a drug or the basis of a drug. For each product: what is the plant that they were isolated from, what is the effect, and what is the drug?

6. Describe three classes of pain medications that act by different molecular mechanisms.

7. Haloperidol and olanzapine are both used as antipsychotics. Explain how they differ.

8. Why is targeting specific neurotransmitters as an approach to CNS drug discovery particularly challenging?

9. Give examples of two different classes of drugs of abuse and an example of each.

10. Name two different drugs that are approved to treat Alzheimer's disease. Choose one and explain how it works. Describe recent approaches to develop drugs to treat the underlying cause of the disease.

11. Based on the examples in this chapter, identify one drug that is a positive allosteric modulator, one that is a partial agonist, and one that is an antagonist. Draw the structure of each, and name the receptor at which it acts.

APPLICATION QUESTIONS

1. Listed in the table are some binding values for reuptake inhibition for (R)- and (S)-citalopram. Referring back to Chapter 3 and Figure 3.4, what is the eudismic ratio for (S)-citalopram versus (R)-citalopram for each symporter?

compound	IC$_{50}$ (nM)		
	SRI[a]	NRI	DRI
(S)-citalopram	2.1	2500	65,000
(R)-citalopram	275	6900	54,000

[a]SRI = serotonin, NRI = norepinephrine, DRI = dopamine.

(Data from Hyttel J [1994] *Int Clin Psychopharmacol* 9[Suppl 1]:19–26. In Textbook of Drug Design and Discovery, 3rd ed, p 320. CRC Press.)

2. Referring to the model of hSERT shown in Figure 13.9 and the binding values in question 1, explain why the S-enantiomer is more potent than the R-enantiomer.

3. Three analogs of citalopram are shown. For each one, on the basis of Figure 13.9 and the binding values in question 1, would you predict it to be more or less active than citalopram? Explain what binding interactions may be gained or lost.

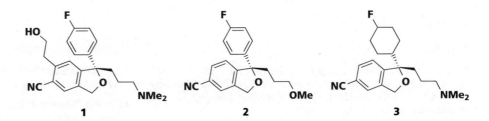

1   2   3

4. During testing of vilazodone, an assay for the effect on binding of radiolabeled GTPγS to cells expressing 5-HT$_{1A}$ receptors gave the curves shown. This is a functional assay measuring potency and intrinsic activity at the 5-HT$_{1A}$ receptor. SB-224289 is a selective 5-HT$_{1B}$ antagonist and was coadministered so that activity was due only to 5-HT$_{1A}$. Comparison was done with serotonin, 8-OH-DPAT, and buspirone.

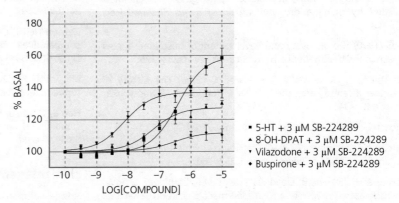

Reference: Hughes ZA, Starr KR, Langmead CJ et al. [2005] Neurochemical evaluation of the novel 5-HT$_{1A}$ receptor partial agonist/serotonin reuptake inhibitor, vilazodone. *Eur J Pharmacol* 510:49–57.

Referring back to Section 6.3, answer the following questions:

(a) What are the structures of 8-OH-DPAT, serotonin, and buspirone?

(b) Based on the graph, identify whether each of these three compounds is a full agonist, a partial agonist, or an antagonist at 5-HT$_{1A}$.

(c) Which is the most potent?

(d) Which has the highest intrinsic activity?

5. Memantine (used for Alzheimer's) and PCP (drug of abuse) are both NMDA antagonists. Research both compounds and explain why memantine does not have the psychosis-inducing effects of PCP.

6. Using examples in this chapter, identify four instances where conformational constraint was used as a medicinal chemistry strategy.

7. Using examples in this chapter, identify two compounds where an isosteric replacement was used. Compare the isostere to the original compound.

8. Several drugs of abuse that are cannabinoid agonists are described in this chapter. Propose a pharmacophore that is consistent with three of the structures.

9. Compound CTS-21166 is a BACE1 inhibitor that was not successfully advanced. Research the structure of this compound. Does this compound adhere to Lipinski's rules? Would you expect this compound to be brain-penetrant, given what you know about the physical properties required for BBB penetration?

10. Figure 13.28 shows the binding of rivastigmine to AChE. Given what you know about designing serine proteases, design two new analogs of rivastagmine that contain different warheads.

11. Identify five drugs in this chapter that contain a privileged structure. At least three of them should be different privileged structures.

FURTHER READING

General

Ornstein P (2015) Some thoughts on the past 50 years of central nervous system therapeutic research. In 2015 Medicinal Chemistry Reviews (Desai MC ed) Vol 50, pp 31–61. Medicinal Chemistry Division, American Chemical Society.

Pajouhesh H & Lenz GR (2005) Medicinal chemical properties of successful central nervous system drugs. *NeuroRx* 2:541–553.

Anti-anxiety/antidepressant

Sieghart W (1992) GABA$_A$ receptors: ligand gated Cl⁻ channels modulated by multiple drug-binding sites. *Trends Pharmacol Sci* 13:446–450.

New JS (1990) The discovery and development of buspirone: a new approach to the treatment of anxiety. *Med Res Rev* 10:283–326.

Lopez-Munoz F, Ucha-Udabe R & Alamo C (2005) The history of barbiturates a century after their clinical introduction. *Neuropsychiatr Dis Treat* 1:329–343.

Sternbach L (1979) The benzodiazepine story. *J Med Chem* 22:1–7.

Calcaterra NE & Barrow JC (2014) Classics in chemical neuroscience: diazepam (Valium). *ACS Chem Neurosci* 5:253–260.

Depoortere H, Zivkovic B, Lloyd KG et al. (1986) Zolpidem, a novel nonbenzodiazepine hypnotic. I. Neuropharmacological and behavioral effects. *J Pharmacol Exp Ther* 237:649–658.

Heinrich T, Bottcher H, Gericke R et al. (2004) Synthesis and structure–activity relationship in a class of indolebutylpiperazines as dual 5-HT$_{1A}$ receptor agonists and serotonin reuptake inhibitors. *J Med Chem* 47:4684–4692.

Dawson LA & Watson JM (2009) Vilazodone: a 5-HT$_{1A}$ receptor agonist/serotonin transporter inhibitor for the treatment of affective disorders. *CNS Neurosci Ther* 15:107–117.

Antipsychotics

Moghaddam B & Javitt D (2012) From revolution to evolution: the glutamate hypothesis of schizophrenia and its implication for treatment. *Neuropsychopharmacology* 37:4–15.

Chappie TA, Helal CJ & Hou X (2012) Current landscape of phosphodiesterase 10A (PDE10A) inhibition. *J Med Chem* 55:7299–7331.

Rowley M, Bristow LJ & Hutson PH (2001) Current and novel approaches to the drug treatment of schizophrenia. *J Med Chem* 44:477–501.

Ban TA (2007) Fifty years chlorpromazine: a historical perspective. *Neuropsychiatr Dis Treat* 3:495–500.

Pain and migraine

Max MB & Stewart WF (2008) The molecular epidemiology of pain: a new discipline for drug discovery. *Nat Rev Drug Discovery* 7:647–658.

Chen R & Chung S-H (2013) Complex structures between the N-type calcium channel (Ca$_v$2.2) and ω-conotoxin GVIA predicted by molecular dynamics. *Biochemistry* 52:3765–3772.

de Lera Ruiz M & Kraus RL (2015) Voltage-gated sodium channels: structure, function, pharmacology, and clinical indications. *J Med Chem* 58:7093–7118.

Bagal SK, Chapman ML, Marron BE et al. (2014) Recent progress in sodium channel modulators for pain. *Bioorg Med Chem Lett* 24:3690–3699.

Hansen-Tfelt P, De Vries P & Saxena PR (2000) Triptans in migraine: a comparative review of pharmacology, pharmacokinetics and efficacy. *Drugs* 60:1259–1287.

Maryanoff BE (2016) Phenotypic assessment and the discovery of topiramate. *ACS Med Chem Lett* 7:662–665.

Han S, Thatte J, Buzard DJ & Jones RM (2013) Therapeutic utility of cannabinoid receptor type 2 (CB$_2$) selective agonists. *J Med Chem* 56:8224–8256.

Neurodegenerative

Atta-ur-Rahman & Choudhary MI (eds) (2014) Enzyme inhibitors involved in the treatment of Alzheimer's disease. In Drug Design and Discovery in Alzheimer's Disease, pp 142–199. Bentham Science.

Connolly BS & Lang AE (2014) Pharmacological treatment of Parkinson disease: a review. *J Am Med Assoc* 311:1670–1683.

Oehlrich D, Prokopcova H & Gijsen HJM (2014) The evolution of amidine-based brain penetrant BACE1 inhibitors. *Bioorg Med Chem Lett* 24:2033–2045.

Case studies

Dawson LA & Watson JM (2009) Vilazodone: a 5-HT$_{1A}$ receptor agonist/serotonin transporter inhibitor for the treatment of affective disorders. *CNS Neurosci Ther* 15:107–117.

Heinrich T, Böttcher H, Gericke R et al. (2004) Synthesis and structure–activity relationship in a class of indolebutylpiperazines as dual 5-HT$_{1A}$ receptor agonist/serotonin reuptake inhibitors. *J Med Chem* 47:4684–4692.

Sugimoto H, Ogura H, Arai Y et al. (2002) Research and development of donepezil hydrochloride, a new type of acetylcholinesterase inhibitor. *Jpn J Pharmacol* 89:7–20.

Sugimoto H, Iimura Y, Yamanishi Y & Yamatsu K (1995) Synthesis and structure-activity relationships of acetylcholinesterase inhibitors: 1-benzyl-4-[(5,6-dimethoxy-1-oxoindan-2-yl)methyl]piperidine hydrochloride and related compounds. *J Med Chem* 38:4821–4829.

Answers to End of Chapter Review Questions

Chapter 1

Answer 1.1

Major advances in the field of medicinal chemistry during the period from 1700 to 1900 include the following:

- Development of procedures to isolate pure compounds from natural sources or complex mixtures

- Attributing biological activity to specific substances

- Understanding of functional group arrangements in complex natural products and early structure elucidation

- Development of procedures to modify isolated substances through semisynthesis in order to generate new compounds and introduction of the first semisynthetic drugs

Answer 1.2

Two examples of semisynthetic drugs and their corresponding natural products are (1) aspirin (acetylsalicylic acid), derived from salicin, and (2) heroin, derived from morphine.

Answer 1.3

Ehrlich and Langley pioneered the idea that drug activities are the result of compounds interacting with a specific entity on or in the cell. Ehrlich proposed the receptor theory in 1897 as an explanation of the interaction between bacterial toxins and antitoxins, which led to his development of Salvarsan. Langley expanded on the receptor theory to describe the receptor as a specific receptive substance that can be activated or antagonized with small molecules after observation of the agonist and antagonist effects of pilocarpine and atropine on heart rate of frogs.

Answer 1.4

Some reasons for development of a total synthesis of a bioactive natural product include the following:

- Isolations can be time-consuming and expensive, often giving variable results.

- Very large amounts of materials (kilograms) may be required to produce milligrams of the desired product.

- Access to materials may be restricted due to climatic or political conditions.

- Independent synthesis of the natural product serves to confirm the structure.

- Synthesis provides reliable access to new and unnatural analogs.

- Synthesis can be a source of large quantities of material that are not available otherwise.

Answer 1.5

Due to advances in small-molecule NMR and MS, only very small quantities of material are required in order determine the presence of functional groups, molecular weight, and molecular connectivity. This drastically reduces the time required for total structure elucidation (down significantly from the 30 years it took to elucidate the structure of compounds such as morphine in the early 1900s) and enhances the degree of confidence in the structures elucidated. Having knowledge of the structures of isolated medicinal compounds allows for advances in total synthesis and opens the door to the development of structural analogs that may have improved activity and reduced toxicity compared to the natural product.

Answer 1.6

Small-molecule X-crystallography provides even more confidence than NMR and MS in structural elucidation of complex molecules. In addition, protein X-ray crystallography has allowed medicinal chemists to "see" a drug as it interacts with a specific enzyme or protein. Often this allows for the design of new drugs based on observable interactions. Medicinal chemists can use these findings to design new analogs and to streamline the process of drug discovery.

Answer 1.7

In order to isolate a product containing an acid functional group, the crude plant preparation could first be partitioned between benzene and aqueous acid (instead of a base for an amine). The organic phase would contain the acid, and would then be extracted with aqueous base to move the deprotonated acid into the aqueous layer. Finally, partition between an acid aqueous layer and an organic layer would move the protonated acid to the organic layer, from which it could be isolated in pure form.

Chapter 2

Answer 2.1

Some naturally occurring sources of hits and leads are as follows:

- Plants (for example, paclitaxel isolated from the yew tree)

- Microbes (for example, doxorubicin isolated from soil fungus *Streptomyces peucetius*)

- Higher animals (for example, ziconotide isolated from cone snails)

- Natural ligands (for example, cimetidine derived from histamine)

Answer 2.2

Split-pool combinatorial synthesis and parallel synthesis are two general approaches to combinatorial synthesis. Split-pool synthesis involves repetitive combine, divide, and couple sequences of molecular building blocks that are often assembled on resin beads. For example, a mixture containing different building blocks is coupled to a second group of building blocks to give dimers. These dimers are then combined, divided, and coupled with a third set of building blocks to give trimers, and so on. Parallel synthesis involves separate preparation of different building block combinations. For example, different building blocks are placed in separate vessels and a second group of building blocks is added to each well, then a third group, and so on. In this method, each individual compound is prepared separately, rather than as part of a mixture as in split-pool synthesis, where deconvolution of any active compounds may be required.

In split-pool synthesis, fewer reaction steps are required compared to parallel synthetic methods to make the same number of compounds. Using the example of a two-step synthesis: In a split-pool synthesis, three building blocks reacted with three different reagents in the first step and then three different reagents in the second step $= 3 \times 3 \times 3 = 27$ products in six reactions. In a parallel synthesis, three starting materials would be reacted individually with three different reagents (nine reactions) and then those nine products would be reacted individually with three reagents. It requires 27 reactions to generate 27 products.

Finally, parallel synthesis usually generates larger quantities of material than split-pool synthesis.

Answer 2.3

Conventional HTS uses various types of assays, and can usually detect activity of compounds in the 1–20 μM range. An isolated protein target is not required. Large numbers of compounds (>100,000) in the 300–500 MW range are usually screened. The specific mode of action of the hit may not be known, nor its binding site. HTS often results in a large number of false positives that must then be identified and eliminated.

FBS relies on an assay where direct interaction between a small molecule and the isolated target can be detected. Smaller numbers of compounds are screened compared to traditional HTS campaigns, the compounds themselves are of lower molecular weight, and binding at very high concentrations (up to millimolar) can be detected. Few false positives occur since direct binding is detected, and in some cases specific binding modes are elaborated. Evolving low-potency FBS hits to high-potency leads may take significant effort.

Answer 2.4

Biochemical assays allow thorough characterization of the kinetics of an enzymatic reaction by monitoring formation of the product, allowing identification of inhibitors and activators. Data from a biochemical assay reflect only the effects of the hit on the specific target; therefore, structure–activity relationship data are relatively straightforward to interpret. However, hits in a biochemical assay may not have the appropriate physical and pharmaceutical properties, such as cell permeability, or may be toxic, and therefore may need significant optimization.

Phenotypic assays can measure phenotypic changes in complex systems, regardless of the specific molecular target, which may not be known. However, it is likely that hits already have some desirable properties such as permeability and lack of toxicity. Phenotypic assays are useful when diseases are poorly understood and no specific target has been identified.

Answer 2.5

A hit is any compound of defined structure and biological activity at some defined threshold. A lead is a compound, usually resulting from structural optimization of the biological, physical, and pharmaceutical properties of a hit, and has the potential to become a drug candidate. Properties of a high-quality lead include potency, selectivity, lack of promiscuity, evidence of emerging SAR, appropriate physical and pharmaceutical properties, and accessibility.

Answer 2.6

Candidates from a drug discovery program based on clinical observation often have the advantage of progressing through clinical trials more rapidly than candidates from other drug discovery programs because they have already overcome various safety and regulatory hurdles required for administration to humans. Additionally, if patients observe a beneficial side effect, it is often robust enough to be a true effect. Overall, the time to approval and market may be shorter than for typical discovery programs.

Answer 2.7

Pros	Cons
Structures derived from natural ligands are likely to be active.	Structures derived from natural ligands will also act similarly to the ligand and could affect all receptor subtypes, resulting in low specificity.
There may be considerable knowledge regarding how the natural ligand binds and affects the protein target.	Strategy is not useful if the target substrate or ligand is not known.

Answer 2.8

Structure-based virtual screening is most appropriate to apply to hit identification when a three-dimensional protein structure, co-structures of the protein and a binding partner, or homology models are available (often determined by or derived from X-ray crystallography, NMR, or other methods). This approach is relatively low in cost and screening time, compared to other methods, and is useful for identifying a small library of compounds when physically screening larger libraries is not feasible. In addition to the structure or a model, a virtual library is also required. Disadvantages are that false positives are common and any hits must still be experimentally verified.

Answer 2.9

Ligand-based virtual screening is an appropriate screening strategy when multiple ligands that bind to the target with a range of affinities have been described. It is particularly useful when the structure of the target has not been elucidated. This strategy requires a computational description of the ligand's structure or conformation in regard to size, polarity, H-bond capabilities, and hydrophobicity. In addition to high-quality data on various ligands, a computationally derived small-molecule virtual library is also required for screening. As in all virtual screens, all hits must be experimentally verified, and there is a high false-positive rate.

Answer 2.10

Three categories of compounds that often cause false positives in high-throughput screens include (1) aggregate-forming compounds, (2) compounds containing reactive functional groups, and (3) redox-active compounds.

Answer 2.11

A Tanimoto coefficient is a value between 0 and 1 that measures the relative similarity between two structures. Structures with a high degree of similarity will have a Tanimoto coefficient close to 1, whereas, structures with a low degree of similarity will have a Tanimoto coefficient close to 0. Tanimoto coefficients are used to evaluate the structural diversity of hits or leads. They are often used during the hit triage process to identify compounds that have structural similarities to each other and those that are structurally diverse.

Chapter 3

Answer 3.1

The proton in the amine (NH-R) and the acid proton (COOH) can act as H-bond donors. The nitrogen and oxygen atoms can act as H-bond acceptors. The carbonyl group (C=O) can participate in dipole–dipole and ion–dipole interactions. The acid functional group, if it is deprotonated, can participate in ion–ion and ion–dipole interactions. The CH_2 can be involved in van der Waals interactions.

Answer 3.2

Aspartic acid contains multiple atoms and functional groups (N, O, N–H, O–H) that are capable of forming H-bonds with water, and is a highly polar compound. Therefore, it will be highly solvated with a shell of water molecules making strong H-bonds to it. Desolvation is generally energetically favorable when nonpolar molecules interact with non-polar binding sites, but as the polarity of the small molecule increases, desolvation becomes more and more energetically unfavorable. Thus, it can be assumed that the desolvation of aspartic acid would be a highly energetically unfavorable process.

Answer 3.3

Property	Specific parameters
electronic properties (electron-donating or -withdrawing)	σ (Hammett)
lipophilicity	$\log P$, π (Hansch)
size	Verloop, MR, E_s (Taft)

Answer 3.4

Receptor-excluded volume and receptor-essential area are two concepts applied to the active-analog approach to three-dimensional pharmacophore models. The receptor-excluded volume is the binding pocket area occupied by a small molecule binder, whereas the receptor-essential volume is the area occupied by the macromolecule. The receptor-excluded volume is determined from the superimposition of the lowest energy conformation of all active compounds containing the pharmacophore, while the receptor-essential area is based on the volume map of the superimposition of inactive compounds containing the pharmacophore, which are assumed to extend into the area occupied by the receptor. A comparison between the volume of active and inactive analogs, all containing the correct pharmacophoric elements, provides a rough three-dimensional map of the size and shape of the binding pocket within a target protein, as well as its boundaries.

Answer 3.5

A pharmacophore describes the three-dimensional orientation of specific steric and electronic features that are necessary for optimal binding interactions with a biological target in order to trigger a desired response. Most pharmacophores have at least three binding elements, and the elements are not specific functional groups or atoms but the feature (e.g. H-bond donor; hydrophobe) they display.

Answer 3.6

Structure-based drug design (SBDD) requires information on the structure of the biomolecular target. Ideally, an X-ray, NMR, or other high-resolution structure of the protein, perhaps bound to a small-molecule ligand, is used to understand the pharmacophore. When such a structure is not available, a homology model—a model of the desired target based on a high resolution structure of a closely related target—is used.

Answer 3.7

Biological activity, physical properties, and pharmaceutical properties (druglike properties) are all optimized during the lead optimization process.

Answer 3.8

The dissociation constant (K_d) is proportional to the concentrations of drug and protein divided by the concentration of drug–protein complex at equilibrium:

$$D{-}P \rightleftharpoons D{+}P \quad \text{and} \quad K_d = \frac{[D][P]}{[D{-}P]}$$

K_d can be related to ΔG according to $\Delta G = -RT \ln K_d$.

Note that K_d is the inverse of the association constant K_a, which relates to ΔG by the equation $\Delta G = -RT \ln K_a$

Answer 3.9

The eudismic ratio is the ratio of biological activity of two enantiomers: the more potent enantiomer (eutomer) divided by the less potent enantiomer (distomer). A higher eudismic ratio indicates a higher degree of stereoselectivity in the interaction.

Answer 3.10

Although hydrophobic interactions themselves are relatively weak, they play an important role in drug-protein binding. Binding of a non-polar small molecule to a non-polar binding site results in water being displaced from unfavorable interactions with nonpolar areas within the protein. In addition, the drug-solvent shell (desolvation) is disrupted, and these interactions are also entropically favorable.

Chapter 4
Answer 4.1

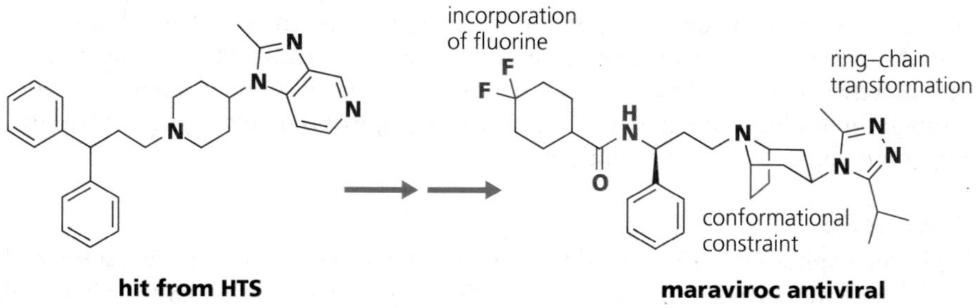

incorporation of fluorine

ring–chain transformation

conformational constraint

hit from HTS

maraviroc antiviral

Answer 4.2

factor Xa inhibitor   roscovitine CDK inhibitor   caspase inhibitor

Answer 4.3

The primary difference between a prodrug approach and a targeting approach is the specificity of their design. A prodrug approach is generally applied in order to address issues of poor permeability or solubility in order to improve the oral bioavailability of the drug. The problem functionalities of the active drug that are identified as responsible for the poor properties are masked as an inactive form of the drug that allows the drug to be better absorbed. The active form is then released (often through hydrolysis catalyzed by nonspecific enzymes). The targeting approach applies the same general premise of the prodrug approach in that the active moiety is modified, but the goal is to concentrate the drug at a specific location within the body. This approach has been used in the development of anti-cancer therapies to generate high drug concentrations at tumor sites, and avoid exposure to other cells. The targeting moiety needs to be specifically designed so that it is recognized by the cells to which it is targeted—by relying on recognition of specific receptors or enzymes, or even a specific feature of the cell such as pH or oxidative environment. In this way the active moiety is generated only at or near its intended target.

Answer 4.4

In compound A, addition of a fluorine atom meta to the aryl sulfonamide may decrease metabolism, increase lipophilicity and gain additional interactions with the target, such as a hydrogen-bonding interaction. In compound B, introduction of a fluorine atom at the α position to the carboxylic acid would reduce the pK_a of the acidic hydrogen. (A second fluorine atom at the α position would further decrease the pK_a). It may also change lipophilicity, and make additional binding interactions with the target.

Answer 4.5

An acid isostere should contain ionizable hydrogens within a pK_a range of 4–5 and/or have hydrogen-bonding donor or acceptor capabilities in order to mimic a carboxylic acid. In addition, it should be as soluble as the acid. By incorporation of an isostere, improvements in permeability and metabolic stability are anticipated.

Answer 4.6

The CF_3 group is highly lipophilic. This property may contribute to the molecules' crossing the blood–brain barrier, where it needs to act.

Answer 4.7

The appropriate lipophilicity is important property for a drug candidate because a careful balance must be achieved. Molecules that are too lipophilic often have poor solubility and can compartmentalize into the lipid bilayer. They are also known to promiscuously bind to proteins. Both of these can prevent the drug from reaching the target tissue or organ. Conversely, molecules that are not lipophilic enough may not penetrate the cell membrane and may be too highly solvated to allow favorable binding to the target protein.

Answer 4.8

High solubility is an important property of a drug candidate because a compound must be soluble in order to be permeable. Lead molecules are often lipophilic in order to achieve high binding to target proteins and require a degree of lipophilicity to be permeable. However, high lipophilicity usually results in poor aqueous solubility, but acceptable aqueous solubility is also required for high permeability. Improving one parameter often results in diminishing the other.

Answer 4.9

A prodrug strategy might be adopted if the lead compound has poor solubility or lipophilicity that cannot be solved by traditional medicinal chemistry strategies. A prodrug can mask specific functional groups that are responsible for the poor permeability or add a solubilizing group to an insoluble analog. A prodrug strategy could also be adopted to improve safety. Targeting approaches may also rely on prodrugs that can be designed to remain in their inactive form until they are exposed to an enzyme (or environment) that is specific for the target cell. This concentrates the active form of the drug at the target and may help to prevent side effects due to lack of selectivity.

Answer 4.10

Primary assays are relatively simple *in vitro* assays that usually measure the potency of a molecule toward a specific target. Secondary assays are generally more complex *in vitro* assays. They may look for various downstream effects due to interactions with the primary target, or direct effects on the target but in the more relevant environment of a cell. They can also be used to identify certain liabilities such as toxicity and poor absorption. A molecule may exhibit a high degree of potency against an isolated target enzyme in a primary assay, but if the molecule is incapable of crossing the cell membrane, if cellular enzymes quickly metabolize it, if the compound has higher affinity for unrelated targets in the cell, or if it cannot access its target, then the potency may drop significantly or all activity could be lost upon testing in a secondary assay.

Chapter 5
Answer 5.1

- Pure Food and Drug Act of 1906: required accurate labeling of medicines and required listing of "addictive and/or dangerous" substances (for example, morphine, cannabis, alcohol)

- Food, Drug, and Cosmetic Act (1938): required testing in animals in order to prove safety

- Kefauver–Harris Amendment (Drug Efficacy Amendment, 1962): required FDA approval of a drug before it could be marketed, clinical trials establishing efficacy in humans, and reporting of serious side effects observed after the drug was approved and marketed

Answer 5.2

Phase I metabolism typically takes place in the liver and involves modification of functional groups of the parent drug. The most common reactions are oxidation, reduction, and hydrolysis. Phase II metabolism involves conjugation of the drug or one of its metabolites to small endogenous molecules. Reactions usually occur on functional groups such as carboxylic acids, alcohols, and amines and include glucuronidation, amino acid conjugation, and N-acetylation. When an electrophile is present in the drug or its metabolite, glutathione conjugation can occur.

Answer 5.3

1. Cytotoxicity assays measure cell viability after treatment with a compound to identify general toxicity to cells. No specific mechanism is implied, but it is a prediction of general toxicity.

2. CYP inhibition or induction assays measure the potential of a compound to inhibit or induce the drug-metabolizing cytochrome P-450 enzymes. Activity in this assay would indicate the compound has the potential to cause drug–drug interactions, meaning the compound could cause the effects of a different drug to be altered because it disrupted the metabolic activity of cytochrome P-450. In some cases, too much of the other drug could result because it wasn't metabolized normally (CYP inhibition); in cases of CYP induction, too little of the drug would be present.

3. hERG channel inhibition assays evaluate the ability of a compound to inhibit an ion channel involved in coordinating the heartbeat. Since inhibition of the hERG channel can result in sudden death, this assay evaluates the potential to cause this specific toxicity.

4. An Ames test measures the potential of a compound to cause mutations in DNA. Mutated DNA has been linked to cancer; therefore, this assay is used to flag compounds that may be mutagenic.

Answer 5.4

A process synthesis must be:

- Capable of producing kilogram quantities
- Cost-effective
- Safe
- Efficient (minimal number of synthetic steps)
- Highly reproducible
- Consistent in yield and impurity profile

A process synthesis must produce much larger quantities than the original synthesis. Therefore, many of the deficiencies of the original synthesis that could be tolerated on a small scale must be addressed a larger scale—specifically cost, safety, and efficiency. Regulatory agencies require limits on impurities, so a consistent impurity profile is required.

Answer 5.5

1. Segment I testing is done in male and female animals to evaluate effects of the drug on fertility and reproductive ability.

2. Segment II testing is done in pregnant mothers and tests for embryonic toxicity (teratogenicity).

3. Segment III testing is done in pregnant animals and mothers during the final stages of pregnancy and after birth; it looks at effects of the drug on delivery and lactation.

Answer 5.6

1. A composition of matter patent covers novel compounds with a proven utility that is not obvious to one skilled in the art. These can cover a specific chemical entity and/or structurally related series with specified modifications.

2. A method of use patent can protect known compounds for which a new, unobvious use has been discovered.

3. A process patent can protect a process or synthesis that is used to manufacture a drug and prevents others from using that same process or synthesis.

Answer 5.7

- Lipophilicity: highly lipophilic compounds accumulate in fatty tissue
- pK_a: pH differences in tissues and organs can affect where it accumulates.
- Permeability: how permeable a compound is will affect where it is absorbed
- Ability to bind to plasma proteins: affects diffusion across membranes and into target organs
- Ability to be recognized by transporter proteins: compounds that are recognized by transporters can reach high concentrations in specific organs and cells. Conversely, compounds recognized by efflux pumps can be prevented from accumulating in certain cells or organs.

Answer 5.8

Three main reasons why a highly bioavailable drug is preferable to a poorly bioavailable drug include safety, cost, and compliance.

1. Safety: The PK of a highly bioavailable drug is often less variable, therefore unexpected side effects due to higher or lower levels of drug than expected are limited. Moreover, lower doses are possible, which can minimize off-target effects compared to less bioavailable drugs.

2. Cost: A highly bioavailable drug requires less active ingredient per dosage form, which can help lower the cost of materials and manufacturing.

3. Compliance: A highly bioavailable drug allows smaller and/or less frequent dosing, which can be more readily accepted by patients.

Answer 5.9

- Pharmacokinetics is what the body does to the drug. including how it is absorbed, distributed, metabolized, and eliminated. All of these processes affect how much of the drug will be able to reach its target.
- Pharmacodynamics is the correlation between efficacy and drug concentration.
- Toxicokinetics describe the correlation between toxicity and concentration of the drug in blood.

Answer 5.10

A drug might have excellent potency in *in vitro* assays but poor activity in *in vivo* animal models due to unfavorable PK properties. Specifically, poor absorption of the compound would prevent it from being absorbed into the bloodstream or into cells. Rapid metabolism and elimination would cause the compound to be degraded or eliminated before it could reach its biological target. Unfavorable distribution properties, due to high plasma protein binding, efflux by transporters, or other mechanisms, would prevent the compound from reaching its target *in vivo*.

Chapter 6

Answer 6.1

Muscarinic acetylcholine receptors are G protein-coupled receptors that, upon binding to an agonist, relay a signal to the interior of the cell through activation of secondary messaging systems. Nicotinic acetylcholine receptors (nAChR) are Cys-loop ligand-gated ion channels that open upon binding of an agonist in order to allow passage of ions into the cell. nAChR is one of several LGICs whose action triggers a wave of depolarization down the length of nerve or muscle cells, allowing for electrochemical signaling within the nervous system.

Answer 6.2

The homologation of the phenol in isoprenaline to a benzylic alcohol and the increased steric bulk of the *tert*-butyl group (compared to the isopropyl group) contribute to the longer half-life of salbutamol due to reduced metabolism.

Answer 6.3

The three major families of ligand-gated ion channels are as follows:

1. Cys-loop receptors (pentameric)
2. Ionotropic glutamate receptors (tetrameric)
3. Purinergic ATP-gated or P2X channels (trimeric)

Answer 6.4

The class 1 (steroid) nuclear receptor superfamily includes (1) estrogen, (2) androgen, (3) progesterone, and (4) glucocorticoid receptors.

Answer 6.5

1. Na_v voltage-gated sodium ion channels are blocked by local anesthetics such as lidocaine.
2. L-type Ca_v voltage-gated calcium channels in the heart are acted upon by blockers such as nifedipine.
3. $Ca_v2.2$ channels are blocked by analgesics such as ziconotide.

Answer 6.6

Nuclear receptors share a highly conserved DNA binding domain (a zinc finger), characterized by a pattern of residues that coordinate to two zinc atoms.

Answer 6.7

1. G-protein coupled receptors (GPCR): an example is A_{2A} adenosine receptor
2. Ion channels: an example is $GABA_A$ receptor, a ligand-gated ion channel (LGIC)
3. Nuclear receptors: an example is peroxisome proliferator-activated receptor γ (PPARγ)
4. Transporters: an example is serotonin transporter

Answer 6.8

The primary difference between an agonist and an antagonist is the effect the ligand has on the activity of the receptor upon binding. After binding, an agonist will elicit a physiological response similar to that of the natural ligand. When an antagonist binds, there is no physiological response. The antagonist serves to block the natural ligand from eliciting the typical response of the receptor.

Answer 6.9

LGICs and VGICs differ on the basis of what initiates their opening and closing:

- Opening of LGICs are triggered by binding of a ligand.
- VGICs respond to changes in membrane potential.
- Neurotransmitter transporters respond to binding of the ligands they transport.

Answer 6.10

Hit identification strategies are differentiated as follows:

- Those for GPCR targets generally rely on ligand-based drug design derived from known small molecules, or screening of focused libraries, using competition binding assays. Ligand based design has the advantage of using a highly potent small molecule as a starting point. Structure-based drug design is not as common since the structures of only a few GPCRs have been solved, and the lack of understanding of the structural requirements for drugs that activate versus inactivate a receptor.

- Those for ion channel targets commonly rely on high-throughput screening, or ligand-based design (for LGICs), Screening natural products has also been productive. Like GPCRs, the lack of many high resolution structures, and challenges in understanding how binding affects activity of the channel makes SBDD a little more complex. However, as new structural information evolves, structure-based design has also become more common.

- Those for nuclear receptor targets rely on ligand-based drug design, high-throughput screening, and structure-based drug design. The availability of high resolution structures of nuclear receptors bound to ligands makes SBDD a common approach.

- Those for transporter targets rely on ligand-based drug design. Like GPCRs, the advantage of this approach is that ligands provide potent small molecule starting points. SBDD for transporters is still an emerging field.

Chapter 7

Answer 7.1

An allosteric inhibitor binds at a location on the enzyme other than the active site. It may produce a change in the shape of the protein, which then interferes with normal activity, or it can stabilize an inactive form of the protein. An active-site inhibitor binds to the active site of the enzyme, preventing substrates from binding. Active-site inhibitors are often designed to either mimic the natural substrate or take advantage of the enzyme's mechanism of action, and while this leads to a high degree of potency, it also risks a low degree of selectivity against enzymes of similar mechanism. Allosteric inhibitors, on the other hand, offer the advantage of binding at a location that is likely unique to the target enzyme, which can result in a high degree of selectivity, but this quality also makes allosteric inhibitors hard to design since each allosteric site may be unique and only evident after small molecule allosteric binders are identified. In addition, allosteric sites are prone to mutations since they are not essential for enzymatic activity.

Answer 7.2

Aspartyl proteases (and proteases in general) catalyze the hydrolysis of a substrate peptide by nucleophilic attack by water on an sp^2 carbon to generate an sp^3-hybridized tetrahedral intermediate transition state. This transition state is stabilized in the active site. Effective inhibitors that mimic the features of this transition state but are stable, transition state mimetics, are recognized by the enzyme and bind tightly to it, preventing substrate from binding. For example, a series of HIV protease inhibitors, including darunavir, lopinavir, saquinavir, and indinavir, are all transition-state mimetics.

Answer 7.3

Transition-state mimetics are not often used as a strategy for kinase inhibitor design, because the transition state of the kinase mechanism involves a pentavalent phosphate carrying multiple negative charges. This is not a structure that can be easily mimicked by standard organic small molecules.

Answer 7.4

Serine proteases are characterized by a Ser-His-Asp catalytic triad that activates the serine. Shown below is a serine protease (black) that forms a covalent bond to an aldehyde inhibitor (red), with the tetrahedral intermediate stabilized in the oxyanion hole of the enzyme.

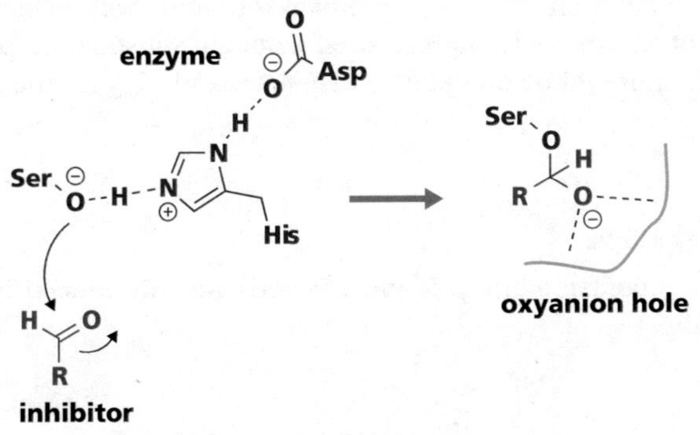

Answer 7.5

Enzymes are druggable targets for the following reasons:

1. Assay development for hit identification and optimization is generally straightforward due to the ability to isolate pure enzymes in significant quantities.

2. Established enzyme kinetics principles allow for thorough characterization of mechanism of action and kinetic parameters of inhibitors and activators.

3. Existing knowledge of the natural substrates and mechanisms of reaction of enzymes can be used to design substrate mimics and transition-state analogs, and are usually promising starting points for hit- and lead-based drug discovery.

4. The structures of enzymes and enzyme–inhibitor complexes can often be solved by various crystallographic or spectroscopic methods that provide opportunities for virtual screening and structure-based approaches to drug design and discovery.

Answer 7.6

The lock and key model proposes that enzymes and their substrates are of rigid, precise complementary shapes, such that only substrates (keys) of precise shapes and sizes will fit into the active sites (locks) to allow the enzymatic reactions to occur. In contrast, the induced-fit model proposes that enzymes and substrates are both flexible and that, as a substrate begins to bind and make specific interactions with an enzyme, the active site repositions to accommodate it until the catalytic groups are poised for reaction. The dynamic nature of proteins and the concept that enzymes stabilize transition states both support the induced-fit model. Additionally, X-ray crystallography often shows considerable conformational changes of protein structures after substrate binding, again supporting the induced-fit model.

Answer 7.7

The ATP-binding site of a kinase has three main features: the hinge region that contains the 'gatekeeper' residue, a hydrophilic pocket, and an activation loop consisting of two amino acid triads. The hinge region forms a series of hydrogen bonds with the adenine base, while the hydrophilic pocket holds the furanose and triphosphate of the ATP molecule. The activation loop acts as a door that controls the flow of substrate and can be opened and closed through phosphorylation of the kinase. Most kinases are more efficient upon phosphorylation of the activation loop.

Answer 7.8

Proximity and orientation effects are two global strategies whereby enzymes accelerate reaction rates. Bringing reactants together (proximity) and in optimal alignment for reaction (orientation) in the active site of an enzyme leads to considerable rate enhancement compared to a nonenzymatic reaction. Understanding these strategies can help in developing inhibitors that can prevent substrate binding to an enzyme.

Answer 7.9

The measured inhibition of a competitive inhibitor will decrease when the concentration of substrate is increased. If enough substrate is present, then a competitive inhibitor will be completely displaced and V_{max} for the enzyme can be reached.

Answer 7.10

- Solubilizing groups:

An N-methyl piperazine group (shown in red) was introduced into imatinib to improve solubility.

imatinib

- Isosteres: The pyridine rings in piclamilast and roflumilast are isosteric replacements for the pyrrolidinone in rolipram (shown in red). Additionally, roflumilast contains a CHF_2 isosteric replacement for a CH_3 substituent in rolipram (shown in blue).

rolipram   **piclamilast**   **roflumilast**

- Privileged structures: Dasatanib contains a heteroarylpiperidine (shown in green), and nevirapine contains a pseudo-benzodiazepine (shown in red).

dasatanib   **nevirapine**

Chapter 8

Answer 8.1

Many of the physiological effects of enzymes and receptors are mediated by small druglike molecules (natural substrates and ligands), and therefore, these targets contain high affinity binding sites that can be occupied by small molecule drugs. These binding sites, often a deep pocket that can accommodate specific polar and hydrophobic interactions, have characteristics that favor binding by small molecules.

In contrast, large flat hydrophobic surfaces mediate the biological effects of lipids and PPIs. Interrupting or mimicking these interfaces by a small molecule can be challenging.

Answer 8.2

When a protein is isolable, common biophysical methods used to detect binding of a small molecule include those that measure differences in size or other physical characteristics between bound and unbound complex. These include surface plasmon resonance (SPR), which detects refractive indices, and can be used to monitor changes in size of a protein when it is bound to a small molecule vs. free, and can determine binding constants. Mass spectrometry (MS) can also detect the molecular mass of a protein complexed to a small molecule. Isothermal calorimetry (ITC) measures the heat given off when a small molecule binds to a protein, and can be used to calculate ΔH and ΔS of binding interactions. Other methods include nuclear magnetic resonance spectroscopy, which detects changes in resonances of one or both of the binding partners upon binding due to changes in their environment, and X-ray crystallography and cryo-electron microscopy, which can provide an atomic scale view of the small molecule bound to the protein.

Answer 8.3

Protein–protein interfaces are relatively flat with large surface areas. High affinity binding between two proteins is usually the result of numerous weak interactions.

Answer 8.4

Fragment-based screening has been successful since it can detect low affinity binders, and these can be further optimized. Structure based design, whereby the structure and bioactive conformation of one of the binding partners is mimicked (often through conformational constraint strategies) by a small molecule is another successful approach. Finally, screening of natural products has led to many examples of small molecules that modulate PPIs.

Answer 8.5

Hot spots are areas of the binding interface or specific residues that contribute more to the binding energy of a protein–protein interaction compared to other sites/residues. When a PPI contains a hot spot, there is a greater potential that small molecules that bind to these regions can compete for binding with the larger protein partner. Identification of hot spots by computational methods can suggest specific regions of the large PPI surface to target.

Answer 8.6

Drug design to target lipids is particularly challenging due to a lack of understanding of how lipid composition affects membranes and proteins, as well as the dynamic nature of the lipid bilayer. In addition much of the interactions involve general (vs. specific) hydrophobic interactions. Many of the drugs that target lipid structures are poorly understood, so applying common strategies to other lipid targets is not possible, and few methods are available to study the highly dynamic lipid bilayers in their natural setting. Without this understanding, it is difficult to design drugs that target lipids as well as to understand their mechanism of action.

Answer 8.7

An interfacial binder is a small molecule that forms a ternary complex with the two protein partners at their interface, and locks the proteins in a nonproductive conformation.

Answer 8.8

See figure on next page and Figure 8.5.

COMPOUNDS INCORPORATING CONFORMATIONAL CONSTRAINT
(CONSTRAINING RING SHOWN IN RED)

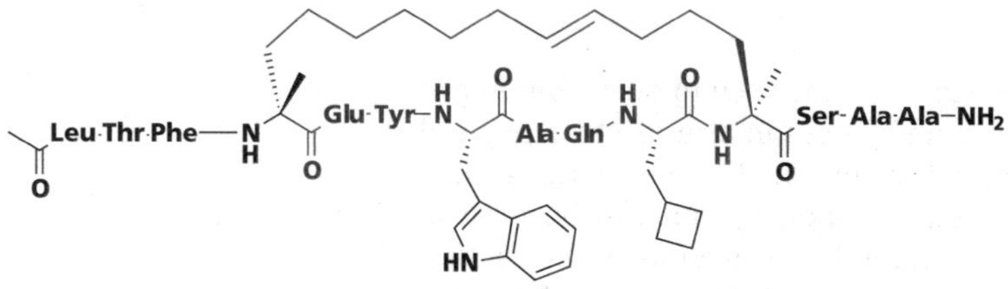

COMPOUNDS CONTAINING A PRIVILEGED STRUCTURE
(PRIVILEGED STRUCTURE SHOWN IN RED)

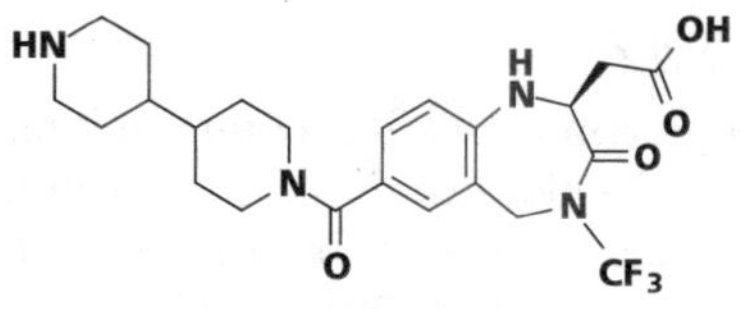

stapled peptide ATSP-7041

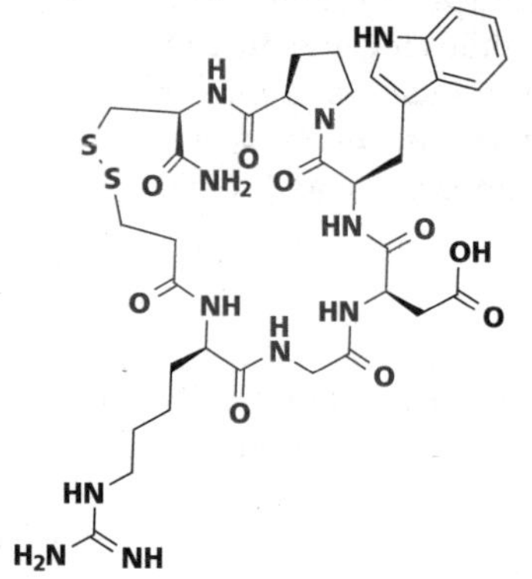

lotrafiban

eptifibatide

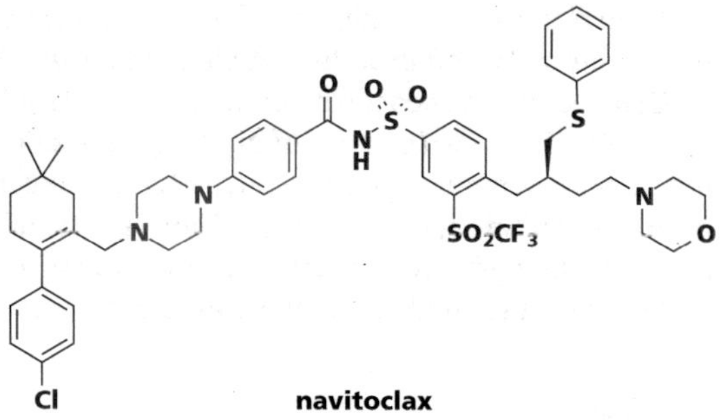

navitoclax

Answer 8.9

A stapled peptide refers to a short peptide constrained by a hydrocarbon bridge or other synthetic "staple" that connects the two ends of the peptide. The staple maintains the short peptide in a helical conformation that is required for bioactivity. It will often improve the protease stability of the compound, compared to the linear peptide, as well as other properties such as cellular penetration.

Answer 8.10

The only structural differences between ergosterol and cholesterol are the incorporation of a double bond to form a conjugated π-system within the ring system and the incorporation of an olefin and a methyl group within the aliphatic chain. These differences are highlighted in red.

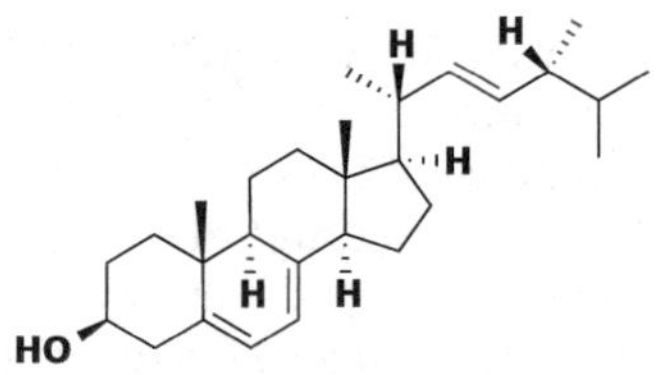

ergosterol

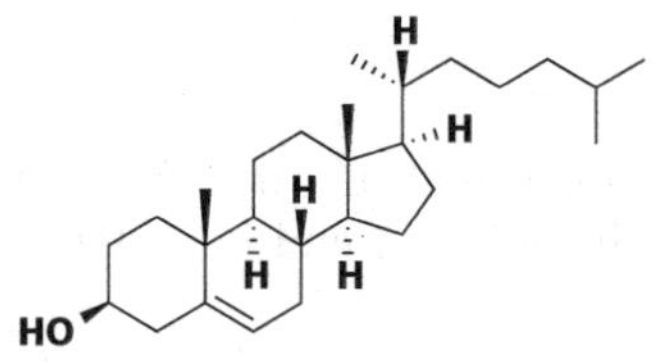

cholesterol

Chapter 9
Answer 9.1

1. Intercalation: Intercalators insert between the DNA base pairs. They exhibit little sequence specificity and bind primarily through π–π stacking with the nucleobases. Intercalators are typically planar aromatic structures.

2. Groove binding: Groove binders sit in one of the grooves of the DNA double helix, most frequently the minor groove. Minor-groove binders hydrogen-bond with the bases making up the floor of the groove and utilize other electrostatic and hydrophobic interactions with the sugar–phosphate backbone. They are typically bent in shape and contain a number of H-bond donors and acceptors. As a class, groove binders may exhibit some sequence specificity compared to intercalators.

Answer 9.2

Classes of DNA alkylators can be characterized by their reactive electrophiles.

1. Nitrogen mustards generate an aziridinium ion.

$$\text{DNA} \diagup\diagdown \overset{\overset{\text{R}}{|}}{\underset{\text{R}}{\text{N}}}$$

2. Nitrosoureas generate a diazonium ion.

$$\text{DNA} \diagup \text{R}$$

3. Sulfonates are electrophilic and don't require further activation.

$$\text{DNA} \diagup \text{R}$$

4. Aziridines are electrophilic and don't require further activation.

$$\text{DNA} \diagup\diagdown \overset{\overset{\text{H}}{|}}{\text{N}}{-}\text{R}$$

5. Triazines generate a diazonium ion.

$$\text{DNA} \diagup \text{R}$$

Answer 9.3

Upon alkylation of the nucleobase, the adduct is electrophilic and can react with water, which generates additional labile adducts, that then go on to ring opening of the base and eventual cleavage of the furanose, resulting in DNA strand breaking.

Answer 9.4

The middle structure has the aromatic, planar character typically associated with intercalators. Intercalators insert between DNA base pairs and make noncovalent interactions, primarily π-stacking interactions. The first compound, while possessing one aromatic ring, does not have the extended π-system that is typical of intercalators.

Answer 9.5

Drugs that bind to, alkylate, cleave, or nick DNA usually do not discriminate between DNA in healthy cells and DNA in disease-affected cells. Therefore, they will have the same effects on all proliferating cells including immune cells, cells in the gastrointestinal tract, and hair follicles as they do on abnormal cancer cells. This lack of discrimination produces toxicity in addition to anti-cancer effects. In addition, sometimes binding to DNA causes the DNA to mutate and results in cancer years later.

Answer 9.6

DNA strand breakers and nicking agents both bind to DNA and cause a break in the DNA strand. A nicking agent results in single-strand cleavage, while a strand breaker results in double-strand cleavage; both lead to incomplete duplication, transcription, and translation. Bleomycin is an example of a strand breaker.

Answer 9.7

The mechanism of sulfur mustards is analogous to the reaction of nitrogen mustards. A highly reactive sulfonium ion is formed, and reacts with nucleophilic nitrogen atoms in nucleobases. After one reaction with DNA occurs, a second sulfonium ion can form, and a second reaction can occur to cross-link the DNA.

Answer 9.8

1. Melting temperature reflects the stability of a nucleic acid double helix; as temperature is increased the helix denatures and the temperature at which half the helix is denatured is the Tm. When a small molecule binds to DNA, it will change its Tm. Changes in the melting temperature are observed and reflect either stabilization (higher melting Tm) or destabilization (lower melting Tm) when compounds bind.

2. Fluorescent assays use a fluorescent probe that binds to the nucleic acid. If the small molecule disrupts the binding of the probe, changes in fluorescence are noted.

Answer 9.9

Antisense drugs must be recognized by complementary RNA strands and often by RNA-degrading enzymes; therefore, they must mimic RNA. In order to be selective, they must consist of at least ~20 nucleotides. However, they also need to be permeable and stable, characteristics that traditional nucleic acid oligomers do not possess. Therefore in designing antisense molecules one must maintain sufficient similarity to the natural nucleotides so that the compounds are recognized by the template and relevant enzymes, but modify them so they do not carry the same instability and lack of permeability as typical nucleotide oligomers.

Answer 9.10

DNA alkylating agents are often delivered as prodrugs to prevent the active form of the drug from reacting with other nucleophiles in the body before it reaches the site of action. If it reacts nonspecifically with proteins or nucleophiles, rather than the intended target, higher toxicity usually results, as does lack of efficacy.

Chapter 10

Answer 10.1

Drugs that target DNA directly are intrinsically more toxic because DNA is found in all cells: cancer cells, normal replicating cells such as immune cells and those found in the GI tract, and cells that do not replicate. Therefore, depending on their mechanism, these drugs have the potential to damage all cells, not just cancer cells. On the other hand, drugs that target oncogenic proteins usually interact only with mutated proteins that drive a cancer phenotype and have less affinity for native proteins. Because of this high selectivity, drugs that target oncogenic proteins exhibit fewer toxic side effects compared to drugs that target DNA directly.

Answer 10.2

MG 132 in chymotrypsin-like site

MG 132 in caspase-like site

Answer 10.3

Kinase inhibitors are specifically amenable to structure-based design because the co-structures of many kinase targets have already been solved by X-ray crystallography. These enzymes are often easy to isolate and therefore are amenable to characterization and structure elucidation. Furthermore, there is high homology among kinases and the ATP-binding sites are often highly conserved, so inhibitor design can be based on what is known about other kinases even when the structure is not known.

Answer 10.4

The ethynyl moiety in ponatinib allows it to be effective against an important resistance mutation, Bcr-Abl(T315I), often observed after treatment with other Bcr-Abl kinase inhibitors such as imatinib. The mutation changes a Thr to an Ile. This change eliminates an important H-bond between Thr and the inhibitors and also introduces steric bulk that blocks access to a binding pocket. The small ethynyl moiety can accommodate the larger Ile side chain and allows access to the binding pocket. It also makes favorable binding interactions with both Thr315 and Ile315, found in native and mutant Bcr-Abl, respectively, and constrains the molecule into a favorable binding pose, providing gains in entropy.

Answer 10.5

Natural products are a frequent source of cancer drugs for two primary reasons: the simplicity of cytotoxicity assays and the innate optimization that occurs within the organisms of origin for properties such as permeability and potency. Cell-based anti-proliferative and cytotoxicity assays are readily applied to bioassay-guided fractionation, a method used to identify the active components of crude natural product extracts, due to the simplicity of the assays. Furthermore, cytotoxicity assays are frequently used as primary assays in cancer drug discovery programs. Because the production of these active compounds evolved as defense mechanisms for the organism, they also are typically already optimized for cell permeability and toxicity, which accelerates the process between lead discovery and clinical drug development. While there are a number of possible examples in the chapter, the table below describes five cancer drugs that were derived from natural products.

Drug	Mechanism
Taxol (paclitaxel)	tubulin stabilizer
doxorubicin	DNA intercalator
topotecan (derived from camptothecin)	topoisomerase I inhibitor
carfilzomib (derived from epoxomicin)	proteosome inhibitor
temsirolimus (derived from rapamycin)	mTOR inhibitor

Answer 10.6

1. FdUMP (derived from administering 5-FU) acts as a suicide inhibitor of the enzyme thymidylate synthase (TS). The presence of a fluorine atom prevents elimination, thus terminating the reaction pathway.

2. 5-Azacytidine, once incorporated in the DNA chain, serves as a suicide inhibitor of the enzyme DNA methyltransferase. It contains an unnatural base and forms a stable covalent bond to the enzyme, rendering it ineffective.

Answer 10.7

For cancers that exhibit hormone-responsive tumors, hormone receptor antagonists can act to reduce tumor growth. Hormone replacement therapy (HRT) raises the overall concentration of the hormone in the body and can promote the growth of tumor cells responsive to the hormone.

Answer 10.8

Temsirolimus and everolimus are semisynthetic ester and ether analogs of rapamycin, respectively, with improved physical properties. They bind to the protein FKBP12, and the resulting macromolecular complex binds to and inhibits a mammalian target of rapamycin (mTOR) protein. This prevents mTOR, a kinase, from phosphorylating downstream proteins and halts the signaling pathway.

Answer 10.9

Anti-cancer agents that target cell proliferation are sometimes also useful anti-inflammatory and immunosuppressant agents. Nonselective anti-proliferative agents prevent the growth of all proliferating cells, including immune cells. Diseases characterized by an inappropriate immune response and/or strong inflammatory response such as multiple sclerosis and rheumatoid arthritis can be treated by certain anti-proliferative agents since they stop the growth of immune cells.

Answer 10.10

Given are four possible examples:

1. 5-FU is an analog of the natural substrate uracil that contains a fluorine atom in place of a hydrogen.

uracil   **5-FU**

2. 5-Azacytidine contains a nitrogen as an isosteric replacement of the carbon in cytidine.

cytidine   **5-azacytidine**

3. Aminopterin, a DHFR inhibitor, contains a secondary amine. Pemetrexed incorporates a -CH$_2$- group as an isosteric replacement.

aminopterin   **pemetrexed**

4. Bortezomib, a proteasome inhibitor, contains a boronic acid, which is a non-classical isostere for an aldehyde.

aldehyde   **bortezomib**

Chapter 11

Answer 11.1

Valacyclovir and sofosbuvir are antiviral prodrugs. The prodrug portion of each compound is highlighted in red. Valacyclovir is an ester prodrug that improves the oral bioavailability of acyclovir. Sofosbuvir is a phosphoramide that is converted *in vivo* to the monophosphate. The monophosphate itself would not be absorbed due to its charged nature. By delivering the monophosphate, the slow monophosphorylation step catalyzed by kinases is bypassed.

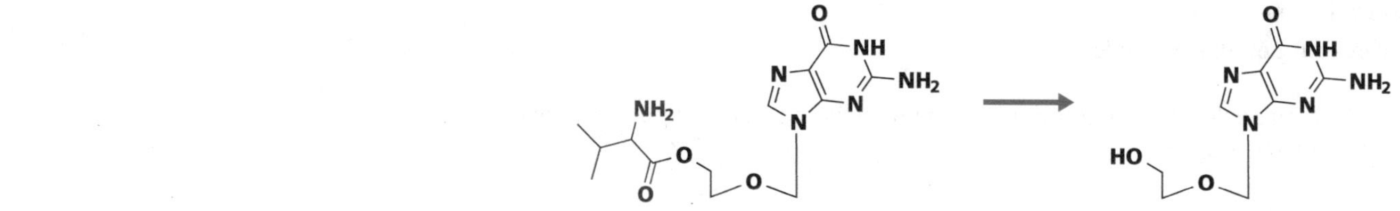

valacyclovir
(prodrug)
HSV, VZV

acyclo-guanosine
(acyclovir)

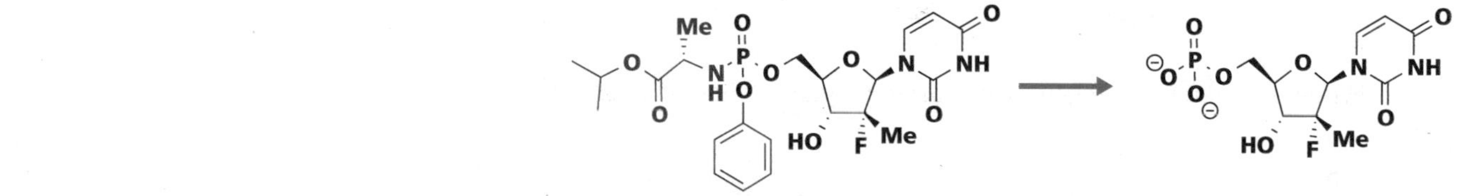

sofosbuvir
(prodrug)
HCV

sofosbuvir
(monophosphate)

Answer 11.2

Nucleoside reverse transcriptase inhibitors (NRTIs) are nucleoside analogs that, once converted to the triphosphate, target the viral enzyme reverse transcriptase. NRTIs are considered competitive inhibitors that act by becoming incorporated in the growing viral DNA chain and causing chain termination. Azidothymidine (AZT) is an example of an NRTI used to treat HIV.

Nonnucleoside reverse transcriptase inhibitors (NNRTIs) also inhibit the viral enzyme reverse transcriptase; however, NNRTIs are allosteric inhibitors that do not bind to the active site. This mechanism often leads to the rapid emergence of resistance to many NNRTIs. Nevirapine is an example of an NNRTI.

Answer 11.3

Three possible answers are maraviroc, which is an entry/fusion inhibitor; azidothymidine, which inhibits HIV reverse transcriptase; and elvitegravir, an inhibitor of the viral integrase.

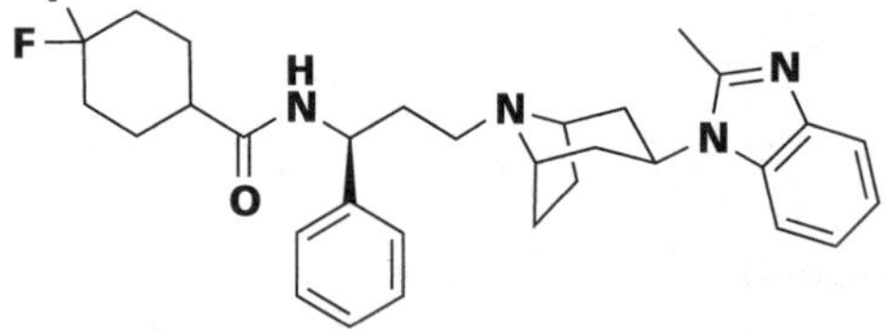

maraviroc
(HIV)

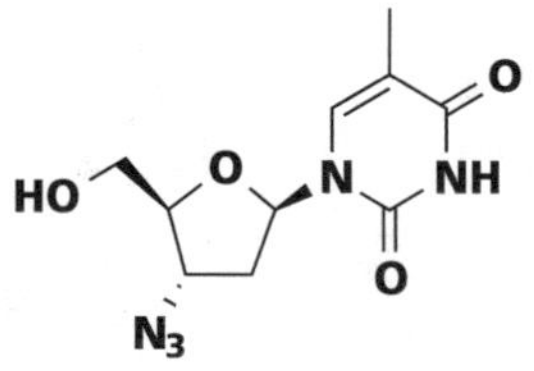

azidothymidine
(HIV)

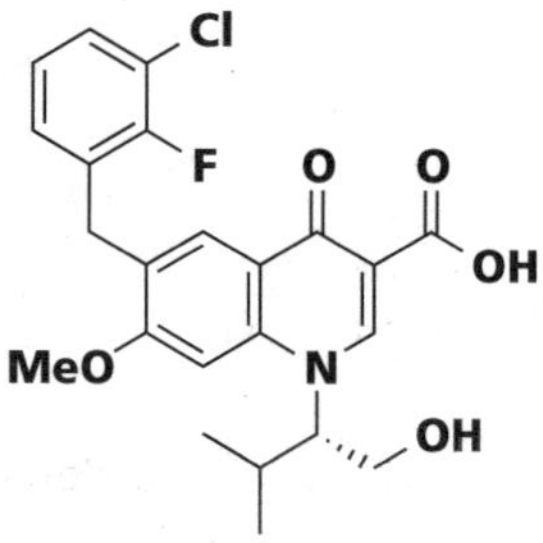

elvitegravir
(HIV)

Answer 11.4

The mechanism of action of polyene antifungal drugs involves a selective lipid–lipid interaction with ergosterol, a steroid found in the inner cell membrane of fungi. This interaction causes sequestration of ergosterol, ultimately leading to cell death.

Azole antifungal drugs also act at the fungal cell membrane; however, the mechanism of action involves inhibition of ergosterol biosynthesis. Azole antifungal drugs inhibit the enzyme sterol 14α-demethylase, a key enzyme in the biosynthesis of ergosterol.

Answer 11.5

The protein target, HS5A, exists as as symmetrical dimer, and it is believed that the symmetrical nature of inhibitors is based on their binding to the dimeric protein target.

Answer 11.6

One reason there are fewer small-molecule drugs to treat viral and fungal infections than bacterial infections is because there are fewer drug targets. Viruses often use host enzymes to replicate and therefore there are fewer viral-specific drug targets compared to bacteria. Fungal cells are very similar to human cells, and have even fewer unique enzymes, and therefore potential fungal drug targets are limited.

Answer 11.7

Nucleoside drugs are often toxic because they have low selectivity in targeting viral polymerases over the host polymerase. Acyclovir is surprisingly nontoxic as a nucleoside drug because it is selectively activated in virally infected cells. Acyclovir is phosphorylated by viral thymidine kinase but not by mammalian kinases, and thus its triphosphate is generated only in virally infected cells.

Answer 11.8

Amantadine is approved for the treatment of influenza A. It binds to the viral M2 protein, which forms a proton ion channel specific to influenza A that is involved in the early stages of viral uncoating. Amantadine physically blocks the pore of the M2 ion channel.

Answer 11.9

Maraviroc has been approved for the treatment of HIV. It prevents binding between of surface glycoprotein gp120 and co-receptor CCR5, preventing the HIV viral membrane from fusing with the host T-cell membrane.

maraviroc
(HIV)

Answer 11.10

Amphotericin B is a polyene antifungal drug used to treat serious fungal infections. Its mechanism of action involves a selective lipid–lipid interaction with ergosterol, a steroid found in the inner cell membrane of fungi. This interaction results in the sequestration of ergosterol, which compromises the protective nature of the membrane, ultimately resulting in cell death.

Answer 11.11

Examples of natural products include griseofulvin, amphotericin B, and echinocandin B (antifungals) and spongothymidine (antiviral). Griseofulvin and amphotericin B are used clinically. Echinocandin B and spongothymidine were the inspiration for approved drugs.

NATURAL PRODUCT

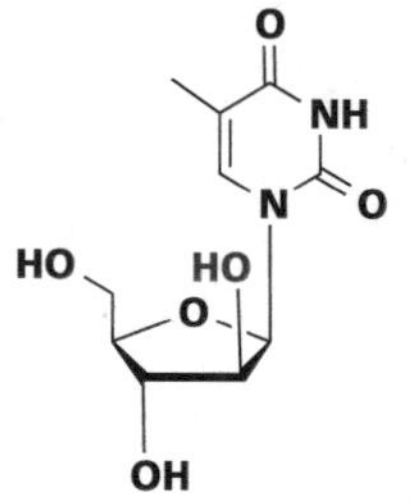

spongothymidine:
related to acyclovir

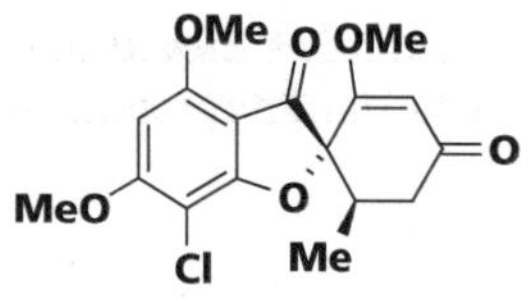

griseofulvin

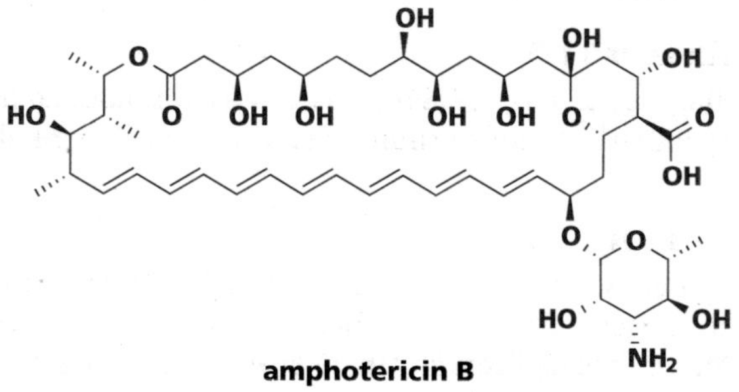

amphotericin B

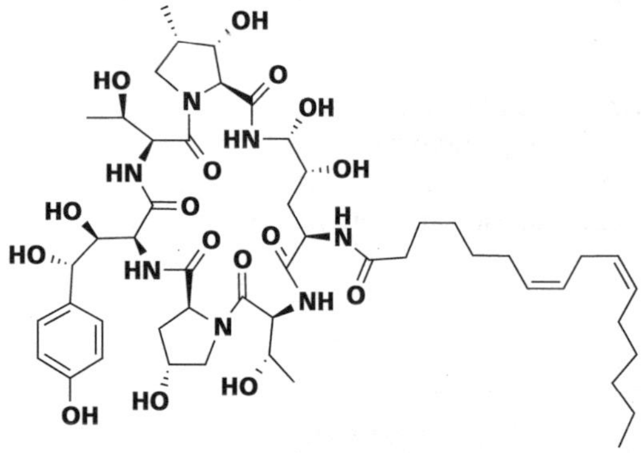

echinocandin B:
related to anidulafungin

Chapter 12

Answer 12.1

Three mechanisms of antibacterial agents include inhibition of cell-wall biosynthesis, inhibition of bacterial protein synthesis, and interfering with cell membrane permeability.

1. The bacterial cell wall is made of cross-linked peptidoglycan strands. Blocking bacterial cell-wall biosynthesis weakens the cell wall, eventually killing the bacteria. Drugs working through this mechanism include the β-lactam antibacterial agents, such as penicillins and cephalosporins. These directly inhibit penicillin-binding protein, an essential bacterial enzyme involved in cell-wall biosynthesis that catalyzes the cross-linking of peptidoglycan strands. Another mechanism by which drugs inhibit cell-wall biosynthesis is through binding to the peptidoglycan substrate. Vancomycin and its related analogs act in this manner.

2. Bacterial protein synthesis inhibitors act on the bacterial ribosome and interfere with protein synthesis. Compounds that work via this mechanism include aminoglycosides, tetracyclines, erythromycins, and oxazolidinones. They bind to the ribosome and this leads to an accumulation of inaccurately synthesized bacterial proteins, arrest of protein synthesis, and eventual cell death.

3. Drugs that affect cell membrane permeability include the polymyxins and daptomycin. Both classes interact with the lipid bilayer of the cell membrane, causing leakage of cellular components.

Answer 12.2

Quinolones inhibit DNA gyrase, which is a topoisomerase responsible for cleaving DNA to release coiling as well as introducing negative superhelical turns. The enzyme is required during DNA replication. Quinolones target DNA gyrase by binding to the DNA–DNA gyrase complex to form a ternary complex, which poisons the enzyme.

Sulfonamides prevent DNA synthesis by interfering with the biosynthesis of required coenzymes. They are alternate substrates for dihydropteroate synthase, an enzyme required for the synthesis of the coenzyme tetrahydrofolic acid. The sulfonamides mimic the natural substrate, p-aminobenzoic acid (PABA), and displace the diphosphate of dihydropteroate diphosphate. With a sulfonamide group in place of an acid moiety, the subsequent steps of the synthesis cannot take place and tetrahydrofolic acid is not formed.

Answer 12.3

Three classes of cell-wall synthesis inhibitors that act by covalent binding are penicillins, cephalosporins, and monobactams. All inhibit penicillin-binding protein by reaction of the β-lactam with the active-site serine and contain a β-lactam moiety.

1. Penicillins are bicyclic β-lactams with the lactam ring fused to a five-membered thiazolidine ring.

2. Cephalosporins differ from penicillins in replacement of the five-membered thiazolidine ring with a six-membered dihydrothiazine ring.

3. Monobactams are monocyclic β-lactams. In each case, the β-lactam structure is shown in red.

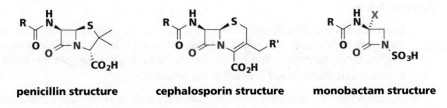

penicillin structure   **cephalosporin structure**   **monobactam structure**

Answer 12.4

Two mechanisms used by bacteria to resist penicillins are production of β-lactamase and production of mutant PBPs. β-Lactamase is an enzyme whose sole purpose is to hydrolyze the β-lactam warhead of penicillin and render the drug inactive. It serves no physiological role in the enzyme. Mutant PBPs maintain the capabilities to catalyze cell-wall biosynthesis but they have a reduced affinity for penicillins, which allows bacteria to avoid effects of the drug.

Answer 12.5

Compared to Gram-positive bacteria, Gram-negative bacteria have an additional outer membrane that contains lipopolysaccharide (LPS) and pore proteins (porins). Both have a peptidoglycan layer, but in Gram-positive bacteria, this is larger. In Gram-negative bacteria, this is a thinner layer (about 10% peptidoglycan) and sits below the outer membrane.

Drugs might be effective against one and not the other due to differences in their ability to penetrate the different cell walls. Some antibacterial drugs can easily cross Gram-positive cell walls but not Gram-negative cell walls; some enter Gram-negative cells through porins, which are not present in Gram-positive bacteria. Resistance may develop differently in Gram-positive versus Gram-negative bacteria, which may also account for differences. Mutations in porins may reduce the efficacy of some drugs toward Gram-negative bacteria, but they may still be effective toward Gram-positive bacteria if they have an alternate mechanism for cell penetration.

Answer 12.6

Neglected tropical diseases are diseases that often affect those living in poverty, in close contact with infectious vectors, and without adequate sanitation. They are neglected because these diseases are nearly eradicated in more developed parts of the world where access to clean water and safe food, and exposure to infectious vectors is not a primary concern. Because of the specific environments where these diseases are prevalent, drug discovery programs geared toward neglected tropical diseases must consider that the cost should be low, the length of treatment short, and administration of the drug convenient so as to assure compliance.

Answer 12.7

Two classes of drugs used to treat malaria are those based on quinine and those based on artemisinin.

1. Quinine-based antimalarial drugs inhibit hemozoin crystallization in the blood, which results in toxic buildup of heme, ultimately killing the parasite.

2. The mechanism of action of artemisinin-based antimalarial drugs, although not fully understood, involves bioactivation by heme iron to generate reactive oxygen species (ROS), which inhibit hemozoin formation and damage cellular targets in the parasite.

Answer 12.8

Advances in genome sequencing of parasitic organisms and an increase in private–public partnerships to support drug discovery for neglected tropical diseases are both responsible for an increase in the efforts to identify drugs to treat parasitic diseases.

Answer 12.9

1. Ivermectin is a semisynthetic derivative of the natural product avermectin, differing only by reduction of a double bond. It is used to treat river blindness and elephantiasis. Its mechanism involves modulation of parasite-specific chloride ion channels, which leads to death of the organism.

2. Pentamidine can be traced to bisguanidines that were present in a plant used for medicinal purposes in medieval Europe. It is used to treat African trypanosomiasis and leishmaniasis. Its mechanism has not been clarified.

3. Artemisinin, a natural product, and the reduced semisynthetic analog artemether are used to treat malaria. The mechanism of action is still not fully defined but involves bioactivation by heme iron to generate reactive oxygen species (ROS). The free radicals inhibit hemozoin formation and damage cellular targets in the parasite.

Answer 12.10

Drugs targeting bacterial DNA replication are often similar to those used in anti-cancer drug discovery because the bacterial enzymes being targeted have human homologs. For example, quinolones inhibit DNA gyrase, a topoisomerase involved in the bacterial replication process. Inhibitors of the homologous human topoisomerase are effective anti-cancer agents. Another example is the sulfonamides, which inhibit dihydropteroate synthase, an enzyme in the bacterial folic acid biosynthesis pathway. Inhibitors of the related human dihydrofolate reductase are also effective anti-cancer agents and work by preventing the synthesis of a key coenzyme.

Chapter 13

Answer 13.1

The blood–brain barrier (BBB) is a unique barrier between the brain and bloodstream, made up of tightly packed endothelial cells that are denser than the membranes surrounding other cell structures. This barrier protects the brain from toxins and infectious agents and also adds an additional barrier for CNS agents to penetrate. Many drugs that can penetrate cells from other organs cannot penetrate the BBB; therefore, CNS drug discovery must take into account these stricter permeability constraints. Some drugs that do penetrate the BBB are substrates for the P-glycoprotein transporter. These drugs are effluxed out of the brain by the transporter.

Answer 13.2

CNS-active drugs must be able penetrate the BBB. They generally exhibit a lower molecular weight, higher lipophilicity, contain fewer H-bond donors/acceptors, and have a smaller polar surface area than drugs acting at other organ systems.

Answer 13.3

Three classes of antidepressants with different mechanisms of action are SSRIs, SNRIs, and 5-HT$_{1A}$ partial agonists. An example of a drug from each class is shown: citalopram is an SSRI, reboxetine is an SNRI and buspirone is a 5-HT$_{1A}$ partial agonist.

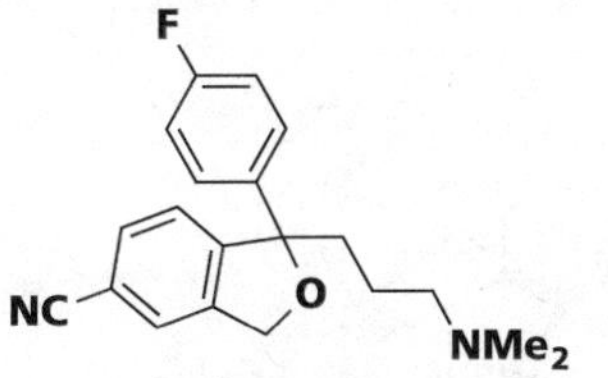

citalopram

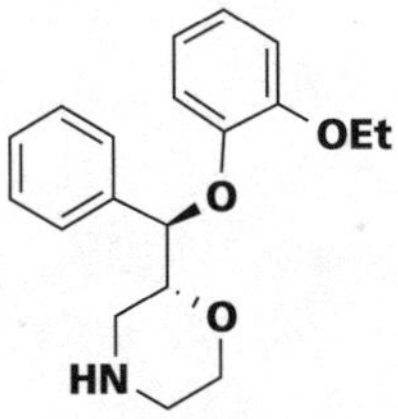

reboxetine

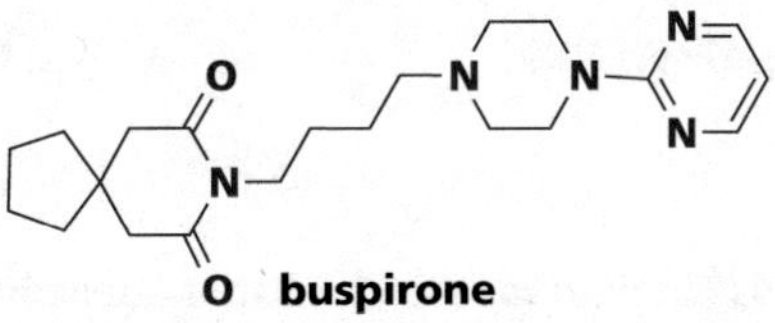

buspirone

Answer 13.4

Five possible examples of neurotransmitters are (1) serotonin (5-HT, 5-hydroxytryptamine), (2) dopamine, (3) epinephrine, (4) glutamic acid, and (5) γ-aminobutyric acid (GABA):

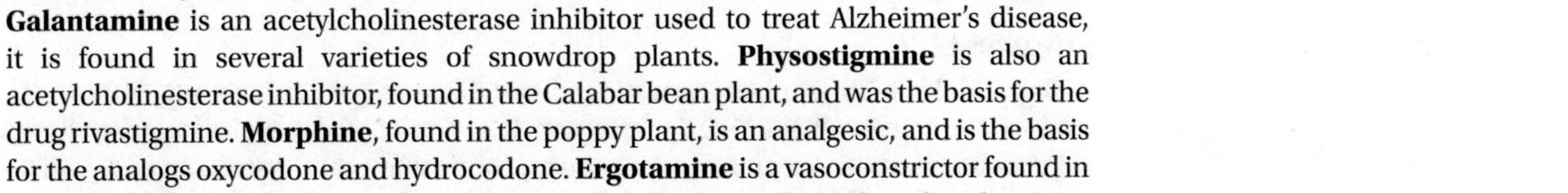

serotonin (5-HT)   **dopamine**   **epinephrine**   **glutamic acid**   **γ-aminobutyric acid (GABA)**

Answer 13.5

Several examples of natural products that have significant CNS effects are given. **Galantamine** is an acetylcholinesterase inhibitor used to treat Alzheimer's disease, it is found in several varieties of snowdrop plants. **Physostigmine** is also an acetylcholinesterase inhibitor, found in the Calabar bean plant, and was the basis for the drug rivastigmine. **Morphine**, found in the poppy plant, is an analgesic, and is the basis for the analogs oxycodone and hydrocodone. **Ergotamine** is a vasoconstrictor found in the ergot fungus, and was used to treat migraines. **Apomorphine**, found in the water lily, is a dopamine agonist used to treat Parkinson's disease. **Tetrahydrocannabinol** (THC) is found in *Cannabis sativa*, and has been used to treat nausea.

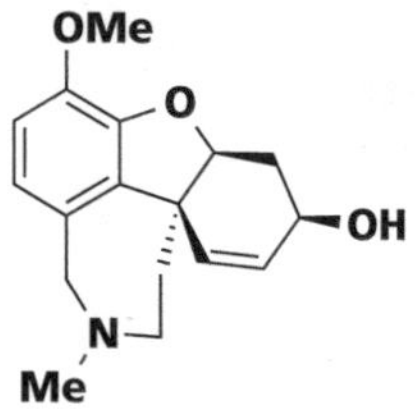

galantamine

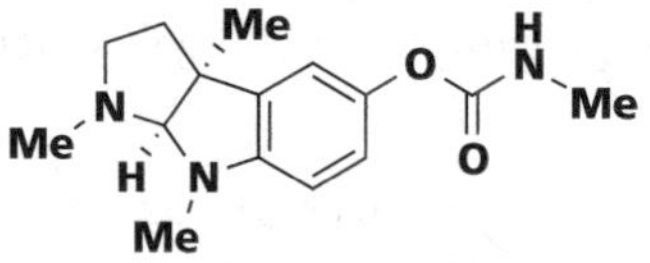

physostigmine

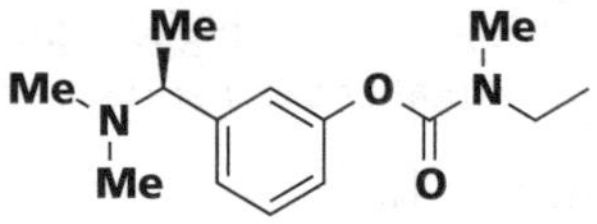

rivastigmine

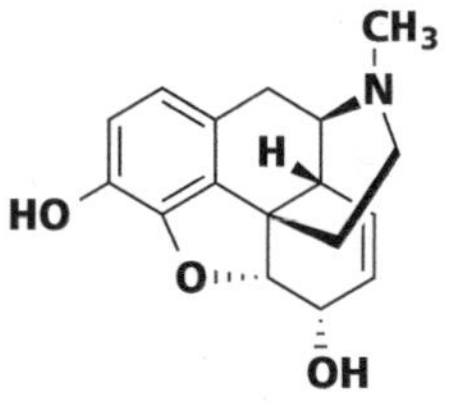

morphine

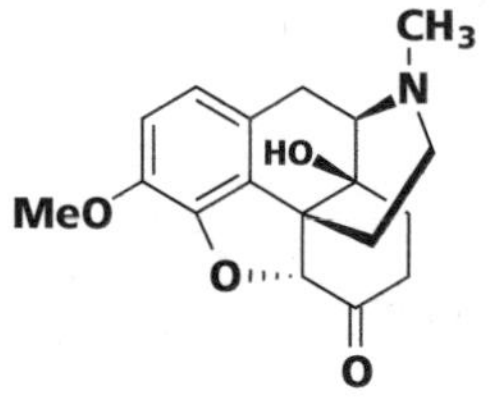

oxycodone

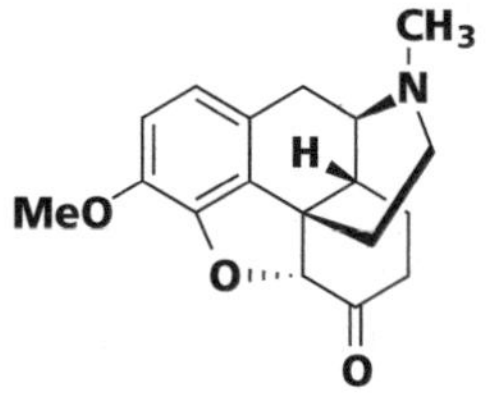

hydrocodone

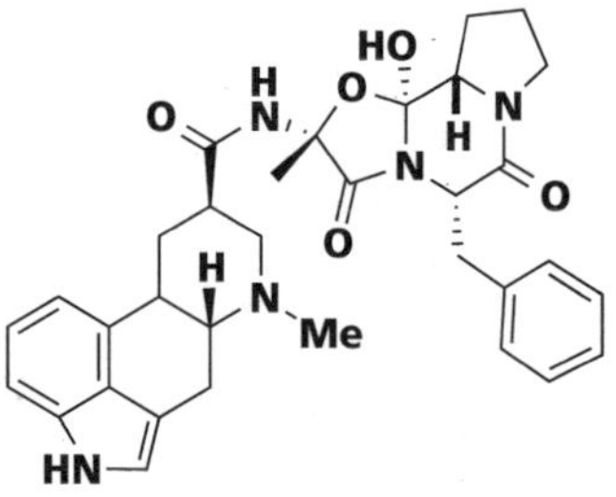

ergotamine

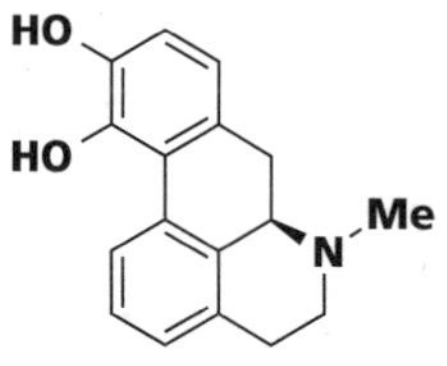

apomorphine

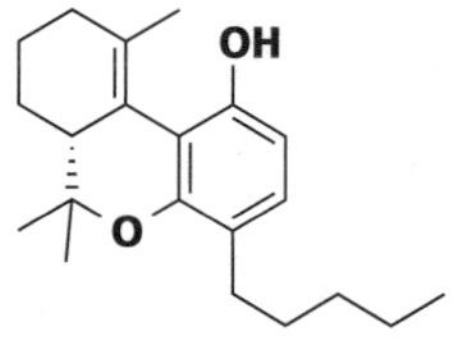

Δ^9-THC (tetrahydrocannabinol)

Answer 13.6

1. Opiates are one class of pain medications that are agonists at the opioid receptors, which are GPCRs. There are three subtypes of opioid receptors, μ, δ, and κ, and agonism of the μ receptor is principally responsible for pain reduction. Activity at the other subtypes leads to additional effects including addiction; thus, efforts to develop subtype-specific drugs have been made.

2. Nonsteroidal anti-inflammatory Drugs (NSAIDs) are another class of pain medications used to treat nociceptive pain. NSAIDs inhibit cyclooxygenase (COX), which is an enzyme involved in prostaglandin H_2 synthesis, thus leading to their anti-inflammatory properties.

3. Selective ion-channel blockers are a newer class of pain medications. One example is ziconotide, a peptide isolated from the cone snail that is administered intrathecally. It blocks the N-type calcium channel $Ca_v2.2$. Other channel blockers are currently under investigation for treatment of neuropathic pain. Several agents that selectively target subtype 1.7 of the voltage-gated sodium channel ($Na_v1.7$) are in clinical trials.

Answer 13.7

Haloperidol is a butyrophenone antipsychotic that acts primarily as a D_2 antagonist, with some activity at the 5-HT$_{2A}$ receptor. It is considered a typical antipsychotic. Olanzapine is a benzazepine atypical antipsychotic that exhibits stronger antagonism against D_4 than D_2 receptors, as well as antagonism of the 5-HT$_{2A}$ receptor. The advantage of olanzapine over haloperidol is that it presents a much lower incidence of EPS while also providing more effective treatment of both negative and positive symptoms of schizophrenia. It is considered an atypical antipsychotic.

Answer 13.8

Targeting specific neurotransmitters as an approach to CNS drug discovery is particularly challenging due to the complexity of signaling pathways in the brain. The concentration and effects of NTs in the synapse is controlled by multiple factors including activity at receptors, down-regulation of receptors and transporters. Furthermore, there is interplay between individual NTs. In addition, the role of a neurotransmitter in a disease state may be specific to one location in the brain. Challenges include targeting one specific neurotransmitter receptor without also affecting the levels of other neurotransmitters, as well as their activity in other signaling pathways. The multiple subtypes of each NT receptor, which all recognize the same neurotransmitter, make it challenging to design CNS drugs selective for one subtype versus another or drugs selective for the NT receptor in a particular brain region.

Answer 13.9

1. Stimulants (both legal and illegal): Caffeine, nicotine, and methamphetamine (derived from ephedrine) are examples of compounds or drugs that are abused.

2. Hallucinogens: LSD (lysergic acid diethylamine) is a semisynthetic derivative of a naturally occurring alkaloid that is abused.

Answer 13.10

Donepezil and memantine are two drugs currently used to treat Alzheimer's disease. Donepezil is a noncompetitive reversible inhibitor of AChE. Inhibition of AChE helps to maintain acetylcholine levels, by preventing the degradation of AChE. It has been shown to improve cognitive function in Alzheimer's patients. Memantine is a low-affinity noncompetitive antagonist of the NMDA receptor. The natural ligand, glutamate, is excitatory and, in excess, can lead to neurotoxicity. Memantine reduces the excitatory effects of glutamate.

Some recent approaches to develop new Alzheimer's treatments aim to modify the course of the disease by focusing on decreasing amyloid plaque production. There are two proteases, γ-secretase and BACE, that are responsible for cleaving APP to generate peptides that aggregate to form the characteristic plaques seen in AD brains. Compounds that inhibit these proteases are being evaluated to see if they can change the course of the disease by reducing the amount of plaques formed.

Answer 13.11

- Diazepam (Valium) is a positive allosteric modulator (PAM) at the $GABA_A$ receptor that is used to treat anxiety and seizures.

- Vilazodone is a partial agonist of the $5\text{-}HT_{1A}$ receptor that is used as an antidepressant.

- Chlorpromazine is a dopamine antagonist that is effective on the positive symptoms of schizophrenia.

diazepam (Valium)   vilazodone   chlorpromazine

Glossary

γ-aminobutyric acid (GABA)
an inhibitory neurotransmitter, which balances the excitatory neurotransmitters

π–π interactions
noncovalent interactions between the π systems of aromatic rings

5-hydroxytryptamine (5-HT)
an inhibitory neurotransmitter that regulates mood as well as sleep, appetite, memory, body temperature, and sexual function (also known as serotonin)

absorption
the mechanism by which a drug moves into the bloodstream from the site of administration

acetylcholine
a neurotransmitter that affects muscle contraction and has a role in memory

acid–base catalysis
a common mechanism used by enzymes that involves proton transfer and relay between amino acid side chains in the active site, substrates, and products

activators
a protein or small molecule that results in increase in the activity of some biological event, such as transcription or enzyme activity

active pharmaceutical ingredient (API)
the active drug substance in a medicine

active transport
an energy-consuming process by which molecules are moved across membranes against a concentration gradient

active-analog approach
strategy for pharmacophore identification that uses low-energy conformers of both active and inactive compounds that bind at a specific protein site

active-site inhibitors
compounds that bind at the reaction site of an enzyme and prevent substrate from binding

acute toxicity
studies of a drug done in animals where increasing doses are administered until signs of toxicity are observed

additivity method
quantitative structure–activity relationship approach that assesses the occurrence of additive substituent effects and estimates their magnitude

affinity
the propensity of a compound to bind to its target

aggregates
noncovalent complexes formed by certain compounds that bind to proteins through nonspecific interactions and interfere with binding assays

agonist
a compound, like the natural ligand, that binds at a receptor, resulting in a physiological response

alkaloid
general term for a nitrogen-containing bioactive compound found in plants

allosteric modulators
compounds that bind at a site remote from the active site of an enzyme and affect enzymatic activity

allosteric sites
binding sites that are remote from where the natural ligand binds

Ames test
assessment of *in vitro* genetic toxicity of a drug that uses a mutant form of the bacterium *Salmonella*

amino acid conjugation
phase II metabolic reaction that couples an amino acid to a drug or its metabolite through amide bond formation

aminoglycosides
antibacterial agents characterized by one or more amino sugars and an aminocyclitol, which is a cyclohexane substituted with amino and hydroxyl groups

amyloid hypothesis
proposal that inhibiting production of the β-amyloid plaques found in the brains of Alzheimer's patients would modify the course of the disease

antagonist
a compound that binds to the receptor and prevents the natural ligand from eliciting a response

antibacterial agents
compounds, natural or synthetic, that inhibit bacterial growth

antibiotic
an antibacterial agent that is derived from microorganisms

antibody–drug conjugates (ADCs)
anti-cancer agents that consist of a compound (known as a payload) linked to an antibody that recognizes epitopes selectively expressed on cancer cells

antifolates
drugs that inhibit enzymes in the folate pathway, thus eliminating key coenzymes required for the synthesis of nucleotide building blocks

antimetabolites
compounds that compete with the natural substrate of an enzyme and are accepted as substrates

antisense therapy
use of an oligonucleotide or modified analog with a complementary sequence to the mRNA produced by a disease-causing gene

antiseptics
compounds that do not have a defined mechanism but are used topically on skin and tissue to inhibit growth of microorganisms

area under the curve (AUC)
measure of total drug exposure over a set time period, measured in *in vivo* pharmacokinetic assays

aspartyl proteases
enzymes that catalyze amide bond cleavage, using aspartic acids residues in the active site and water as a nucleophile

atypical antipsychotics
antipsychotic drugs characterized by a binding profile that includes stronger antagonism at D_4 than at D_2 receptors, as well as 5-HT_{2A} antagonism; they have a lower incidence of extrapyramidal symptoms

bactericidal
describes antibacterial agents that kill bacteria

bacteriostatic
describes antibacterial agents that inhibit replication but do not kill bacteria

barbiturates
a class of sedatives and hypnotics based on barbituric acid

benzamides
a class of atypical antipsychotics with a benzamide core, including amisulpride and sulpiride

benzazepines
a class of atypical antipsychotics with a benzazepine core, including clozapine and olanzapine

benzisoxazoles
a class of atypical antipsychotics, including risperidone, ziprasidone, and lurasidone

benzodiazepines (BZs)
a family of drugs with a benzodiazepine core, such as valium, that are used to treat anxiety

binding assays
experimental procedures to determine the affinity of interaction between two molecules

bioavailability
the fraction of a molecule absorbed after a specific route of administration, compared to what is theoretically possible

bioisosteres
compounds or functional groups that possess near-equal molecular shapes and volumes and approximately the same distribution of electrons and exhibit similar biological properties

biologics
protein and antibody therapeutics that either inhibit a protein–protein interaction or supplement one of the protein partners involved in such an interaction

biomolecular recognition
specific binding interactions between a drug and target macromolecule

bis-alkylating agents
compounds that form two separate covalent bonds to DNA, forming cross-links

blood–brain barrier (BBB)
a layer of tightly packed endothelial cells in the brain that is denser than other membrane structures; it protects the brain from toxins and infectious agents but also provides an additional barrier for drugs to penetrate

butyrophenones
a class of antipsychotic drugs, exemplified by haloperidol

cation–π interactions
interactions that occur between the π system of an aromatic ring and a cation

cephalosporins
a class of β-lactam antibacterial agents that differ from penicillins by replacement of the thiazolidine five-membered ring with a six-membered dihydrothiazine ring

chain branching
addition of alkyl branching points to an alkyl chain

chain terminators
polymerase inhibitors that are incorporated into a growing nucleic acid strand but lack a 3′-hydroxyl group, thus blocking further chain elongation

channel activators
compounds that act to open an ion channel

channel blockers
compounds that act to close an ion channel

cholinergic hypothesis
proposal that low levels of the neurotransmitter acetylcholine in Alzheimer's patients contribute to cognitive decline

chronic testing
toxicity assessment of drug candidates that lasts for longer than 3 months and should have at least the same duration as the proposed clinical trials

classical irreversible inhibitors
compounds that bind through covalent interactions and do not dissociate from the enzyme, thus decreasing enzyme activity

classical isosteres
atoms, ions, and molecules with identical peripheral layers of electrons

clearance (CL)
the volume of plasma cleared of a drug per unit time, usually expressed in mL/min or L/hr

cleavage-dependent mechanism
means of action used by antisense agents that relies on endonuclease-mediated cleavage of RNA

clinical candidate
a compound with activity and safety levels sufficient for testing in humans and that is appropriate for development into a drug

clinical trials
testing that proves the efficacy and safety of a drug candidate in human subjects; required for regulatory approval by a government agency such as the U.S. Food and Drug Administration

C_{max}
maximum concentration: peak plasma concentration of a drug after administration

combinatorial chemistry
method for synthesizing collections of molecules, each containing the same number of subunits, typically accomplished via a modular approach to join subunits together

combinatorial libraries
relatively large libraries (>100) of structurally related compounds, synthesized in multiple combinations with similar reactions and varying building blocks

competition binding assays
procedures to evaluate the ability of a test compound to compete with a known, labeled compound (typically either radiolabeled or fluorescently labeled) for binding to a macromolecular target; after incubation, the ligand–receptor complex is isolated and quantified

competitive inhibitors
molecules that block the functioning of an enzyme by displacing a naturally occurring ligand

composition of matter patent
a patent that protects the specific compounds claimed in the patent

congeners
compounds with similar core structures but varying functional group appendages

covalent binding
type of binding in which the interaction energy is dominated by the interaction of filled orbitals with unfilled orbitals

covalent catalysis
a common mechanism used by enzymes that involves formation of a covalent bond between amino acid side chains in the active site and the substrate

C_{ss}
steady-state concentration: equilibrium concentration of drug in plasma after a number of doses

cysteine proteases
enzymes that catalyze amide bond cleavage, using the thiol of a cysteine residue in the active site as a nucleophile

cytochrome P-450 inhibition or induction
toxicity assays that can predict drug–drug interactions due to inhibition or induction of important metabolic enzymes

cytostatic
describes compounds that stop proliferation of cells

cytotoxic
describes compounds that kill cells

cytotoxicity assays
procedures that involve treating cells with a small molecule for some period of time and then measuring specific biological readouts of cell viability to determine if the compound causes cell death

deconvolution
isolation and identification of the active component in a combinatorial library synthesized by a split-pool method

desolvation
removal of a polar chemical group, such as an amino, hydroxy, or a phosphate group, from water, which is energetically unfavorable

dipole–dipole interactions
interactions between permanent dipoles where the partial positive charge on one atom is attracted to the partial negative charge on the other

distomer
the less potent enantiomer of a drug

distribution
the process through which a drug is dispersed from the bloodstream to various compartments of the body, including tissues, brain, and other organs

diversity-oriented syntheses (DOS)
synthetic approach to libraries of a series of compounds with diverse structural scaffolds

DNA alkylating agents
molecules that bind to DNA through covalent bonds

DNA-encoded libraries (DEL)
a combinatorial chemistry approach where, at each synthetic step, a DNA oligomer is co-synthesized and serves as a barcode for the ultimate identification of active hits

DNA minor groove binders
compounds that act primarily through interacting with the minor groove of DNA

docking
the process of computationally fitting sets of compounds into a model of the binding site of a protein

dopamine
a neurotransmitter that plays roles in motor behavior, motivation, and emotion

dopamine reward system
a mechanism in the brain that mediates responses to rewards such as food and sex (also known as the mesolimbic dopamine system)

dose ratio (r)
amount of agonist required to give an effect at a defined antagonist concentration compared to the amount of agonist required to give the same effect without a competitive antagonist present

dose-dependent
describes activity of a drug where there is a change in potency with a change in drug concentration

double-blind
describes a clinical trial where neither the patient nor the clinician knows if the patient is receiving drug or placebo

drug
a compound that has advanced through clinical trials and received regulatory approval to be used as a medicine

drug development
the process involved in the later stages of advancing a drug into clinical trials that involves characterization of a clinical candidate in a series of animal tests, as well as optimization of its synthesis and development of an appropriate formulation

drug targets
macromolecules, most often proteins or nucleic acids, that a drug affects in the body

druglike
describes molecules that contain functional groups and/or have physical properties consistent with the majority of known drugs

druglike properties
features for a compound that are correlated with successful drugs; they include chemical and metabolic stability, solubility, lipophilicity, and safety

ED_{50}
Effective Dose; median dose of a drug that causes 50% of maximal response

effector system
an enzyme or ion channel linked to a G protein-coupled receptor that is activated or deactivated in response to ligand binding to the receptor

efficacy
degree of effect of a compound, usually measured as a percentage compared to a standard

electronic properties
physicochemical parameters used in quantitative structure–activity relationship studies, usually with Hammett coefficients

electrostatic (ionic) interactions
noncovalent forces that occur between two oppositely charged ions

elimination
removal of a drug or its metabolites from the bloodstream, usually in urine or feces (also called excretion)

enthalpy
the energetics of a drug–target system, related to the specific interactions between compound and target

entropy
a measure of disorder in a system: the greater the number of equivalent rearrangements of the molecules, the greater the entropy value

enzymatic or biochemical assays
procedures that typically monitor the reaction of an isolated macromolecule, often detecting formation of the product of an enzymatic reaction

enzyme (E)
a protein capable of catalyzing a chemical transformation

epigenetics
study of heritable factors that are not encoded by the organism's DNA sequence; for example, DNA methylation or modification of histones can influence otherwise identical sequences of DNA

epinephrine
an excitatory neurotransmitter involved in regulation of sleep and alertness in the central nervous system and in the periphery; it also has roles in controlling heart rate and bronchodilation

ethnopharmacology
use of plants to treat diseases in native populations

eudismic ratio
potency of the more active enantiomer of a drug (eutomer) compared to that of the less active enantiomer (distomer)

eutomer
the more potent enantiomer of a drug

excitatory neurotransmitters
compounds that increase the concentration of cations, causing depolarization and relay of an electrical signal (the action potential) along the axon

excretion
removal of a drug or its metabolites from the bloodstream, usually in urine or feces (also called elimination)

extended ternary complex (ETC)
model for G protein-coupled receptor action that takes into account inactive, active, and active/bound to G protein forms of the receptor

focused screening
strategy where compounds assayed are not random but in fact are known or predicted to have some activity against the biological target

formulation
combination of the active pharmaceutical ingredient with other components, known as excipients

fraction unbound (f_u)
proportion of a drug that is not bound to plasma proteins in the blood

fragment-based screening (FBS)
strategy based on the concept of identifying small fragments (up to molecular weight about 300) that can bind to a specific protein target, even with only modest affinity

Free–Wilson method
classical quantitative structure–activity relationship procedure that assesses the occurrence of additive substituent effects and estimates their magnitude

functional assays
procedures that generally measure downstream effects of a binding event

G protein-coupled receptors (GPCRs)
a common class of receptors with seven transmembrane domains that transduce extracellular hormone signals into intracellular actions like contraction, secretion, or mitotic proliferation

generic drugs
drugs that are sold by commercial organizations other than the original patentor or licensee, after patent expiration

genetic toxicity assays
studies to establish the mutagenic potential of a drug; that is, whether or not it causes DNA damage

glucuronidation
phase II metabolic reaction that couples a glucuronic acid moiety to a drug or its metabolite through addition of a nucleophile to the anomeric carbon

glutamic acid
an excitatory neurotransmitter with roles in synaptic plasticity, which refers to changes in the connections between neurons

glutathione conjugation
phase II metabolic reaction that adds the thiol of glutathione to a drug or its metabolite through addition to an electrophilic center on the drug

glycine
an inhibitory neurotransmitter that plays a role in movement

half-life ($t_{1/2}$)
time for the concentration of a compound to drop to half of its initial value

herbals
written collections of descriptions of plants useful for medicinal purposes

hERG channel
ion channel encoded by the human ether-à-go-go related gene that transports potassium ions in heart muscle and is critical for coordinating the heart's beating

high-throughput screening (HTS)
strategy for examining up to millions of compounds to detect those that have a defined effect: it relies on miniaturized in vitro assays, performed robotically

hit
a small molecule of confirmed structure and purity that exhibits biological activity at some defined threshold (typically <20 µM) in a particular biological test

hit triage
process of evaluating hits, eliminating some and validating others

hit-to-lead process
evaluation of attributes and liabilities of validated hits to identify and prioritize those most likely to be improved further during the optimization process

homologation
process of lead modification by adding a methylene unit to an alkyl chain

hot spots
small subsets of residues that often contribute disproportionately to binding energies in protein–protein interactions

hydrogen-bonding interactions
interactions that take place between a hydrogen donor that is covalently bound to an electronegative atom, such as oxygen or nitrogen, and an electronegative atom acceptor, such as oxygen, nitrogen, or fluorine

hydrophobic interactions
interactions that occur between nonpolar groups and involve temporary dipoles

induced-fit model
a representation of binding where the enzyme and substrate are both flexible, and as the substrate starts to bind and make specific interactions with the enzyme, the active site moves to accommodate it until the catalytic groups are in the appropriate orientation for reaction, much like a hand fitting into a glove

inhibitors
drugs acting on enzymes that decrease the function of the enzyme

inhibitory neurotransmitters
compounds that decrease the concentration of cations, causing polarization and blocking relay of an electrical signal (action potential) along the axon

interactome
map of the network of molecular interactions within a particular cell or organism

intercalators
planar aromatic molecules that bind to DNA by inserting between base pairs via π-stacking and additional hydrophobic and electrostatic interactions

interfacial binders
compounds that form a ternary complex with two protein partners at their interface and lock the proteins in a nonproductive conformation

intrinsic activity
degree to which a drug, by binding to a receptor, has the capacity to result in a biological response

inverse agonist
a compound that binds and results in a decrease in the response of a constitutively active receptor

Investigational New Drug Application (IND)
an extensive report filed with the U.S. FDA that includes preclinical data for a clinical candidate, including method of synthesis, formulation plan, and results of pharmacokinetic and toxicity studies in multiple animal species, as well as a plan for clinical trials

ion channels
a class of proteins that form pores in cell membranes; after opening in response to a regulatory signal, these proteins allow the passage of ions through the pore (includes both ion-specific and nonspecific channels)

ion–dipole interactions
interactions between the negative end of a permanent dipole and a cation

isosteres
compounds or groups that possess near-equal molecular shapes and volumes and approximately the same distribution of electrons and exhibit similar physical properties

kinases
a class of transferase enzymes responsible for transferring a phosphoryl group to a hydroxyl group, using ATP as the phosphate donor

lead
a compound with desirable potency, target selectivity, lack of target promiscuity, evidence of structure–activity relationships, and appropriate pharmaceutical and physical properties

lead optimization
process of modifying the structure of a lead compound in an effort to improve activity and selectivity, reduce toxicity, and optimize physical and pharmaceutical properties; when successful, this process leads to a clinical candidate

lead series
a set of structural analogs that have a defined set of characteristics, based on potency and properties, and are deemed to be promising starting points for medicinal chemistry optimization

legacy libraries
compounds that have been synthesized in the past, often as part of a medicinal chemistry optimization effort, and retained for testing in the future; these have historically provided some important hits and/or drugs

library screening
testing of many compounds simultaneously to identify starting points for drug discovery

ligand efficiency (LE)
assessment of how efficiently a compound binds, calculated by determining the ratio of a molecule's affinity to the number of heavy (non-H) atoms: LE = $-\Delta G$/HAC (heavy atom count)

ligand lipophilic efficiency (LLE)
gauge of how the lipophilicity of a compound contributes to its potency, defined as activity minus cLogP (either experimental or calculated)

ligand-based drug design
medicinal chemistry approach that relies on analysis of low-energy conformers of compounds that are known to bind to a specific target

ligand-based virtual screening
hit identification strategy that relies on computational chemistry: knowledge of ligands that bind to a particular target is used to develop a model, and then compound libraries (virtual or real) are screened *in silico* to identify those that adhere to the model

Lipinski rules
a set of guidelines, based on molecular weight, numbers of H-bond donors and acceptors, and log P, that predict oral absorption (also known as the rule of five)

lipophilicity
affinity of a molecule for lipids or nonpolar media

lock and key hypothesis
proposal by Emil Fischer to explain how a substrate interacts with an enzyme by fitting into a specific geometric shape as a key (substrate) does in a lock (enzyme)

lock and key model
a representation of ligand–receptor interactions in which both molecules are assumed to be rigid

macromolecular target
a protein, enzyme, receptor, or nucleic acid (DNA or RNA) that interacts with a small molecule or drug to cause a physiological effect

magic bullet
a concept introduced by Paul Ehrlich that suggests the possibility of a drug that is precisely targeted to only one macromolecular target, with no effects on any other protein

maximum tolerated dose (MTD)
the highest dose of a drug that does not show significant toxicity

mechanism-based inactivator
a specific type of irreversible enzyme inhibitor that binds to the enzyme and is acted upon by it; the modified inhibitor then covalently modifies the enzyme, resulting in irreversible inhibition (also called suicide inhibitor)

medicinal chemistry
branch of chemistry that focuses on the design and synthesis of new medicines or drugs

metabolism
chemical modification of a substance in the body, used as a mechanism to remove toxic and/or foreign substances (xenobiotics)

metabolites
compounds that are formed as a result of metabolic transformation of a drug molecule

metal ion catalysis
a common mechanism used by enzymes, whereby metal ions are essential for coordinating, activating, or shielding substrates and/or products to allow the enzymatic reaction to occur

metalloprotease
any proteolytic enzyme that requires a metal ion for activity; drugs for cardiovascular disease (angiotensin-converting enzyme inhibitors) target this class of enzymes

metastasis
development of tumors at a site remote from the primary site

method of use patent
a patent that covers the use of a compound, often already known in the literature or patented, to treat a specific disease

minimum effective dose (MED)
the lowest dose that produces a statistically significant desirable effect

mixed inhibitors
compounds that bind with unequal affinity to both the free enzyme and the enzyme–substrate complex

molecular fingerprints
results of a computational method to describe a molecule, where a binary code is used to represent the presence or absence of a specific structural feature

monoamine neurotransmitters
a subclass of small molecules that modulate neurotransmission, usually consisting of serotonin, dopamine, and norepinephrine

monobactams
a class of antibacterial agents characterized by a monocyclic β-lactam structure

N-acetylation
phase II metabolic reaction whereby an amine is converted to an N-acetate

natural ligands
physiologically relevant compounds, often peptides or small molecules, that bind to or interact with a macromolecule to initiate a biological response

negative allosteric modulators (NAM)
compounds that bind at an allosteric site of a receptor and decrease the affinity of the natural ligand for the receptor

neuropathic pain
describes pain resulting from injury to nerves

neutral antagonist
a compound that binds to a receptor and prevents the natural ligand (or an agonist) from binding but elicits no biological effect when the natural ligand is not present (also called an antagonist)

New Drug Application (NDA)
an extensive report filed with the U.S. Food and Drug Administration that details the results of clinical trials and animal studies and the process by which a drug will be manufactured; it is required to initiate the drug approval process

nicking agents
molecules that bind to duplex DNA and cause one strand to break

nociceptive pain
describes pain resulting from injury to muscle or bone tissue

nonclassical bioisostere
a functional group, atom, or groups of atoms that can replace a functional group, atom, or group of atoms in a bioactive molecule while allowing the resultant molecule to still retain activity

noncompetitive inhibitors
compounds that bind to an allosteric site and do not compete directly with the natural substrate for binding

norepinephrine
an excitatory neurotransmitter; along with serotonin and dopamine, considered one of the monoamine neurotransmitters

occupancy-only mechanism
one of the mechanisms by which antisense nucleotides work; their binding to the translation initiation site on mRNA blocks movement of the ribosome and prevents protein synthesis

occupation theory
proposal by Ariens and Stephenson that the biological activity of a molecule is not only directly proportional to the fraction of occupied receptors but also dependent on the molecule's intrinsic activity; this theory helps explain the phenonemon of partial agonism

oncogenes
genes that have the potential to cause cancer; they are often mutated versions of normal genes and code for aberrant proteins that contribute to the development of cancer

oral bioavailability
exposure of drug in the blood after oral dosing, as compared to exposure after intravenous dosing; often indicated as fraction absorbed (FA)

orphan GPCRs
G protein-coupled receptors for which the natural ligand is unknown

orthosteric sites
locations on a protein (receptor) where the natural ligand binds

oxazolidinones
a class of antibacterial agents characterized by the presence of an oxazolidinone heterocycle that acts by inhibiting protein synthesis; examples include linezolid and tedizolid

pan-assay interference compounds (PAINS)
compounds that are frequently identified as active in high-throughput screens; their promiscuous activity, through a variety of mechanisms, is considered artifactual

parallel synthesis
combinatorial setup where each reaction is run on an individual compound in parallel and in separate vessels

partial agonist
a compound that binds to a receptor but gives less than a full response in relation to some defined response by a full agonist or the natural ligand, regardless of increasing concentration

passive diffusion
movement of molecules via passive transport, along a gradient; in contrast, in active transport, movement of molecules in cells is driven by chemical energy, usually the hydrolysis of ATP or other nucleoside triphosphates

patent
an exclusive right granted by a government that excludes others from making, using, or selling an invention for a specific time in exchange for public disclosure

penems and carbapenems
broad-spectrum antibacterial agents characterized by the presence of a beta-lactam fused to an unsaturated five-membered ring (an all-carbon ring in the case of carbapenems and a sulfur-containing ring in the case of penems)

penicillin-binding protein
a serine protease that catalyzes the cross-linking of peptidoglycan units during the synthesis of bacterial cell walls; it is the target of many antibacterial agents including β-lactams, cephalosporins, penems, carbapenems, and monobactams

penicillins
an important class of antibacterial agents, characterized by the presence of a β-lactam fused to a five-membered thiazolidine ring, that inhibit cell wall biosynthesis; the first examples were isolated by Alexander Fleming from mold and ushered in the antibiotic age

peptide mimetics
fragments of molecules that mimic the characteristics of a peptide bond, such as H-bonding capacity and polarity, but are more stable (also called peptidomimetics)

peptidoglycan
polymer consisting of carbohydrates and amino acid residues that is a building block of bacterial cell walls; it is a substrate for penicillin-binding proteins

peptidomimetic
a small molecule or fragment that has many of the structural features of a peptide but is more stable (also called peptide mimetic)

permeability
ability of a small molecule to cross a lipophilic membrane, measured as a rate of transport across the membrane

peroxisome proliferator-activated receptors (PPARs)
nuclear receptors involved in carbohydrate and lipid metabolism and adipose tissue differentiation; they are targets of fibrates and glitazones, which are important classes of diabetes drugs

pharmaceutical properties
specific characteristics of a small molecule related to its suitability as a drug, including metabolic stability, permeability, and oral bioavailability, among others; most often related to its absorption, distribution, metabolism, and excretion characteristics

pharmacodynamics (PD)
relationship between the concentration of a drug at the site of action and its biological effect

pharmacokinetics (PK)
study of how the body is affected by a drug, encompassing absorption, distribution, metabolism, and excretion

pharmacology
study of drug action

pharmacopeias
written collections of descriptions of plants or drugs, their effects, and directions for their use

pharmacophore
steric and electronic features of a molecule and their spatial relationship to each other, which defines the characteristics of a molecule that displays a specific biological effect; an abstract concept that considers common interaction capacities rather than particular atoms or groups of atoms

phase I clinical trials
first of four steps to evaluate a drug in humans, which assesses safety and pharmacokinetics of the drug when administered to a small number of healthy patients for a short duration

phase I metabolic reactions
processes for drug metabolism that involve modifying a functional group of the compound administered, usually through oxidation, reduction, or hydrolysis

phase II metabolic reactions
processes for drug metabolism that involve conjugating the drug or its metabolite to a small molecule such as glucuronic acid, glutathione, or an amino acid.

phase II studies
second of four steps to evaluate a drug in humans, which assesses efficacy in a group (100–300) of carefully selected patients compared to a placebo or comparison drug

phase III studies
third of four steps to evaluate a drug in humans, which assesses efficacy in a large number of patients to determine optimal dosing, most responsive patient population, and tolerability, among other parameters

phase IV studies
studies of a drug in humans after it is approved for use, *see also* **postmarketing surveillance**

phenothiazines
a class of drugs used to treat psychosis, termed typical antipsychotics; chlorpromazine is a prototypical example

phenotypic assays
biological tests that measure changes in a characteristic or effect (phenotype) in a complex system, regardless of the specific molecular target; they can be performed in cells and even in higher organisms such as yeast, zebrafish, and flies

physicochemical parameters
characteristics of a molecule, such as lipophilicity that can be correlated with biological activity; used in early quantitative structure–activity relationship models

PK studies
pharmacokinetic studies: experiments that determine the concentration of drug in plasma (or other organs and tissues) over a specific time period after a specific administered dose

plasma proteins
macromolecules present in the blood in high levels, such as albumin, that can bind to drug molecules and modify their biological effects and/or pharmacokinetic characteristics

positive allosteric modulators (PAM)
compounds that bind at an allosteric site of a receptor and increase the affinity of the natural ligand for the receptor

postmarketing surveillance
monitoring of the safety of the drug after it has been approved, *see also* **phase IV studies**

potency
concentration of a compound that results in the desired biological effect

privileged structures
structural motifs that are capable of binding to a variety of biological targets

probability model
description of the effects of small molecules on G protein-coupled receptors, based on the existence of large ensembles of receptor conformations, which states that binding of a ligand shifts the overall distribution, increasing some states and decreasing others

process chemistry research
development of a method to synthesize multikilogram quantities of a drug candidate that takes into account safety, efficiency, cost, reproducibility, and consistency

process patent
a specific type of patent that protects syntheses and processes for making a drug

prodrug
a molecule, typically inactive, that affords the active drug molecule upon being metabolized within the body

prophylaxis
therapeutic intervention in healthy invididuals to prevent disease

protein–protein interactions (PPIs)
physical contacts between two or more proteins that mediate a biological event

proto-oncogenes
normal genes that promote cell division; upon mutation, they become oncogenes and contribute to the development of cancer

proximity and orientation effects
in enzymatic reactions, bringing the reactants together (proximity) in the appropriate alignment (orientation) to facilitate reaction

quantitative structure–activity relationship (QSAR)
computational model that correlates physical properties of a compound with its biological effects, used to predict the biological activity of untested compounds

range-finding studies
toxicology testing that evaluates several different doses of a compound in animals over several weeks to establish the range of doses that can be administered without significant toxicity

rate theory
hypothesis developed by Paton and Rang, stating that activity of a small molecule at a receptor is a function of the rates of association and dissociation, not just the number of occupied receptors

reactive functional groups
parts of a molecule that can react nonspecifically with assay components by forming covalent bonds; compounds containing these are usually considered poor starting points for drug discovery

receptor
a macromolecule that propogates a signal or initiates subsequent events in response to some stimulus; broadly includes G protein-coupled receptors, ion channels, nuclear receptors, and transporters

redox-active compounds
molecules that can generate free radicals under assay conditions and initiate a redox cycle, thereby appearing to inhibit enzymes and/or proteins; they are usually considered poor starting points for drug discovery

reproductive toxicity studies
a series of studies that evaluates, in animals, whether the drug will have effects on fertility, the ability to maintain a pregnancy, and the health of progeny of the tested species

repurposed
describes an approved drug (or a drug in advanced clinical trials) used for a different disease than was originally intended

reuptake
process by which neurotransmitters that are released into the synapse are taken up back into the presynaptic cell by monoamine transporters; this process is important for maintaining the appropriate concentration of neurotransmitters in the synapse

reversible inhibitors
compounds that can be recovered intact after binding to a protein; enzymatic activity can also be restored after removal of the inhibitor

ring–chain transformations
medicinal chemistry strategies that increase or decrease the size of a ring system, convert a ring to an acyclic system, or convert an acyclic system to a ring

RNase H
an endonuclease that recognizes RNA–DNA duplexes, cleaves the RNA, and releases the DNA; it is important for the activity of antisense oligonucleotides that work through a cleavage-

dependent mechanism, as it also recognizes the RNA–antisense duplex and cleaves the RNA sense strand

rule of five
a set of guidelines based on molecular weight, numbers of H-bond donors and acceptors, and log P that predict oral absorption (also known as Lipinski rules)

rule of three
a variation of the Lipinski rule (rule of five), most often applied during fragment-based screening and hit triage, in which all parameters are factors of three

saturation curve
graph used to describe enzymatic activity that plots velocity of the reaction versus substrate concentration; above some concentration of substrate (saturation), the velocity will no longer change

scaffold hopping
medicinal chemistry strategy that involves replacement of the nonpharmacophoric core of a molecule with a different core that displays the pharmacophoric elements in the same orientation

scissile bond
the peptide bond that is cleaved by a protease enzyme; often replaced to design protease inhibitors

screening
testing or assaying a specific collection (library) of small molecules

second messenger
usually an ion or small molecule that, once modulated by the action of a G protein-coupled receptor, activates enzymes or affects ion channels, resulting in a specific physiological effect; a component of signal transduction

segment I testing
evaluates fertility and reproductive performance in both male and female animals after administration of a drug

segment II testing
evaluates embryonic toxicity (teratogenicity) of a drug in female animals during early pregnancy

segment III testing
evaluates in animals whether there are any effects of a drug on the final stage of pregnancy, as well as delivery and lactation, when administered to a pregnant female or mother

selective estrogen receptor modulators (SERMs)
a class of drugs that targets the estrogen receptor; their activity toward the receptor varies in different tissues

selective serotonin reuptake inhibitors (SSRIs)
a class of drugs widely used to treat neuropsychiatric disorders such as depression; they work by inhibiting the reuptake of serotonin and causing levels of the neurotransmitter to be maintained in the synapse

selectivity
activity of a compound toward the desired target versus its effect on another, usually undesired, target

semisynthetic compound
compound that is derived from a natural product but undergoes additional chemical modification, usually requiring only a few synthetic steps

semisynthetic drugs
drugs prepared by chemical derivatization of natural products

serine/threonine proteases
enzymes that cleave a peptide bond by using the hydroxyl group of a serine or threonine as a nucleophile in the reaction; drugs that target serine/threonine proteases include antibacterial cell-wall biosynthesis inhibitors and proteasome anti-cancer agents

serotonin
an inhibitory neurotransmitter that regulates mood as well as sleep, appetite, memory, body temperature, and sexual function (also known as 5-hydroxytryptamine)

signal transduction
conversion of one type of signal in a chemical or physical form into another type of chemical signal, often involving transmission from the outside of a cell to the inside

slow tight-binding inhibitors
compounds that bind to enzymes reversibly but are so strongly bound and have such a slow off-rate that they act like irreversible inhibitors

solubility
ability of a compound to dissolve in a specific liquid, usually water

split-pool synthesis
a combinatorial chemistry method where compounds are synthesized by a repetitive sequence of combine, divide, and couple (react)

stabilization of the transition state
a means by which enzymes accelerate a reaction by binding to and lowering the energy of the transition state of the reaction

stapled peptides
small peptides constrained by a macrocyclic carbon-based ring that allows them to maintain an active conformation (usually an α-helix) and increases their stability

steroid receptors
a class of nuclear receptors (class I) that respond to binding by small-molecule hormones such as estrogen, testosterone, cortisol, and aldosterone; they are targeted by a number of drugs that treat various disorders such as breast cancer, osteoporosis, prostate cancer, and inflammation

strand breakers
molecules that bind to duplex DNA and result in both strands being broken

structure–activity relationships (SAR)
effects of a change in the structure of a molecule on its biological activity

structure-based drug design
a medicinal chemistry strategy that can be applied when a structure of the macromolecular target, or a closely related homolog, is available; it relies on observed interactions between the small molecule and the protein target

structure-based virtual screening
a hit identification strategy that relies on computational chemistry and knowledge of the structure of the biological target: small molecules are computationally fitted into the target and evaluated for how well they bind to the target

subchronic testing
phase of animal toxicity assessment where animals (either rodents or nonrodents) are dosed daily for 3 months and monitored for signs of toxicity, including weight loss or gain; after completion of the study, tissues are harvested and examined for histological changes compared to control animals

suicide inhibitor
a specific type of irreversible enzyme inhibitor that binds to the enzyme and is acted upon by it; the modified inhibitor then covalently modifies the enzyme, resulting in irreversible inhibition (also called mechanism-based inactivator)

Tanimoto coefficient
a measure of similarity between compounds, where highly similar compounds are assigned numbers close to 1 and dissimilar compounds are assigned numbers close to 0

tetracyclines
a class of broad-spectrum antibacterial agents characterized by four fused six-membered rings; they inhibit protein synthesis by preventing tRNA from binding to the A site in the ribosome

therapeutic index (TI)
ratio of maximum tolerated dose to minimum effective dose, which is a reflection of the safety of the drug (higher TI values are preferred)

threading intercalators
molecules that bind between DNA base pairs and also make interactions with the major and minor grooves of the DNA duplex

t_{max}
in a pharmacokinetic study, the time, after dosing, when the maximum concentration of drug is achieved

topoisomerase poison
a type of inhibitor of the enzyme topoisomerase that works by binding to and stabilizing the topoisomerase–DNA complex but does not bind to either enzyme or DNA in isolation

total synthesis
complete preparation of a natural product from simple starting materials

toxicity studies
testing performed in multiple animal species to evaluate the safety of a drug

toxicokinetics (TK)
study of the relationship between the concentration of a compound in blood (or tissues or organs) and the observed toxicity

transition-state mimetics
molecules that have many of the same features as the transition state of an enzymatic reaction but are stable; frequently utilized to develop enzyme inhibitors

transporters
membrane-bound proteins that bind and transport certain small molecules such as neurotransmitters, amino acids, and carbohydrates; drugs that target transporters include antidepressants, diuretics, and anti-diabetic agents

tricyclic antidepressant
a class of drugs used to treat depression that are nonselective reuptake inhibitors; they have largely been replaced with selective serotonin reuptake inhibitors

tumor suppressor genes
genes that encode proteins that negatively regulate cell growth; when mutated, they can contribute to the development of cancer

two-hit hypothesis
theory proposed by Alfred Knudson to explain how a specific cancer can develop in both individuals who carry cancer susceptibility genes and those with normal genes, proposing that two events are required for cancer to develop; individuals who inherit a mutated gene will require only one additional event, while individuals born with normal genes will require two events

typical antipsychotics
drugs that are antagonists at dopamine receptors used to treat schizophrenia (the prototype is chlorpromazine); they have largely been replaced with atypical antipsychotics

uncompetitive inhibitors
compounds that bind to the enzyme–substrate complex at an allosteric site and decrease enzyme activity

validated hit
a term sometimes used to describe a molecule that has reproducible, dose-dependent biological activity after its resynthesis and that works through a desirable mechanism of action

van der Waals forces
very weak interactions between hydrophobic regions of molecules; when present in a drug–target complex, they can result in significantly higher binding

Veber rules
a set of guidelines to predict oral bioavailabilty that incorporate molecular flexibility (rotatable bonds) and polar surface area; these factors were meant to account for the unexpected oral bioavailability of certain larger molecular weight drugs

viral-specific proteins
proteins that are uniquely present in viruses but not in humans

virions
particles representing the complete form of a virus, containing nucleic acid and essential proteins

virtual screening (VS)
assaying by computer and predicting activity, rather than experimentally screening genuine compounds to identify potential hits (also called in silico screening)

virulence
the pathogenicity of an organism (for example, viruses, fungi, or bacteria)

volume of distribution (V_d)
this number, calculated from pharmacokinetic studies, assesses the amount of drug distributed throughout the organism compared to the amount present in plasma: compounds with high volumes of distribution will exhibit low concentrations in plasma

warhead
an electrophilic moiety in an enzyme inhibitor that covalently reacts with a nucleophile in the enzyme, thereby preventing the reaction from proceeding; most often used to inhibit serine/threonine or cysteine proteases

xenobiotics
substances that are not naturally found in the body, such as most drugs

Index

Note: Page numbers followed by f refer to figures, and those followed by t refer to tables.